Pain Control in Ambulatory Surgery Centers

Kanishka Rajput • Nalini Vadivelu
Alan David Kaye • Rinoo Vasant Shah
Editors

Pain Control in Ambulatory Surgery Centers

Springer

Editors
Kanishka Rajput
Department of Anesthesiology
Yale University
New Haven, CT
USA

Nalini Vadivelu
Department of Anesthesiology
Yale University
New Haven, CT
USA

Alan David Kaye
Departments of Anesthesiology and Pharmacology, Toxicology, and Neurosciences
Louisiana State University Health Science Center
Shreveport, LA
USA

Rinoo Vasant Shah
Department of Anesthesiology
Louisiana State University Health Science Center
Shreveport, LA
USA

ISBN 978-3-030-55261-9 ISBN 978-3-030-55262-6 (eBook)
https://doi.org/10.1007/978-3-030-55262-6

This Springer imprint is published by the registered company Springer Nature Switzerland AG
The registered company address is: Gewerbestrasse 11, 6330 Cham, Switzerland

Kanishka Rajput: Dedicated to my parents, without whom I wouldn't be who I am; to my husband Karthik, for all his encouragement; and to my little children, Neel and Naira, who gave me time to do this.

Nalini Vadivelu: I wish to dedicate this book to my husband Mr. Thangamuthu Kodumudi and our sons Dr. Gopal Kodumudi, MD, and Vijay Kodumudi, MBA student, for all their support and encouragement.

Alane Kaye: I dedicate this book to my colleagues within the LSU Healthcare systems who work to help others each day. I also dedicate this book to my wife Dr. Kim Kaye, MD, for everything she does for me and my family.

Rinoo Shah: I dedicate this book to my loving and dedicated wife, Kejal; mom and dad, Rajul and Vasant; and children, Dev, Diyaa, and Maaya. I love them!

Foreword

Advances in surgical and anesthetic techniques have resulted in dramatic increases in both the volume and scope of ambulatory surgical cases. Patients presenting for surgery in the ambulatory setting come with significant comorbid diseases and offer unique challenges for both intra and postoperative anesthesia care. In addition, the rapid expansion of interventional techniques now makes it possible to care for patients in the ambulatory setting who would have traditionally required care in a hospital-based setting.

One of the most challenging aspects of ambulatory anesthetic care is ensuring adequate postoperative pain management. The opioid epidemic and other associated substance use disorders have further highlighted the importance of effective perioperative pain management.

Opportunities for further expanding care in the ambulatory setting will require the ability to provide novel and innovative pain management techniques.

Pain Control in Ambulatory Surgery Centers provides a contemporary and evidence-based approach to optimizing pain management in a broad array of patient conditions and procedures now being performed in the ambulatory setting. This text gives the reader an opportunity to become familiar with invasive as well as noninvasive and multi model management techniques.

The approach provided in this text is one which highlights the importance of developing a patient-focused care plan which is informed by patient disease, planned procedure, and the most contemporary approaches to pain management. The reader's clinical repertoire will be enriched and expanded by the text's content. Most importantly, patients' care will be significantly advanced from the approaches presented.

Roberta Hines
Nicholas M. Greene Professor of Anesthesiology
Department Chair and Chief, Anesthesiology
Yale University School of Medicine
New Haven, CT, USA

Preface

The number of surgeries being performed in ambulatory settings has skyrocketed in the last two decades, so has the diversity and acuity of cases. In parallel, the opioid epidemic has necessitated changes in the way we practice anesthesia. The push towards minimizing exposure to opioids around the time of surgery has led to increasing use of alternative modalities for pain control. Despite this, poor pain control remains one of the leading reasons for delayed discharge and unplanned admission following ambulatory surgery. Ambulatory patients often do not get the same level of thought put into their pain management regimens. The biggest motivation for us to write this book was to provide an easy reference for ambulatory providers working in a busy setting to devise optimal pain control strategies, while minimizing side effects and maintaining efficiency.

Within this book, we have made every effort to collate the latest evidence available for an ambulatory setting in an easy-to-read format for a variety of special situations and patient populations.

The book begins with an introduction to ambulatory surgery centers (ASCs) and hospital outpatient departments (HOPDs), describes the challenges faced by anesthesiologists for relatively short yet painful cases, and explains how to best optimize available resources for formulating perioperative analgesic plans with multimodal analgesia.

With the proliferation of non-operating room anesthesia (NORA) locations, hospitals are scrambling to find good pain-management regimens for this complex group of patients. We've incorporated chapters on unique considerations in NORA locations within ASCs and HOPDs (such as GI, bronchoscopy suite, IR, and interventional pain) as well as chapters on perioperative pain control for special populations such as patients on medication-assisted treatment (e.g., methadone, suboxone, and naltrexone), those with active substance abuse, with indwelling devices such as intrathecal pumps and spinal cord stimulators, with obstructive sleep apnea, and pediatric patients. Pain management can be especially challenging in these subsets of patients in the outpatient world. To make it comprehensive, we also included recovery-room concerns to be addressed before discharge and examples of weaning protocols after discharge.

The book is divided into parts with similar chapters grouped together. Each chapter, however, can be perused independent of other chapters since relevant key concepts required for a thorough understanding of the topic are introduced at the beginning of each chapter.

The book is intended to educate trainees, practicing anesthesiologists, nurse anesthetists, surgeons, interventionalists, and nurses who work in ambulatory settings as a guide to optimizing pain management.

We would like to acknowledge the mentorship of Dr. Viji Kurup, professor of anesthesiology at Yale University School of Medicine, an accomplished educator and author herself, who was a constant source of wisdom and knowledge during the writing of this book.

New Haven, CT, USA — Kanishka Rajput
New Haven, CT, USA — Nalini Vadivelu
Shreveport, LA, USA — Alan David Kaye
Shreveport, LA, USA — Rinoo Vasant Shah

Contents

Contributors

Newaj Abdullah, MD Department of Anesthesiology, Baylor College of Medicine, Houston, TX, USA

Nitish Aggarwal, MD Department of Anesthesiology, Yale University School of Medicine, New Haven, CT, USA

Anwar Alinani, MD Department of Anesthesiology and Perioperative Medicine, Penn State College of Medicine, Milton S. Hershey Medical Center, Hershey, PA, USA

Suwarna Anand, MD Department of Anesthesiology, University of Mississippi Medical Center, Jackson, MS, USA

Prathima Anandi, MD Department of Anesthesiology, LSU Health Shreveport, Shreveport, LA, USA

Alexander Bautista, MD, FASA Department of Anesthesiology and Perioperative Medicine, University of Louisville, Louisville, KY, USA

Colin Beals, MD Department of Anesthesiology, Yale University School of Medicine, New Haven, CT, USA

Sarah C. Bertrand, BS LSU Health Shreveport School of Medicine, Shreveport, LA, USA

Harley J. Bordelon, BS Louisiana State University Health Sciences Center Shreveport, Shreveport, LA, USA

Andrew Paul Bourgeois, MD Department of Anesthesiology, Louisiana State University Health Sciences Center, New Orleans, LA, USA

Raquel E. Candal, MD Department of Surgery, Louisiana State University Health Sciences Center Shreveport, Shreveport, LA, USA

Ellise Cappuccio, MD Montefiore Medical Center, Department of Anesthesiology, Bronx, NY, USA

Sam Carlson, BS Medical College of Wisconsin, Wauwatosa, WI, USA

Michelle A. Carroll Turpin, PhD Department of Biomedical Sciences, College of Medicine, University of Houston, Houston, TX, USA

Veronica P. Carullo, MD, FAAP University of Mississippi Medical Center, Jackson, MS, USA

Debbie Chandler, MD, MBA Department of Anesthesiology, Louisiana State University Health Shreveport, Shreveport, LA, USA

Jianguo Cheng, MD, PhD Department of Pain Management, Cleveland Clinic Foundation, Cleveland, OH, USA

Robert Chow, MD Department of Anesthesiology, Yale University School of Medicine, New Haven, CT, USA

Lindsey Cieslinski, DO Department of Anesthesiology, Tulane University School of Medicine, New Orleans, LA, USA

Peter Clapp, PhD Regis University School of Pharmacy, Denver, CO, USA

Elyse M. Cornett, PhD Department of Anesthesiology, Louisiana State University Health Shreveport, Shreveport, LA, USA

Katherine Cox, MD Department of Anesthesiology, Tulane University School of Medicine, New Orleans, LA, USA

Rajeev Dalal, MD Department of Anesthesiology and Perioperative Medicine, Penn State Milton S. Hershey Medical Center, Hershey, PA, USA

Yi Deng, MD Department of Anesthesiology, Baylor College of Medicine, Houston, TX, USA

Randi E. Domingue, BS LSU Health Shreveport School of Medicine, Shreveport, LA, USA

Laura Edwards, MD Department of Anesthesiology, Tulane University School of Medicine, New Orleans, LA, USA

Levin Fairchild, BS Louisiana State University Health Shreveport, Shreveport, LA, USA

David Fanelli, MD Department of Anesthesiology and Perioperative Medicine, Penn State College of Medicine, Milton S. Hershey Medical Center, Hershey, PA, USA

Alexandra Fonseca, MD Department of Anesthesia, Critical Care, and Pain Medicine, Beth Israel Deaconess Medical Center, Harvard Medical School, Boston, MA, USA

Paul Fontanez, MBA, RN Yale New Haven Hospital, Perioperative Services, New Haven, CT, USA

Katie Frith, BS Louisiana State University Health Shreveport, Shreveport, LA, USA

Mitchell C. Fuller, BS Medical College of Wisconsin, Wauwatosa, WI, USA

Clifford Gevirtz, MD, MPH LSU New Orleans, New Orleans, LA, USA

Somnia, Inc, Harrison, NY, USA

Meredith L. Gioe, BS Louisiana State University Health New Orleans, School of Medicine, New Orleans, LA, USA

Brook Girma, MD Department of Anesthesiology, LSU Health Shreveport, Shreveport, LA, USA

Nirmal Gosalia, MD Department of Internal Medicine, AMITA Health Saint Francis Hospital, Evanston, IL, USA

Tanith Graham, MD Department of Anesthesiology and Pain, University of Mississippi Medical Center, Jackson, MS, USA

Daniel Haddad, MD Department of Anesthesiology, Yale University School of Medicine, New Haven, CT, USA

Kyleigh Harrison, BS Medical College of Wisconsin, Wauwatosa, WI, USA

Alec Hendon, MD Department of Anesthesiology, Baylor College of Medicine, Houston, TX, USA

Sarahbeth Howes, Medical student LSU Medical School, Shreveport, LA, USA

Taylor R. Jeansonne, BS LSU Health Shreveport School of Medicine, Shreveport, LA, USA

Mark R. Jones, MD Beth Israel Deaconess Medical Center, Harvard Medical School, Department of Anesthesia, Critical Care, and Pain Medicine, Boston, MA, USA

Department of Anesthesiology, Weill Cornell Medical College, New York-Presbyterian Hospital, New York, NY, USA

Department of Anesthesia, Critical Care, and Pain Medicine, Beth Israel Deaconess Medical Center, Harvard Medical School, Boston, MA, USA

Weill Cornell Medical College, Department of Anesthesia, New York, NY, USA

Lukas J. Kandler, MD University Hospital Zurich, Zurich, Switzerland

Alan David Kaye, MD, PhD Departments of Anesthesiology and Pharmacology, Toxicology, and Neurosciences, Louisiana State University Health Shreveport, Shreveport, LA, USA

Sathya Kikkeri, BA Alabama College of Osteopathic Medicine, Dothan, AL, USA

Gopal Kodumudi, MD Department of Anesthesiology, Louisiana State University Health Shreveport, Shreveport, LA, USA

Jonathan B. Kozinn, MD University of Missouri-Kansas City School of Medicine, Kansas City, MO, USA

Saint Luke's Health System, Department of Anesthesiology, Saint Luke's Hospital, Kansas City, MO, USA

Shreedhar Kulkarni, MD Ochsner LSU Health – Shreveport, Shreveport, LA, USA

Olabisi Lane, MD, PharmD Department of Anesthesiology/Pain Medicine, Emory University Hospital, Atlanta, GA, USA

Maxwell Laurans, MD Department of Neurosurgery, Yale University School of Medicine, New Haven, CT, USA

Jinlei Li, MD, PhD Department of Anesthesiology, Yale University School of Medicine, New Haven, CT, USA

Robert Liu, DO Department of Anesthesiology and Perioperative Medicine, University of Louisville, Louisville, KY, USA

Henry Liu, MD, MS, FASA Department of Anesthesiology and Perioperative Medicine, Penn State College of Medicine, Milton S. Hershey Medical Center, Hershey, PA, USA

Jonathan S. McDougal, MD University of Missouri-Kansas City School of Medicine, Kansas City, MO, USA

Saint Luke's Health System, Department of Radiology, Saint Luke's Hospital, Kansas City, MO, USA

Patrick McQuillan, MD Department of Anesthesiology and Perioperative Medicine, Penn State Milton S. Hershey Medical Center, Hershey, PA, USA

Vanessa Moll, MD, PhD, FCCM, FASA Department of Anesthesiology, Division of Critical Care Medicine, Emory University School of Medicine, Atlanta, GA, USA

University Hospital Zurich, Zurich, Switzerland

Luke Mosel, DO Department of Anesthesiology, LSU Health Shreveport, Shreveport, LA, USA

Chizoba Mosieri, MD, FFARCSI Department of Anesthesiology, Louisiana State University Health Shreveport, Shreveport, LA, USA

Anh L. Ngo, MD MBA Pain Specialty Group, Newington, NH, USA

Melissa Annette Nikolaidis, MD Department of Anesthesiology, Baylor College of Medicine, Houston, TX, USA

Chikezie N. Okeagu, MD Department of Anesthesiology, LSU Health Sciences Center, New Orleans, LA, USA

Justin Pachuski, MD Department of Anesthesiology and Perioperative Medicine, Penn State Milton S. Hershey Medical Center, Hershey, PA, USA

Aimee Pak, MD Department of Anesthesiology, The University of Oklahoma Health Sciences Center, Augusta, GA, USA

Shilpadevi S. Patil, MD Department of Anesthesiology, LSU Health Shreveport, Shreveport, LA, USA

Shilpa Patil, MD Department of Anesthesiology, Louisiana State University Health Shreveport, Shreveport, LA, USA

Alex D. Pham, MD, PGY1 Department of Anesthesiology, Louisiana State University Health New Orleans, New Orleans, LA, USA

Melissa E. Phuphanich, MD, MS Department of Physical Medicine and Rehabilitation, UCLA/Greater Los Angeles VA Health Care System, Los Angeles, CA, USA

David Geffen School of Medicine at UCLA, University of California, Los Angeles, CA, USA

Petra Piccolruaz, MD University Hospital Zurich, Zurich, Switzerland

Amit Prabhakar, MD MS Department of Anesthesiology, Division of Critical Care Medicine, Emory University School of Medicine, Atlanta, GA, USA

Anand M. Prem, MD Department of Anesthesiology, University of Mississippi Medical Center, Jackson, MS, USA

Kanishka Rajput, MD Department of Anesthesiology and Pain Medicine, Yale University School of Medicine, New Haven, CT, USA

Rhett M. Reynolds, Medical Student Louisiana State University Shreveport Health Science Center, Shreveport, LA, USA

Sasha A. Ridgell, MD Department of Anesthesiology, LSU Health Shreveport, Shreveport, LA, USA

Anna C. Rogers, BS Louisiana State University Health Shreveport, School of Medicine, Shreveport, LA, USA

Praveen N. Sankrithi, BS Kansas City University of Medicine and Biosciences, Kansas City, MO, USA

Anitha Senthil, MBBS, DNB Department of Anesthesiology, Lahey Hospital & Medical Center, Burlington, MA, USA

Rinoo Vasant Shah, MD, MBA Louisiana State University Health Science Center – Shreveport School of Medicine, Shreveport, LA, USA

Achal Shah, MD Department of Anesthesiology, Yale University School of Medicine, New Haven, CT, USA

Kelley L. Sharp, BSN, MA Frank H. Netter School of Medicine – Quinnipiac University, North Haven, CT, USA

Harish Siddaiah, MD Department of Anesthesiology, LSU Health Shreveport, Shreveport, LA, USA

Kunal R. Sinha, MD Department of Physical Medicine and Rehabilitation, UCLA/Greater Los Angeles VA Health Care System, Los Angeles, CA, USA

David Geffen School of Medicine at UCLA, University of California, Los Angeles, CA, USA

Taylor Smith, Medical Student Department of Anesthesiology, Louisiana State University Health Shreveport, Shreveport, LA, USA

Sadie Smith, MD Department of Anesthesiology and Perioperative Medicine, Penn State College of Medicine, Milton S. Hershey Medical Center, Hershey, PA, USA

Warren Southerland, MD Department of Anesthesia, Critical Care, and Pain Medicine, Beth Israel Deaconess Medical Center, Harvard Medical School, Boston, MA, USA

Allyson L. Spence, PhD Department of Pharmaceutical Science, Regis University, Denver, CO, USA

Gabriel Stapleton, MD Department of Internal Medicine, Tulane University School of Medicine, New Orleans, LA, USA

Cain W. Stark, BS Medical College of Wisconsin, Wauwatosa, WI, USA

Nick Stiles, MD Department of Anesthesiology and Perioperative Medicine, Penn State College of Medicine, Milton S. Hershey Medical Center, Hershey, PA, USA

Max Antonio Thomasius, MD University Hospital Zurich, Zurich, Switzerland

Matthew Torre, DO Virginia Commonwealth University, Richmond, VA, USA

Mason E. Triay, BS Louisiana State University Health Shreveport, School of Medicine, Shreveport, LA, USA

Erin Tullis, BS Medical College of Wisconsin, Wauwatosa, WI, USA

Dirk Ubmann, MD University Hospital Zurich, Zurich, Switzerland

Nalini Vadivelu, MD Department of Anesthesiology, Yale University School of Medicine, New Haven, CT, USA

Steven D. Waldman, MD, JD University of Missouri – Kansas City School of Medicine, Kansas City, MO, USA

Dennis J. Warfield Jr., MD Department of Anesthesiology and Perioperative Medicine, Penn State College of Medicine, Milton S. Hershey Medical Center, Hershey, PA, USA

Brandt C. Wible, MD University of Missouri-Kansas City School of Medicine, Kansas City, MO, USA

Saint Luke's Health System, Department of Radiology, Saint Luke's Hospital, Kansas City, MO, USA

Ethan Williamson, MD University of Missouri – Kansas City School of Medicine, Kansas City, MO, USA

Jill Zafar, MD Department of Anesthesiology, Yale University School of Medicine, New Haven, CT, USA

Naema Zarish, MD Department of Anesthesiology, LSU Health Shreveport, Shreveport, LA, USA

Part I

Introduction

Academic and Non-academic Ambulatory Surgery Centers and Hospital Outpatient Departments

1

Tanith Graham

Abstract

Ambulatory surgery centers (ASCs), both academic and non-academic, have steadily increased in numbers since the 1970s when the first ASCs were started. ASCs offer surgeons the opportunity to perform procedures more efficiently and conveniently than hospital-based operating rooms. ASCs operate exclusively to provide surgical services to patients not requiring hospitalization and where the expected duration of services would not exceed 24 hours following admission. ASCs include those that provide service for specific indications such as orthopedics or eye surgery, as well as those that provide ambulatory surgery for a wide variety of procedures. They also vary widely in whether the ASC is physician owned, connected to a hospital, or part of an academic institution. Hospital outpatient departments (HOPDs) provide services similar to ASCs but are controlled more by hospital rules and processes than freestanding ASCs. These include hospital rules for physician privileges, restrictions on which patients can be included, and differing reimbursement rates from insurers.

Adequate pain management in an ASC requires communication among providers, patient education, preoperative multimodal medication use, judicious intraoperative narcotic use, and use of regional anesthesia when indicated. Some hurdles to provide ideal care involve the elaborate and different payment schemes from insurers and the lack of providers educated in current acute pain management techniques.

T. Graham (✉)
Department of Anesthesiology and Pain, University of Mississippi Medical Center, Jackson, MS, USA
e-mail: tgraham2@umc.edu

Introduction

Ambulatory surgery centers (ASCs), both academic and non-academic, have steadily increased in numbers since 1970 when Ford and Reed established the first modern non-hospital-associated ASC in Phoenix, Arizona [1]. ASCs offer surgeons the opportunity to perform procedures more efficiently and conveniently than hospital-based operating rooms. ASCs operate exclusively to provide surgical services to patients not requiring hospitalization and for whom the expected duration of services would not exceed 24 hours following admission. ASCs include those that provide service for specific indications such as orthopedics or eye surgery and those that provide ambulatory surgery for a wide variety of procedures. They also vary widely in whether the ASC is physician owned, con-

K. Rajput et al. (eds.), *Pain Control in Ambulatory Surgery Centers*,
https://doi.org/10.1007/978-3-030-55262-6_1

nected to a hospital, or part of an academic institution. Hospital outpatient departments (HOPDs) also provide services similar to ASCs but are controlled more by hospital rules and processes than ASCs. These include hospital rules for physician privileges and restrictions on which patients can be included.

Since the 1970s, increasing numbers of surgeries have been performed in ambulatory surgery centers (ASCs) that are increasingly less homogeneous. According to the Agency for Healthcare Research and Quality, almost 75% of all operations in the United States are done on an ambulatory basis, with many done in an ASC [2]. ASCs were originally started by physicians that wanted less hospital interference in day-to-day operations while being convenient for patients. ASCs may serve a single specialty such as ophthalmology, gastrointestinal (GI) procedures, or orthopedics, but most have evolved to cover almost all specialties. For example, neurosurgeons used ASCs in the 1980s and 1990s to perform carpel tunnels or minor nerve transfers, but now larger procedures such as laminectomies, general surgeries such as cholecystectomies, and joint replacements are commonly performed in ASCs.

Hospital outpatient departments (HOPDs) also take care of a large number of outpatient procedures and include surgery, GI, interventional radiology, radiation oncology, bronchoscopy, dialysis, and interventional pain services. Sometimes procedures done in these sites could easily be done in an ASC but for the burden of specialized equipment (such as CT scanners and robots) needed that can be budgeted better across both inpatients and outpatients. Both academic and non-academic institutions depend on these departments.

Organizations such as the Society for Ambulatory Anesthesia (SAMBA) and the International Association for Ambulatory Surgery (IASS) have formed to provide guidance and promote ambulatory surgery across the globe. The American Society of Anesthesiologists (ASA) offers guidelines for ambulatory anesthesia and surgery; these are summarized in Table 1.1. These guidelines state that all ASA standard practices should be maintained and set expectations in regard to staffing [3]. Government oversight is through agencies such as the The Joint Commission (JCAH) or the American Association for Accreditation of Ambulatory Surgery Facilities.

Definitions

Ambulatory Surgery Center (ASC) *An independent financial entity where procedures are done for patients that are expected to go home postoperatively, certainly within 24 hours.*

For purposes of Medicare, "an ASC is a distinct entity that operates exclusively for the purpose of providing surgical services to patients not requiring hospitalization and in which the expected duration of services would not exceed 24 hours following an admission [2]." An ASC has its own Medicare agreement that complies with the ASC Covered Procedures List, which is aimed at ensuring that procedures with appropriate risk are performed in these freestanding centers.

Occasionally, an ASC will be located within a hospital, but it is required to have a separate operational and financial structure.

Academic ASC An ASC that operates under the auspices and management of an educational entity whether within or outside the institution's buildings.

Hospital Outpatient Department (HOPD) Outpatient center owned and typically attached to a hospital. Most are physically attached to a hospital but can still be classified as a HOPD if it is within a 35-mile radius of the hospital and falls under the same financial and administrative contracts [4].

Table 1.1 An outline of ASA guidelines for ambulatory anesthesia and surgery [3]

I. ASA Standards, Guidelines and Policies should be adhered to in all settings except where they are not applicable to outpatient care.
II. A licensed physician should be in attendance in the facility, or, in the case of overnight care, immediately available by telephone, at all times during patient treatment and recovery and until the patients are medically discharged.
III. The facility must be established, constructed, equipped, and operated in accordance with applicable local, state, and federal laws and regulations. At a minimum, all settings should have a reliable source of oxygen, suction, resuscitation equipment, and emergency drugs. Specific reference is made to the ASA "Statement on Nonoperating Room Anesthetizing Locations."
IV. Staff should be adequate to meet patient and facility needs for all procedures performed in the setting and should consist of: A. Professional staff 1. Physicians and other practitioners who hold a valid license or certificate are duly qualified. 2. Nurses who are duly licensed and qualified. B. Administrative staff C. Housekeeping and maintenance staff
V. Physicians providing medical care in the facility should assume responsibility for credentials review, delineation of privileges, quality assurance, and peer review.
VI. Qualified personnel and equipment should be on hand to manage emergencies. There should be established policies and procedures to respond to emergencies and unanticipated patient transfer to an acute care facility.
VII. Minimal patient care should include: A. Preoperative instructions and preparation. B. An appropriate pre-anesthesia evaluation and examination by an anesthesiologist, prior to anesthesia and surgery. In the event that nonphysician personnel are utilized in the process, the anesthesiologist must verify the information and repeat and record essential key elements of the evaluation. C. Preoperative studies and consultations as medically indicated. D. An anesthesia plan developed by an anesthesiologist and discussed with and accepted by the patient and documented. E. Administration of anesthesia by anesthesiologists, other qualified physicians, or nonphysician anesthesia personnel medically directed by an anesthesiologist. Non-anesthesiologist physicians who are administering or supervising the administration of the continuum of anesthesia must be qualified by education, training, licensure, and appropriately credentialed by the facility. F. Discharge of the patient is a physician responsibility. G. Patients who receive other than un-supplemented local anesthesia must be discharged with a responsible adult. H. Written postoperative and follow-up care instructions. I. Accurate, confidential, and current medical records.

Trends

Ownership of ASCs involves physician-owned, hospital -owned, and joint venture models. Private physicians originally started ASCs to provide efficient service to outpatients while retaining control of management and better renumeration. These early centers were almost always controlled by the doctor-owners. With the strong competitive forces in many areas, physicians are drawn to consider a joint venture with another organization, such as a hospital or health maintenance organization (HMO), as a way to protect their practice without selling out entirely. With a partner, risk as well as planning and management can be shared. The advantages of a joint venture are the ability to collaborate with other partners, the ability to enter markets that require more capital, and accessing expertise without needing to hire more staff. Disadvantages are setting unrealistic objectives, coping with differing cultures as far as management styles, and managing communication with all the parties. The success of a joint venture requires thorough research and analysis by both parties. In joint ventures with a hospital, the ASC may use the hospital's greater buying power and the managerial expertise to bring a balance that benefits both the physician owners and the hospital. Many times, the hospital sees a joint venture as a good investment to keep doctors in their system. Of course, with the hospital governance comes more rules and credentialing issues than if solely physician owned. Quite often the hospital will acquire at least a 51% stake and a clear ASC board makeup that protects their investment. The ASC can share equipment and personnel with the hospital, lowering overheads. Facility fees that are separate from physician fees will then be shared with the hospital. New markets can be entered successfully that may have been prohibitive by the ASC alone, with the fiscal and marketing power of the hospital [5].

Now there are more than 9000 ASCs with incredible variety in procedures done in each and equally varied ownership schemas.

Non-academic ASC, as mentioned above, can be physician owned, hospital owned, or, more frequently, a joint venture between a doctor group and hospital. Although some teaching may occur, it is not the main focus of the ASC.

Academic institutions also own ASCs. Payment models of insurers, including private, Medicare, and Medicaid, are quite complex involving payment for physicians separate from the institutions. For these ASCs, payments are less than for the same procedures done at hospitals, but the cost of supplies and labor may be less, so complicated analysis is required when attempting to predict profitability.

Low-risk surgical procedures can be performed more efficiently in ASCs than in hospitals [6]. Because most ASCs are designed to deliver a narrow range of outpatient services, they can be more efficient than hospitals in ways such as faster OR turnover and lower facility overhead costs. By shifting certain cases that are repetitive and use the same supplies, hospitals can save cost by using ASCs for these cases. Another reason hospitals invest in ASCs is to regain their market share or to head off potential threats from future ASCs built in their catchment areas [7].

Improved patient convenience is an important reason for the shift to an ASC. Improved patient satisfaction, greater accessibility, easier parking, and a more peaceful environment are often mentioned in marketing quoted by ASCs, but there is little published research to confirm these opinions [8].

Improved access to meet community needs is often mentioned by hospitals as a reason to invest in ASCs in communities. Some health systems view local population health as part of their core mission. In some low-income and uninsured populations, ASCs may provide a lower-cost way to provide care. Often, care is complicated in these populations involving additional needs such as transportation, pharmacy, and follow-up visits, to make this transition work. The lower cost of the procedures might be offset by higher associated costs. In some situations, especially where the health system's status and value are tied to treating those populations, the additional cost can be justified [9].

Difference in Academic and Non-academic ASCs and HOPDs

There are major differences in academic and non-academic ASCs. In non-academic ASCs, management can be hired and directed by a physician board if privately owned. This gives the physician owners some control over who joins the ASC and control over cost containment. Often there is give and take over what procedures are done so as to limit the capital costs and overhead expenses just as in any other private enterprise. Of course, the ASC must follow Medicare and Medicaid guidelines if these patients are included [10].

Hospitals may decide to build an ASC either within their buildings or as a separate entity. As was earlier mentioned, some health systems want to provide an ASC as an efficient way to enter certain markets either as a profit center or as a service to populations that is unique.

Either way, the hospital usually manages the ASC as a department and uses their credentialing for physicians that utilize the ASC. In addition to Medicare and Medicaid guidelines, JCAHO inspections may be required. If students, residents, and fellows are involved, then academic accreditation reviews will also be required.

Hospital outpatient departments (HOPDs) also take care of a large number of outpatient procedures which include surgery, GI, interventional radiology, radiation oncology, bronchoscopy, dialysis, and interventional pain services. Sometimes, procedures done in these sites could easily be done in an ASC but for the burden of specialized equipment (such as CT scanners or robots) needed that can be budgeted better across both inpatients and outpatients. Both academic and non-academic institutions depend on these departments. Hospital outpatient departments also serve patients that will return home after procedures which makes comparison research with ASCs difficult.

In an academic ASC, whether in the main hospital or remote, management is a subdivision of the main university, credentialing is more regimented, and accommodation is usually necessary for resident and student education. Despite these limitations, academic ASCs abound as academic hospitals compete for the same outpatients as non-academic institutions and try to create the same efficiencies in lowering cost and improving patient satisfaction. One example of how academic medical centers have approached managing ASCs is the Johns Hopkins model [11]: Johns Hopkins University (JHM) has developed and used this model since 2014, using a *Surgery Coordinating Council* to integrate its eight ASCs with its HOPDs. This *Council* has several functions, namely, (1) promoting multidisciplinary interactions among JHM-employed and non-JHM-employed physicians; (2) setting strategy for ASC quality and safety efforts; and (3) identifying, implementing, and evaluating best practices. By including selected members from all the ASCs and the medical center within this Council, JHM feels that they have been successful in managing which patients should go to HOPDs versus ASCs and have managed quality measures that are difficult to assess individually at disparate ASCs. This has occurred despite a large increase in their ASC utilization and large increase in number of providers involved. For example, hospital transfer data highlighted differences between freestanding and hospital-based ASCs. Preliminary data demonstrated higher transfer rates at hospital-based ASCs. After more specific data was reviewed, it was found that a more severe case mix existed at these hospital-based centers, with overflow "inpatient" cases also scheduled in the hospital-based ASCs due solely to proximity. Therefore, the data had to be adjusted for appropriate and fair comparison among sites.

Funding

A major difference in funding for ASCs is in the way insurance companies, Medicare and Medicaid, pay for physician and facility fees. For ASCs in general, payment is 10–40% less for the same procedure done in an ASC versus a hospital outpatient department (HOPD). This is true even if the procedure is an identical outpatient procedure. For example, Medicare payment for colonoscopy (code 45380) in ASC is $405 and in HOPD setting is $803. Medicare payment for knee arthroscopy with repair of fractures (code 29851) is $570 in ASC, versus $1084 at HOPD. This is true for most procedures [12]. In addition, insurers tie increases in fees paid to ASCs to the overall Consumer Price Index for All Urban Consumers which rises slower than what is used for HOPDs, which is the hospital market basket for medical care services that is based solely on cost of medical care.

It gets complicated when certain areas of hospitals (or remote buildings) are considered HOPD versus ASC. This inequity has caused some hospitals to invest in outpatient facilities that are considered HOPD despite being quite remote from the original hospital buildings. In other situations, it makes more sense for a hospital to convert or buy an ASC.

Patient Selection

When choosing patients for ambulatory surgery, it is important to remember the expectation that the patient is to return home (or prior living situation) the same day or certainly within 24 hours. It is expected that there is no need for complex postoperative care or ongoing blood loss at a minimum. Patients with difficult airway history are usually scheduled for surgery at a hospital. Obstructive sleep apnea (OSA) patients require additional planning and examination but can be done safely on an ambulatory basis if capabilities of the facility and need for post-op opioids are taken into account. In OSA patients, the anesthesiologist should expect increased likelihood of difficult intubation, higher requirements for vasopressors, and possible need for supplemental oxygen in the PACU (postanesthesia care unit) [13]. Cardiovascular disease is incredibly prevalent even in ambulatory patients, and the American Heart Association (AHA), along with the American College of Cardiology (ACC), have practice guidelines that aid physicians in predicting perioperative complications and the need for further testing prior to ambulatory surgery. Patients who are known to be at risk for malignant hyperthermia are usually done at a hospital, but all ASCs must keep dantrolene on hand and have a "Malignant Hyperthermia Plan," including transportation to the nearest intensive care unit, for patients triggered without warning [14].

It is clear that all patients should have a preoperative evaluation with as much lead time as possible. For some healthy patients, a telephone assessment is appropriate, but in older patients with comorbidities, a face-to-face evaluation is advisable. Despite historically reserving ASCs for ASA I and II patients, procedures for ASA III and IV patients are safely done currently in ASCs provided their comorbid diseases are optimized and stable [15].

Intraoperative Management Technique

Choice of anesthetic technique is guided by multiple patient and surgery specific factors that may compete with each other [16]. Most anesthetists aim to provide great surgical conditions with rapid emergence. To make sure the patient can leave on time, postoperative nausea and vomiting (PONV) and pain must be controlled in a way that does not delay discharge. Controlling anxiety is important as up to 80% of patients presenting for a surgical procedure have preoperative anxiety [17], and several methods from preoperative benzodiazepines to allowing the patient to listen to music have been found to be effective [18]. General and/or regional anesthesia may be used depending on the particular surgery and patient's preference.

An exhaustive list of anesthetics will not be included, but just about all anesthetics that have ever been used have been used in an ambulatory setting. In general, most anesthetists follow the mantra, "Keep it Simple!" For small, short procedures, total intravenous anesthesia (TIVA) with propofol and/or local anesthetic is used. For more invasive procedures, TIVA or general anesthesia with pretreatment for nausea and vomiting along with pain medications may be used. Regional anesthesia may be substituted or added if the anesthetist is adept. A meta-analysis comparing discharge time from an ambulatory center among patients receiving peripheral nerve blocks, neuraxial technique, or general anesthesia showed no significant difference [19], although in another study [20], it was found that patients that received peripheral nerve blocks had less PONV and less pain and were discharged earlier.

Recovery should use the Aldrete scoring system (or its variant) until the patient is in phase I, when he is alert, able to maintain an airway, and hemodynamically stable; this may occur in the OR. In phase II, the patient is ready for discharge and can sit up, take oral input, and void.

Risk factors for PONV include female sex, use of postoperative opioids, prior history of PONV, and intraoperative use of volatile anesthetic agents and opioids. Dewinter and colleagues showed that a simple algorithm could be effective in preventing and treating PONV. This algorithm utilizes two anti-emetics for men and either three anti-emetics or two anti-emetics + propofol TIVA for women. This strategy has shown to result in a 33% decrease in incidence of PONV [21].

Postoperative pain management will be discussed in later chapters in more detail. It should be mentioned that a plan for postoperative pain management must be in place prior to induction of anesthesia. Multimodal analgesia is the use of two or more pain relieving agents that target pain pathways at different levels. This approach has been shown to reduce opioid use and its associated side effects [22]. Also, local anesthesia placed by surgeon or regional anesthesia blocks placed by anesthesiologist can add to patient's comfort while minimizing opioids.

Discharge

Patient safety is paramount when deciding to discharge a patient. Prior to surgery, living arrangement and home support, need to not drive for 24 hours, written discharge instructions, and how to contact a provider should be carefully discussed with the patient. These instructions should be reviewed again with patient and caregiver just prior to discharge.

Outcomes of Surgeries Performed in ASCs and HOPDs

Although attempts have been made to compare quality of care in ASC versus HOPD, it has been difficult due to the difference in patient characteristics at different institutions. Despite ASCs tending to do repetitive surgeries on relatively healthy patients, with HOPD patients tending to be unhealthier in general and in training environments, there have been some comparative studies done.

Grisel and Arjmand (2009), in a retrospective review of 486 cases, measured quality of ENT outpatient surgery done in an ambulatory surgery center (ASC) compared to a hospital-based facility (HOPD). The ASC had no unexpected safety events (0/211) compared to nine events at the HOPD (9/211). Patient satisfaction was similar between the facilities. Cases finished "on time" 77% of time at ASC and 38% of time at HOPD. Limitations of the retrospective study included slightly worse ASA classification and the use of surgery residents at the HOPD [23].

Ohsfeldt et al. (2017) used a multivariable logistic regression model to compare the risk-adjusted probability of hospitalization among a million patients across physician offices, ASCs, and HOPDs. The authors studied hospitalization rates at 7 and 30 days for 88 different procedures and 12 CPT groupings based on standard body system categories such as cardiovascular, GI, and genitourinary. The study found that ASCs had a slightly lower risk of hospitalization than HOPDs which was expected due to higher-risk patients at HOPDs [24].

Fleisher et al. (2004), in an observational study of claims analysis in Medicare patients undergoing 16 different surgical procedures for rates for mortality, ER visits, and hospital admissions within 7 days after outpatient surgery at HOPDs and ASCs. Risk-adjusted 7-day mortality rate was 25 per 100,000 procedures at an ASC and 50 per 100,000 procedures at HOPDs. Similar values were found for ER visits and hospital admissions [25].

Advantages of an ASC

ASCs have been shown to have greater efficiency with either no difference or fewer complications compared to HOPDs. A narrower scope of procedures performed at ASCs allows for more specialized care and high patient satisfaction. Selection of technology and scheduling preferences can be tailored to subspecialties and can place ASCs at an advantage [25]. Physicians who have ownership in an ASC may be more motivated to change or comply with cost-saving or quality improvement measures that would improve value of care. Even when ASCs are owned by academic institutions, many of these same advantages are applicable due to a smaller group of staff and comradery found when working with the same colleagues day in and day out.

Advantages of a HOPD

With a HOPD, physicians avoid the financial risks and loss of investment that they can suffer when investing in an ASC. Conflicts of interest can be avoided when the surgeon does not have a financial incentive to operate. More predictable payments for surgical care may be possible, although without ownership, fees may be lower. Currently, despite insurers improving disparity between ASC and HOPD fee schedules, HOPDs have advantage of higher reimbursement for most procedures. And finally, HOPD can be convenient for those patients that may need unexpected overnight or possibly longer stays [26].

Pain Relief in ASCs and HOPDs

Pain relief will be discussed in more detail in later chapters. One of the major challenges at ASCs, academic ASCs, and HOPDs is communication. It is imperative for the perioperative team including surgeon, anesthesiologist, and nurses to inquire into patient's expectations for pain control, previous experiences, and current medication regimens. With this knowledge, a plan can be formulated to successfully treat the expected pain from each procedure. Often, this plan includes multimodal medications such as anticonvulsants, acetaminophen, and even narcotics on occasion. Local anesthesia can be infiltrated by the surgeon or nerve block performed by the anesthesiologist to supplement more painful cases.

As an example, for mastectomy, patients are often prescribed pre-emptive analgesics such as gabapentin and Tylenol prior to surgery. An anesthesiologist may perform either a paravertebral block or Pecs (Pectoralis) block, in addition to using narcotics to aid in post-op pain relief. To arrange this scenario, the physician's office would have to order the gabapentin preoperatively and explain any side effects. An anesthesiologist trained in regional anesthesiology would have to be present to perform the block. Such planning takes time and effort requiring processes to be established in an ASC/HOPD setting but in the long run is expected to improve outcomes and patient satisfaction scores.

Summary

In this chapter, academic and non-academic ambulatory surgery centers have been described and compared with hospital outpatient departments. Ownership is varied and depending upon whether the center is physician owned or part of a hospital system either totally or as part of a joint venture; the management system and financial arrangements can be quite complex. If part of an academic institution, the management hierarchy will also control the ASC, and teaching is an important part of the mission. ASC reimbursement and increase in fees over time are less than that for HOPDs for the same procedures. Patient disease severity is greater in both HOPDs and hospital ASCs making quality comparisons difficult among academic ASCs, non-academic ASCs, and HOPDs.

Patient selection, discharge plans, and communication among providers are extremely important parts of a successful outpatient experience and probably more important than the specific anesthetic used for a particular case [27].

References

1. Ambulatory Surgical Care Association. 2020. www.ascassociation.org. Accessed May 30, 2020.
2. Wier LM, Steiner CA, Owens PL. Surgeries in hospital-owned outpatient facilities, 2012, Healthcare cost and utilization project statistical brief #188. Rockville: Agency for Healthcare Research and Quality; 2015. www.hcup-us.ahrq.gov/reports/statbriefs/sb188-Surgeries-Hospital-Outpatient-Facilities-2012.jsp. Accessed March 1, 2020.
3. American Society of Anesthesiologists. Guidelines for ambulatory anesthesia and surgery. Amended October 2016. www.asahq.org/quality-and-practice-management/standards-guidelines-and-related-resorces/guidelines-for-ambulatory-anesthesia-and-surgery?_ga=2.43925733.13287440.15194871618824.1416088195. Accessed May 1, 2020.
4. Tanaka MJ. Ambulatory surgery centers versus hospital-based outpatient departments: what's the difference? American Academy of Orthopedic Surgeons Practice Management. September 2019.
5. Marlow K, Sagraves B. In: Peisert KC, editor. The hospital joint venture book. San Diego: The Governance Institute; 2015. Governanceinstitute.com. Accessed June 1, 2020.
6. Mitchell JM, Carey K. A comparison of ambulatory surgery center production costs and Medicare payments: evidence on colonoscopy and endoscopy. Med Care. 2016;54(2):126–32.
7. O'Neill SM, Frencher SK, Pellegrini CA, Flum DR. Should your health care system invest in an ambulatory surgery center? A decision-making framework.

The Bulletin. November 1, 2017. https://bulletin.facs.org/2017/11/should-your-health-care-system-invest-in-an-ambultory-surgery-center-a-decision-making-framework/.
8. Gardner TF, Nnadozie MU, Davis BA, Kirk S. Patient anxiety and patient satisfaction in hospital based and freestanding ambulatory surgery centers. J Nurs Care Qual. 2005;20(3):238–43.
9. Hayanga AJ, Kaiser HE, Sinha R, Berenholtz SM, Makary M, Chang D. Residential segregation and access to surgical care by minority populations in U.S. counties. J Am Coll Surg. 2009;208(6):1017–22.
10. Urman RD, Philip BK. Accreditation of ambulatory facilities. Anesthesiol Clin. 2014;32:551–7.
11. Ishii L, Pronovost PJ, Demski R, Wylie G, Zenilman M. A model for integrating ambulatory surgery centers into an academic health system using a novel ambulatory surgery coordinating council. Acad Med. 2016;91(6):803–6.
12. Medicare.gov: Price Procedure Lookup. Available at: https://www.medicare.gov/procedures-price-lookip/cost/. Accessed May 1, 2020.
13. Stierer TL, Wright C, George A, et al. Risk assessment of obstructive sleep apnea in a population of patients undergoing ambulatory surgery. J Clin Sleep Med. 2010;6:467–72.
14. Litman RS, Joshi GP. Malignant hyperthermia in the ambulatory surgery center: how should we prepare? Anesthesiology. 2014;120(6):1306–8. https://doi.org/10.1097/ALN.0000000000000256.
15. Ansell G, Montgomery J. Outcome of ASA III patients undergoing day case surgery. Br J Anaesth. 2004;92:71–4.
16. Dibble JE, Calimaran AL. Ambulatory and office based surgery. In: Fox CJ, Cormett EM, Ghali GE, editors. *Castastrophic perioperative complications and management: a comprehensive textbook*. Cham: Springer; 2019.
17. Sheen MJ, Chang FL, Ho ST. Anesthetic premedication: new horizons of an old practice. Acta Anaesthesiol Taiwanica. 2014;52:134–42.
18. Hole J, Hirsch M, Ball E, et al. Music as an aid for postoperative recovery in adults: a systemic review and meta-analysis. Lancet. 2015;386:1659–71.
19. Liu S, Strodtbeck W, Richman J, et al. A comparison of regional versus general anesthesia for ambulatory anesthesia: a meta-analysis of randomized controlled trials. Anesth Analg. 2005;101:1634–42.
20. Hadzic A, Arliss J, Kerimoglu B, et al. A comparison of infraclavicular nerve block versus general anesthesia for hand and wrist day-case surgeries. Anesthesiology. 2004;101:127–32.
21. Dewinter G, Staelens W, Veef E, Teunkens A, Van de Velde M, Rex S. Simplified algorithm for the prevention of PONV: a before and after study. Br J Anaesth. 2018;120:156–63.
22. Halawi MS, Grawl SA, Bolognesi MP. Multimodal analgesia for total joint arthroplasty. Orthopedics. 2015;38:c615–25.
23. Grisel J, Arjmand E. Comparing quality at an ambulatory surgery center and a hospital-based facility: preliminary findings. Otolaryngol Head Neck Surg. 141:701–9. PubMed: https://journals.sagepub.com/doe/10.1016/j.otohns.2009.09.002.
24. Ohsfeldt RL, Pengxiang L, Schneider JE, Stojanovic I, Scheibling CM. Outcomes of surgeries performed in physician offices compared with ambulatory surgery centers and hospital outpatient departments in Florida. Health Serv Insights. 2017;10:1178632917701025. https://doi.org/10.1177/1178632917701025.
25. Fleisher LA, Pasternak LR, Herbert R, Anderson GF. Inpatient hospital admission and death after outpatient surgery in elderly patients: importance of patient and system characteristics and location of care. Arch Surg. 2004;139(1):67–72. https://doi.org/10.1001/archsurg.139.1.67.
26. Shafrin J. A study in quality: ambulatory surgery centers versus hospital outpatient departments. *Healthcare Economist*. January 7, 2008. https://www.healthcare-economist.com/2008/01/07/a-study-in-quality-ambulatory-surgery.
27. Lee JH. Anesthesia for ambulatory surgery. Korean J Anesthesiol. 2017;70(4):398–406. https://doi.org/10.4097/kjae.2017.70.4.398. Accessed June 8, 2020.

Opioid Epidemic

2

Our Current Opioid Epidemic in the United States: Prevalence, Physiology, Mechanisms, and Clinical Implications

Michelle A. Carroll Turpin, Allyson L. Spence, Brook Girma, Peter Clapp, Anitha Senthil, Harish Siddaiah, Mark R. Jones, Elyse M. Cornett, and Alan David Kaye

Abstract

Opioid medications prescribed to treat acute pain may become misused and lead to opioid use disorder or death from overdose. The successful management of moderate or severe acute pain, which involves a complex network of signaling molecules and receptor types and is physiologically distinct from other forms of pain, has historically relied on the administration of potent opioids. A variety of non-opioid pharmacotherapies, including non-steroidal anti-inflammatory agents, anticonvulsants, and glutamate channel blockers, receive attention from prescribers as safer alternatives to opioid analgesics. Additionally, nonpharmacologic approaches may provide effective pain relief and can also improve functional performance and hasten recovery from injury. This chapter will provide an in-depth examination of acute pain treatment in the context of the ongoing opioid misuse epidemic, including physiologic

Theme of chapter: Linkage to opioids given for acute pain management, what is the evidence

M. A. Carroll Turpin
Department of Biomedical Sciences, College of Medicine, University of Houston, Houston, TX, USA
e-mail: macarrol@central.uh.edu

A. L. Spence
Department of Pharmaceutical Science, Regis University, Denver, CO, USA
e-mail: aspence002@regis.edu

B. Girma · H. Siddaiah
Department of Anesthesiology, LSU Health Shreveport, Shreveport, LA, USA
e-mail: bgirma@lsuhsc.edu; hbanga@lsuhsc.edu

P. Clapp
Regis University School of Pharmacy, Denver, CO, USA
e-mail: pclapp@regis.edu

A. Senthil
Department of Anesthesiology, Lahey Hospital & Medical Center, Burlington, MA, USA

M. R. Jones
Department of Anesthesiology, Weill Cornell Medical College, New York-Presbyterian Hospital, New York, NY, USA

Weill Cornell Medical College, Department of Anesthesia, New York, NY, USA

E. M. Cornett (✉)
Department of Anesthesiology, Louisiana State University Health Shreveport, Shreveport, LA, USA
e-mail: ecorne@lsuhsc.edu

A. D. Kaye
Departments of Anesthesiology and Pharmacology, Toxicology, and Neurosciences, LSU Health Shreveport, Shreveport, LA, USA
e-mail: akaye@lsuhsc.edu

K. Rajput et al. (eds.), *Pain Control in Ambulatory Surgery Centers*,
https://doi.org/10.1007/978-3-030-55262-6_2

mechanisms of acute pain, alternate pharmacologic therapies to target acute pain, and pain management through multimodal analgesic approaches.

Introduction

The United States is in the midst of an opioid epidemic that has manifest in the overdose deaths of approximately 47,000 Americans in 2018, the latest year available since the President declared a public health emergency in the fall of 2017. The drugs responsible for these deaths include natural and semi-synthetic opioids (e.g., oxycodone, morphine), heroin, and synthetic opioids (e.g., fentanyl). The involvement of synthetic opioids has been steadily increasing since the start of 2017, and these drugs were present in more than 70% of opioid-related deaths in 2019 [1]. The opioid crisis affects broad segments of the population, including over two million persons 12 years and older who report meeting criteria for an opioid use disorder (OUD) in the past 12 months [2].

The epidemic is complex, much as the history of opioid medication use in pain management is complex, and involves competing interests and changing perceptions of responsible treatment goals [3]. It is important to recognize the delicate balance between the need to effectively treat pain and the potential consequences of repeated exposure to psychoactive opioid medications. Prescription opioids remain an important treatment option for pain management, particularly for the treatment of postprocedural or perioperative pain within a controlled setting and short-term neuropathic pain and cancer pain. Adequate pain control is a goal of physicians and hospital systems. Effective management often requires treatment combinations (including an opioid) that target multiple pathways or high potency medications to reduce pain significantly [4]. In this regard, all states have created laws limiting opioid prescriptions for acute pain such as after surgical procedures to be limited to approximately seven days in an attempt to curb the opioid epidemic since many of those patients previously were prescribed opioids for months leading to dependence and addiction.

The risks of long-term opioid use (i.e., the development of an opioid use disorder (OUD) or lethal overdose) have been most closely associated with treating chronic or persistent pain. It should be noted that any person who takes exogenous opioids will shut down their endogenous opioid production over weeks and months. When exogenous opioids are then stopped, central nervous system hyperarousal, e.g., withdrawal, is seen.

Furthermore, although evidence of effectiveness is lacking, well-intended physicians have prescribed opioids for chronic noncancer pain for years believing that the risk of addiction was low [5]. Opioids produce positive subjective effects, including euphoria and pain relief through overlapping pathways in the central nervous system. Extended exposure can produce a physical dependence that is characterized by tolerance and an aversive withdrawal syndrome. The potential for abuse among related compounds, such as prescription opioid medications like oxycodone and illicit opioids like heroin, is related to the potency of the compound, route of administration, and the pharmacokinetic properties of the drug formulation. However, a significant cross-tolerance may develop, allowing individuals to substitute different opioids to achieve similar subjective effects [6].

Although short-term opioid use alone, in the setting of acute pain treatment, is less likely to promote dependence or OUD, opioid therapy prescribed for acute pain has been associated with a greater likelihood of long-term use [7]. Acute injuries, such as those due to sporting or motor vehicle accidents, may be treated in the short term with opioids prescribed by an emergency department for outpatient use. Opioid use in this context can establish a pattern of chronic use in some patients.

In the context of this ongoing epidemic, strategies for reducing misuse of prescription and illicit opioids and preventing new cases of overdose, death, and diagnosis of OUD include reductions in supply, demand, and harms caused by misuse [8]. Specifically, policies to reduce the opioid supply may involve regulations on the types of products approved by the Federal Drug Administration for use (e.g., abuse-deterrent formulations) and restricting lawful access through the Controlled Substances Act. Furthermore, the provision of prescribing guidelines and provider education initiatives may influence prescribers to reduce the legal supply in the patient's hands. Demand may be reduced through patient education on the risks associated with opioid use and by increasing access to treatment for OUD. Harm reduction strategies include increasing access to rescue medications such as naloxone to prevent overdose deaths and establishing needle exchange programs for those who administer opioids by injection.

Providers treating patients for acute pain have additional strategies to prevent increasing patterns of misuse. Guidelines for acute pain management, including dosage and dosing intervals, may be developed and adopted by state medical boards and professional associations to promote safer prescribing practices that minimize reliance on opioids in favor of non-opioid alternatives and nonpharmacologic interventions. Each patient may be assessed before opioid therapy to determine the risk of developing behavior patterns of misuse or abuse. This strategy involves screening patients for abuse potential using an interview-based method during the initial visit, including a review of medical records, signs of existing substance abuse, point of care urine drug testing, and other approaches [9]. The decision to prescribe opioids can also be informed by utilizing a prescription drug monitoring program (PDMP). These statewide databases collect information on controlled substances that have been prescribed and dispensed to individuals over time and allow for the detection of high-risk patterns of use, and unsafe drug combinations and inappropriate prescribing practices [10].

The remainder of this chapter will provide a more in-depth examination of acute pain treatment in the context of the ongoing opioid misuse epidemic. Following a description of the current knowledge on the physiologic mechanisms of acute pain, we will discuss alternate pharmacologic therapies to target acute pain, including pain management through multimodal analgesic approaches. Finally, a discussion of how nonpharmacologic approaches may be utilized in practice, and the importance of patient and provider education on the effectiveness of nonpharmacologic treatments will be presented.

Opioid Epidemic

The United States has been the epicenter for an epidemic of opioid abuse and overdose death for over 20 years. The flashpoint for this crisis is often assigned paradoxically as the legitimate realization, in the mid-1990s, that pain went frequently unrecognized and undertreated, which inspired a well-intentioned campaign that characterized pain as the "fifth vital sign" [11]. This was accompanied by relaxed regulatory oversight of narcotic prescriptions [12] and a pharmaceutical marketing bonanza for new drug formulations lauded as less risky, when they were highly addictive. Prescriptions for the popular extended-release oxycodone OxyContin® increased approximately tenfold from 1997 to 2002 [13]. Meanwhile, visits to the nation's emergency departments due to opioid overdose more than tripled [14], and the Drug Abuse Warning Network medical examiner and coroner surveillance system reported a 96% increase in overdose deaths due to opioid analgesics, with a concurrent mind-boggling 728% rise in oxycodone-related fatalities [15], during that time.

Looking back over the data on drug overdoses for this time, it has become clear that the epidemic was comprised of three waves: the first initial increase in prescription opioid abuse, the second a rise in heroin use, and the third terrifyingly steep wave of synthetic opioid overdose [16]. The number of deaths due to synthetic opioid overdose has dwarfed the numbers previous waves have been responsible for, and the fatalities continue to climb. In 2017, two out of every three drug overdose deaths was attributed to an opioid [17].

Nationally, the rate at which opioids were prescribed peaked in 2012, and fell to the lowest rate in over ten years in 2018 [18]. It is important to note that this trend is not ubiquitous – hot spots still remain in certain areas of the country, where some counties have reported prescription rates up to six times higher than the national average [18]. While a general downward trend in prescribing may help reduce the availability of drugs for diversion and abuse, there is ample evidence that many users switch to illicit drug use. Eighty percent of heroin users surveyed in one study reported starting with prescription opioids [19].

Despite the mounting concern over the prevalence of opioid abuse, 38% of US adults reported having been prescribed an opioid in 2015 [20]. To limit the availability of prescription opioids, more than half of state legislatures have responded to this public health crisis by passing laws to provide guidance and limitations on the dosage and duration of opioid prescription for acute pain [21]. Many such laws focus on restricting the number of days an initial prescription can be written for acute, noncancer pain – no more than seven days' worth, in most cases [22] – as the likelihood of chronic opioid use is related to the length of the first prescription. However, some research would suggest that this timeframe is problematic, as the probability for long-term opioid use was found to be most highly correlated to 5 (and 31) days of use [23], and notably, the average length of initial opioid therapy was found to be 5.1 days in a 2017 study [24].

Another attempt at state-level prescription opioid control has been the development of prescription drug monitoring programs (PDMPs), databases maintained by a state which records all prescriptions of scheduled substances. Many state laws enacted to control prescription opioid use include a stipulation that a prescriber must reference the PDMP before providing a patient a prescription for a narcotic. As of the year 2020, 49 states and the District of Columbia have developed PDMPs. Data on the effectiveness of PDMP use is limited but promising. The state of Wisconsin passed a law in 2017 requiring review of the PDMP before an opioid prescription could be written. A study conducted by the Mayo Clinic Health System in Wisconsin looked at opioid prescribing rates over time starting before the law went into effect. The amount of opioids prescribed per patient encounter went down 33%, with a 13% reduction in the number of patient encounters resulting in an opioid prescription [25]. These data would suggest required PDMP review is helpful in reigning in opioid use. However, as it represents only one healthcare system in a single state, the reproducibility of these results across states, where PDMP requirements vary and cannot be easily predicted.

Healthcare providers have likewise responded to the burgeoning epidemic with their programs and policy changes. Ninety-eight percent of hospitals surveyed in a 2018 study reported having developed new policies and procedures related to opioid prescription. The most commonly implemented action was provider education, followed by improved technological oversight of prescribing and the use of alternative, non-narcotic options for acute pain management [26]. Other responses included prescription limitations, safe disposal programs, and the addition of new staff specifically to support opioid crisis response efforts. Although the new policies and strategies were deemed as least "moderately effective" by the majority of respondents, there was wide variability among which actions were described as "very" and "extremely" effective. Notably, although prescriber education was the most popular implementation, only 24% characterized it as "very" or "extremely" effective. Conversely, very few respondents added new staff; however, 67% of those who did describe the change as "very" effective [26]. Perhaps the most startling takeaway from the study was, despite the collective national recognition of the scope and severity of the opioid epidemic, 40% of survey respondents reported their organization had not increased spending to support new opioid-related policies, and procedures and 34% were unsure.

While broad oversight at the state and healthcare systems level may help curtail the current opioid crisis, a significant challenge remaining is the lack of standardized recommendations to inform the prescription of narcotics for acute pain. Although the CDC published guidelines chronic pain management in 2016 [27], acute pain management remains largely splintered, varying widely among prescribers and hospitals, and guided mostly by professional opinion and anec-

Table 2.1 Types of acute pain [33]

	Types of pain	Symptom	Mechanism
1a	Somatic nociceptive pain	Short pricking pain, well-localized pain (Aδ-myelinated fibers) Dull pain sensation, poor localization (C fibers-unmyelinated)	Response of nociceptors to stimuli Superficial structures-Aδ and C Deep structures -C fibers Aδ-thermal and mechanical stimuli C-thermal, mechanical, or chemical stimuli
1b	Visceral nociceptive pain	Vague, colicky, pressure, achy, poorly localized pain	Silent nociceptors stimulated by chemical inflammatory mediators
2	Neuropathic pain	Associated allodynia due to repetitive non-painful stimulation of receptors	Peripheral and central sensitization Increased expression of Na_v channel Nerve injury due to trauma, toxins, and inflammation from herpes zoster infections
3	Inflammatory pain	Hyperalgesia, allodynia (Aδ fibers)	Release of inflammatory mediators

dotal evidence. A systemic review published in 2018 identified four sets of guidelines for the management of acute, nonmalignant pain, which generally agree on several commonly accepted actions, including the restriction of narcotic use for pain that has not responded to previous non-opioid therapy, reference to a PDMP before prescribing an opioid, starting with the lowest effective dose, and placing a limitation on the duration of opioid use. Guidelines lack consensus when it came to strategies to avoid opioid-related adverse events [28].

Ultimately, the majority of the American public views prescription opioid addiction as a belief that increased education for medical students and physicians would be a very effective method of preventing prescription drug addiction. Additionally, it would appear that increased patient/public education is necessary, considering very few Americans (7%) express concern that they might become addicted to pain killers [29].

Acute Pain

Acute pain is an unpleasant subjective sensation, which is a physiological response provoked by tissue injury resulting from mechanical, chemical, or thermal insult. Acute pain differs from other types of pain as it is sudden in onset and time-limited and influences behaviors to avoid potential or actual tissue injury [30]. Plasticity demonstrated by pain pathways to noxious stimuli is initially protective and beneficial, but with persistent changes, acute pain can transform into chronic pain [31]. Acute pain could last up to 3 months [32] and can result in functional impairment limiting mobility, self-care [30], and sleep deprivation and hinder social interactions (Table 2.1).

Acute pain can be precipitated by various factors such as:

1. Tissue injury due to surgery or trauma
2. Burns
3. Acute illness
4. Acute exacerbation of chronic disease, for example, sickle cell crisis, multiple sclerosis, trigeminal neuralgia, pancreatitis, or acute pain related to cancer or cancer treatment
5. Labor pain

Pain Pathway and Molecular Mechanisms

Pain is perceived when a noxious stimulus activates myelinated Aδ fibers and unmyelinated C-fibers. The impulse transmits from the peripheral nervous system to the central and autonomic nervous systems through the dorsal horn of the spinal cord via the lateral spinothalamic tract to the thalamus and spinoreticulothalamic tract to the thalamus via the brainstem. From the thalamus, the information is transferred to the ipsilateral postcentral gyrus and subcortical regions, including the amygdala, hypothalamus, periaqueductal grey, and basal ganglia. The output from the spinal cord is regulated by the descending inhibitory pathways from the midbrain [33].

Pain transmission involves a variety of excitatory and inhibitory receptors and neurotransmitters. Transduction molecules expressed on the nociceptors like transient receptor potential ion channels {TRPV1, TRPM8, TRPA1}, sodium channels (such as NaV 1.8 and 1.9), and potassium channel (such as TRAAK and TREK-1) modulate the nociceptor excitability [31]. Activation of nociceptors by noxious stimulus and chemical inflammatory mediators transmits information via excitatory neurotransmitter glutamate. The chemical mediators released from the site of injury are prostaglandins, leukotrienes, 5-hydroxy-tryptamine, histamine, bradykinin, protons, nerve growth factors, and nitric oxide (NO) to name a few, which activates nociceptors to produce neurotransmitter substance P [34]. Transmission of signal from spinoreticulothalamic tract results in the release of norepinephrine from the locus coeruleus neurons of the brainstem, which has an important role in pain modulation along with endogenous opioid peptides like enkephalins, dynorphins, and β-endorphins, which stimulate the opioid receptors in the neurons of the dorsal horn of spine and periaqueductal grey matter of the midbrain [34]. Other chemical mediators that modulate pain perception are non-inflammatory mediators like gamma-aminobutyric acid (GABA) and calcitonin gene-related peptide [33]. Expression of (tyrosine kinase) TrkA neurotrophin receptor on the nociceptor responds to nerve growth factor (NGF) [31].

Treatment of Acute Pain

Individuals differ in their ability to cope with the sudden onset of pain, and it is a challenging situation for a clinician to strike the delicate balance between adequate pain relief and avoidance of possible abuse risk. In addition to the options discussed below, it is essential to diagnose and treat the underlying cause of pain. To achieve maximum patient comfort while minimizing the risks, multimodal analgesia is strongly recommended by the American Pain Society and American Society of Anesthesiologists. This approach involves the simultaneous use of various analgesic medications and techniques with different mechanisms of action, targeting pain pathways with or without additional nonpharmacologic interventions [35, 36]. Various techniques such as epidural analgesia, patient-controlled analgesia, and peripheral nerve blocks including continuous local anesthetic-based peripheral regional techniques can be used to achieve optimum pain control and allow a reduction in opioid dosage. Treatment plans usually require close monitoring and adjustments depending on the response, prevailing clinical situation, and development of adverse events.

1. Pharmacologic therapies (see Table 2.2)
   - Opioids and non-opioids
2. Nonpharmacologic interventions
   - Cognitive-behavioral modalities, namely, relaxation methods, distraction techniques [32]
   - Application of cold/heat, immobilization
   - Transcutaneous electrical nerve stimulation [38]

     Delivery of pulsed electrical currents across intact skin surface to stimulate peripheral nerves for pain relief [38]
   - Others: acupuncture, exercise, guided motor imagery, psychosocial interventions, and rehabilitation
3. Interventional procedures
   - Regional and neuraxial blocks

Pain therapy is individualized after a thorough assessment of the patient. Strategies for planning require careful risk stratification based on the nature of the disease or injury resulting in pain, individual patient preferences, age, gender of patient, and associated risk factors like allergies; alcohol, tobacco, and substance abuse; concomitant medications; preexisting pain; anxiety; depression; severity of pain; and existing comorbidities [35]. The center for disease control recommends using the lowest effective opioid dose and shortest duration appropriate for the pain condition that balances benefits, risks, and

Table 2.2 Pharmacologic therapies for acute pain [4, 36]

Medications	Mechanism of action	Indication	Concern	Comments
Acetaminophen {intravenous (IV), oral, or rectal}	Inhibits cyclooxygenase and prostaglandin H2 synthase	Mild to moderate pain Opioid-sparing effects	Hepatotoxicity Renotoxicity	Have been used in addition to opioids Not to exceed 4000 mg/day
Non-steroidal anti-inflammatory drugs {NSAIDS, including cyclooxygenase-(COX)-2 inhibitors}	Inhibits the enzyme, cyclooxygenase, and decreases prostaglandin synthesis	Mild to moderate pain	Bronchospasm, bleeding, anastomotic leaks [32], acute kidney injury Cardiovascular events	Have been used in addition to opioids
Tramadol	(μ, κ, δ agonist) Also inhibits reuptake of norepinephrine and serotonin	Moderate to severe acute pain	Serotoninergic and noradrenergic effects, risk of misuse and dependence	Caution on use with SSRI (selective serotonin reuptake inhibitor)
Opioids, for example, hydrocodone, oxycodone, morphine, fentanyl, tapentadol (IV, oral, subcutaneous, transdermal, transmucosal)	Act on central and peripheral μ, κ, and δ opioid receptors in the nervous system	Moderate to severe acute pain	Respiratory depression, sedation, pruritus, addiction, withdrawal, constipation, nausea, vomiting	Opioids used with regional anesthetic techniques and patient-controlled analgesia (PCA) Caution regarding serotonin syndrome while using tapentadol with serotonergic medications
Antidepressants, for example, duloxetine	Serotonin-norepinephrine reuptake inhibitor, blocks voltage-gated sodium channels	Acute neuropathic pain	Gastrointestinal side effects	
Ketamine	*N*-methyl-D-aspartate (NMDA) receptor antagonist	Postoperative pain	Psychotomimetic effects, nausea, vomiting	Dampens central sensitization [37]
Anticonvulsants – gabapentin, pregabalin (oral)	Calcium channel α-2-δ1 and α-2-δ2 antagonists	Opioid-sparing effect	Sedation, dizziness	Reduces release of serotonin, glutamate, norepinephrine, dopamine, and substance P
Alpha-2 agonists – clonidine, dexmedetomidine		Opioid-sparing effect	Sedation, hypotension Bradycardia	
Magnesium	NMDA receptor antagonist	Opioid-sparing effect and reduced pain scores		Synergistic effect with ketamine
Glucocorticoids (dexamethasone) Oral and IV	Anti-inflammatory	Postoperative pain, nausea, vomiting	Delayed wound healing and hyperglycemia	Side effects more of concern with prolonged use

adverse reactions. Ideally, opioid prescription for less than seven days could help prevent unintentional chronic use [39, 40]. Clinicians should individualize dose based on a carefully monitored medication trial. Clear instructions on tapering of analgesics are very important to prevent the continuation of use.

Treatment goals include alleviation of fear and anxiety, reduce incidence of adverse effects, facilitate early mobilization, and enhance recovery, restoration of function, and overall patient satisfaction.

Engagement of the patients in the decision-making process, reassurance, and timely intervention are the key for successfully implementing interventions targeted at acute pain relief [35]. Patient and family education about realistic goals and expectations have to be discussed at length. Interdisciplinary team involvement including pain specialists, nurses, physiotherapists, and pharmacists is important for safe and effective management of pain relief.

Multimodal Analgesia and Opioid Alternatives

The consequences of the opioid epidemic have spurred the development of non-opioid modalities for the treatment of acute pain. Many of the negative effects contributing to the tragic death toll seen in the epidemic are also encountered by clinicians frequently in the acute setting, including respiratory depression, gastrointestinal dysmotility, hyperalgesia, over-sedation, and more. Entire surgical protocols and pathways are now devoted to, in large part, limiting the deleterious effects of opioids. These protocols, deemed enhanced recovery after surgery or ERAS pathways, incorporate multimodal analgesia as a foundational principle without exception.

Multimodal analgesic theory derives from the multifactorial physiology of pain and nociception. As our understanding of pain mechanisms has evolved, it has become clear that an array of biochemical receptors and pathways coalesce into the ultimate subjective pain experience. No single therapeutic intervention can extend an effect over all the various receptors. Furthermore, overreliance on one modality increases the risk of the side effects from that particular therapy, as seen with opioids. By understanding the multifaceted nature of pain, clinicians can simultaneously target the array of individual components with additive or synergistic effects to achieve an acceptable level of analgesia while avoiding or minimizing opioids [41]. Many institutions now employ standardized multimodal regimens for specific surgical subtypes, with all patients, barring contraindications, receiving the same combination of analgesic options. Similarly, many societies have introduced procedure-specific guidelines for postoperative pain control.

Three main pillars make up the approach to multimodal analgesia; see Table 2.3. The first component, systemic analgesia, comprises the extensive pharmacologic options available to a clinician treating a patient in acute pain. Table 2.2 lists the most frequently encountered analgesic medications utilized in multimodal regimens. A typical regimen will include a combination of NSAIDs, acetaminophen, gabapentinoids, and NMDA antagonists, with opioids reserved for breakthrough analgesia. Preoperative administration of oral medications, such as gabapentinoids, promotes sustained analgesia that extends into the postoperative period, reducing the reliance on opioids both intra- and postoperatively. It is important to recognize that a synergistic analgesic benefit is reached by delivering a formulation that acts on multiple receptor subtypes

Table 2.3 Example of multimodal analgesic pathway for total knee arthroplasty [42]

Multimodal analgesia for total knee arthroplasty	
Preoperative nonpharmacologic	Compression
	Cryotherapy
	Acupuncture
	Electrical stimulation
Preoperative pharmacologic	Acetaminophen
	Pregabalin
	Gabapentin
Neuraxial anesthesia	Spinal vs. epidural
Intraoperative medications	Dexamethasone
	Ketorolac
	Ketamine
	Magnesium
Local and regional anesthesia	Femoral nerve ± sciatic nerve
	Adductor canal block
	Lumbar plexus ± sacral plexus
	Femoral nerve ± LIA
	Adductor canal ± LIA
	Adductor canal ± IPACK
	LIA only
PACU analgesia	Repeat acetaminophen
	Oxycodone
	Hydromorphone
	Rescue regional anesthesia (i.e., sciatic block for refractory knee pain)

LIA ¼ local infiltration analgesia, *IPACK* ¼ infiltration between the popliteal artery and capsule of the knee simultaneously. In that respect, multimodal analgesic regimens should be utilized as needed for an extended period postoperatively to provide continued pain relief and limit reliance on opioids.

Neuraxial anesthesia serves as the second component of multimodal analgesia. By accessing the epidural or intrathecal space of the spinal canal, a clinician may administer local anesthetic via an epidural catheter or a single shot spinal dose. Continuous epidural infusion of local anesthetic has been shown to provide postoperative analgesia superior to opioids, and decreased perioperative pulmonary-cardiac morbidity, and promote earlier return of gastrointestinal tract function [43]. Employed for thoracoabdominal surgeries with large incisions, continuous epidural analgesia effectively controls pain without reliance on opioids but is limited by side effects such as hypotension, sensory deficits, motor weakness, and urinary retention. As an adjunct, opioids such as hydromorphone and fentanyl are commonly added to an epidural infusion or intrathecal spinal dose and can impart significant analgesia. Similar to systemic opioids, side effects include nausea, vomiting, pruritus, or respiratory depression.

Regional anesthetic techniques, representing the final arm of multimodal analgesia, have in recent decades improved drastically in scope, safety, and efficacy and are now considered a critical aspect of most multimodal regimens. Regional anesthesia may be defined as applying local anesthetic around a target nerve plexus to inhibit the sensation of painful surgical stimuli in a specific dermatomal distribution. Techniques exist for upper extremity, lower extremity, thoracoabdominal, and head and neck surgeries.

The advent of ultrasound has allowed for considerable improvements in the technical safety profile of nerve blocks, allowing a larger range of anesthesiologists to provide regional anesthesia capably [44]. This is of considerable importance as it not only allows for relief from acute pain and reduces opioid consumption but enables significant improvements in overall patient outcomes as well. In hip and knee arthroplasty, regional anesthesia has demonstrated reductions in mortality, major morbidity such as pulmonary complications and transfusion requirements, and improvements in economic outcomes such as hospital length of stay [45, 46]. The potential benefits extend to oncologic surgery, whereby mechanistic evidence suggests that regional anesthesia may inhibit tumor cell seeding and growth [47]. Moreover, the risk of chronic, postoperative pain states such as post-thoracotomy syndrome is also reduced by applying regional techniques [48]. The optimal analgesic strategy likely prophylactically inhibits the nociceptive impulse by utilizing pre-incisional rather than postoperative nerve blockade, in combination with other multimodal techniques [49].

In addition to ultrasound guidance, several other recent advances have allowed expansion of the scope of practice. The main drawback of regional anesthesia is the finite duration of single-injection techniques. Patients typically enjoy 12–16 hours of effective analgesia but are caught off guard by powerful rebound pain once the block wears off. One solution to this challenge has been to prolong the duration of effect by using sustained-release local anesthetics or utilizing continuous catheter techniques. Liposomal bupivacaine is currently the only sustained-release local anesthetic formulation commercially available in the United States. By encasing standard bupivacaine in liposomes, local anesthetic release duration may be prolonged as the liposomes break down and emit the active medication [50]. While it theoretically should provide pain relief for several days, current evidence suggests only a mild benefit that does not warrant the increased cost [44]. Alternatively, perineural catheters may be left following the block that continuously infuses local anesthetic. These may be left for several days and effectively reduce the risk of rebound pain from a single shot. However, catheters are more complex to perform and resource-intensive to care for, and incur the additional risks of undesirable side effects from prolonged conduction block, infection, and catheter entrapment, and added mechanical problems such as catheter migration, dislodgement, leakage, pump malfunction, or suboptimal dosing regimens [44].

One report suggested that problems resulting from perineural catheter placement included technical problems (17%), failure of pain relief (3.2%), and transient paresthesia and dysesthesia (1.4%) [51]. Colonization of bacteria was also present in 28% of cases [51]. Furthermore, a 2018 study found adverse effects of a continuous pain pump (On-Q) for total knee arthroplasty [52]. Patients displayed decreased ambulation and had an increased length of stay, suggesting that pain catheters can yield the opposite of the intended effect for patients. Another 2018 study found an increased length of stay in patients who received the On-Q pump and further reported that the pump was no more effective at improving postoperative pain compared to a single-shot nerve block [53]. Finally, there is also evidence to suggest that Exparel is more effective at decreasing the need for oral pain medication following surgery when compared to the On-Q pump [54]. Overall, these studies suggest that perineural catheters may not be the best choice for extended pain control in all patients.

An alternative to neuraxial anesthesia, fascial plane blocks are an interesting group of regional anesthetic techniques that have developed over recent years. Fascial plane blocks are performed by injecting local anesthetic into fascial planes rather than directly around discrete nerves and are primarily applied as simpler and safer truncal analgesia alternatives than thoracic epidurals and paravertebral blocks. The transversus abdominis plane (TAP) block was the first to enter mainstream practice, but today fascial plane blocks encompass a diverse range of techniques that provide analgesia for surgeries of the thorax and abdomen and include the rectus sheath block, quadratus lumborum (QL) block, and erector spinae plane (ESP) block [55, 56].

The tools available for providing multimodal analgesia in the acute setting are wide-ranging and impactful. Extensive knowledge of pharmacology and fine technical skill is required to utilize multimodal analgesia to its full extent. Already a powerful alternative to opioids, the regimens of medications, neuraxial anesthesia, and regional anesthesia will continue to refine as the medical field combats the perils of the opioid epidemic. By approaching acute pain with the several-pronged spear that is multimodal analgesia, clinicians can more deftly apply pain relief that is personalized to the individual patient while avoiding the negative consequences of opioids.

Nonpharmacologic Treatments for Acute Pain

Research has demonstrated that nonpharmacologic interventions provide a safer alternative for the treatment of acute pain compared to opioids. Importantly, these nonpharmacologic treatment regimens have also demonstrated efficacy in relieving acute pain, improving function and quality of life, and increasing patient compliance [57, 58]. Systematic reviews and meta-analyses suggest that manual therapy, exercise therapy, and acupuncture may be viable treatment alternatives for acute pain (See Table 2.4) [1, 3].

The current data surrounding the effectiveness of manual therapy, or hands-on therapy, is inconsistent. While several studies have touted

Table 2.4 Nonpharmacologic treatments for acute pain[a]

Massage therapy	Light, moderate, or deep pressure that is applied to the soft tissues, particularly the muscle [59]
Chiropractic and osteopathic manipulation	Manual therapy technique that involves the manipulation of muscles, bones, and joints [60]
Physical therapy	A branch of rehabilitative health that includes manual forms of therapy (such as massage) with exercise therapy to alleviate pain and improve movement and function [61]
Exercise therapy	Activities that require physical effort, such as aerobic conditioning and muscle strengthening [62]
Acupuncture	Traditional Chinese treatment that involves the strategic insertion of thin needles through a patient's skin [63]

[a]This list does not encompass all of the many nonpharmacologic treatment options that are available to provide acute pain relief. Other viable treatment options include, but are not limited to, yoga, Tai Chi, cognitive behavioral therapy, mindfulness mediation, and the locus of control technique [64]

the efficacy of these treatment regimens, other researchers argue that positive responses to these interventions are simply due to the placebo response [65–67]. Sports injuries, falls, and car accidents are a few of the most common causes of acute musculoskeletal pain that can be treated with manual therapy [68]. Interestingly, evidence indicates that manual therapy can be as effective and even more effective, in treating musculoskeletal pain compared to oral analgesics [69]. Careers that employ manual therapies have significantly grown in popularity in recent years. The number of practicing osteopathic physicians, who engage in manual therapies such as osteopathic manipulation, has grown more than 60% in the past decade and almost 300% over the past three decades [70]. Similarly, physical therapists have seen substantial job growth in the past decade, and the Bureau of Labor Statistics predicts that this growth is not expected to slow down any time soon [71]. The increased popularity of manual therapies to treat acute pain is important since many of these therapies, such as spinal manipulations and mobilizations, not only have proven to be effective in reducing pain but have also demonstrated efficacy in increasing functional performance [72, 73]. The underlying mechanisms responsible for the efficacy of these manual therapies in providing pain relief include enhancing neuromuscular function while also improving biomechanical balance [73].

Further studies point to the increased benefit of combining manual therapy, such as massage therapy, with analgesic pharmacotherapies to alleviate the acute postoperative pain. Patients receiving massage therapy combined with pharmacotherapies reported significantly less pain than patients who only received analgesic medications [74]. A similar study found that massage therapy significantly reduced postoperative acute pain and opioid administration [75]. Another study conducted in the acute care setting found massage therapy positively impacted patients' overall pain level, emotional well-being, and ability to sleep [76]. Several mechanisms are thought to be responsible for the ability of massage therapy to provide acute pain relief, including the stimulation of competing nerve fibers, anxiolytic effects, and the relaxation of painful muscles, joints, and tendons [77].

Among the nonpharmacologic treatment options available for pain, exercise therapy has the strongest evidence supporting its efficacy in reducing pain symptoms [78, 79]. Similar to massage therapy, regular exercise alleviates pain through the stimulation of competing nerve fibers. High-intensity exercise also stimulates the release of beta-endorphins and neurotransmitters correlated with increased mood and reduced pain [80]. However, most of this research emphasizes the role that exercise therapy plays in reducing chronic pain, and research involving exercise therapy and acute pain is limited and often inconsistent [81, 82]. Researchers remain hopeful that exercise may still be a viable option for the acute pain associated with surgeries, as physical activity is a key factor in contributing to a faster recovery with fewer symptoms of pain [41].

Acupuncture is a nonpharmacologic, traditional Chinese treatment that involves the strategic insertion of thin needles through a patient's skin [63]. This commonly used form of therapy has provided a significantly greater pain reduction compared to both sham groups and groups receiving traditional analgesic injections [83]. Researchers have proposed that acupuncture may relieve pain by targeting pain-modulating neurotransmitters, specifically met-enkephalin and substance P [84]. Although acupuncture has been around for thousands of years and demonstrates high efficacy in alleviating pain, many clinicians still claim that its ability to reduce pain is no different than the placebo effect, and thus, more research should be done to strengthen its use in the clinical setting [83, 85].

These nonpharmacologic treatments have two important similarities with pharmacological treatments. First, research has shown that these regimens should be administered at proper "doses" for optimal effectiveness. For example, low doses of exercise (i.e., defined as three times per week) did not sufficiently reduce symptoms of acute pain, whereas moderate to high doses of exercise (i.e., defined as five to ten times per week) significantly reduced patients' pain ratings

[86]. Likewise, massage therapy reduces chronic pain when administered for at least 60 minutes, as 30-minute massages did not provide pain relief [87]. Although more research needs to be done to see if these same dosing regimens are required to alleviate acute pain, these findings are particularly interesting because they may explain the inconsistencies found in the efficacy of nonpharmacologic interventions for pain relief.

Also similar to pharmacological treatments, the outcomes of these nonpharmacologic treatments depend on patient compliance, which can be improved by implementing several key factors [88]. One of the most effective ways to increase patient adherence is to "prescribe" these nonpharmacologic treatment strategies [89]. This "prescription" can ensure that patients receive the proper "dose" and fully understand the recommended treatment regimen. Furthermore, patients are more likely to take these treatment regimens more seriously when they are prescribed by doctors, thus leading to increased patient adherence [90].

In summary, these nonpharmacologic treatments for acute pain possess many benefits, as they reduce the need for opioid administration, diminish symptoms of pain, improve functionality, are easily accessible, and are cost-efficient for patients [57, 64, 91, 92].

Summary

The ongoing US opioid epidemic has taken many lives and impacted millions of Americans' health and well-being. Although illegal narcotics such as heroin are partially responsible for the epidemic, the role of prescription opioid pain medications is of critical importance to understanding how patterns of misuse and abuse develop over time. Opioid medications prescribed to treat acute pain may become misused and lead to opioid use disorder or death from overdose. Patients, prescribers, and manufacturers all share the burden of responsibility for the developing epidemic that has steadily increased in mortality since the mid-1990s. Changes in approval policies and treatment guidelines and increased vigilance of healthcare providers and hospital systems may stem the flow of opioids. Enhanced education for medical professionals and the American public, supported by rigorous biomedical research, may ultimately be the most effective strategy for changing practice.

The successful management of moderate or severe acute pain, which involves a complex network of signaling molecules and receptor types and is physiologically distinct from other forms of pain, has historically relied on the administration of potent opioids. Acute pain has numerous causes and different presentations that make it difficult for many patients to manage. A variety of non-opioid pharmacotherapies including non-steroidal anti-inflammatory agents, anticonvulsants, and glutamate channel blockers, receive attention from prescribers as safer alternatives to opioid analgesics. Improved understanding of the pathways in the nervous system that transmit pain signals has led to multimodal regimens of therapy that aim to provide effective analgesia and at the same time minimize the harmful side effects of each monotherapy. Combining systemic analgesia with epidural and regional anesthetic techniques has empowered clinicians to apply precise and scalable pain relief in a controlled, acute setting. Nonpharmacologic approaches may provide effective pain relief and can also improve functional performance and hasten recovery from injury. Evidence is growing to support the use of manual therapy, exercise, and acupuncture in addition to more traditional medicine for pain management. In all cases, caution must be taken so that treatments for acute pain are administered at appropriate doses and for a safe and effective duration of time.

Pain is a real and life-changing phenomenon that must be a priority for healthcare providers to improve their patients' well-being. At the same time, the powerful effect of opioids to reduce the sensation of pain is inextricably tied to the activation of reward pathways in the brain that reinforce the continued use of these drugs. To move away from practices that have contributed to the opioid epidemic will require creative and evidence-based approaches that reduce our reliance on opioids as the sole solution to the problem of pain.

References

1. CDC. Vital statistics rapid release: provisional drug overdose death counts. Centers for Disease Prevention and Control. 2020.
2. CDC. Annual surveillance report of drug-related risks and outcomes – Usnited States surveillance special report. Centers for Disease Control and Prevention, U.S. Department of Health and Human Services. 2019.
3. Jones MR, Viswanath O, Peck J, Kaye AD, Gill JS, Simopoulos TT. A brief history of the opioid epidemic and strategies for pain medicine. Pain Ther. 2018 Jun;7(1):13–21.
4. Blondell RD, Azadfard M, Wisniewski AM. Pharmacologic therapy for acute pain. Am Fam Physician. 2013;87(11):766–72.
5. Krashin D, Murinova N, Sullivan M. Challenges to treatment of chronic pain and addiction during the "opioid crisis". Curr Pain Headache Rep. 2016;20:65.
6. Dunn KE. Promoting a comprehensive understanding of the opioid epidemic. Int Rev Psychiatry. 2018;30:89.
7. Dowell D, Haegerich TM, Chou R. CDC guideline for prescribing opioids for chronic pain – United States, 2016. JAMA [Internet]. 2016 Apr 19 [cited 2017 Nov 1];315(15):1624. Available from: http://jama.jamanetwork.com/article.aspx?doi=https://doi.org/10.1001/jama.2016.1464.
8. Bonnie RJ, Ford MA, Phillips JK. Pain management and the opioid epidemic: balancing societal and individual benefits and risks of prescription opioid use. Washington, DC: The National Academies Press; 2017 [cited 2020 Jun 8]. Available from: https://doi.org/10.17226/24781.
9. Kaye AD, Jones MR, Kaye AM, Ripoll JG, Jones DE, Galan V, et al. Prescription opioid abuse in chronic pain: an updated review of opioid abuse predictors and strategies to curb opioid abuse (part 2) – PubMed. Pain Physician [Internet]. 2017 Feb [cited 2020 Jun 8];20(2S):S111–33. Available from: https://pubmed.ncbi.nlm.nih.gov/28226334/.
10. Patrick SW, Fry CE, Jones TF, Buntin MB. Implementation of prescription drug monitoring programs associated with reductions in opioid-related death rates. Health Aff. 2016;35:1324.
11. Morone NE, Weiner DK. Pain as the fifth vital sign: exposing the vital need for pain education. Clin Ther. 2013;35(11):1728–32.
12. Joranson DE, Gilson AM, Dahl JL, Haddox JD. Pain management, controlled substances, and state medical board policy: a decade of change. J Pain Symptom Manage. 2002;23(2):138–47.
13. Hwang CS, Chang H-Y, Alexander GC. Impact of abuse-deterrent OxyContin on prescription opioid utilization. Pharmacoepidemiol Drug Saf. 2015;24:197–204.
14. Hasegawa K, Espinola JA, Brown DFM, Camargo CA. Trends in U.S. emergency department visits for opioid overdose, 1993-2010. Pain Med. 2014;15(10):1765–70.
15. Paulozzi LJ. Opioid analgesic involvement in drug abuse deaths in American metropolitan areas. Am J Public Health. 2006;96(10):1755–7.
16. Centers for Disease Control and Prevention. Opioid overdose. 2020.
17. Wilson N, Kariisa M, Seth P, Smith H, Davis NL. Drug and opioid-involved overdose deaths – United States, 2017-2018. MMWR Morb Mortal Wkly Rep. 2020;69(11):290–7.
18. Centers for Disease Control and Prevention. US opioid prescribing rate maps. 2020.
19. Muhuri PK, Gfroerer JC, Davies MC. Associations of nonmedical pain reliever use and initiation of heroin use in the United States. CBHSQ Data Review. 2013.
20. Han B, Compton WM, Blanco C, Crane E, Lee J, Jones CM. Prescription opioid use, misuse, and use disorders in U.S. adults: 2015 national survey on drug use and health. Ann Intern Med. 2017;167(5):293–301.
21. National Conference of State Legislatures. Prescribing policies: states confront opioid overdose epidemic. 2019.
22. Davis CS, Lieberman AJ, Hernandez-Delgado H, Suba C. Laws limiting the prescribing or dispensing of opioids for acute pain in the United States: a national systemic legal review. Drug Alcohol Depend. 2019;194:166–72.
23. Shah A, Hayes CJ, Martin BC. Characteristics of initial prescription episodes and likelihood of long-term opioid use – United States, 2006–2015. Morb Mortal Wkly Rep. 2017;66(10):265–9.
24. Zhu W, Chernew ME, Sherry TB, Maestas N. Initial opioid prescriptions among U.S. commercially insured patients, 2012-2017. N Engl J Med. 2019;380(11):1043–52.
25. Derleth BM, Dexter DD, Arndt R, Lea CM, Dierkhising RA, Dow JF. Effect of a statewide controlled-substance monitoring requirement on the opioid prescribing practice for treatment of acute pain. WMJ. 2020;119(1):33–6.
26. The opioid epidemic – a view from the front lines survey results. 2018. p. 1–11.
27. Dowell D, Haegerish TM, Chou R. CDC guidelines for prescribing opioids for chronic pain – United States, 2016. MMWR Morb Mortal Wkly Rep. 2016;65:1–49.
28. Herzig SJ, Calcaterra SL, Mosher HJ, Ronan MV, Van Groningen N, Shek L, et al. Safe opioid prescribing for acute noncancer pain in hospitalized adults: a systematic review of existing guidelines. J Hosp Med. 2018;13(4):256–62.
29. Blendon RJ, Benson JM. The public and the opioid-abuse epidemic. N Engl J Med. 2018;378(5):405–7.

30. Kent ML, Tighe PJ, Belfer I, Brennan TJ, Bruehl S, Brummett CM, et al. The ACTTION–APS–AAPM Pain Taxonomy (AAAPT) multidimensional approach to classifying acute pain conditions. Pain Med Off J Am Acad Pain Med. 2017;18(5):947.
31. Basbaum AI, Bautista DM, Scherrer G, Julius D. Cellular and molecular mechanisms of pain. Cell. 2009;139(2):267–84.
32. Small C, Laycock H. Acute postoperative pain management. Br J Surg. 2020;107(2):e70–80.
33. Yam MF, Loh YC, Tan CS, Adam SK, Manan NA, Basir R. General pathways of pain sensation and the major neurotransmitters involved in pain regulation. Int J Mol Sci. 2018;19(8):2164.
34. Garland EL. Pain processing in the human nervous system: a selective review of nociceptive and biobehavioral pathways. Prim Care. 2012;39(3):561–71.
35. Chou R, Gordon DB, de Leon-Casasola OA, Rosenberg JM, Bickler S, Brennan T, et al. Management of postoperative pain: a clinical practice guideline from the American Pain Society, the American Society of Regional Anesthesia and Pain Medicine, and the American Society of Anesthesiologists' Committee on Regional Anesthesia, Executive Committee, and Administrative Council. J Pain. 2016;17(2):131–57.
36. Helander EM, Menard BL, Harmon CM, Homra BK, Allain AV, Bordelon GJ, et al. Multimodal analgesia, current concepts, and acute pain considerations. Curr Pain Headache Rep. 2017;21(1):3.
37. Wardhan R, Chelly J. Recent advances in acute pain management: understanding the mechanisms of acute pain, the prescription of opioids, and the role of multimodal pain therapy. F1000Res. 2017;6:2065.
38. Johnson MI, Jones G, Paley CA, Wittkopf PG. The clinical efficacy of transcutaneous electrical nerve stimulation (TENS) for acute and chronic pain: a protocol for a meta-analysis of randomised controlled trials (RCTs). BMJ Open. 2019;9(10):e029999.
39. Shah A, Hayes CJ, Martin BC. Characteristics of initial prescription episodes and likelihood of long-term opioid use – United States, 2006–2015. MMWR Morb Mortal Wkly Rep. 2017;66(10):265–9.
40. Dowell D, Haegerich TM, Chou R. CDC guideline for prescribing opioids for chronic pain – United States, 2016. MMWR Recomm Rep [Internet]. 2016 Mar 15 [cited 2017 Nov 13];65(1):1–49. Available from: http://www.cdc.gov/mmwr/volumes/65/rr/rr6501e1er.htm.
41. Beverly A, Kaye AD, Ljungqvist O, Urman RD. Essential elements of multimodal analgesia in enhanced recovery after surgery (ERAS) guidelines. Anesthesiol Clin [Internet]. 2017 Jun [cited 2019 Oct 7];35(2):e115–43. Available from: http://www.ncbi.nlm.nih.gov/pubmed/28526156.
42. Kandarian BS, Elkassabany NM, Tamboli M, Mariano ER. Updates on multimodal analgesia and regional anesthesia for total knee arthroplasty patients. Best Pract Res Clin Anaesthesiol. Bailliere Tindall Ltd. 2019;33:111–23.
43. Wick EC, Grant MC, Wu CL. Postoperative multimodal analgesia pain management with nonopioid analgesics and techniques: a review. JAMA Surg. American Medical Association. 2017;152:691–7.
44. Albrecht E, Chin KJ. Advances in regional anaesthesia and acute pain management: a narrative review. Anaesthesia. Blackwell Publishing Ltd. 2020;75:e101–10.
45. Perlas A, Chan VWS, Beattie S. Anesthesia technique and mortality after total hip or knee arthroplasty. Anesthesiology. 2016;125(4):724–31.
46. Memtsoudis SG, Sun X, Chiu YL, Stundner O, Liu SS, Banerjee S, et al. Perioperative comparative effectiveness of anesthetic technique in orthopedic patients. Anesthesiology. 2013;118(5):1046–58.
47. Cata JP. Outcomes of regional anesthesia in cancer patients. Curr Opin Anaesthesiol. 2018;31:593–600.
48. Weinstein EJ, Levene JL, Cohen MS, Andreae DA, Chao JY, Johnson M, et al. Local anaesthetics and regional anaesthesia versus conventional analgesia for preventing persistent postoperative pain in adults and children. Cochrane Database Syst Rev. 2018;6(6):CD007105.
49. Holmberg A, Sauter AR, Klaastad Ø, Drægni T, Ræder JC. Pre-operative brachial plexus block compared with an identical block performed at the end of surgery: a prospective, double-blind, randomised clinical trial. Anaesthesia. 2017;72(8):967–77.
50. Ilfeld BM, Gabriel RA, Eisenach JC. Liposomal bupivacaine infiltration for knee arthroplasty: significant analgesic benefits or just a bunch of fat? Anesthesiology. Lippincott Williams and Wilkins. 2018;129:623–6.
51. Boezaart AP. Perineural infusion of local anesthetics. Anesthesiology [Internet]. ASA Publications. 2006 [cited 2020 Jun 16];104:872–80. Available from: https://anesthesiology.pubs.asahq.org/article.aspx?articleid=1923431.
52. O'Neil S, Danielson K, Johnson K, Matelic T. ON-Q infusion pump linked to increased hospital stay after total knee arthroplasty. J Orthop. 2018;15(2):666–70.
53. Ganta A, Ding D, Fisher N, Lavery J, Jain S, Tejwani NC. Continuous infraclavicular brachial block versus single-shot nerve block for distal radius surgery. J Orthop Trauma [Internet]. 2018 Jan [cited 2020 Jun 16];32(1):22–6. Available from: http://journals.lww.com/00005131-201801000-00005.
54. Tecce MG, Bae A, Familusi OT, Lanni MA, Weissler JM, Carney MJ, et al. Abstract 60. Exparel versus the On-Q pump. Plast Reconstr Surg Glob Open. 2017;5(2 Suppl):52–3.
55. Chin KJ, Mcdonnell JG, Carvalho B, Sharkey A, Pawa A, Gadsden J. Essentials of our current understanding: abdominal wall blocks. Reg Anesth Pain Med. 2017;42:133–83.
56. Chin KJ. Thoracic wall blocks: from paravertebral to retrolaminar to serratus to erector spinae and back again – a review of evidence. Best Pract Res Clin Anaesthesiol. Bailliere Tindall Ltd. 2019;33:67–77.

57. Bonnie RJ, Ford MA, Phillips JK. Pain management and the opioid epidemic: balancing societal and individual benefits and risks of prescription opioid use, A consensus study report of the National Academies of Sciences, Engineering, Medicine. Washington, DC: The National Academies Press; 2017.
58. Haneline MT, Cooperstein R. Chiropractic care for patients with acute neck pain: results of a pragmatic practice-based feasibility study. J Chiropr Med. 2009;8(4):143–55.
59. Field T. Massage therapy research review. Complement Ther Clin Pract. 2016;24:19.
60. Rist PM, Hernandez A, Bernstein C, Kowalski M, Osypiuk K, Vining R, et al. The impact of spinal manipulation on migraine pain and disability: a systematic review and meta-analysis. Headache. 2019;59:532.
61. Chimenti RL, Frey-Law LA, Sluka KA. A mechanism-based approach to physical therapist management of pain. Phys Ther. 2018;98:302.
62. Ambrose KR, Golightly YM. Physical exercise as non-pharmacological treatment of chronic pain: why and when. Best Pract Res Clin Rheumatol. 2015;29:120.
63. Zhuang Y, Jing-jing X, Li J, Zeng BY, Liang F. History of acupuncture research. Int Rev Neurobiol. 2013;111:1–23.
64. Kaye AD, Granier AL, Garcia AJ, Carlson SF, Fuller MC, Haroldson AR, et al. Non-opioid perioperative pain strategies for the clinician: a narrative review. Pain Ther. 2020;9(1):25–39.
65. Wong JJ, Shearer HM, Mior S, Jacobs C, Côté P, Randhawa K, et al. Are manual therapies, passive physical modalities, or acupuncture effective for the management of patients with whiplash-associated disorders or neck pain and associated disorders? An update of the Bone and Joint Decade Task Force on Neck Pain and Its Associated Disorders by the OPTIMa collaboration. Spine J. 2016;16:1598–630.
66. Bialosky JE, Beneciuk JM, Bishop MD, Coronado RA, Penza CW, Simon CB, et al. Unraveling the mechanisms of manual therapy: modeling an approach. J Orthop Sports Phys Ther. 2018;48:8.
67. Bialosky JE, Bishop MD, Penza CW. Placebo mechanisms of manual therapy: a sheep in Wolf's clothing? J Orthop Sports Phys Ther. 2017;47:301.
68. Geri T, Viceconti A, Minacci M, Testa M, Rossettini G. Manual therapy: exploiting the role of human touch. Musculoskelet Sci Pract. 2019;44:102044.
69. Qaseem A, Wilt TJ, McLean RM, Forciea MA. Noninvasive treatments for acute, subacute, and chronic low back pain: a clinical practice guideline from the American College of Physicians. Ann Intern Med. 2017;166(7):514.
70. American Osteopathic Association. Osteopathic medical profession report. 2019.
71. U.S. Bureau of Labor Statistics. Physical therapists. 2019.
72. Carpino G, Tran S, Currie S, Enebo B, Davidson BS, Howarth SJ. Does manual therapy affect functional and biomechanical outcomes of a sit-to-stand task in a population with low back pain? A preliminary analysis. Chiropr Man Therap. 2020;28:5.
73. Bodine WA. Osteopathic manipulative treatment: a primary care approach. Am Fam Physician. 2019;99(4):214.
74. Boitor M, Gélinas C, Richard-Lalonde M, Thombs BD. The effect of massage on acute postoperative pain in critically and acutely ill adults post-thoracic surgery: systematic review and meta-analysis of randomized controlled trials. Heart Lung. 2017;46:339.
75. Miladinia M, Pishgooie AH, Aliyari S, Nouri EM. The comparison of the effect of two complementary medicine methods (music therapy and massage therapy) on postoperative acute pain after abdominal surgery: a randomized clinical trial study. Iran Red Crescent Med J. 2017;19 https://doi.org/10.5812/ircmj.14974.
76. Adams R, White B, Beckett C. The effects of massage therapy on pain management in the acute care setting. Int J Ther Massage Bodywork. 2010;3:4–11.
77. Zhong H, Wang C, Wan Z, Lei J. The possible mechanisms of massage therapy. Biomed Res. 2019;30(5):1–6.
78. Cohen SP, Hooten WM. Advances in the diagnosis and management of neck pain. BMJ. 2017;358:j3221.
79. Furlan AD, Yazdi F, Tsertsvadze A, Gross A, Van Tulder M, Santaguida L, et al. Complementary and alternative therapies for back pain II. Evid Rep Technol Assess. 2010;194:1–764.
80. Martins DF, Mazzardo-Martins L, Soldi F, Stramosk J, Piovezan AP, Santos ARS. High-intensity swimming exercise reduces neuropathic pain in an animal model of complex regional pain syndrome type I: evidence for a role of the adenosinergic system. Neuroscience. 2013;234:69–76.
81. Gross A, Kay TM, Paquin JP, Blanchette S, Lalonde P, Christie T, et al. Exercises for mechanical neck disorders. Cochrane Database Syst Rev. 2015;1:CD004250.
82. Casser H-R, Seddigh S, Rauschmann M. Acute lumbar back pain. Dtsch Arztebl Int. 2016;113:223–34.
83. Xiang A, Cheng K, Shen X, Xu P, Liu S. The immediate analgesic effect of acupuncture for pain: a systematic review and meta-analysis. Evid Based Complement Alternat Med [Internet]. 2017 [cited 2019 Oct 2];2017:3837194. Available from: http://www.ncbi.nlm.nih.gov/pubmed/29234385.
84. Cheng KJ. Neurobiological mechanisms of acupuncture for some common illnesses: a clinician's perspective. J Acupunct Meridian Stud. 2014;7:105.
85. Zhu D, Gao Y, Chang J, Kong J. Placebo acupuncture devices: considerations for acupuncture research. Evid Based Complement Alternat Med. 2013;2013:628907.
86. Polaski AM, Phelps AL, Szucs KA, Ramsey AM, Kostek MC, Kolber BJ. The dosing of aerobic exercise therapy on experimentally-induced pain in healthy female participants. Sci Rep. 2019;9:14842.
87. Sherman KJ, Cherkin DC, Hawkes RJ, Miglioretti DL, Deyo RA. Randomized trial of therapeutic massage for chronic neck pain. Clin J Pain. 2009;25:233.

88. Walters-Salas T. The challenge of patient adherence. Bariatr Nurs Surg Patient Care. 2012;7(4):186.
89. Seth A. Exercise prescription: what does it mean for primary care? Br J Gen Pract. 2014;64:12.
90. Maiorana A, Levinger I, Davison K, Smart N, Coombes J. Exercise prescription is not just for medical doctors: the benefits of shared care by physicians and exercise professionals. Br J Sports Med. 2018;52:879.
91. Miyamoto GC, Lin CWC, Cabral CMN, Van Dongen JM, Van Tulder MW. Cost-effectiveness of exercise therapy in the treatment of non-specific neck pain and low back pain: a systematic review with meta-analysis. Br J Sports Med. 2019;53:172.
92. Hidalgo B, Hall T, Bossert J, Dugeny A, Cagnie B, Pitance L. The efficacy of manual therapy and exercise for treating non-specific neck pain: a systematic review. J Back Musculoskelet Rehabil. 2017;30:1149–69.

Current US Policy for Opioid Prescribing

3

Achal Shah, Daniel Haddad, Nalini Vadivelu, and Kanishka Rajput

Abstract

The United States is in the throes of a prescription opioid epidemic responsible for more than 150,000 deaths over the past decade. In many ways, this is a historical retread of a story told previously in the late nineteenth-century United States, one of rampant prescription drug abuse and the sharp professional and governmental correction that ensued. Since that time, numerous federal regulations, treatment guidelines, and programs to reduce opioid-related harm have been established. In addition to federal initiatives, individual states have also relied on medical practice standards and prescription drug monitoring programs to curb addiction and misuse at a local level.

To ensure best practice with regard to opioid prescribing, prescribers must be familiar with guidelines and keep abreast of recent developments in opioid policy. This would ensure improved patient outcomes and reduced risk of diversion and addiction while protecting providers from disciplinary action. This chapter provides an overview of the historical groundwork of opioid laws and the present-day role of regulatory bodies such as the DEA, FDA, and state medical boards. We will also discuss recent policy initiatives regarding opioid prescribing as well as the outlook of those likely destined for fruition.

Introduction

Pain management in the midst of an enduring opioid epidemic cannot be practiced in a silo. Judicious prescribing of opiates must not only weigh the patient specific risks against their analgesic benefits but also integrate the public health externalities that result from their misuse and abuse. Opioid prescribing practices have come under scrutiny due to a number of alarming trends, most notably a fourfold increase in the rate of death from prescription opioid overdose from 1999 to 2017 (from 1.3 to 5.4 deaths per 100,000 persons) [1]. Figure 3.1 illustrates this disturbing trend, with prescription opioid deaths rising in accordance with increased prescription use from 1999 to 2010 (a period which saw the quadrupling of morphine milligram equivalents prescribed per capita) and subsequently plateauing with increased opioid pre-

A. Shah · D. Haddad · N. Vadivelu
Department of Anesthesiology, Yale University School of Medicine, New Haven, CT, USA
e-mail: achal.shah@yale.edu; daniel.haddad@yale.edu

K. Rajput (✉)
Department of Anesthesiology and Pain Medicine, Yale University School of Medicine, New Haven, CT, USA
e-mail: kanishka.rajput@yale.edu

K. Rajput et al. (eds.), *Pain Control in Ambulatory Surgery Centers*,
https://doi.org/10.1007/978-3-030-55262-6_3

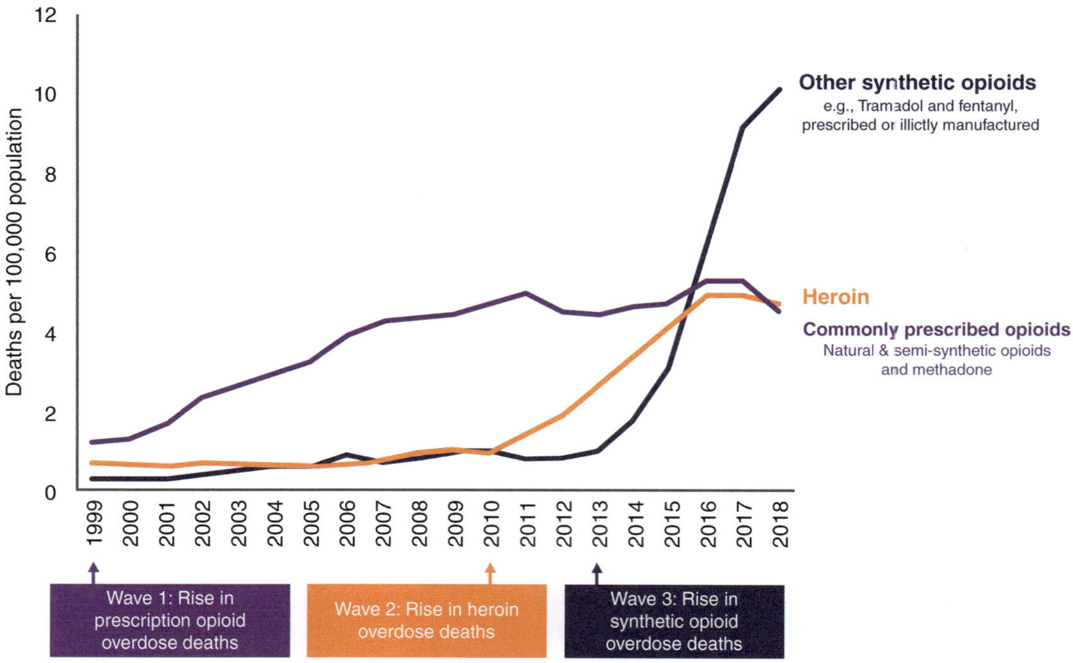

Fig. 3.1 Rise in opioid overdose deaths from 1999 to 2018. (Source: National Vital Statistics System Mortality File)

scription surveillance instituted from 2011 onward at the national, state, and clinical levels that curbed opioid prescriptions [2, 3]. The rise in prescriptions occurred in spite of only a 25% increase in reported pain prevalence from 1997 to 2014, effectively demonstrating an incommensurate rise in opioid prescriptions [4]. To complicate matters further, during this same time period, drug and alcohol poisoning contributing to the increase in midlife mortality disproportionately affected white non-Hispanic populations, especially those with lower education levels more so than their Hispanic and Black counterparts, perhaps pointing to racial disparities even in the increased opioid prescriptions [5]. Though prescription opioids constitute only about a third of overdose deaths due to any opioid, their outsized culpability in the epidemic's mortality can be inferred, given that about 80% of people who use heroin first misused prescription opioids [6, 7]. The end result has been a tragedy with widespread public health and socioeconomic repercussions that have devastated communities and stymied rural prosperity.

The national response to mitigate the crisis has involved multiple fronts – curbing opioid demand, reducing opioid-related harm, and limiting opioid supply. The former two strategies are focused on the patient level and are employed by various programs that provide treatment for opioid addiction as well as chronic pain using nonopioid and interventional approaches. At the prescriber level, opioid supply is broadly restricted by federal regulations that dictate which drugs can be brought to market and their approved indications for use, as well as by the issuance of guidelines and mandates to influence prescribing practices. Acknowledging that unintended consequences can arise from regulations applied unmindfully, national and state policies have ultimately proved necessary for a coordinated response to address adverse health outcomes on a population level. Knowledge of opioid legislative edicts and regulatory stipulations has become essential in the clinical setting. This promotes best practices in patient care and helps prevent undesired practice patterns, ranging from the gross undertreatment of pain due to an excessive aversion to prescribing opioids when indicated to unsafe prescribing that could lead to professional disciplinary actions or criminal investigations. Moreover, an understanding of the historical context of opioid regulation and the modes of operation of present-day regulatory bodies enables one to anticipate and help shape the future of opioid prescribing through both practice and advocacy. Much of the scope of this topic relates to the management of chronic pain, but this chapter will also make mention of the public health sequelae of opioids prescribed in the postoperative setting and the implications of current policy on their future use.

History of Opioid Prescriptions

Parallels abound between the inception of the original US opioid epidemic in the late nineteenth century and our present straits. Opioid consumption and addiction increased throughout the nineteenth century, tripling over the 1870–1880s and peaking in the 1890s [8]. Here too, the proximate cause is deemed to be iatrogenic – the rising curve directly follows the proliferation of the hypodermic syringe in the 1870s, which incidentally was developed for the very administration of morphine itself [8]. Injectable morphine fulfilled the medical community's dire need for a therapy that was effective in the treatment of a wide range of maladies. Such immediately acting symptomatic relief was unprecedented, and unsurprisingly, given the physician's limited pharmacopoeia at the time, it became prone to overuse. This compounded with the spread of widely available narcotic-based "patent medicines" (heavily advertised over-the-counter remedies) to result in a rampant opioid addiction affecting an estimated 150,000 persons, not including those who were afflicted due to smoking opium [9].

Despite similar origins, the resolution of our respective opioid epidemics diverges in course. Whether warranted or not, the perception remains that the medical community was caught flat-footed by today's opioid crisis, obliging governmental directives to drive the response. This was not so at the close of the nineteenth century. A growing body of medical literature, starting in the 1870s, cautioned physicians against the use of opioids, highlighting their attendant risks of addiction, disability, as well as losing efficacy over time. Such teachings began to take hold in medical school curricula in the 1890s [9]. Physicians, along with pharmacists, advocated for state and local laws that restricted the sale of narcotics, and medical consensus repudiated those who liberally prescribed them. This reform movement succeeded in effecting a sustained yearly decrease in medicinal opiate consumption from 1895 to 1914 before any national level response was mustered [8].

A federal response did ultimately arrive in the form of the Harrison Act of 1914, notable for being the first federal foray into drug policy. Though largely written with the anodyne aim of limiting the sale of non-medical narcotics through their taxation and registration, it is now also a noteworthy example of well-intentioned regulation begetting adverse health consequences. Interpretation of the law by the Treasury found the prescription of maintenance opioid therapy to addicted patients to be a "non-medical" use and resulted in the prosecution and imprisonment of many physicians [10]. This served to entrench a bias against maintenance therapy into legal code, establishing a precedent that would impede medical efforts at harm reduction for many years to come.

US opioid policy continued to be driven by the Treasury as well as the Food and Drug Administration (FDA) until passage of the Controlled Substances Act (CSA) of 1970, which classified most commonly prescribed opioids as Schedule II substances, denoting their high potential for abuse but also legitimizing their use as medical therapy [11]. The CSA created a robust structure for federal regulation of all drugs with potential for abuse, unifying previously disparate responsibilities of public health oversight, prescription drug control, and drug enforcement under one banner [12]. With such broad regulatory power being granted, it sought to fulfill equally manifold aims, ranging from the control of illegal street drugs to the implementation of public health policies on drug abuse and addiction. For prescribers, it sought to reconcile the legitimate medical use of certain drugs with the harms of their oversupply and overprescription, which it accomplished with prescription refill restrictions, production limits, security standards, and various documentation and monitoring requirements for the provision and dispensing of controlled substances [12]. Unlike the Harrison Act, however, the CSA was not created in response to an upsurge of unsafe prescribing practices of the time. In fact, as the twentieth century progressed, there had been little to challenge the dogma established in medical education that discouraged the use of opioids to manage chronic non-cancer pain (CNCP).

In the 1990s and early 2000s, a number of developments brought that time-honored precedent into question, and a new course of increased opioid prescribing was charted. The development of new formulations of traditional opioids (e.g., OxyContin or controlled-release oxycodone) was paired with aggressive marketing campaigns by pharmaceuticals that sought to broaden their compass beyond the traditional, smaller chronic cancer pain market while misrepresenting and minimizing their drugs' harms [13]. Furthermore, concerns in the medical community about the undertreatment of chronic pain and its seriousness as a public health problem were conveyed by professional societies to regulators, ultimately leading to policy shifts at the state and federal level that expanded opioid indications to include CNCP and eased restrictions on prescribers [14].

These attempts to raise internal awareness about the inadequate management of chronic pain were adopted as national policy and reshaped as a patient rights issue by the Joint Commision, which issued standards in 2001 that promoted the consideration of pain as a "fifth vital sign" and emphasized assessment of quantitative self-reported pain intensity scores. The reporting of numeric values was then used to evaluate institutional compliance with standards and as the sole measure for grading the "quality" of inpatient pain care [15]. These were adapted into clinical protocols by large healthcare organizations like the Veterans Health Administration, which increased interventions for pain but without evident improvement in the quality of pain management [16]. Though patient satisfaction scores increased, their rise was accompanied by undesirable repercussions, as studies demonstrated that titrating analgesia to one-dimensional numerical pain scores doubled adverse opioid reactions and led to dangerous levels of postoperative sedation [17, 18]. Another misguided national operation introduced perverse incentives for prescribing opioids by associating surveys of patient satisfaction with pain management to provider compensation and promotion, specifically the Hospital Values-Based Program of the Centers for Medicare and Medicaid Services [19]. The end result was the sharp increase in opioid prescribing in every setting – from chronic pain managed as an outpatient to acute pain treated in the emergency department and after surgery.

Federal Oversight

Given the worrisome trends outlined thus far, the federal government has increasingly exercised its broad authority over the healthcare sector in an attempt to reverse their course. These powers are exerted largely by means of federal administrative agencies, which themselves derive their jurisdiction from organic statutes enacted by Congress. They are tasked with interpreting, implementing, enforcing, and prescribing rules and policies that fall under the legislative intent of their originating statute. Administration of current federal opioid regulation lies at the nexus of two statutes in particular, the Controlled Substances Act (CSA) and the Food, Drug, and Cosmetic Act (FDCA), which, respectively, confer enforcement powers to the Drug Enforcement Administration (DEA) and the FDA. Other agencies, such as the Centers for Disease Control and Prevention (CDC) and the Office of National Drug Control Policy (ONDCP), have diverse non-enforcement functions, including data collection, scientific and public health research, and coordination of federal funds (Table 3.1).

The DEA falls within the purview of the Department of Justice (DOJ) and was estab-

Table 3.1 Roles of federal agencies in opioid regulation and policy

Centers for Disease Control	Publishes evidence-based prescribing guidelines
	Collects and analyzes data on opioid-related overdoses
	Educates public with awareness campaigns
	Evaluates state policies/programs on preventing opioid misuse
Centers for Medicare and Medicaid Services	Reviews Part D enrollees for potential opioid overutilization
	Provides access to treatment for opioid use disorder
Drug Enforcement Administration	Investigates diversion of opioids
	Controls production, distribution, and dispensing of prescription opioids
	Schedules opioids as controlled substances based on potential for misuse
Food and Drug Administration	Ensures safety of marketed opioids
	Controls opioid approval and manufacturing standards
	Implements REMS for opioids
National Institute on Drug Abuse	Funds/supports research on opioid abuse and addiction
Office of National Drug Control Policy	Formulates plans to execute national opioid policies
	Coordinates across government agencies to ensure implementation and funding
Substance Abuse and Mental Health Services Administration	Addresses mental health and opioid abuse with treatment/recovery services
	Supports service delivery and policy research on pain and addiction
	Develops resources for clinical education/support for prescribers

lished in 1973 to be the administrative body of the CSA, enforcing both its criminal laws and noncriminal regulations [14]. Although the DEA is more publicly known for its role in curtailing the supply and distribution of narcotics illicitly produced both at home and abroad, it also seeks to achieve these goals through criminal inquiries and administrative actions against physicians with questionable prescribing practices [20]. In order to prescribe or administer opioids, a clinician must register with the DEA and assent to their rules on drug security and reporting. The most elemental of these legal requirements are delineated in the Code of Federal Regulations and United States Code, which specify that in each instance where a physician prescribes a controlled substance to a patient, the physician must establish a "legitimate medical purpose," act "in the usual course of his professional practice," and maintain "effective control against diversion" of said controlled substance [21, 22]. Therefore, it is incumbent upon the physician to practice reasonable measures to identify signs of abuse, which falls outside legitimate medical use, and signs of diversion. What procedure constitutes the minimum standards for such "reasonable measures" or what degree of negligence meets certain grounds for prosecution, however, is not further illustrated by the DEA. The extent of physician oversight practiced is thus individually tailored to one's setting, patient, and reasoned medical judgment that coincides with recognized professional standards.

The FDA can credit its origins, in part, to opioid medications. The Pure Food and Drug Act of 1906 followed the efforts of muckraking journalists such as Samuel Hopkins Adams who exposed the patent medicine industry for underhanded practices like advertising "Soothing Syrup" for colicky infants while neglecting to inform the public of its major ingredient – morphine [23]. At its inception, the administrative priority of the FDA was the truthful labeling of contents and dosages of medications. The modern FDA's focus on premarket approval of safety and efficacy of drugs derives from the expanded scope afforded to it with the passage of the 1938 FDCA and its many subsequent amendments [24]. The FDA has approved numerous new opioids and reformulations since its installation, including short-acting combination products like Percocet in 1976 (oxycodone/acetaminophen), long-acting formulations like MS Contin in 1985 (morphine), and opioids with purported abuse-deterrent properties like Nucynta ER in 2011 (tapentadol extended release) [14]. Its capacity in confronting the opioid epidemic entails not only this gatekeeping activity but also its role in post-approval monitoring of the use of opioid products. This is exercised through spontaneous adverse event reporting, active post-market surveillance of safety outcomes, post-market requirements imposed on manufacturers (e.g., clinical trials, observational studies, patient registries, risk evaluation and mitigation strategies, etc.), communicating drug safety information via labeling, and regulating industry marketing.

State Oversight

Although federal law imposes broad limits on opioid prescribing, it does so while recognizing their legitimate medical use and does not attempt to govern medical judgment by fiat. Neither the CSA nor the FDCA proscribes opioid prescriptions to suggested doses or labeled indications, nor do they restrict the quantity or duration of prescriptions. Even the manner by which diversion and abuse monitoring should be conducted is left undefined. Such constraints are deferred by the federal government because the regulation of the practice of medicine is an area traditionally under the jurisdiction of the states. Regulation of opioid prescribing at the state level is determined principally by the intersection of their own controlled substance laws with professional standards set by medical boards and practice guidelines issued by states themselves [25]. Should state and federal law disagree, the more rigorous obligations take precedence, which more often than not are levied by the state.

Although an exhaustive framework of the many multitudes of state regulations in current use is out of the scope of this chapter, two ubiquitous privileges wielded by states are worth expounding – determination of medical practice standards and ordination of prescription drug monitoring programs (PDMPs). Regarding the former, many states and medical boards have modeled their policies on iterations of the "Guidelines for the Chronic Use of Opioid Analgesics" published by the Federation of State Medical Boards, which comprises best practice recommendations for various aspects of opioid prescribing, including patient evaluation and risk stratification, ongoing assessment, periodic and unannounced drug testing, and medical recordkeeping [26]. Although treatment guidelines are meant to do just that – guide – they may be put forward in court as standard of care and, if adopted by states, can bear the force of law. A consequential example is the guideline produced in 2007 by Washington state, of which the chief recommendation was that daily doses greater than 120 MME should only be prescribed after specialty pain consultation [27]. Since its institution, the dosage ceiling has evolved from a guidance to a requisite and has proliferated to multiple other states. Moreover, the creation of PDMPs is a paradigm of how state governments have advanced creative defenses that pinpoint irregular prescribing practices and impede diversion in order to pare down prescription opioid supply in the community. Widely applied in 49 US states (Missouri being the exception), PDMPs are statewide electronic databases that compile data on prescribed controlled substances, including prescriber, patient, dose, amount dispensed, and pharmacy [24]. This information can prove instrumental in ascertaining problematic patient behavior (i.e., "doctor shopping") as well as improper prescribing patterns, helping effectuate the state's goal to alter prescriber behavior. Lastly, other state-level authorities that also deserve mention include insurance oversight and medical licensure.

Recent Policy Initiatives

Historically, policies to address pain management and the opioid epidemic were largely the domain of individual states. Only recently has the federal government attempted enterprises that sought to map cohesive approaches to pain and opioid policy.

The National Pain Strategy is one such example, released in 2016 by a federal advisory committee created by the Department of Health and Human Services [28]. The document submits a comprehensive public health approach to pain and emphasizes specific areas of improvement: population research, prevention and care, disparities, service delivery and payment, professional education and training, and public education and communication. It lays out a blueprint that acknowledges the hazards accompanying opioid use in chronic pain and alternatively accentuates the biopsychosocial determinants of pain and the evidence base behind integrative treatment strategies [11].

The CDC, with its charge of bettering population health, also responded to the opioid epidemic with a seminal, evidenced-based "Guideline for Prescribing Opioids for Chronic Pain" in 2016. Targeted at primary care physicians in outpatient settings treating CNCP, the guidelines address the matters of (1) determining when to initiate or continue opioids for chronic pain; (2) opioid selection, dosage, duration, follow-up, and discontinuation; and (3) assessing risk and addressing harms of use [29]. With 12 recommendations in total, they are notable for being more restrictive and more circumspect than preceding opioid prescribing guidelines. The overarching objective to reduce the prevalence of opioid dependence by limiting patients' initial exposure forms the bedrock of these guidelines. To that end, the CDC stresses nonopioid and nonpharmacologic therapies as first-line treatment for pain. When opioids are necessary for acute pain, they suggest the lowest effective dose of short-acting agents for the shortest duration of time, noting that 3 days or less will often be sufficient. A credit to the CDC's national reach is how the impact of these guidelines can be appreciated on every level, from hospitals utilizing them in institutional protocols to large-scale education of the public and prescribers.

Complementing these initiatives, the FDA introduced its own Opioid Action Plan in 2016. The agenda drafted a number of undertakings involving changes to strengthen immediate-release opioid labeling, increasing requirements for manufacturer post-market surveillance of ER/long-acting (LA) opioids, updating risk evaluation and mitigation strategy (REMS) program requirements, expanding access to abuse-deterrent formulations (ADFs), and making naloxone more accessible [14]. Since their enactment, however, evidence for some of these strategies has proved to be meager or conflicting. For instance, REMS programs are post-marketing requirements imposed on manufacturers that seek to shape prescribing practices and ensure safe use. Though they can take many forms, the FDA has required a REMS for opioids that compels drug companies to impart training to prescribers that educate them in the proper use of opioids. Be that as it may, their effectiveness has been limited in the face of their voluntary nature – prescribers may simply abstain, which more than two-thirds do [24]. Second, ADFs have physical or chemical properties that thwart misuse, and the FDA has expended considerable resources into their investigation. In spite of this, their expansion remains cautiously limited, as evidence has yet to show improved public health outcomes with their use, possibly due to users substituting them with illicit heroin or fentanyl. In addition, should deterrence fail, risks are still inherent with their misuse, as exhibited when injection abuse of reformulated Opana ER (oxymorphone hydrochloride) caused an outbreak of HIV and HCV as well as cases of thrombotic microangiopathy, prompting the FDA to remove it from the market [14]. The FDA's attempts at improving naloxone access, on the other hand, show more promise. They hold the power to revise its prescription status to that of over-the-counter (OTC), which they have advanced by aiding the development of OTC naloxone products [30]. In the meantime, states have been spearheading naloxone access efforts with legislation that allows pharmacists to dispense naloxone without a prescription and laws that grant legal immunity to laypeople who administer naloxone to those who have overdosed [31].

Future Directions

Just as no one individual or group is free from culpability in the genesis of today's opioid epidemic, each will have to shoulder responsibility as we move toward resolving these issues. One can be buoyed by early signs that the prescription opioid crisis is slowing – in 2018, the opioid prescribing rate had fallen 37% since 2012, having steadily decreased each year [32]. This welcome trend demonstrates the collective impact of federal, state, and local initiatives deployed against the epidemic. To continue this encouraging trajectory toward higher-quality pain management while avoiding an inadvertent exacerbation of the public health burden of pain or addiction, it will be imperative to build, review, and eventually publicize the evidence base behind both our present interventions and novel approaches to pain management. A successful outcome hinges on concerted actions by government agencies, professional societies, healthcare organizations, payers, prescribers, and most importantly patients.

Before discussing the future application of policies with the potential to improve outcomes, it is prudent to review the sheer breadth of what we still don't know and, accordingly, targets for future research. Opioids have been an attractive therapy for pain since the debut of hypodermic morphine, precisely due to a lack of better alternatives. The opioid epidemic, then, reflects a failure in our understanding and management of pain. Despite substantial research into the basic science and neurobiology of pain, most newly approved analgesics in the past 30 years have acted upon established targets [33]. The lack of novel analgesics hence indicates a need for improved research methods and preclinical models of pain. By the same token, our continued reliance on opioids demonstrates a need for further research into new pain treatment modalities and nonpharmacologic therapies. That being said, opioids have a distinct utility in the management of acute pain, particularly in the emergency department and postoperative settings, and the vast majority of patients who are prescribed opioids do not use them habitually or misuse them [34]. Safer prescribing could be facilitated if patients who are at risk for opioid use disorder could be reliably identified in those environments. Yet, a systematic review of screening tools for opioid addiction when initiating prescription opioids found that they had little value in distinguishing high- vs. low-risk patients and none were useful for patients with an initial presentation of previously untreated pain [35]. Given ostensible deficiencies in all aspects of pain, from physiology to assessment to treatment, support for further research should be a paramount policy goal.

Though research can be funded by federal bodies like the National Institutes of Health, it does need to be complemented by institutions that can give teeth to the policies they influence. At the federal level, the FDA is best poised to do so, as it has a robust regulatory apparatus already in place that can guide further progress. Nonetheless, it must be engaged shrewdly to avoid requirements that are too burdensome or, worse, detrimental. Much of the untapped potential lies in the FDA's broad license to oversee post-approval monitoring. This can entail bolstering active surveillance on opioid misuse to improve latencies in regulatory response, reevaluating opioid approvals periodically based on public health outcomes, and further restricting opioid marketing, all of which are recommended approaches in a report commissioned by the FDA [14].

An uncustomary sphere where the FDA's post-market powers may provide the largest dividends, however, is that of pain and opioid education. This has been applied in the form of opioid REMS, which in its present form requires manufacturers to provide continuing medical education on the safe prescribing of opioids. As previously discussed, the major obstacle to their success is that prescriber participation is voluntary. Recall that the eighteenth-century prescription opioid epidemic was quelled, in large part, by education of physicians in medical school and academic literature. With further study of the effectiveness of REMS enabling us to determine which aspects demonstrably improve prescribing practices, the FDA should then embrace its mandate to maximize prescriber education. One way to do so is outlined in the 2011 ONDCP plan that recommends passing legislation to make training about appropriate opioid prescribing compulsory as part of the DEA registration process [36]. Another possibility includes using REMS to educate not only about opioid pharmacovigilance but also about pain management broadly, particularly nonopioid and interventional alternatives for chronic pain. Equally important is targeting the education to prescribers who would benefit from it the most, which can be facilitated by professional societies and evidence-based guidelines. For example, primary care physicians (PCPs) manage the overwhelming majority of patients burdened with acute and chronic pain, but surveys have demonstrated their dissatisfaction with their training on pain management [37]. Common gaps in knowledge and clinical practice that education can bridge include poor comprehension of how to assess chronic pain and reassess it in the context of opioid use, inappropriate selection and dosing of opioids, and an inadequate understanding of tolerance and addiction [38]. The FDA's REMS programs have also been adapted to address the woefully lacking pain curricula of medical schools with initiatives such as Boston University School of Medicine's SCOPE (Safe and Competent Opioid Prescribing Education) of Pain [39]. By continuing to expand beyond the prescriber level and reinforcing multidisciplinary pain care, particularly nonpharmacological strategies, as a fundamental aspect of medical education, REMS may prove to be one of the more versatile tools in opioid policy.

Opioid education was similarly furthered by the CDC through the dissemination of their comprehensive 2016 guidelines. Nevertheless, if prior research on the impact of clinical practice guidelines can be extrapolated to the CDC's work, then it appears that guidelines alone cannot be expected to substantially alter prescribing practices. For instance, circulating opioid guidelines in Stanford clinics improved the usage of urine drug testing, but otherwise had no impact on recommended prescriber behaviors like specialty referrals (PT, pain, psychiatry) and routine follow-up [40]. This implies that, short of making them mandatory, guidelines need to be accompanied by supplementary training to improve prescriber compliance. At the other end of the spectrum, steps need to be taken to ensure that guidelines aren't hamfistedly adopted to meet bureaucratic benchmarks for opioid reduction while support for chronic pain patients and access to integrated pain management are neglected [41].

While the CDC guidelines provide a road map for the future directions of chronic pain, no such standard exists for postoperative opioid prescribing. Any approach to systematize or even better inform appropriate postoperative prescribing practices must seek to address two complementary goals – reducing opioid addiction and diversion. Thus, efforts are being made to limit exposure and overprescription.

The importance of exposure is highlighted in research that has shown that half of all postoperative patients who are prescribed opioids are actually opioid-naive and as many as 6.5% of these patients go on to have new and persistent opioid use [42, 43]. Strategies to reduce postoperative opioid use have largely centered on incorporating regional anesthesia and nonopioid adjuncts under the umbrella of "multimodal analgesia." However, these techniques are applied with significant variation across the United States, indicating the need for further research that delineates which one, alone or in combination, best prevents prolonged opioid use after surgery [44]. Moreover, to maximize their utility, such preventative endeavors should be targeted to patients who are most vulnerable to developing postoperative chronic opioid use. Several predictive factors for this have been identified, including lower socioeconomic status, thoracic surgical procedures, younger age, and comorbid anxiety or depression [43]. These have been incorporated into risk indices that attempt to predict a patient's risk of developing chronic post-surgical pain [45]. Proposed methods of targeted intervention include perioperative cognitive behavior therapy (CBT) and distraction techniques for those with preoperative depression [46]. Though CBT has been shown to be useful in improving functional disability for chronic low back pain, further research is needed to evaluate the effect of such interventions on postoperative opioid use [47]. Broadly instituting preoperative CBT to every surgical patient with depression may not be financially viable. The importance of support for research into recognizing patients most likely to benefit from such interventions is therefore further underscored. With further characterization of high-risk predictive factors and individualized interventions, surgeons may be able to safely provide access to postoperative opioid analgesia for low-risk patients while still allaying the risk of postoperative opioid addiction overall.

The focus on curbing overprescription of postoperative opioids is an acknowledgement of its role in driving diversion. This is borne out by studies that have reported that less than 30% of prescribed postoperative opioids are taken and the majority of patients hold on to these unused opioids instead of properly discarding them after surgery [48, 49]. This disparity between consumption and prescription opens up avenues to establish guidelines for postoperative prescribing targets. Incorporating the desire to assuage postoperative pain and minimize the number of visits for refills, one proposed approach recalls the Pareto principle and suggests prescribing the number of pills that would sufficiently satisfy the opioid requirements of 80% of patients undergoing a given operation (e.g., 10 pills of oxycodone 5 mg for a partial mastectomy with sentinel lymph node biopsy) [49]. By combining this practice with strategies to reduce opioid use in high-risk patients, it is hoped that only some fraction of the other 20% will actually present for a refill. In fact, a follow-up study that instructed patients to take acetaminophen and nonsteroidal antiinflammatory drugs prior to opioids allowed for a reduction of the recommended prescription for partial mastectomy with sentinel lymph node biopsy to just five pills, and only 1 out of 224 patients studied required an opioid refill [50]. Other strategies developed to educate surgeons and inform them on an optimal pain management approach throughout the entire postoperative course include the RIGHTT guide, which is an acronym standing for risk for adverse event, insight into pain, going over pain plan, halting opioids, tossing unused opioids, and trouble identification [51]. Yet, it bears repeating that only with evidence generated by future prospective clinical trials can the value of these proposals and strategies be assessed.

While federal regulations and national guidelines portend the large-scale shifts in opioid prescribing that are to come, state-level initiatives may be more germane in directing immediate clinical practice and shaping future opioid policy. One example discussed previously is the creation of PDMPs, which have so far demonstrated benefit in tempering opioid misuse and abuse trends, albeit with several limitations [52]. These will likely continue to evolve and play a prevalent role as research into their effectiveness has identified several potential opportunities for improvement. One constraint is the availability of data. The information is typically restricted to physicians, pharmacists, and law enforcement of a given state. Controls on sharing data across state lines can result in crucial gaps in a patient's opioid history and introduce openings for abuse [24]. In addition, the data largely is not displayed in real time [20]. Naturally, such delays in data reporting can misinform a clinician who is tasked with making real-time decisions. A potential solution is a nationwide database paired with mandatory electronic prescribing for scheduled substances that would allow for the most up-to-date information to be rendered on demand [24]. Another limitation in some states' PDMPs is that their use is not mandated, despite access being made available [14]. Though arguably vexing to an established workflow, requiring their use prior to prescribing opioids would serve to improve provider participation, and in fact, PDMPs have been shown to be effective *only* if accessing them is a prescriber obligation [53]. Yet, this remains only one of many interventions one can conceive of being implemented by states, as they will retain the ability to incubate innovative solutions, apply them on a relatively smaller scale, compare them to their neighbors, and readily modify them as they see fit.

Although the supply-side interventions discussed above are most relevant to prescribers, equally important is the work being done to reduce opioid harms and demand by improving access to overdose treatment (i.e., naloxone) and opioid use disorder (OUD) treatment, respectively. Policies to improve naloxone availability were previously described at the pharmacy level, but these must be complemented with similar efforts at the provider and community level. For prescribers, the CDC guidelines recommend naloxone coprescription for patients who are at high risk for opioid overdose [29]. However, even with improved access by way of coprescription and the independent dispensing of naloxone by pharmacists, one obvious impediment remains – to respond to opioid overdose, someone other than the victim needs to be able to recognize the signs and know how to administer naloxone. To facilitate this, there are programs in the community that function in overdose education, specifically training drug users and their family members on how to identify likely overdose and appropriately treat it with naloxone [54]. Between the expansion of such programs and the FDA's pursuit of an OTC designation for naloxone, barriers to opioid harm reduction should continue to fall.

A fundamental aspect of broadening access to any kind of treatment in the United States is insurance coverage, which remains a major obstacle for naloxone and various nonopioid chronic pain treatments. This principle applies especially so for medication-assisted treatment (MAT) for OUD (e.g., methadone, buprenorphine), as one-third of people needing treatment for substance use disorder cite lack of health insurance as their primary barrier [55]. This can be partially remedied by further Medicaid expansion, an Affordable Care Act provision expanding eligibility criteria which was adopted by only certain states. Improved access to MAT drugs for low-income individuals followed for these states, particularly Medicaid-reimbursed prescriptions for buprenorphine. There are other state-level Medicaid restrictions that hamper MAT utilization as well, such as those observed in the states who do not include all MAT drugs on their preferred drug lists and those who require a prior authorization for buprenorphine-naloxone treatment [56]. Given how grossly underutilized treatment for OUD has been, policy changes to secure the availability of MAT may ultimately prove to be the most valuable future directive in reducing opioid misuse.

Limitations

Some caution must be exercised when implementing opioid policies that have a disproportionate focus on supply-side intervention, which is the case for the United States today. Though we have witnessed a downtrend in the rate of prescription opioid deaths, an asymmetric focus on opioid prescribers can neglect treating the causes of the opioid epidemic while patching up the symptoms. In other words, an approach that targets only low-hanging fruit by restricting opioid prescriptions may accordingly reduce opioid morbidity and mortality but can result in unintended consequences by exacerbating the burden of chronic pain on our patients. Even well-intentioned, evidence-based guidelines like those issued by the CDC in 2016 can harm patients. A consensus panel report notes various prescriber behaviors that reflect a clumsy application of recommendations without regard for the individual patient [57]. Examples include setting hard dosage ceilings and prescription duration limits, abrupt tapering of chronic opiate prescriptions to meet recommended thresholds, as well as misapplying guidelines intended for chronic non-cancer pain onto patients with malignancies and acute pain [57].

These demonstrate a tendency for prescribers to "opt-out" of individually treating pain when faced with perceived external edicts. Though imperfect, this sort of management is understandable given the pressures that prescribers (surgeons included) face while carrying the brunt of repercussions and liability for opioid-related harms. Numerous factors can contribute to the development of a patient's opioid addiction, be it chronic conditions like sickle cell disease, musculoskeletal sequelae of physical trauma, comorbid psychiatric illness, or socioeconomic disparities. A national pain strategy that seeks to erect barriers to opioid prescriptions without offering better treatment for chronic pain or addressing social inequalities leaves the prescriber with few tools to adequately treat their patient. Thus, these encumbrances may lead physicians to continue "opting-out" of treating chronic pain, aggravating established disparities in the process. These disparities in access to pain treatment can occur due to bias (e.g., racial, ethnic), stigmatization (e.g., people with substance use disorders, HIV), inability to communicate (e.g., infants, elderly), and other discrimination [28]. By solely focusing on regulating the prescriber, these populations can be disproportionately harmed in the process. These limitations underscore the importance of a comprehensive approach to the opioid epidemic that also seeks effective treatment for chronic pain, improved access to said treatment, as well as efforts to treat the harms caused by opioids before they can result in mortality.

Summary

Policies addressing pain and opioid prescribing have impacts that far surpass any one individual's approach to pain management. Indeed, the number of opioid prescriptions continues to decline with the maturation of modern strategies. Nonetheless, policies that focus on prescription control to the exclusion of delivering safe, effective analgesia or expanding OUD treatment run the risk of ameliorating the associated symptoms but not the causes of the opioid epidemic. In other words, system-level failures have been responsible for creating the current crisis, demanding an equally encompassing response in return. Thus, stronger regulation must be supplemented with scientifically grounded clinical guidelines, research examining nonopioid alternatives for pain, and support for all aspects of pain care. By continuing to reevaluate our opioid prescribing policies and advancing the field of pain management, we are poised to turn a corner in our approach to treating pain and finally siphon away the fuel that has long inflamed this crisis.

References

1. Hedegaard H, Miniño AM, Warner M. Drug overdose deaths in the United States, 1999–2018. Hyattsville: National Center for Health Statistics; 2020.
2. Knight KR, et al. Opioid pharmacovigilance: a clinical-social history of the changes in opioid prescribing for patients with co-occurring chronic non-cancer pain and substance use. Soc Sci Med. 2017;186:87–95.
3. National Academies of Sciences, Engineering, and Medicine. Framing opioid prescribing guidelines for acute pain: developing the evidence. Washington, DC: National Academies Press; 2020.
4. Nahin RL, et al. Eighteen-year trends in the prevalence of, and health care use for, noncancer pain in the United States: data from the medical expenditure panel survey. J Pain. 2019;20(7):796–809.
5. Case A, Deaton A. Rising morbidity and mortality in midlife among white non-Hispanic Americans in the 21st century. Proc Natl Acad Sci. 2015;112(49):15078–83.
6. Muhuri PK, Gfroerer JC, Davies MC. CBHSQ data review. Center for Behavioral Health Statistics and Quality. SAMHSA. 2013;1:17.
7. Centers for Disease Control and Prevention. Wonder: CDC; 2020. https://wonder.cdc.gov/.
8. Courtwright DT. Preventing and treating narcotic addiction—a century of federal drug control. N Engl J Med. 2015;373(22):2095–7.
9. Courtwright DT, editor. Dark paradise: a history of opiate addiction in America (Enl. ed.). Cambridge, MA: Harvard University Press; 2001.
10. Musto DF. The American disease: origins of narcotic control. New York: Oxford University Press; 1999.
11. Gross J, Gordon DB. The strengths and weaknesses of current US policy to address pain. Am J Public Health. 2019;109(1):66–72.
12. Spillane J, McAllister WB. Keeping the lid on: a century of drug regulation and control. Drug Alcohol Depend. 2003;70(3):S5–S12.
13. Van Zee A. The promotion and marketing of oxycontin: commercial triumph, public health tragedy. Am J Public Health. 2009;99(2):221–7.
14. National Academies of Sciences, Engineering, and Medicine. Pain management and the opioid epidemic: balancing societal and individual benefits and risks of prescription opioid use. Washington, DC: National Academies Press; 2017.
15. Franklin G, et al. A comprehensive approach to address the prescription opioid epidemic in Washington state: milestones and lessons learned. Am J Public Health. 2015;105(3):463–9.
16. Mularski RA, et al. Measuring pain as the 5th vital sign does not improve quality of pain management. J Gen Intern Med. 2006;21(6):607–12.
17. Taylor S, Voytovich AE, Kozol RA. Has the pendulum swung too far in postoperative pain control? Am J Surg. 2003;186(5):472–5.
18. Vila H, et al. The efficacy and safety of pain management before and after implementation of hospital-wide pain management standards: is patient safety compromised by treatment based solely on numerical pain ratings? Anesth Analg. 2005;101(2):474–80.
19. Adams J, Bledsoe GH, Armstrong JH. Are pain management questions in patient satisfaction surveys driving the opioid epidemic? Am J Public Health. 2016;106(6):985.
20. Webster LR, Grabois M. Current regulations related to opioid prescribing. PM&R. 2015;7:S236–47.

21. US Department of Justice, Drug Enforcement Administration. Title 21 Code of federal regulations: purpose of issue of prescription. Part 1306. 2005. 1306.4.
22. Legal Information Institute. Title 21: Food and drugs. Chapter 13: Drug abuse prevention and control. Subchapter I: Control and enforcement. Part C: Registration of manufacturers, distributors, and dispensers of controlled substances. Section 823: Registration requirements. Oct 2018.
23. Cassedy JH. Muckraking and medicine: Samuel Hopkins Adams. Am Q. 1964;16(1):85–99.
24. Soelberg CD, et al. The US opioid crisis: current federal and state legal issues. Anesth Analg. 2017;125(5):1675–81.
25. Gilson AM, Joranson DE. US policies relevant to the prescribing of opioid analgesics for the treatment of pain in patients with addictive disease. Clin J Pain. 2002;18(4):S91–8.
26. Federation of State Medical Boards. Guidelines for the chronic use of opioid analgesics. 2017.
27. Ziegler SJ. The proliferation of dosage thresholds in opioid prescribing policies and their potential to increase pain and opioid-related mortality. Pain Med. 2015;16(10):1851–6.
28. U.S. Department of Health and Human Services. National pain strategy: a comprehensive population health-level strategy for pain. Washington, DC: National Institutes of Health (U.S.); 2016.
29. Dowell D. CDC guideline for prescribing opioids for chronic pain. 2016.
30. U.S. Food and Drug Administration and Norman E. "Ned" Sharpless. Statement on continued efforts to increase availability of all forms of naloxone to help reduce opioid overdose deaths. FDA Statement. 2019.
31. Abouk R, Pacula RL, Powell D. Association between state laws facilitating pharmacy distribution of naloxone and risk of fatal overdose. JAMA Intern Med. 2019;179(6):805–11.
32. Centers for Disease Control and Prevention. US opioid prescribing rate maps. Atlanta: Centers for Disease Control and Prevention; 2018.
33. Woolf CJ. Overcoming obstacles to developing new analgesics. Nat Med. 2010;16(11):1241–7.
34. Shah A, Hayes CJ, Martin BC. Characteristics of initial prescription episodes and likelihood of long-term opioid use—United States, 2006–2015. MMWR Morb Mortal Wkly Rep. 2017;66(10):265.
35. Klimas J, et al. Strategies to identify patient risks of prescription opioid addiction when initiating opioids for pain: a systematic review. JAMA Netw Open. 2019;2(5):e193365.
36. Ray JB. Implications of the extended-release/long-acting opioid REMS for managed care. Am J Manag Care. 2015;21:S177a–87a.
37. Upshur CC, Luckmann RS, Savageau JA. Primary care provider concerns about management of chronic pain in community clinic populations. J Gen Intern Med. 2006;21(6):652.
38. Murnion BP, Gnjidic D, Hilmer SN. Prescription and administration of opioids to hospital in-patients, and barriers to effective use. Pain Med. 2010;11(1):58–66.
39. Alford DP, et al. SCOPE of pain: an evaluation of an opioid risk evaluation and mitigation strategy continuing education program. Pain Med. 2016;17(1):52–63.
40. Chen JH, et al. Effect of opioid prescribing guidelines in primary care. Medicine. 2016;95(35):e4760.
41. Bonnie RJ, et al. Pain management and opioid regulation: continuing public health challenges. Am J Public Health. 2019;109(1):31–4.
42. Brummett CM, et al. New persistent opioid use after minor and major surgical procedures in US adults. JAMA Surg. 2017;152(6):e170504.
43. Clarke H, et al. Rates and risk factors for prolonged opioid use after major surgery: population based cohort study. BMJ. 2014;348:g1251.
44. Ladha KS, et al. Variations in the use of perioperative multimodal analgesic therapy. Anesthesiology. 2016;124(4):837–45.
45. Althaus A, et al. Development of a risk index for the prediction of chronic post-surgical pain. Eur J Pain. 2012;16(6):901–10.
46. Dunn LK, et al. Influence of catastrophizing, anxiety, and depression on in-hospital opioid consumption, pain, and quality of recovery after adult spine surgery. J Neurosurg Spine. 2018;28(1):119–26.
47. van Tulder MW, et al. Behavioral treatment for chronic low back pain: a systematic review within the framework of the Cochrane Back Review Group. Spine. 2000;25(20):2688–99.
48. Bartels K, et al. Opioid use and storage patterns by patients after hospital discharge following surgery. PLoS One. 2016;11(1):e0147972.
49. Hill MV, et al. Wide variation and excessive dosage of opioid prescriptions for common general surgical procedures. Ann Surg. 2017;265(4):709–14.
50. Hill MV, et al. An educational intervention decreases opioid prescribing after general surgical operations. Ann Surg. 2018;267(3):468–72.
51. Yorkgitis BK, Brat GA. Postoperative opioid prescribing: getting it RIGHTT. Am J Surg. 2018;215(4):707–11.
52. Reifler LM, et al. Do prescription monitoring programs impact state trends in opioid abuse/misuse? Pain Med. 2012;13(3):434–42.
53. Ayres I, Jalal A. The impact of prescription drug monitoring programs on US opioid prescriptions. J Law Med Ethics. 2018;46(2):387–403.
54. Clark AK, Wilder CM, Winstanley EL. A systematic review of community opioid overdose prevention and naloxone distribution programs. J Addict Med. 2014;8(3):153–63.
55. Sharp A, et al. Impact of Medicaid expansion on access to opioid analgesic medications and medication-assisted treatment. Am J Public Health. 2018;108(5):642–8.
56. Mark TL, et al. Medicaid coverage of medications to treat alcohol and opioid dependence. J Subst Abus Treat. 2015;55:1–5.
57. Kroenke K, et al. Challenges with implementing the centers for disease control and prevention opioid guideline: a consensus panel report. Pain Med. 2019;20(4):724–35.

4 Rationale and Goals for Optimal Pain Control in Ambulatory Surgical Centers

Nick Stiles, Sadie Smith, Dennis J. Warfield Jr., David Fanelli, Jinlei Li, Alan David Kaye, and Henry Liu

Abstract

More and more complicated surgical and diagnostic procedures are being performed in ambulatory surgery centers (ASCs). It can be a daunting task to provide adequate analgesia while minimizing side effects. Anesthesia providers are increasingly facing higher social, financial, and administrative pressures to decrease opioid consumption, shorten operating room turnaround time, avoid anesthetic side effects and complications, and ensure timely discharge. Multimodal analgesia strategy, including non-opioid analgesic drugs and measures such as nerve blocks, has gained widespread recognition to provide perioperative analgesia. The analgesic goals in ASCs include cost-effectiveness, efficiency, patient satisfaction, minimizing drug side effects, and anesthetic complications. This chapter will discuss these analgesic goals and their rationales.

N. Stiles · S. Smith · D. J. Warfield Jr
D. Fanelli · H. Liu (✉)
Department of Anesthesiology and Perioperative Medicine, Penn State College of Medicine, Milton S. Hershey Medical Center, Hershey, PA, USA
e-mail: ssmith38@pennstatehealth.psu.edu; dwarfield@pennstatehealth.psu.edu; dfanelli@pennstatehealth.psu.edu

J. Li
Department of Anesthesiology, Yale University School of Medicine, New Haven, CT, USA

A. D. Kaye
Departments of Anesthesiology and Pharmacology, Toxicology, and Neurosciences, Louisiana State University Health Shreveport, Shreveport, LA, USA

Introduction

Ambulatory/outpatient surgical centers (ASCs) primarily focused on elective ASA I or II patients about 20 years ago for surgical procedures of short duration, not requiring intensive and invasive monitoring and expecting a rapid patient recovery. Now, majority of surgeries in the United States are performed in ASCs, accepting patients with advanced ASA statuses [1]. As of 2018, a large proportion of registered community hospitals in the United States are either nongovernmental not-for-profit hospitals (56.5%) or state and local government hospitals (18.6%), without physician ownership [1]. There has been more than a 100% increase in the total number of ambulatory surgery centers since 1990 in the United States [2]. By having ownership interests in surgical centers, the degree of anesthesia involvement can potentially be affected by their relationships with physician owners [2]. More and more complex procedures are increasingly performed in ASCs by almost all surgical subspecialties and other nonsurgical medical specialties. This uptrend in procedure volume and

K. Rajput et al. (eds.), *Pain Control in Ambulatory Surgery Centers*,
https://doi.org/10.1007/978-3-030-55262-6_4

surgical complexity is contributed by multiple factors. Physician ownership of ASCs is just part of the reason [3]. The ability to return home the same day after undergoing a procedure is appealing to many patients and healthcare facilities. In addition, patients having surgery at ASCs may avoid some of the risks associated with hospital admission, such as hospital-acquired infections [4]. Complicated surgical and diagnostic procedures demand intensive perioperative monitoring and management. Satisfactory perioperative pain management is pivotal to the successful and safe discharge of surgical patients from ASCs. However, it can be challenging to provide optimal pain treatment in ASC settings for potentially painful and complicated surgeries, yet the ambulatory surgical patients in ASCs are expected to be discharged home within 24 hours after surgery. Maintaining a delicate balance between adequate pain control and minimizing adverse effects of opioids, especially respiratory complications and urinary retention, are only some of the challenges faced by anesthesia providers in ambulatory surgery settings [2, 4] (Fig. 4.1).

Without any doubt, it is extremely challenging to provide adequate analgesia to patients in ASCs especially when the United States, like many other countries, has witnessed a steep increase in narcotic-related mortality from both prescription and illegal opioids in the past three decades [5]. Misuse and addiction have been and will continue to be one of the major public health crisis, which not only requires national preventative measures but also therapeutic strategies focused on overdose reversal agents as well as safe, innovative, and effective nonaddictive pain treatments [2, 5]. More than 90 Americans die every day from opioid overdose, leading to greater than 33,000 deaths per year [2, 5, 6]. The healthcare system is commonly viewed as a gateway to addiction; however, individuals entering drug treatment programs are more likely to report their opioid abuse beginning with heroin rather than a prescription analgesic [5, 6]. Between 2013 and 2016, the fatalities attributed to synthetic opioids such as fentanyl and carfentanil spiked as much as 540% with pronounced regional increases [6, 7]. This rapid acceleration of mortality has led to the opioid crisis being designated as a national public health emergency and the immediate call for alternative approaches to provide analgesia in surgical and nonsurgical patients. The implementation of guidelines from federal agencies and prescription drug monitoring programs (PDMPs) is crucial in reducing opioid-associated deaths and promoting appropriate medical use of opioids.

An enhanced recovery after surgery (ERAS) protocol has been increasingly adopted by many hospitals and ASCs. Multimodal analgesia is a pivotal part of the ERAS pathway designed to provide evidence-based perioperative management via limiting opioids and reducing major complications associated with surgery and opioid administration [8–10]. A recent meta-analysis showed that ERAS programs were associated with lower morbidity rates and shorter hospital stays after colorectal surgery [11]. Patients in ERAS protocol were able to recover faster while reducing the need for hospital stays by about 30% or more than 2 days after major abdominal surgeries [11].

Status of Pain Control in Ambulatory Surgery Centers

ASCs generally provide better efficiency for many surgical procedures compared to a hospital setting. ASCs require lower costs from Medicare and private insurance companies as well as out-of-pocket payments for patients [12, 13]. The

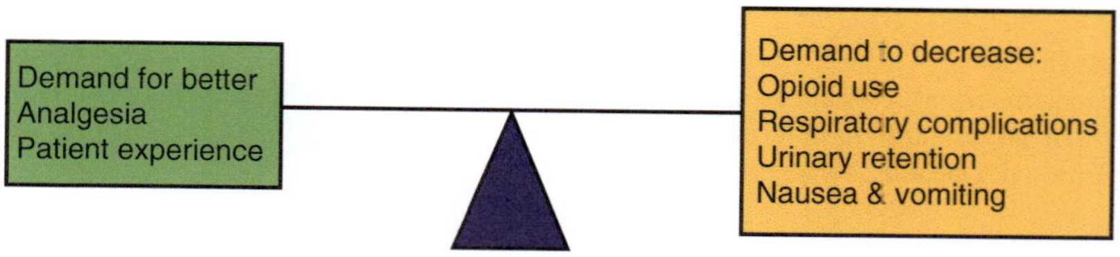

Fig. 4.1 Challenges in providing analgesia in ambulatory surgery centers

average procedure time can be decreased by about 30 minutes across all surgical specialties when the same procedure is performed at ASCs rather than hospital operating rooms [13]. Thus, the total number of ASC operating rooms has increased by 60% in the United States [14]. Moreover, the spectrum of surgical procedures has also been expanding in ASCs nationally [15].

Pain is the most common complication after surgical procedures and accounts for many unplanned hospital admissions after ambulatory surgery [16, 17]. Inadequate postoperative pain management and the adverse effects of overtly aggressive analgesia with increasing opioids are both important factors determining as to which procedures can be performed in an ambulatory setting [2, 15, 18]. Therefore, the management of perioperative pain often requires the employment of a multimodal approach and interventions facilitated by pain specialists. Effective analgesia can often be achieved in ambulatory surgery with opioid-sparing practices and the utilization of regional anesthesia techniques [9, 19]. A multimodal approach to adequate analgesia usually combines a variety of medications and non-pharmacologic techniques which target different mechanisms of action in the peripheral and central nervous system in order to provide synergistic/additive pain relief when compared to a single-modality intervention [9, 19, 20]. Certain types of surgeries, as well as higher body mass index, young males, and longer duration of anesthesia, have been shown to have a higher incidence of severe pain [19, 20]. Despite multimodal approaches, widespread prevalence of inadequate analgesia in ASCs is validated by many studies [2, 3, 19, 21]. A prospective study aimed to evaluate postoperative pain in ASC in patients receiving multimodal analgesia found that despite receiving multimodal analgesia, patients' reported postoperative pain scores were ≥4/10. A multimodal analgesic approach consisting of infiltration of local anesthetics and multiple oral analgesic agents was insufficient for certain patient groups after ambulatory anorectal surgery [22]. A significant proportion of patients experienced inadequate analgesia at home or days after discharge in most ASCs leading to additional unwarranted costs and medicolegal implications [23]. Gan et al. reported that 75% of ambulatory patients experience pain in the recovery phase with over half of those patients describing the pain as moderate to severe [24]. This results in patient dissatisfaction, recurrent visits to family practitioners or emergency departments, and even readmissions [17, 25]. Evidence suggests that more than 80% of patients who undergo surgical procedures experience some form of acute postoperative pain. However, less than half of these patients report adequate postoperative pain relief [21]. Severe postoperative pain is also associated with potential cardiopulmonary complications and longer recovery times following surgical procedures and is the most common cause of unanticipated admissions to the hospital after ambulatory surgery [19, 26, 27] (Table 4.1). It is important to acknowledge that there are several predictive factors for severe postoperative pain in the ambulatory setting that could be used to provide tighter pain control and prevent unanticipated complications [28]. The growing demand for improvements in pain management techniques and regimens in ASCs is apparent [2].

Analgesic Goals in Ambulatory Surgery Centers

Standard of care for the treatment of postoperative pain in ASCs should include a cost-effective multimodal analgesia protocol, identification of patients at increased risk of developing severe postoperative pain, rescue interventions when the implemented analgesic plan is unsuccessful, and ensuring a safe discharge [29] (Table 4.2). The American Pain Society and American Society of Anesthesiologists have collaborated to promote evidence-based, effective, and safe postoperative pain management in adults and children [30]. The groups recommend that clinicians provide individualized goal-driven education to each patient on treatment options for their management of surgical pain and document the plan and goals for postoperative pain management. In order to formulate an appropriate perioperative management plan, clinicians should conduct a detailed preoperative evaluation. This should

Table 4.1 Negative clinical outcomes associated with postoperative pain [2, 19]

System	Effect	Result
Cardiovascular	Tachycardia Hypertension ↑ Myocardial O_2 demand and workload	Myocardial ischemia or infarct Cardiac failure
Pulmonary	↓ Tidal volume and ventilation due to abdominal and chest muscle splintingInhibition of coughing and secretion mobilization	Atelectasis Pulmonary infections
Gastrointestinal	Slowing gut motility, gastric distension, and intestinal dilatation	Postoperative ileus
Urological	Imbalance of ANS smooth muscle	Urinary retention
Endocrine	↑ Catabolism ↑ Antidiuretic hormone ↑ Aldosterone, cortisol, and adrenaline	Sodium and water retention Hyperglycemia
Immunological	Altered immune system	Infection-related complications
Hematological	Restriction in mobility ↑ Cortisol and catecholamine secretion	DVT and pulmonary embolism ↑ Blood viscosity and clotting ↑ Fibrinolysis and platelet aggregation
Neurological	↑ Peripheral and central sensitization	Chronic pain, sleep deprivation, anxiety, fatigue

ANS autonomous nervous system, *DVT* deep vein thrombosis

include the assessment of medical and psychiatric comorbidities, concomitant medications, chronic pain history, substance abuse, and previous treatment regimens [30]. Parents of children who undergo surgery should receive appropriate methods for assessing pain as well as counseling on appropriate administration of analgesics and modalities. Recognizing high-risk patients in the preoperative assessment will help minimize the risk of inadequate pain control postoperatively, avoid hospital admissions, and prevent delayed discharges [28]. Patients at risk include females, preoperative anxiety, history of chronic pain, and younger individuals [28, 31]. Postoperative pain can be effectively minimized in ASCs with the addition of preemptive multimodal techniques involving centrally and peripherally acting analgesics and other non-pharmacologic techniques [30, 31]. The American Society of Anesthesiologists' Task Force on Acute Pain Management recommends the use of regional blocks and a scheduled regimen of opioid-sparing medications as part of the multimodal approach [31]. Peripheral nerve blocks and the infiltration of local anesthetics can facilitate the recovery process in the postoperative period allowing for earlier ambulation and discharge home [32]. Acetaminophen, nonselective NSAIDs, and COX-2 selective NSAIDs have become the mainstay of background analgesia to control postoperative pain in all surgical settings [2, 19, 33]. Gabapentin and pregabalin also have become key components to providing multimodal analgesia. These anticonvulsants offer preoperative sedation and anxiolysis and reduce the overall opioid requirements, which then decrease the various adverse effects from opioids [23, 34].

Table 4.2 Analgesic goals in ambulatory surgery centers [2, 10, 29]

Cost-effectiveness	The analgesic approaches should not add too much financial burden to the ASCs
Efficiency	The analgesic approaches should be efficient and not delay scheduled procedure and/or increase the OR turnaround time in ASCs
Adequate analgesia and patient satisfactory	The analgesic approaches should provide adequate analgesia and ensure patient satisfaction in ASCs
Minimized drug side effects	Avoidance of large dose-related side effects from individual drugs. Adoption of "lower dose and multi-mechanism drugs" approach
Minimized anesthetic complications	Respiratory, urinary, digestive, and other complications should be avoided

OR operating room, *ASC* ambulatory surgery center

It is essential in ASCs to have a postoperative rescue strategy in case of inadequate pain control. Opioids do have an imperative role as rescue analgesia, but it is important to remember the increased risks of impaired ventilation, particularly when used in obese patients and those with sleep-disordered breathing. Laying out plans for additional medications in the recovery room and the use of postoperative regional anesthetics are all valuable components that can aid in patient recovery. Lastly, it is important to educate the patient and family about surgical expectations and managing postoperative pain at home.

Summary

It can be extremely challenging to provide optimal analgesia to surgical patients in ASCs. On the one side, ASCs need to offer adequate analgesia to the patients; on the other side, ASCs and healthcare providers are facing increasingly higher social pressure to decrease opioid consumption. Adoption of multimodal analgesic strategy seems to be the best solution to the dilemma. The analgesic approaches should serve the following goals: cost-effectiveness, efficiency, adequacy, patient satisfaction, and minimal drug side effects and anesthetic complications. The best approach should be tailored based on individual patient needs and available ASC resources.

References

1. American Hospital Association. Fast facts on U.S. hospitals. 2020. https://www.aha.org/statistics/fast-facts-us-hospitals. Accessed 28 June 2020.
2. Vadivelu N, Kai AM, Kodumudi V, Berger JM. Challenges of pain control and the role of the ambulatory pain specialist in the outpatient surgery setting. J Pain Res. 2016;9:425–35. Published 2016 Jun 17. https://doi.org/10.2147/JPR.S86579. Mitchell JM. Effect of physician ownership of specialty hospitals and ambulatory surgery centers on frequency of use of outpatient orthopedic surgery. Arch Surg. 2010;145(8):732–8. https://doi.org/10.1001/archsurg.2010.149.
3. Rana MV, Desai R, Tran L, Davis D. Perioperative pain control in the ambulatory setting. Curr Pain Headache Rep. 2016;20(3):18. https://doi.org/10.1007/s11916-016-0550-3.
4. Volkow ND, Collins FS. The role of science in addressing the opioid crisis. N Engl J Med. 2017;377(4):391–4. https://doi.org/10.1056/NEJMsr1706626.
5. Blanco C, Volkow ND. Management of opioid use disorder in the USA: present status and future directions. Lancet. 2019;393(10182):1760–72. https://doi.org/10.1016/S0140-6736(18)33078-2.
6. Dart RC, Surratt HL, Cicero TJ, et al. Trends in opioid analgesic abuse and mortality in the United States. N Engl J Med. 2015;372(3):241–8. https://doi.org/10.1056/NEJMsa1406143. Schug SA, Chandrasena C. Postoperative pain management following ambulatory anesthesia: challenges and solutions. Ambul Anesth. 2015;2:11–20.
7. Prekupec MP, Mansky PA, Baumann MH. Misuse of novel synthetic opioids: a deadly new trend. J Addict Med. 2017;11(4):256–65. https://doi.org/10.1097/ADM.0000000000000324.
8. Kehlet H, Jensen TS, Woolf CJ. Persistent postsurgical pain: risk factors and prevention. Lancet. 2006;367(9522):1618–25.
9. Baboli KM, Liu H, Poggio JL. Opioid-free postoperative analgesia: is it feasible? Curr Probl Surg. 2020;57(7):100795. https://doi.org/10.1016/j.cpsurg.2020.100795.
10. Liu H, Emelife PI, Moll V, Kendrick J, Parr A, Hyatali F, Pankaj T, Li J, Cornett EM, Prabhakar A, Urman RD, Fox CJ, Kaye AD. Regional anesthesia for cardiac surgery. Best Pract Res Clin Anaesthesiol. 2019;33(4):387–406. Elsevier. https://doi.org/10.1016/j.bpa.2019.07.008.
11. Greco M, Capretti G, Beretta L, Gemma M, Pecorelli N, Braga M. Enhanced recovery program in colorectal surgery: a meta-analysis of randomized controlled trials. World J Surg. 2014;38(6):1531–41. https://doi.org/10.1007/s00268-013-2416-8.
12. Munnich EL, Parente ST. Procedures take less time at ambulatory surgery centers, keeping costs down and ability to meet demand up. Health Aff (Millwood). 2014;33(5):764–9. https://doi.org/10.1377/hlthaff.2013.1281.
13. Kadhim M, Gans I, Baldwin K, Flynn J, Ganley T. Do surgical times and efficiency differ between inpatient and ambulatory surgery centers that are both hospital owned? J Pediatr Orthop. 2016;36(4):423–8. https://doi.org/10.1097/BPO.0000000000000454.
14. Hollenbeck BK, Dunn RL, Suskind AM, Zhang Y, Hollingsworth JM, Birkmeyer JD. Ambulatory surgery centers and outpatient procedure use among Medicare beneficiaries. Med Care. 2014;52(10):926–31. https://doi.org/10.1097/MLR.0000000000000213.
15. Gologorsky Y. Outpatient spine surgery: transition to the ambulatory surgery center. World Neurosurg. 2018;114:369–70. https://doi.org/10.1016/j.wneu.2018.04.119.

16. Segerdahl M, Warrén-Stomberg M, Rawal N, Brattwall M, Jakobsson J. Clinical practice and routines for day surgery in Sweden: results from a nation-wide survey. Acta Anaesthesiol Scand. 2008;52(1):117–24. https://doi.org/10.1111/j.1399-6576.2007.01472.x.
17. Mattila K, Hynynen M, Intensium Consortium Study Group. Day surgery in Finland: a prospective cohort study of 14 day-surgery units. Acta Anaesthesiol Scand. 2009;53(4):455–63. https://doi.org/10.1111/j.1399-6576.2008.01895.x.
18. Prabhakar A, Cefalu JN, Rowe JS, Kaye AD, Urman RD. Techniques to optimize multimodal analgesia in ambulatory surgery. Curr Pain Headache Rep. 2017;21(5):24. https://doi.org/10.1007/s11916-017-0622-z.
19. Kaye AD, Urman RD, Rappaport Y, et al. Multimodal analgesia as an essential part of enhanced recovery protocols in the ambulatory settings. J Anaesthesiol Clin Pharmacol. 2019;35(Suppl 1):S40–5. https://doi.org/10.4103/joacp.JOACP_51_18.
20. Li J, Lam D, King H, Credaroli E, Harmon E, Vadivelu N. Novel regional anesthesia for outpatient surgery. Curr Pain Headache Rep. 2019;23(10):69. Published 2019 Aug 1. https://doi.org/10.1007/s11916-019-0809-6.
21. Apfelbaum JL, Chen C, Mehta SS, Gan TJ. Postoperative pain experience: results from a national survey suggest postoperative pain continues to be undermanaged. Anesth Analg. 2003;97(2):534–40. https://doi.org/10.1213/01.ane.0000068822.10113.9e.
22. Ceulemans A, De Looze D, Van de Putte D, Stiers E, Coppens M. High post-operative pain scores despite multimodal analgesia in ambulatory anorectal surgery: a prospective cohort study. Acta Chir Belg. 2019;119(4):224–30. https://doi.org/10.1080/00015458.2018.1500802.
23. Schug SA, Chong C. Pain management after ambulatory surgery. Curr Opin Anaesthesiol. 2009;22(6):738–43. https://doi.org/10.1097/ACO.0b013e32833020f4.
24. Gan TJ, Habib AS, Miller TE, White W, Apfelbaum JL. Incidence, patient satisfaction, and perceptions of post-surgical pain: results from a US national survey. Curr Med Res Opin. 2014;30(1):149–60. https://doi.org/10.1185/03007995.2013.860019.
25. Englbrecht JS, Pogatzki-Zahn EM. Ambulante Schmerztherapie – Optimierung der Schmerztherapie nach ambulanten Operationen [Pain management after ambulatory surgery in Germany]. Anasthesiol Intensivmed Notfallmed Schmerzther. 2010;45(1):44–55. https://doi.org/10.1055/s-0029-1243378.
26. Tasmuth T, Kataja M, Blomqvist C, von Smitten K, Kalso E. Treatment-related factors predisposing to chronic pain in patients with breast cancer – a multivariate approach. Acta Oncol. 1997;36(6):625–30. https://doi.org/10.3109/02841869709001326.
27. Shea RA, Brooks JA, Dayhoff NE, Keck J. Pain intensity and postoperative pulmonary complications among the elderly after abdominal surgery. Heart Lung. 2002;31(6):440–9. https://doi.org/10.1067/mhl.2002.129449.
28. Gramke HF, de Rijke JM, van Kleef M, et al. Predictive factors of postoperative pain after day-case surgery. Clin J Pain. 2009;25(6):455–60. https://doi.org/10.1097/AJP.0b013e31819a6e34.
29. Dickerson DM. Acute pain management. Anesthesiol Clin. 2014;32(2):495–504. https://doi.org/10.1016/j.anclin.2014.02.010.
30. Gordon DB, de Leon-Casasola OA, Wu CL, Sluka KA, Brennan TJ, Chou R. Research gaps in practice guidelines for acute postoperative pain management in adults: findings from a review of the evidence for an American Pain Society clinical practice guideline. J Pain. 2016;17(2):158–66. https://doi.org/10.1016/j.jpain.2015.10.023.
31. American Society of Anesthesiologists Task Force on Acute Pain Management. Practice guidelines for acute pain management in the perioperative setting: an updated report by the American Society of Anesthesiologists Task Force on Acute Pain Management. Anesthesiology. 2012;116(2):248–73.
32. Kampitak W, Tanavalee A, Ngarmukos S, Amarase C. Opioid-sparing analgesia and enhanced recovery after total knee arthroplasty using combined triple nerve blocks with local infiltration analgesia. J Arthroplast. 2019;34(2):295–302. https://doi.org/10.1016/j.arth.2018.10.009.
33. Kandarian BS, Elkassabany NM, Tamboli M, Mariano ER. Updates on multimodal analgesia and regional anesthesia for total knee arthroplasty patients. Best Pract Res Clin Anaesthesiol. 2019;33(1):111–23. https://doi.org/10.1016/j.bpa.2019.02.004.
34. Wick EC, Grant MC, Wu CL. Postoperative multimodal analgesia pain management with nonopioid analgesics and techniques: a review. JAMA Surg. 2017;152(7):691–7. https://doi.org/10.1001/jamasurg.2017.0898.

Challenges of Pain Control in Ambulatory Surgery Setting

5

David Fanelli, Dennis J. Warfield Jr., Sadie Smith, Anwar Alinani, Alan David Kaye, and Henry Liu

Abstract

Ambulatory surgery centers (ASCs) are prevalent throughout the United States and provide benefits to both patients and healthcare systems. Accordingly, ASCs have anesthetic challenges that are unique from hospitals in providing optimal patient care. Success of these centers is predicated on same-day patient discharge while maintaining patient safety and comfort. Adequate control of analgesia and postoperative nausea and vomiting remain two fundamental challenges of achieving this goal. Regional anesthetic techniques in combination with multimodal analgesia and enhanced recovery protocols aid in this process. Failure to meet these objectives may result in delayed discharge or escalation of care resulting in hospital admission. We present an overview of the causes of inadequate analgesia in ASCs, major postoperative concerns, regional anesthetic techniques to aid in recovery and discharge, and fundamentals of appropriate discharge analgesia.

Introduction

Improvements in surgical techniques in combination with adjustments in payment structures for surgical procedures have led to an increased prevalence of ambulatory surgery centers (ASCs) throughout the United States [1]. There are many benefits to ASCs including cost efficacy for healthcare systems, increased efficiency, patient convenience, and decreased risk of surgical site infection [2, 3]. Accordingly, an increasing number of surgical procedures are routinely performed in ASCs. In these settings, patient discharge is expected immediately after the procedure or within 24 hours. However, there are a number of barriers to discharge from ASCs including inadequately controlled postoperative pain, persistent postoperative nausea and vomiting, and a lack of a capable caregiver for post-procedural support. In this chapter we focus on the challenges of pain control in ASCs, the consequences of inadequate analgesia, and methods to keep postoperative pain from becoming a barrier to discharge.

D. Fanelli · D. J. Warfield Jr. · S. Smith · A. Alinani H. Liu (✉)
Department of Anesthesiology and Perioperative Medicine, Penn State College of Medicine, Milton S. Hershey Medical Center, Hershey, PA, USA
e-mail: dfanelli@pennstatehealth.psu.edu; dwarfield@pennstatehealth.psu.edu; ssmith38@pennstatehealth.psu.edu; aalinani@pennstatehealth.psu.edu

A. D. Kaye
Departments of Anesthesiology and Pharmacology, Toxicology, and Neurosciences, Louisiana State University Health Shreveport, Shreveport, LA, USA
e-mail: akaye@lsuhsc.edu

K. Rajput et al. (eds.), *Pain Control in Ambulatory Surgery Centers*,
https://doi.org/10.1007/978-3-030-55262-6_5

Causes of Inadequate Analgesia in ASCs

Pain is an inevitable consequence of a surgical procedure, and treatment of pain is one fundamental responsibility of an anesthesia provider. Pain after surgery remains a top concern among patients [4, 5]. The modern anesthesia provider has numerous tools available to treat intraoperative and postoperative pain. Opioid medications that are routinely utilized for pain management have undesirable side effects such as respiratory depression, sedation, and nausea. With improper opioid dosing, these side effects may prevent patients from meeting commonly used ASC discharge criteria such as the modified Aldrete scoring system and/or the postanesthetic discharge scoring system. As a result, anesthesia providers may be inclined to avoid or under-dose these agents over concern for their side effect profile and fear of delaying discharge. The consequence of this rationale is untreated or under-treated postoperative pain and inadequate analgesia in the post-anesthesia care setting [6, 7]. This remains a common reason for hospital readmission following ambulatory surgery [8].

Patient selection is another key predictor of inadequate analgesia in ASCs. ASCs are designed to accommodate the care needs of specific patient populations, and as a result patient selection is critical. Improper patient selection influences perioperative outcomes and may result in reduced efficiency of ASCs, delayed discharge, unplanned hospital admission or readmission, increased postoperative complications, and patient dissatisfaction. While ASCs have traditionally accommodated ophthalmic, orthopedic, and gynecologic surgeries, advances in minimally invasive surgical techniques have further broadened the variety of procedures that can be safely performed at these centers. As the number of procedures eligible to be performed at ambulatory surgery centers increases, so does the number of patients. A recent meta-analysis found anxiety, preoperative pain, type of surgery, and age to be significant predictors of postoperative pain [9]. Patients with these risk factors may have increased analgesic requirements and are more likely to be inadequately treated. Adequate pain treatment may result in side effects that further delay discharge from ASCs or result in hospital readmissions. Careful assessment of these factors should be performed prior to scheduling patients at ASCs to minimize risk and should be incorporated in standard of care perioperative screening (Table 5.1). Patients who do not meet requirements for surgery at an ASC should appropriately be referred to a main hospital for surgical care.

Table 5.1 Etiologies of inadequate analgesia

Etiologies of inadequate analgesia [10]	Basic features
Side effect profile	Provider concern over opioid side effect profile and potential for delayed discharge from ASCs
History of chronic pain	Higher baseline requirements Reluctance of physicians to prescribe over concerns of regulatory environment [10, 11]
Insufficient provider training	Low rates and emphasis on pain management in medical and postgraduate training [12] Less likely to appropriately prescribe opioids
Patient concerns of abuse	Concerns regarding addictive properties of opioids with reluctance to take them even when prescribed Inadequate counseling from providers regarding safe opioid use

Major Postoperative Concerns in ASCs

Major postoperative concerns in ASCs are centered on the adequacy of postoperative recovery within 24 hours and subsequent discharge home. Controlling postoperative pain and postoperative nausea and vomiting (PONV) is an important aspect of this goal. Furthermore, these remain central concerns to the patients as well [4, 5, 13]. There are several postoperative assessment tools that are available to anesthesia providers to assess recovery. These include the Aldrete consciousness scoring system, modified Aldrete scoring system (Table 5.2), and postanesthetic discharge scoring system (Table 5.3) [14–16]. Patients are

Table 5.2 The modified Aldrete scale

The modified Aldrete scale [15]			
Respiration	2 Able to breathe deeply and cough freely	1 Dyspnea, limited breathing	0 Apneic or on mechanical ventilation
O_2 saturation	2 Able to maintain O_2 saturation >92% on room air needs	1 Needs O_2 inhalation to maintain O_2, saturation >90%	0 O_2, saturation <90% even with O_2 supplement
Consciousness	2 Fully awake	1 Arousable on calling	0 Not responding
Circulation	2 BP ± 20% of pre-anesthetic level	1 BP ± 20% to 49% of pre-anesthetic level	0 BP ± 50% of pre-anesthetic level
Activity	2 Able to move four extremities voluntarily or on command	1 Able to move two extremities voluntarily or on command	0 Unable to move extremities voluntarily or on command

A total modified Aldrete score is 10 with a score ≥9 considered ready for discharge

Table 5.3 Postanesthetic discharge scoring system

Postanesthetic discharge scoring system [18]			
Vital signs	2 Within 20% of preoperative value	1 20%–40% of preoperative value	0 40% preoperative value
Activity and mental status	2 Oriented × 3 and has a steady gait	1 Oriented × 3 or has a steady gait	0 Neither
Pain, nausea, and/or vomiting	2 Minimal	1 Moderate, having required treatment	0 Severe, requiring treatment
Surgical bleeding	2 Minimal	1 Moderate	0 Severe
Intake and output	2 Has had PO fluids and voided	1 Has had PO fluids or voided	0 Neither

A total PADS score is 10 with a score ≥9 considered ready for discharge

scored on a number of parameters such as vital signs with the total indicating whether they may safely leave the post-anesthesia care unit (PACU) and be discharged from the ASC (Table 5.4) [17]. Although pain scoring is not universally utilized within these systems, prolonged and severe postoperative pain will cause derangement of other parameters such as blood pressure and respiratory status ultimately affecting the final score. As a result, postoperative pain control is an important component of promoting rapid recovery and meeting discharge criteria expeditiously. Finding a balance between adequate analgesia to facilitate discharge and over-treating postoperative pain with resultant medication side effects is a principle challenge in the practice of anesthesia within ASCs.

PONV is another significant postoperative concern that factors into speed of recovery and discharge readiness. Some of the previously discussed scoring systems specifically address PONV, while others do not [14–16]. Similar to postoperative pain control, inadequate PONV treatment may disrupt other postoperative assessment parameters and prevent patients from meeting discharge criteria. ASC operating principles rely on rapid postoperative recovery to facilitate discharge. Adequate analgesia and PONV treat-

Table 5.4 American Society of Anesthesiologists Standards for Post-anesthesia Care

Standards for post-anesthesia care [17]	
Standard I	All patients who received monitored anesthesia care, general anesthesia, or regional anesthesia shall have appropriate post-anesthesia management
Standard II	A patient transported to the post-anesthesia recovery unit should be accompanied by a member of the anesthesia team who is knowledgeable of the patient's medical condition. The patient shall be monitored during transport and appropriately supported
Standard III	In the PACU, a verbal report should be given to the PACU nurse who will care for the patient by a member of the anesthesia team
Standard IV	The patient should be continually evaluated in the PACU
Standard V	A physician is responsible for evaluating the patient for discharge from the PACU. Discharge criteria must be approved by the Anesthesiology Department and may vary

ment are two major concerns of anesthesia providers working in ASCs that must be optimized to ensure adequate patient safety, recovery, and discharge.

Consequences of Inadequate Analgesia in ASCs

A fundamental tenet of anesthesia care is the provision of adequate analgesia during the procedure. Failure to achieve analgesic control may manifest as patient movement or hemodynamic derangements that compromise achievement of hemostasis. This can potentially hinder the ability of the surgical team to perform the procedure and subsequently lead to poor outcomes [19–22]. Furthermore, an inadequate operative environment becomes a safety concern for both the patient and the staff.

Not only does inadequate intraoperative analgesia effect the operative environment, but it can quickly become a source of patient distress and subsequent dissatisfaction following procedures [23, 24]. Postoperative pain is consistently rated as a top concern of patients, yet individual satisfaction in postoperative pain relief remains low [5, 25]. While providing optimal care to patients remains the top priority of clinicians, patient satisfaction scores have also been linked to hospital compensation. In a landmark decision in 2012, the Centers for Medicare and Medicaid Services (CMS) instituted Hospital Consumer Assessment of Healthcare Providers and Systems (HCAHPS) surveys that aim to capture essential elements of patient satisfaction including pain management [26, 27]. Results of these surveys were previously tied to institutional compensation from CMS. Patient perceptions of well-managed pain are associated with higher satisfaction scores [28]. In an increasingly complex national healthcare market, maintaining high patient satisfaction remains a priority for insuring the fiscal stability of independent hospital systems.

A final consequence of inadequate analgesia in ASCs is the delayed discharge and/or escalation of care resulting in admission. ASCs rely on discharging patients within 24 hours of their procedure. Postoperative pain and nausea are common causes of unanticipated hospital admission following outpatient surgery [29–31]. Unplanned admissions have negative consequences for the institution including additional utilization of resources as well as increased costs for the patient and the healthcare system. Furthermore, patient satisfaction scores are likely to be negatively impacted by these events.

Unique Aspects of ASC Versus Hospital OR Surgery in Relation to Anesthesia Techniques

Healthcare systems, and by extension ambulatory surgery centers, are increasingly more focused on providing value-based care to patients where quality and service are maximized while costs are minimized [32]. Enhanced recovery after surgery (ERAS) protocols are utilized as one way to continue improving value and outcomes after major operations [33]. Consequently, there has been a proliferation of ERAS protocols that are often specific to a single procedure, although compliance with these protocols remains poor [34]. Comprehensively reviewing each of these protocols is beyond the scope of this chapter. However, these protocols all emphasize the importance of multimodal analgesia within pain management as a major component of enhanced recovery.

More specifically, multimodal analgesia relies on the co-administration of several different medications and adjuncts for the management of pain. This allows increased therapeutic effects with lower dosing requirements and a more favorable side effect profile [33, 35, 36]. Accordingly, these principles are readily applied to anesthetics performed at ambulatory surgery centers [37, 38]. This includes the use of local anesthetics, NSAIDs, gabapentinoids, acetaminophen, alpha-2 agonists, and ketamine among others [37]. Like multimodal analgesia, balanced anesthesia relies on the synergy of multiple anesthetic agents to create a more favorable operative environment while minimizing adverse effects. Multimodal analgesia remains a crucial component of providing a balanced anesthetic. These principles are essential for the successful practice of anesthesia at ASCs where obtaining the appropriate operative conditions while minimizing prolonged pharmacologic side effects is prioritized. Failure of anesthesia providers to utilize these may contribute to delayed discharge from ASCs.

Anesthesia provided at ASCs exists as a continuum from monitored anesthesia care (MAC) through general anesthesia. MAC is often compared to conscious sedation; however a key distinction of MAC is the ability of a MAC provider to convert to general anesthesia [39]. Choosing to perform the case under MAC versus general anesthesia is a multifactorial decision that is contingent on patient, procedural, surgical, and anesthetic factors [40, 41]. Cases performed under MAC have been associated with shorter recovery times and increased satisfaction which aligns with the goals of ASCs [41, 42]. Regardless of the primary anesthetic choice, accompanying use of regional anesthesia promotes rapid recovery and patient satisfaction in ASCs [43].

Regional Anesthesia in ASCs

Multimodal analgesia is the cornerstone of pain management in ASCs in order to minimize adverse effects of any one dominant modality [44]. Regional anesthesia (RA) applications not only expand the options available within this domain but have an analgesic potential that far surpasses what is provided by conventional opioid-centric therapeutics [43]. There is less postoperative nausea and vomiting (PONV) and less need for endotracheal intubation [45, 46]. Multiple randomized control trials (RCTs) have demonstrated reduced time until discharge readiness and overall shortened hospitalization following RA [47]. Similarly, one RCT showed a decrease in total costs by 79% in the early discharge group following RA [48, 49].

The choice of local anesthetic (LA) and RA technique depends on the surgical site, the intensity of the block desired, anticipated length of the procedure, duration of the postoperative pain control, LA allergy, need for postoperative ambulation, need for postoperative neurological examination, and finally the ASC's institutional policies for the duration and discharge from the PACU [50]. Commonly used amide LAs (i.e., lidocaine, bupivacaine, and ropivacaine) are preferred over esters (i.e., procaine, cocaine, chloroprocaine, tetracaine, and benzocaine) secondary to their perceived more favorable allergy profile, but interestingly, there is no definitive evidence that one class is better than the other in terms of hypersensitivity [51]. Another preference within the amides seems to be reliance on more lipid-soluble LAs such as bupivacaine than more hydrophilic agents such as ropivacaine for surgical anesthesia. However, recent RCTs concluded that ropivacaine not only is equipotent but possesses a better cardiotoxicity profile [52]. A technique employed to speed up block onset times is to combine lidocaine with a longer-acting LA (i.e., ropivacaine or bupivacaine) or by the addition of a buffering solution such as bicarbonate [53]. This stems from the relationship of onset times with the dissociation constant (pK_a) of LAs. The lower the pK_a (closer to physiologic pH), the faster the block onset [53]. Lidocaine, having a pK_a around 7.9, therefore has a faster onset than bupivacaine (pK_a of 8.1) and ropivacaine (pK_a of 8.2). However, many studies fail to show any benefit in terms of faster onset, using this practice [54]. Furthermore, mixing lidocaine with other longer-acting LAs can shorten the overall block duration in comparison to when these longer-acting LA are used alone [55].

In terms of duration of the block, many factors come into play such as the amount of protein binding as well as the alkalinity and pK_a of the solution, site of the blockade, metabolism, concentration, and volumes of LA used [56]. These dynamic factors could offset expectations of onset and durations of LAs in daily practice. On average, duration of blockade for commonly used LAs is as follows: 2% lidocaine, 2–5 hours; 0.5% ropivacaine, 4–12 hours; and 0.5% bupivacaine, 5–15 hours [57].

If pain coverage is desired beyond these timelines, use of continuous peripheral nerve block catheters (CPNBCs) can be employed. However, if CPNBCs are not a feasible option, use of adjuncts in conjunction with a LA can be applied to prolong the initial single-injection peripheral nerve block (PNB). Table 5.5 lists the common peripheral nerve blocks utilized in an ASC setting.

Adjuncts

Commonly used adjuncts in ASCs include steroids, epinephrine, alpha-2 agonists, and opiates.

Dexamethasone

Dexamethasone prolongs the duration of the nerve block depending on the site blocked, the type of LA used, and the dose at which it is used. One of the more favorable sites to utilize this adjunct is for an interscalene block where it has been reported to increase the block duration up to 22 hours when combined with ropivacaine [58, 59]. For supraclavicular blocks, when mixed with mepivacaine, reports state duration can last up to 5 hours [60]. Average prolongation of the PNB increases by 8 hours for long-acting and intermediate-acting LAs (bupivacaine and ropivacaine) and by 4 hours for short-acting LAs (lidocaine, mepivacaine, and prilocaine) [61]. The dose-related prolonged effect of LA continues to increase until the ceiling is reached at a dexamethasone adjunct dose of 4 mg [62]. Though transient use of dexamethasone at these doses has not been associated with adverse outcomes in terms of wound healing and systemic infections, the RCTs describing this have been excluding high-risk critically ill populations [63]. More studies are needed to answer the question of its use in diabetic, immunocompromised, and critically ill patient subgroups [63]. For concerned providers, a lower dose of 2 mg is also sufficient to prolong the block by an average of 5.9 hours [64]. Being a potent steroid, it is difficult to pinpoint any one mechanism of action, but several have been described such as (a) stimulation of glucocorticoid receptors leading to increased inhibition of the potassium-gated channels in the nociceptive C fibers, (b) a localized vasoconstrictive effect decreasing the reuptake of the LAs, and (c) a localized or systemic anti-inflammatory effect [65]. Interestingly, some question the use of dexamethasone for perineural application all together as when given parenterally, the administration results in a similar increase in the duration of the block [66].

Epinephrine

Proposed mechanism includes vasoconstriction leading to reduced uptake and metabolism of the LA at the proposed site [67]. Though this effect is seen with most LAs, its inconsistent action with ropivacaine has led some to question this hypothesis [68]. In five RCTs an average increase of 1 hour to the block duration was seen with an epinephrine dose of 5 μg/ml (1:200,000) in the LA solution. In one study there was a decrease in peripheral nerve perfusion by 20% from baseline raising the fear of potential nerve ischemia, though this effect in a healthy adult is clinically negligible and amounts to the same risk as that of a pneumatic tourniquet [69, 70]. However, cau-

Table 5.5 Common peripheral nerve blocks utilized in an ASC setting

Upper extremity block technique	Location	Nerve(s) Blocked	Indications	Considerations
Interscalene	Roots of brachial plexus (BP)	C5–C7 roots	Surgery to shoulder and/or proximal to mid-humerus	Ipsilateral hemidiaphragmatic paresis due to phrenic nerve (C3–C5) blockade. Unsuitable for patients unable to tolerate a 25% reduction in pulmonary function. Larger volumes can cause neuraxial spread [84]
Supraclavicular	Trunks and divisions of BP	Superior, middle, and inferior trunks	Surgery to distal humerus, elbow, forearm, wrist, and/or hand	Risk of pneumothorax requires caution in ambulatory care setting. Phrenic nerve paresis in 30% of cases [84]
Infraclavicular	Cords of BP	Lateral, posterior, and medial cords	Surgery to elbow, forearm, wrist, and/or hand	Less risk of pneumothorax. Catheter site easier to affix and maintain [85]
Axillary	Terminal branches of BP	Radial, ulnar, median, and musculocutaneous nerves	Surgery on forearm, wrist, and/or hand; less suitable for procedures near the elbow	Musculocutaneous nerve needs to be targeted separately. May need to block intercostobrachial nerve additionally for tourniquet pain [85]
Truncal block technique	Location	Nerve(s) blocked	Indications	Considerations
Pectoralis (PECS) I, II	Fascial plane between pectoralis major and minor muscles (PECS I); fascial plane between pectoralis minor and serratus anterior muscle (PECS II)	Medial and lateral pectoral nerves (PECS I); lateral branches of the intercostal nerves and long thoracic nerve (PECS II)	Breast surgery, traumatic chest injuries, and pacemaker and chest drain insertions	Long thoracic nerve blockade causes "winged scapula" and sometimes masks intraoperative damage [86]
Serratus anterior plane (SAP) (PECS III)	Fascial plane between the serratus anterior muscle and underlying rib	Intercostobrachial, thoracodorsal, and long thoracic nerves as well as the lateral cutaneous branches of T3–T9 intercostal nerves	Breast surgery, rib fractures, and anterolateral chest wall surgery or injury	Often supplemented with PECS blocks [87]
Paravertebral (PVB)	Paravertebral space (PVS)	Dorsal and ventral rami of spinal nerves, sympathetic chain and rami communicantes	Breast surgery, traumatic chest injuries, thoracic or abdominal wall procedures, upper and lower abdominal surgery, and hernia repair	Fewer side effects than epidural. Preferential caudal spread. Large volume single injections may produce less reliable anesthesia than multiple small volume injections at individual targeted dermatomal levels [43]

(continued)

Table 5.5 (continued)

Upper extremity block technique	Location	Nerve(s) Blocked	Indications	Considerations
Erector spinae plane (ESP)	Fascial plane between anterior surface of erector spinae muscles and posterior surface of transverse process of thoracic vertebrae	Dorsal rami of spinal nerves and intercostal nerves	Breast surgery, traumatic chest injuries, thoracic or abdominal wall procedures, upper and lower abdominal surgery, hernia repair, and postsurgical neuropathic pain	Cephalocaudal spread unpredictable. Requires high volume. Paravertebral spread inconsistent [88]
Transversus abdominis plane (TAP)	Fascial plane between internal oblique and transversus abdominis muscles	Anterior and lateral cutaneous branches of lower intercostal, ilioinguinal, and iliohypogastric nerves	Upper and lower abdominal surgery including cesarean section	Techniques include subcostal, lateral, posterior, ilioinguinal, and four-quadrant TAP blocks [89]
Lower extremity block technique	Location	Nerve(s) blocked	Indications	Considerations
Femoral	L2–4 terminal branches of lumbar plexus (LP)	Femoral nerve	Anteromedial thigh surgery and surgery of the distal femur and/or knee	Block can cause significant weakness of the quadriceps muscles (vastus lateralis, vastus medialis, vastus intermedius, and rectus femoris)
Adductor canal / saphenous	Adductor canal	Saphenous nerve	Knee surgery and surgery of the distal anteromedial thigh, medial calf, and/or ankle	Considered a sensory block, but varies according to the volume used and the level selected within the adductor canal. Spread can reach the nerve to the vastus medialis as well as the femoral triangle that houses most of the motor divisions of the femoral nerve [90]
Popliteal sciatic	Popliteal fossa	Tibial and common peroneal nerves	Foot, ankle, and/or Achilles tendon surgery	Complete anesthesia for surgeries below the knee can be provided when combined with a saphenous nerve block [44]
Infiltration between the popliteal artery and cof the knee (iPACK)	Tissue plane between the popliteal artery and the posterior capsule of the knee joint	Articular branches arising from the main trunks of the tibial and obturator nerves	Total knee arthroplasty and cruciate ligament surgeries	Recommended to use color Doppler to identify the saphenous branch of the descending genicular artery, prior to needle advancement, in order to avoid inadvertent needle trauma to the saphenous nerve [91]
Ankle block	Various locations at or around the level of the medial and lateral malleoli	Posterior tibial, deep peroneal, superficial peroneal, sural, and saphenous nerves	Foot and/or toe surgery distal to the ankle	Does not provide anesthesia for tourniquet use [43]

tion is needed when dealing with vasculopathic patients and uncontrolled diabetics where 2.5 μg/ml (1:400,000) is noted to be a more acceptable dose when indicated [71].

Alpha-2 (α2) Agonists

Clonidine and dexmedetomidine are both α2 agonists used frequently as PNB adjuncts. Dexmedetomidine has eight times the affinity for α2 receptors than clonidine, yet the effect in prolongation of the block is not proportional to its α2 selectivity. Dexmedetomidine, while having a much greater affinity than clonidine, only increases block duration by 4.5 hours versus 2.5 hours for clonidine [72, 73]. This disproportional effect stems from the fact that α2 receptors have little to do with increasing the block duration as they are completely absent in the peripheral nerves. The mechanism of action is described as the inhibition of the hyperpolarization-activated, cyclic nucleotide-gated membrane channels that restore the action potential from the refractory phase [74]. Alpha-2 agonists are also implicated in pain modulation by augmenting inhibitory synaptic transmission in the superficial dorsal horn through activation of descending noradrenergic control [75]. The mean dose for the proposed prolongation is stated to be 150 μg for clonidine and 50–60 μg for dexmedetomidine, respectively [72]. There have been cases described of bradycardia, arterial hypotension, sedation, and orthostatic hypotension, more so with clonidine than with dexmedetomidine. These adverse effects should preclude the use of these adjuncts in high-risk populations.

Buprenorphine

Studies conducted on opioids such as fentanyl, tramadol, morphine, and hypnotics such as ketamine have either yielded lack of clinical effectiveness or conflicting and inconclusive findings when used as adjuncts with LAs [74]. Buprenorphine, conversely, has shown some effect. A μ receptor agonist and K receptor antagonist, it tends to increase the block duration to an average of 8.5 hours when used perineurally and 7 hours when used intramuscularly [76]. Main adverse effects reported include PONV and pruritus; however in these studies, no prophylaxis was used.

Liposomal Bupivacaine

Liposomal vesicles are a lipid bilayer (phospholipids) that contains internal reservoirs used for the sustained release of drugs, such as LAs. A LA used in this context is liposomal bupivacaine, which has been in development since the 1980s, but not approved for clinical use until 2011 [70]. Studies conducted when used as a sole agent for local infiltration are not so encouraging [77–79]. There is some promise when used for truncal or PNBs, but there too, it has been deemed less potent than plain bupivacaine [80–82]. However, liposomal bupivacaine has been FDA approved for interscalene brachial plexus nerve blocks and has been used along with plain bupivacaine. When combined, the potency needed in the acute phase increases, while the liposomal component provides prolonged analgesia for up to 72 hours [77]. This is a highly controversial subject as the data on its efficacy among PNBs is inconsistent. Where it has shown promise is with the improvement in NRS pain scores, but by only a magnitude of 1–1.5, making it clinically insignificant from much cheaper and well-studied LAs [83]. More RCTs are needed to gauge its potential for PNBs as a substitute, as an adjunct to other LAs, or for potentially replacing CPNBCs.

Continuous Peripheral Nerve Block Catheters

Benefits of PNBs are not only limited to the immediate perioperative setting within ASCs. The advent of CPNBCs has extended these benefits into the postoperative phase as well [92].

Most of the anatomical sites used for single-injection PNBs can incorporate CPNBCs. For blocks such as interscalene or supraclavicular,

CPNBCs may require techniques such as catheter tunneling to obtain more stability. Though first described in 1946, the first prospective RCT including CPNBCs was not performed until 2000 [50]. Since then, nerve block catheters have come a long way in their utility; however, complications are still possible. Perineural loop, catheter migration, leakage, knot, kink, adherence, bleeding and hematoma, infection, local anesthesia systemic toxicity (LAST), neurological damage, and continued risk of fall are a few of the complications that need to be taken into consideration [93–101]. While these adverse events are rare, defining a criteria for better patient selection can further minimize the risks associated with performing CPNBC techniques [102].

Criteria for Patient Selection

- CPNBCs should be considered for surgeries expected to have at least a moderate degree of postoperative pain, lasting more than 24 hours [103, 104]. Notable exceptions to this include patients suffering from chronic pain, cancer-related pain, complex regional pain syndromes, scenarios requiring continuous sympatholysis, ulcer-derived pain, and patients at risk for developing phantom-limb pain.
- Catheter care needs cooperation and a degree of cognition, both for successful infusion and patient safety [105–107]. Patients with learning disabilities or where a basic understanding of the CPNBCs cannot be established should be reconsidered, unless a guardian or caregiver can ensure consent, responsibility, safety, and operability.
- On the first postoperative night, the patient might still be cognitively impaired secondary to the effects of combined general anesthesia. Presence of a caregiver during discharge is important for proper disposition of catheter care instructions [50].
- Patients with renal failure, hepatic failure, and cardiac conduction abnormalities are at a greater risk for LAST [108]. Doses should either be adjusted, or in severe circumstances, regional intervention should be limited to a single-injection PNB only.
- COPD and heart failure patients might not be able to tolerate any reduction in their functional residual capacity (FRC). Blocks such as interscalene and supraclavicular block can cause up to a 25% reduction in FRC. In healthy individuals, this may not be clinically relevant, but in COPD and heart failure patients, this unilateral paralysis of the diaphragm can be life-threatening [109].
- Surgical intervention may require serial neurological examinations postoperatively. Since CPNBCs can lead to both motor and sensory block, they should be avoided in this cohort to ensure an accurate examination.
- In the rehabilitative phases where mobility is paramount and risk of fall great, sites for CPNBCs notorious for causing falls such as the femoral nerve block should be avoided [97].
- Infections close to the site and patients with evidence of sepsis or neurological damage have a relative contraindication for CPNBCs. Judicious use of CPNBCs is advocated after weighing the benefits versus the risks of a regional intervention.

Placement of CPNBCs

With the ease and availability of ultrasonography, catheter failure rates have declined to less than 10% [110, 111]. Though there is little doubt in ultrasound taking over for nerve stimulation guided catheter techniques, there are various scenarios such as deep, non-lucent areas where support by nerve stimulation is warranted [111]. Another technique to decrease the rate of catheter failure is to administer the initial bolus of LA after the catheter has been placed (failure rate 1–8%) versus giving the bolus first and then placing the catheter (failure rate as high as 40%) [110, 111]. While placement protocols differ according to the design and manufacturing of the catheter kit as well as provider preference, every effort should be made in securing the catheter in its optimal position. Use of Opsites™, Tegaderms™, Dermabond™, benzoin, Steri-Strips™, and specialized anchoring devices such as Starlocks™ has been described to assist in achieving this goal [112]. For catheter in situ duration, one retrospective analysis showed the infection risk to increase after day 4 of placement, although there are no RCTs yet to answer this question [113]. There is also no defined upper limit of catheter in situ duration, as case reports have described catheters to be safe up to 88 days post-insertion [114].

Infusate delivery options (continuous infusion versus intermittent auto bolus) and dosage, including patient-controlled analgesia boluses, may differ for each block type and anatomical site. For infusion pump selection, numerous manufacturers with varying programmability options, ergonomics, disposability, and unit cost all factor into the decision when gauging a particular model.

CPNBC Discharge Guidelines

- Care instructions pertaining to the pump, catheter site, and catheter removal need to be communicated verbally as well as in written form with contact information of the primary service, regional and acute pain service responsible, and manufacturer [115].
- Model number and pertinent pump data with troubleshooting instructions needs to be available with the device when it is handed off to the patient along with disposition details of all equipment once the catheter is removed.
- A signs and symptoms checklist for infection, neurological injury, and LAST needs to be provided to the patient and caregiver with contact numbers for emergencies.
- For patients ambulating and having CPNBCs for their lower extremity in place, education about fall prevention and appropriate safety tips need to be elaborated.
- Phone follow-up by the regional and acute pain service should be arranged on a daily basis for the duration of catheter use to inquire about matters such as the patient's current pain control, catheter site appearance, as well as expected completion of the infusion [116].

Post-discharge Analgesia

In addition to having expertise in multimodal analgesia during procedures performed in ambulatory surgical centers, anesthesiologists should also be knowledgeable and acutely aware of the significance for postoperative pain control after discharge. The opioid crisis as we know it began in the 1990s, and it was triggered by an introduction of the notion of "pain as a fifth vital sign" [117]. Medical care, and in turn Medicare compensation, was tied to prioritizing and optimizing pain control. From the late 1990s until the late 2000s, opioid prescription sales and opioid overdose death had a parallel increase of fourfold [118]. Several studies in the 2010s have demonstrated that surgical patients use substantially less opioid than prescribed. Excessive postsurgical opioid prescribing can lead to long-term opioid dependence, misuse, and diversion [119–121].

A meta-analysis from 2018 by Feinberg et al. found that patients who had abdominal procedures took less than 15 opioid pills (they defined "opioid pills" as 5 mg of oxycodone [119]. For orthopedic procedures, the mean number of pills ranged from 9 to 22; patients had more opioid use with procedures that required bone versus soft tissue involvement. Dermatologic and breast lumpectomy procedures require very little or no opioid postoperatively [119]. Although it may be tempting to write a patient more opioid pills postoperatively to avoid refills, this practice can lead to serious unintended side effects of opioids, including opioid dependence and diversion.

It is critical that prescribing physician, whether that be the anesthesiologist or surgeon, prescribes the smallest amount of opioid, accounting for the procedure performed. As procedures performed in ambulatory surgical centers are typically shorter in time, recovery, and blood loss (compared to procedures required inpatient hospital care), prescribing physicians need to take even more caution to prescribe the least amount of opioid required or none at all. Physicians and advance practice providers need to emphasize to patients the importance of utilization of non-opioid analgesics such as acetaminophen and

NSAIDs (as appropriate), as well as rest, ice, heat, physical therapy, and other conservative modalities, in order to avoid the potential harmful consequences of opioid use.

Summary

ASCs provide benefits to both patients and hospital systems. Success of these centers relies on balancing the comfort and safety of patients with optimization for same-day discharge. Regional anesthesia as a component of multimodal analgesia, enhanced recovery protocols, and pharmacologic treatment of PONV are fundamental in achieving this balance. Postoperative pain management with opioid prescriptions remains common but should be minimized to the greatest extent possible. Regional anesthesia and CPNBCs have utility in minimizing opioids as part of a balanced multimodal approach to analgesia. ASCs will continue to grow in popularity as surgical techniques advance. Anesthesiologists must continue to develop practices to aid in this pursuit.

References

1. Hall MJ, Schwartzman A, Zhang J, Liu X. Ambulatory surgery data from hospitals and ambulatory surgery centers: United States, 2010. Natl Health Stat Report. 2017;2017(102):1–15.
2. Edmonston DL, Foulkes GD. Infection rate and risk factor analysis in an orthopaedic ambulatory surgical center. J Surg Orthop Adv. 2010;19(3):174–6.
3. Goldfarb CA, Bansal A, Brophy RH. Ambulatory surgical centers: a review of complications and adverse events. J Am Acad Orthop Surg. 2017;25(1):12–22.
4. Rana MV, Desai R, Tran L, Davis D. Perioperative pain control in the ambulatory setting. Curr Pain Headache Rep. 2016;20(3):1–9.
5. Strassels SA, Chen C, Carr DB. Postoperative analgesia: economics, resource use, and patient satisfaction in an urban teaching hospital. Anesth Analg. 2002;94(1):130–7.
6. Ward S, Guest C, Goodall I, Bantel C. Practice and bias in intraoperative pain management: results of a cross-sectional patient study and a survey of anesthesiologists. J Pain Res. 2018;11:561–70.
7. Gan TJ. Poorly controlled postoperative pain: prevalence, consequences, and prevention. J Pain Res. 2017;10:2287–98.
8. Rosero EB, Joshi GP. Hospital readmission after ambulatory laparoscopic cholecystectomy: incidence and predictors. J Surg Res. 2017;219:108–15. https://doi.org/10.1016/j.jss.2017.05.071.
9. Ip HYV, Abrishami A, Peng PWH, Wong J, Chung F. Predictors of postoperative pain and analgesic consumption: a qualitative systematic review. Anesthesiology. 2009;111(3):657–77.
10. Sinatra R. Causes and consequences of inadequate management of acute pain. Pain Med. 2010;11(12):1859–71.
11. Sinnenberg LE, Wanner KJ, Perrone J, Barg FK, Rhodes KV, Meisel ZF. What factors affect physicians' decisions to prescribe opioids in emergency departments? MDM Policy Pract. 2017;2(1):238146831668100.
12. Loeser JD, Schatman ME. Chronic pain management in medical education: a disastrous omission. Postgrad Med. 2017;129(3):332–5.
13. Cao X, White PF, Ma H. An update on the management of postoperative nausea and vomiting. J Anesth. 2017;31(4):617–26.
14. Aldrete JA, Kroulik D. A postanesthetic recovery score. Anesth Analg. 1970;49(6):924–34.
15. Aldrete JA. The post-anesthesia recovery score revisited. J Clin Anesth. 1995;7(1):89–91.
16. Chung F. Recovery pattern and home-readiness after ambulatory surgery. Anesth Analg. 1995;80(5):896–902.
17. American society of anesthesiologists: committee on standards and practice parameters. Standards for postanesthesia care. 2019.
18. Chung F, Chan VWS, Ong D. A post-anesthetic discharge scoring system for home readiness after ambulatory surgery. J Clin Anesth. 1995;7(6):500–6.
19. Jayasekera PSA, Kai A, Lawrence CM. Preoperative hypertension increases intraoperative bleeding in patients undergoing Mohs micrographic surgery. J Am Acad Dermatol. 2019;80(2):562–4. https://doi.org/10.1016/j.jaad.2018.08.005.
20. Kawaguchi Y, Nomi T, Fuks D, Mal F, Kokudo N, Gayet B. Hemorrhage control for laparoscopic hepatectomy: technical details and predictive factors for intraoperative blood loss. Surg Endosc. 2016;30(6):2543–51.
21. Vázquez-Narvaéz KG, Ulibarri-Vidales M. The patient with hypertension and new guidelines for therapy. Curr Opin Anaesthesiol. 2019;32(3):421–6.
22. Bunick CG, Aasi SZ. Hemorrhagic complications in dermatologic surgery. Dermatol Ther. 2011;24(6):537–50.
23. Odom-Forren J, Reed DB, Rush C. Postoperative distress of orthopedic ambulatory surgery patients. AORN J. 2017;105(5):464–77. https://doi.org/10.1016/j.aorn.2017.03.005.
24. Odom-Forren J, Reed DB, Rush C. Postoperative symptom distress of laparoscopic cholecystectomy ambulatory surgery patients. J Perianesthesia Nurs. 2018;33(6):801–13. https://doi.org/10.1016/j.jopan.2017.12.002.

25. Geisler A, Dahl JB, Karlsen APH, Persson E, Mathiesen O. Low degree of satisfactory individual pain relief in postoperative pain trials. Acta Anaesthesiol Scand. 2017;61(1):83–90.
26. Mehta SJ. Patient satisfaction reporting and its implications for patient care. AMA J Ethics. 2015;17(7):616–21.
27. Strate C. How does patient satisfaction impact reimbursement. Access [Internet]. 2018;2–6. Available from: https://www.accessefm.com/blog/how-does-patient-satisfaction-impact-reimbursement
28. Mazurenko O, Collum T, Ferdinand A, Menachemi N. Predictors of hospital patient satisfaction as measured by HCAHPS: a systematic review. J Healthc Manag. 2017;62(4):272–83.
29. Vadivelu N, Kai AM, Kodumudi V, Berger JM. Challenges of pain control and the role of the ambulatory pain specialist in the outpatient surgery setting. J Pain Res. 2016;9:425–35.
30. Tewfik MA, Frenkiel S, Gasparrini R, Zeitouni A, Daniel SJ, Dolev Y, et al. Factors affecting unanticipated hospital admission following otolaryngologic day surgery. J Otolaryngol. 2006;35(4):235–41.
31. Zulfiquer FA, Pattanayak K. Evaluation of unplanned admission following day surgery at a new surgical centre in London. Ambul Surg. 2009;15(4):1–4.
32. Porter ME. What is value in health care? N Engl J Med. 2010;363:2477–81.
33. Beverly A, Kaye AD, Ljungqvist O, Urman RD. Essential elements of multimodal analgesia in enhanced recovery after surgery (ERAS) guidelines. Anesthesiol Clin. 2017;35(2):e115–43.
34. Joshi GP, Kehlet H. Postoperative pain management in the era of ERAS: an overview. Best Pract Res Clin Anaesthesiol. 2019;33(3):259–67. https://doi.org/10.1016/j.bpa.2019.07.016.
35. Brown EN, Pavone KJ, Naranjo M. Multimodal general anesthesia: theory and practice. Anesth Analg. 2018;127(5):1246–58.
36. Gabriel RA, Swisher MW, Sztain JF, Furnish TJ, Ilfeld BM, Said ET. State of the art opioid-sparing strategies for postoperative pain in adult surgical patients. Expert Opin Pharmacother. 2019;20(8):949–61.
37. Elvir-Lazo OL, White PF. The role of multimodal analgesia in pain management after ambulatory surgery. Curr Opin Anaesthesiol. 2010;23(6):697–703.
38. Elvir-Lazo OL, White PF. Postoperative pain management after ambulatory surgery: role of multimodal analgesia. Anesthesiol Clin. 2010;28(2):217–24.
39. Delegates AH of. Distinguishing Monitored Anesthesia Care ("MAC") From Moderate Sedation/Analgesia (Conscious Sedation). 2018;1–2.
40. Lee JH. Anesthesia for ambulatory surgery. Korean J Anesth. 2017;70(4):398–406.
41. Das S, Ghosh S. Monitored anesthesia care: an overview. J Anaesthesiol Clin Pharmacol. 2015;31(1):27–9.
42. Sá Rêgo MMS, Watcha MF, White PF. The changing role of monitored. 1997;1020–36.
43. Ardon AE, Prasad A, McClain RL, Melton MS, Nielsen KC, Greengrass R. Regional anesthesia for ambulatory anesthesiologists. Anesthesiol Clin. 2019;37(2):265–87.
44. Kopp SL, Horlocker TT. Regional anaesthesia in day-stay and short-stay surgery. Anaesthesia. 2010;65(April):84–96.
45. Liu SS, Strodtbeck WM, Richman JM, Wu CL. A comparison of regional versus general anesthesia for ambulatory anesthesia: a meta-analysis of randomized controlled trials. Anesth Analg. 2005;101(6):1634–42.
46. Liu Y, Su M, Li W, Yuan H, Yang C. Comparison of general anesthesia with endotracheal intubation, combined spinal-epidural anesthesia, and general anesthesia with laryngeal mask airway and nerve block for intertrochanteric fracture surgeries in elderly patients: a retrospective cohort stud. BMC Anesthesiol. 2019;19(1):4–9.
47. Ilfeld BM. Continuous peripheral nerve blocks: a review of the published evidence. Anesth Analg. 2011;113(4):904–25.
48. Ilfeld BM, Vandenborne K, Duncan PW, Sessler DI, Enneking FK, Shuster JJ, et al. Ambulatory continuous interscalene nerve blocks decrease the time to discharge readiness after total shoulder arthroplasty: a randomized, triple-masked, placebo-controlled study. Anesthesiology. 2006;105(5):999–1007.
49. White PF, Issioui T, Skrivanek GD, Early JS, Wakefield C. The use of a continuous popliteal sciatic nerve block after surgery involving the foot and ankle: does it improve the quality of recovery? Anesth Analg. 2003;97(5):1303–9.
50. Ilfeld BM, Enneking FK. Continuous peripheral nerve blocks at home: a review. Anesth Analg. 2005;100(6):1822–33.
51. Weinschenk S, Mergenthaler C, Armstrong C, Göllner R, Hollmann MW, Strowitzki T. Local anesthetics, procaine, lidocaine, and mepivacaine show vasodilatation but no type 1 allergy: a double-blind, placebo-controlled study. Biomed Res Int. 2017;2017:1–9.
52. Kaur A, Bahadur Singh R, Tripathi RK, Choubey S. Comparison between bupivacaine and ropivacaine in patients undergoing forearm surgeries under axillary brachial plexus block: a prospective randomized study. J Clin Diagnostic Res. 2015;9(1):1–6.
53. Buckenmaier C, Kent M, Brookman J, Tighe P, Mariano E, Edwards D. Acute pain medicine. 1st ed. New York: Oxford University Press; 2019. p. 282–3.
54. Ribotsky BM, Berkowitz KD, Montague JR. Local anesthetics. Is there an advantage to mixing solutions? J Am Pod Med Assoc. 1996;86(10):487–91.
55. Cuvillon P, Nouvellon E, Ripart J, Boyer JC, Dehour L, Mahamat A, et al. A comparison of the pharmacodynamics and pharmacokinetics of bupivacaine, ropivacaine (with epinephrine) and their equal volume mixtures with lidocaine used for femoral and sciatic nerve blocks: a double-blind randomized study. Anesth Analg. 2009;108(2):641–9.

56. Becker DE, Reed KL. Local anesthetics: review of pharmacological considerations. Anesth Prog. 2012;59(2):90–102.
57. Gadsden J. Local anesthetics: clinical pharmacology and rational selection. In: Hadzic A, editor. Hadzic's peripheral nerve blocks and anatomy for ultrasound-guided regional anesthesia. 2nd ed. New York: McGraw-Hill; 2012. p. Chapter 2.
58. Cummings KC, Napierkowski DE, Parra-Sanchez I, Kurz A, Dalton JE, Brems JJ, et al. Effect of dexamethasone on the duration of interscalene nerve blocks with ropivacaine or bupivacaine. Br J Anaesth. 2011;107(3):446–53. https://doi.org/10.1093/bja/aer159.
59. Parrington SJ, O'Donnell D, Chan VWS, Brown-Shreves D, Subramanyam R, Qu M, et al. Dexamethasone added to mepivacaine prolongs the duration of analgesia after supraclavicular brachial plexus blockade. Reg Anesth Pain Med. 2010;35(5):422–6.
60. Kirksey MA, Haskins SC, Cheng J, Liu SS. Local anesthetic peripheral nerve block adjuvants for prolongation of analgesia: a systematic qualitative review. PLoS One. 2015;10(9):e0137312.
61. Albrecht E, Kern C, Kirkham KR. A systematic review and meta-analysis of perineural dexamethasone for peripheral nerve blocks. Anaesthesia. 2015;70(1):71–83.
62. Kirkham KR, Jacot-Guillarmod A, Albrecht E. Optimal dose of perineural dexamethasone to prolong analgesia after brachial plexus blockade: a systematic review and meta-analysis. Anesth Analg. 2018;126(1):270–9.
63. Polderman JAW, Farhang-Razi V, Van Dieren S, Kranke P, Devries JH, Hollmann MW, et al. Adverse side effects of dexamethasone in surgical patients. Cochrane Database Syst Rev. 2018;2018(8):CD011940.
64. Schnepper GD, Kightlinger BI, Jiang Y, Wolf BJ, Bolin ED, Wilson SH. A retrospective study evaluating the effect of low doses of perineural dexamethasone on ropivacaine brachial plexus peripheral nerve block analgesic duration. Pain Med. 2018;19(7):1485–93.
65. Witt NJ, Zochodne DW, Bolton CF, Grand'Maison F, Wells G, Young GB, et al. Peripheral nerve function in sepsis and multiple organ failure. Chest. 1991;99(1):176–84. https://doi.org/10.1378/chest.99.1.176.
66. Abdallah FW, Dwyer T, Chan VWS, Niazi AU, Ogilvie-Harris DJ, Oldfield S, et al. IV and perineural dexmedetomidine similarly prolong the duration of analgesia after interscalene brachial plexus block: a randomized, three-arm, triple-masked, placebo-controlled trial. Anesthesiology. 2016;124(3):683–95.
67. Sinnott CJ, Cogswell LP, Johnson A, Strichartz GR. On the mechanism by which epinephrine potentiates lidocaine's peripheral nerve block. Anesthesiology. 2003;98(1):181–8.
68. Weber A, Fournier R, Van Gessel E, Riand N, Gamulin Z. Epinephrine does not prolong the analgesia of 20 mL ropivacaine 0.5% or 0.2% in a Femoral three-in-one block. Anesth Analg. 2001;93(5):1327–31.
69. Neal JM. Effects of epinephrine in local anesthetics on the central and peripheral nervous systems: neurotoxicity and neural blood flow. Reg Anesth Pain Med. 2003;28(2):124–34.
70. Vadhanan P, Tripaty DK, Adinarayanan S. Physiological and pharmacologic aspects of peripheral nerve blocks. J Anaesthesiol Clin Pharmacol. 2015;31(3):384–93.
71. Partridge BL, Phil D. The effects of local anesthetics and epinephrine on rat sciatic nerve blood flow. Anesthesiology. 1991;75(2):243–51.
72. Vorobeichik L, Brull R, Abdallah FW. Evidence basis for using perineural dexmedetomidine to enhance the quality of brachial plexus nerve blocks: a systematic review and meta-analysis of randomized controlled trials. Br J Anaesth. 2017;118(2):167–81.
73. Williams BA, Hough KA, Tsui BYK, Ibinson JW, Gold MS, Gebhart GF. Neurotoxicity of adjuvants used in perineural anesthesia and analgesia in comparison with ropivacaine. Reg Anesth Pain Med. 2011;36(3):225–30.
74. Desai N, Albrecht E, El-Boghdadly K. Perineural adjuncts for peripheral nerve block. BJA Educ. 2019;19(9):276–82. https://doi.org/10.1016/j.bjae.2019.05.001.
75. Funai Y, Pickering AE, Uta D, Nishikawa K, Mori T, Asada A, et al. Systemic dexmedetomidine augments inhibitory synaptic transmission in the superficial dorsal horn through activation of descending noradrenergic control: an in vivo patch-clamp analysis of analgesic mechanisms. Pain. 2014;155(3):617–28.
76. Schnabel A, Reichl SU, Zahn PK, Pogatzki-Zahn EM, Meyer-Frießem CH. Efficacy and safety of buprenorphine in peripheral nerve blocks: a meta-analysis of randomised controlled trials. Eur J Anaesthesiol. 2017;34(9):576–86.
77. Bergese SD, Ramamoorthy S, Patou G, Bramlett K, Gorfine SR, Candiotti KA. Efficacy profile of liposome bupivacaine, a novel formulation of bupivacaine for postsurgical analgesia. J Pain Res. 2012;5:107–16.
78. Langford R, Chappell G, Karrasch J. A single administration of depobupivacaine intraoperatively results in prolonged detectable plasma bupivacaine and analgesia in patients undergoing inguinal hernia repair. In: The Annual Postgraduate Assembly in Anesthesiology of the New York State Society of Anesthesiologists. The Annual Postgraduate Assembly in Anesthesiology of the New York State Society of Anesthesiologists: New York; 2008.
79. White P, Schooley G, Ardeleanu M. Analgesia following a single administration of depobupivacaine intraoperatively in patients undergoing inguinal herniorrhaphy: preliminary dose-ranging studies. Anesth Analg. 2009;108(suppl 3S):S242.

80. Okoroha KR, Lynch JR, Keller RA, Korona J, Amato C, Rill B, et al. Liposomal bupivacaine versus interscalene nerve block for pain control after shoulder arthroplasty: a prospective randomized trial. J Shoulder Elb Surg. 2016;25(11):1742–8.
81. Okoroha KR, Keller RA, Marshall NE, Jung EK, Mehran N, Owashi E, et al. Liposomal bupivacaine versus femoral nerve block for pain control after anterior cruciate ligament reconstruction: a prospective randomized trial. Arthroscopy. 2016;32(9):1838–45.
82. Namdari S, Nicholson T, Abboud J, Lazarus M, Steinberg D, Williams G. Randomized controlled trial of interscalene block compared with injectable liposomal bupivacaine in shoulder arthroplasty. J Bone Jt Surg. 2017;99(7):550–6.
83. Vandepitte C, Kuroda M, Witvrouw R, Anne L, Bellemans J, Corten K, et al. Addition of liposome bupivacaine to bupivacaine HCl versus bupivacaine HCl alone for interscalene brachial plexus block in patients having major shoulder surgery. Reg Anesth Pain Med. 2017;42(3):334–41.
84. Auyong DB, Hanson NA, Joseph RS, Schmidt BE, Slee AE, Yuan SC. Comparison of anterior suprascapular, supraclavicular, and interscalene nerve block approaches for major outpatient arthroscopic shoulder surgery a randomized, double-blind, noninferiority trial. Anesthesiology. 2018;129(1):47–57.
85. Neal JM, Gerancher JC, Hebl JR, Ilfeld BM, McCartney CJL, Franco CD, et al. Upper extremity regional anesthesia. Essentials of our current understanding, 2008. Reg Anesth Pain Med. 2009;34(2):134–70.
86. Miller B, Pawa A, Mariano E. Problem with the Pecs II block: the long thoracic nerve is collateral damage. Reg Anesth Pain Med. 2019;44(8):817–8.
87. Kunigo T, Murouchi T, Yamamoto S, Yamakage M. Spread of injectate in ultrasound-guided serratus plane block: a cadaveric study. JA Clin Rep. 2018;4(1):4–5.
88. Choi YJ, Kwon HJ, Jehoon O, Cho TH, Won JY, Yang HM, et al. Influence of injectate volume on paravertebral spread in erector spinae plane block: an endoscopic and anatomical evaluation. PLoS One. 2019;14(10):e0224487.
89. Tsai HC, Yoshida T, Chuang TY, Yang SF, Chang CC, Yao HY, et al. Transversus abdominis plane block: an updated review of anatomy and techniques. Biomed Res Int. 2017;2017(8284363):1–12.
90. Grevstad U, Jæger P, Sørensen JK, Gottschau B, Ilfeld B, Ballegaard M, et al. The effect of local anesthetic volume within the adductor canal on quadriceps femoris function evaluated by electromyography: a randomized, observer- and infject-blinded, placebo-controlled study in volunteers. Anesth Analg. 2016;123(2):493–500.
91. Tran J, Chan V, Peng P, Agur A. Response to Sebastian et al: the saphenous nerve and iPACK blocks. Reg Anesth Pain Med. 2020;45(3):245–6.
92. Grossi P, Urmey WF. Peripheral nerve blocks for anaesthesia and postoperative analgesia. Curr Opin Anaesthesiol. 2003;16(5):493–501.
93. Gharabawy R, Abd-Elsayed A, Elsharkawy H, Farag E, Cummings K, Eid G, et al. The Cleveland clinic experience with supraclavicular and popliteal ambulatory nerve catheters. Sci World J. 2014;2014:572507.
94. Gurnaney H, Kraemer FW, Maxwell L, Muhly WT, Schleelein L, Ganesh A. Ambulatory continuous peripheral nerve blocks in children and adolescents: a longitudinal 8-year single center study. Anesth Analg. 2014;118(3):621–7.
95. Bures E, Rivet P, Estebe JP. Échec De Retrait De Cathéters Nerveux Périphériques: Les Nœuds, Une Complication À Connaître. Ann Fr Anesth Reanim. 2009;28(5):493–5.
96. Presta MV, Byram SW, Reis CL, Sniderman M. Noninvasive removal of an entrapped supraclavicular catheter. J Clin Anesth. 2012;24(4):350–2.
97. Clendenen SR, Robards CB, Greengrass RA, Brull SJ. Complications of peripheral nerve catheter removal at home: case series of five ambulatory interscalene blocks. Can J Anesth. 2011;58(1):62–7.
98. Warner NS, Duncan CM, Kopp SL. Acute retroperitoneal hematoma after psoas catheter placement in a patient with myeloproliferative thrombocytosis and aspirin therapy. A A Case Rep. 2016;6(2):28–30.
99. Walker BJ, Long JB, De Oliveira GS, Szmuk P, Setiawan C, Polaner DM, et al. Peripheral nerve catheters in children: an analysis of safety and practice patterns from the pediatric regional anesthesia network (PRAN). Br J Anaesth. 2015;115(3):457–62.
100. Bleckner L, Solla C, Fileta BB, Howard R, Morales CE, Buckenmaier CC. Serum free ropivacaine concentrations among patients receiving continuous peripheral nerve block catheters: is it safe for long-term infusions? Anesth Analg. 2014;118(1):225–9.
101. Henningsen MH, Jæger P, Hilsted KL, Dahl JB. Prevalence of saphenous nerve injury after adductor-canal-blockade in patients receiving total knee arthroplasty. Acta Anaesthesiol Scand. 2013;57(1):112–7.
102. Ilfeld BM. Continuous peripheral nerve blocks: an update of the published evidence and comparison with novel, alternative analgesic modalities. Anesth Analg. 2017;124(1):308–35.
103. Ribeiro FC, Georgousis H, Bertram R, Scheiber G. Plexus irritation caused by interscalene brachial plexus catheter for shoulder surgery. Anesth Analg. 1996;82(4):870–2.
104. Rawal N, Allvin R, Axelsson K, Hallén J, Ekbäck G, Ohlsson T, et al. Patient-controlled regional analgesia (PCRA) at home: controlled comparison between bupivacaine and ropivacaine brachial plexus analgesia. Anesthesiology. 2002;96(6):1290–6.
105. Ilfeld BM, Morey TE, Enneking FK. Continuous infraclavicular brachial plexus block for postoperative pain control at home: a randomized, double-blinded, placebo-controlled study. Anesthesiology. 2002;96(6):1297–304.
106. Ilfeld BM, Morey TE, Wang RD, Enneking FK. Continuous popliteal sciatic nerve block for postoperative pain control at home: a random-

ized, double-blinded, placebo-controlled study. Anesthesiology. 2002;97(4):959–65.

107. Ilfeld BM, Morey TE, Wright TW, Chidgey LK, Enneking FK. Continuous interscalene brachial plexus block for postoperative pain control at home: a randomized, double-blinded, placebo-controlled study. Anesth Analg. 2003;96(4):1089–95.
108. Denson DD, Raj PP, Saldahna F, Finnsson RA, Ritschel WA, Joyce TH, et al. Continuous perineural infusion of bupivacaine for prolonged analgesia: pharmacokinetic considerations. Int J Clin Pharmacol Ther Toxicol. 1983;21(12):591–7.
109. Pere P. The effect of continuous interscalene brachial plexus block with 0.125% bupivacaine plus fentanyl on diaphragmatic motility and ventilatory function. Reg Anesth. 1993;18(2):93–7.
110. Borgeat A, Dullenkopf A, Ekatodramis G, Nagy L. Evaluation of the lateral modified approach for continuous interscalene block after shoulder surgery. Anesthesiology. 2003;99(2):436–42.
111. Borgeat A, Blumenthal S, Karovic D, Delbos A, Vienne P. Clinical evaluation of a modified posterior anatomical approach to performing the popliteal block. Reg Anesth Pain Med. 2004;29(3):290–6.
112. Tighe P, Buckenmaier CC, Boezaart AP, Carr DB, Clark LL, Herring AA, et al. Acute pain medicine in the United States: a status report. Pain Med. 2015;16(9):1806–26.
113. Bomberg H, Bayer I, Wagenpfeil S, Kessler P, Wulf H, Standl T, et al. Prolonged catheter use and infection in regional anesthesia: a retrospective registry analysis. Anesthesiology. 2018;128(4):764–73.
114. Pacenta HL, Kaddoum RN, Pereiras LA, Chidiac EJ, Burgoyne LL. Continuous tunnelled femoral nerve block for palliative care of a patient with metastatic osteosarcoma. Anaesth Intensive Care. 2010;38(3):563–5.
115. Macaire P, Gaertner E, Capdevila X. Continuous postoperative regional analgesia at home. Minerva Anestesiol. 2001;67(9 Suppl 1):109–16.
116. Borgeat A, Kalberer F, Jacob H, Ruetsch YA, Gerber C. Patient-controlled interscalene analgesia with ropivacaine 0.2% versus bupivacaine 0.15% after major open shoulder surgery: the effects on hand motor function. Anesth Analg. 2001;92(1):218–23.
117. Huang N, Cunningham F, Laurito CE, Chen C. Can we do better with postoperative pain management? Am J Surg. 2001;182(5):440–8.
118. Paulozzi LJ, Jones CM, Mack KA, Rudd RA. Vital signs: overdoses of prescription opioid pain relievers — United States, 1999–2008. Morb Mortal Wkly Rep. 2011;60(43):1487–92.
119. Feinberg AE, Chesney TR, Srikandarajah S, Acuna SA, McLeod RS. Opioid use after discharge in postoperative patients: a systematic review. Ann Surg. 2018;267(6):1056–62.
120. McDonald DC, Carlson K, Izrael D. Geographic variation in opioid prescribing in the U.S. J Pain. 2012;13(10):988–96.
121. Gomes T, Juurlink D, Moineddin R, Gozdyra P, Dhalla I, Paterson M, et al. Geographical variation in opioid prescribing and opioid-related mortality in Ontario. Healthc Q. 2011;14(1):22–4.

6 Assessment and Optimization of Available Resources for Pain Control (In Ambulatory Surgery Setting)

Alan David Kaye, Sarahbeth Howes, Sarah C. Bertrand, Randi E. Domingue, Taylor R. Jeansonne, Sasha A. Ridgell, Chikezie N. Okeagu, Andrew Paul Bourgeois, Cain W. Stark, Shreedhar Kulkarni, Prathima Anandi, Naema Zarish, and Elyse M. Cornett

Abstract

Ambulatory surgery is increasing in numbers, and deployment of resources is extremely important to ensure safe and adequate delivery of anesthesia and pain medicines. Pain management services must be available to these patients in the ambulatory setting in all phases of care. Management of perioperative pain in the ambulatory surgery setting is becoming increasingly complex and requires the employment of a multimodal approach and interventions facilitated by ambulatory surgery pain specialists.

A. D. Kaye
Departments of Anesthesiology and Pharmacology, Toxicology, and Neurosciences, LSU Health Shreveport, Shreveport, LA, USA
e-mail: akaye@lsuhsc.edu

S. Howes
LSU Medical School, Shreveport, LA, USA
e-mail: srive2@lsuhsc.edu

S. C. Bertrand · R. E. Domingue · T. R. Jeansonne
LSU Health Shreveport School of Medicine, Shreveport, LA, USA
e-mail: sbert5@lsuhsc.edu; rdomi2@lsuhsc.edu; tjean1@lsuhsc.edu

S. A. Ridgell · P. Anandi · N. Zarish
Department of Anesthesiology, LSU Health Shreveport, Shreveport, LA, USA
e-mail: sridg1@lsuhsc.edu; panan4@lsuhsc.edu; nzaris@lsuhsc.edu

C. N. Okeagu
Department of Anesthesiology, LSU Health Sciences Center, New Orleans, LA, USA
e-mail: cokeag@lsuhsc.edu

A. P. Bourgeois
Department of Anesthesiology, Louisiana State University Health Sciences Center, New Orleans, LA, USA
e-mail: abour7@lsuhsc.edu

C. W. Stark
Medical College of Wisconsin, Wauwatosa, WI, USA
e-mail: cwstark@mcw.edu

S. Kulkarni
Ochsner LSU Health – Shreveport, Shreveport, LA, USA
e-mail: skulka@lsuhs.edu

E. M. Cornett (✉)
Department of Anesthesiology, Louisiana State University Health Shreveport, Shreveport, LA, USA
e-mail: ecorne@lsuhsc.edu

K. Rajput et al. (eds.), *Pain Control in Ambulatory Surgery Centers*,
https://doi.org/10.1007/978-3-030-55262-6_6

Introduction

The frequency of ambulatory surgery is increasing within the USA and globally, accounting for over 50% of all surgeries in some countries [1]. Consequentially, postoperative pain is an ever-increasing problem, with the prevalence of severe postoperative pain ranging from 54.3% to 91% [1, 2]. Analysis of perioperative analgesia regimens, workflow, and staffing systems can minimize postoperative pain, unexpected hospital admissions, and emergency room visits. Such investigations and cost reduction analyses followed by implementating available interventions may decrease costs to patients and healthcare systems.

Pain control in the ambulatory care setting is vital, as the consequences of undertreating pain can be serious. Reported sequelae include unplanned admissions, emergency room visits, and chronic pain. Pain is also the most frequent reason for unscheduled contact with healthcare providers in the weeks following ambulatory surgery [3]. Brix et al. found that 9.2% of patients are presented to the emergency room for postoperative pain management, and 2.8% required hospital admission [3]. These extra visits place an undue and costly burden upon patients and the healthcare system, costing several thousand dollars per visit [4].

In addition to the economic burden of uncontrolled pain, chronic pain is a sociopsychobiological problem related to genetic and environmental risk factors. Chronic postoperative pain is present in 11.8% of patients following surgery [5]. Consequences of chronic pain include decreased functionality, work absences, severe depression, and anxiety [6]. In a study surrounding the physiologic effects of pain on the endocrine system, Tennant reports that pain manifests as stress by stimulating the hypothalamic-pituitary-adrenal-thyroid-gonadal system (HPATG) system to secrete hormones that target specific tissues, leading to hormonal dysregulation that can result in enhanced pain and reduced healing [7].

This chapter focuses on methods to improve post-op pain management for ambulatory surgery and recommendations for how hospital systems can optimize the treatment of ambulatory pain to reduce costs and improve patient outcomes. Preoperative evaluations to determine which patients are at high risk for post-op pain issues will allow for better planning of perioperative analgesia. Assessments that document pain history, determine expectations of pain management, and set pain management goals with patients are important for risk stratification before surgery [6]. Intraoperative factors, such as the use of regional analgesic techniques, ketamine, and minimally invasive nerve-sparing techniques, should be considered in pre-planning for minimal post-op pain [8, 9].

Assessment and management of postoperative pain require that physicians consider how to best assess that pain needs treatment and manage complicating factors. Chronic opioid use, drug abuse, and past medical history may complicate analgesic treatments. It is important to remember that control of acute pain with multimodal techniques may preemptively mitigate the development of chronic pain. Recommendations for how hospital systems can optimize treatment of ambulatory pain to reduce costs should center around procedure-specific recommendations and control of acute pain with multimodal techniques for preventing chronic pain [6]. One hospital reported a 58% decrease in readmissions following outpatient surgery by focusing on risk-stratifying patients and improving pain management techniques [10]. Further research, data compilations, and treatment analyses are necessary to see similar decreases in readmissions and cost-effective pain treatment options in ambulatory surgery settings.

Preoperative Setting

Preoperative Screening

A thorough preoperative workup and discussion with the patient are imperative for effective pain management in the ambulatory setting. Several factors are predictive of increased postoperative pain. Some studies have shown that younger patients, males, and those with a higher body mass index tend to have a higher incidence of severe postoperative pain [11]. Certain psychological conditions, including depression, anxiety, and neuroticism, have also been shown to be significant predictors of uncontrolled pain, as have preoperative and chronic use of opioids or pre-existing pain conditions [12]. Lastly, pain can be impacted by the type of surgical insult and anesthesia duration [11]. One study found that orthopedic surgery had the highest incidence of intensified pain, followed by urologic, general, and plastic surgery [11].

Preoperative screening should assess patients for these risk factors. Ideally, information should be gathered early enough before the scheduled surgery to allow ample time for preoperative planning and development of a treatment plan to optimize pain management [12]. Screening tools should include questions regarding the patient's history of depression and anxiety, substance abuse, and pain control [11]. Inquiries about their current pain, frequency and duration, and current medications and dosages taken for the pain will also help risk-stratify patients. Importantly, patients that are chronic opioid consumers should be identified. Special considerations need to be made for these patients with pain management plans that include prophylactic analgesic regimens and multimodal analgesic approaches [13]. These patients should be educated about the possible need for increased opioids postoperatively and a higher risk of severe pain [13, 14]. They should also be counseled to take their regular daily opioid dose on the day of surgery to avoid withdrawal [11, 13].

In addition to questions about history and current pain, multiple scales exist that can be used to assess a patient's individual tolerance for pain. Pain is a subjective experience and largely depends on individual patient characteristics and thresholds for pain. The Pain Catastrophizing Scale is a measure consisting of 13 items, each scored from 0 to 4, that assesses three components: rumination, magnification, and helplessness [15, 16]. A higher score indicates that the patient has more pain catastrophizing thoughts. A score greater than 30 points (out of 52 possible) has been previously associated with clinical relevance. The Pain Anxiety Symptom Scale (PASS) is another metric that can be used [17]. This questionnaire has 20 items designed to measure a patient's fear and anxiety response to pain [17]. Each question is rated on a 5-point scale from 0 (never) to 5 (always), with higher scores denoting greater pain-related anxiety. One study suggested the following cut-offs for determining levels of pain anxiety: mild, 0–34; moderate, 35–67; and severe, 68–100 [18]. Finally, the Fear-Avoidance Components Scale (FACS) is a more recently developed questionnaire that can be used [19]. This tool consists of 20 items scored from 0 (completely disagree) to 5 (completely agree), with higher scores implying higher levels of pain-related fear avoidance. The authors of the questionnaire recommended the following five severity levels to guide clinical interpretation: subclinical (0–20), mild (21–40), moderate (41–60), severe (61–80), and extreme (81–100). While collecting a comprehensive pain-related history and employing the aforementioned validated pain scales are undoubtedly very important, setting expectations with patients and their family members is arguably the most valuable component of the preoperative process.

Pain Management Expectations

Despite centuries of study, the complexity of pain continues to make targeted treatments extremely difficult to engineer, and pain remains one of the most complex sensations experienced by the human body. As such, it has been classified by most professionals involved in the management of pain as multifaceted and extremely complex, manifesting itself as physical, emotional, and/or psychological or sometimes an amalgam of all of these perceptions simultaneously, with the perceived manifestations of pain sometimes being far worse than the physical pain itself.

As the perception of pain has proven to vary greatly between individuals, it should be the goal of pain management to address not only the organic causes of pain but also the emotional and psychological manifestations linked to the perception of pain as well, by discussing the patient's expectations of pain in hopes of providing complete relief.

Studies demonstrate that preoperatively addressing the anticipated level of pain that the patient can expect postoperatively and discussing realistic goals for pain control can achieve better postoperative pain management via patient satisfaction scores. A study published by the *European Journal of Pain* in 2001 found that of 191 randomly sampled surgical patients, 61% had current pain at baseline before the surgical procedure, 91% expected postoperative pain of moderate to severe intensity, and of those 76% reported experiencing such levels [20]. Despite 76% experiencing moderate to severe intensity pain, 81% of the patients claimed to be satisfied with the pain management, while only 8% were dissatisfied [20]. This data serves to reiterate the importance of understanding and addressing patient attitudes and concerns regarding pain prior to management.

Other factors that seemed to influence overall satisfaction versus dissatisfaction among patients during the study included sex, age, and overall prior "pain experience," with the most dissatisfied patients being of younger age and female sex [20]. The study concluded that patients commonly expect moderate-to-severe pain in the postoperative period and that the overall experience is in accordance with the preoperative expectations [20].

Another study published in the *Journal of Clinical Anesthesia* set out to highlight the unrealistic expectations among many patients regarding postoperative pain management. The cross-sectional observation study collected 732 surveys over 5 weeks from inpatients who presented for preoperative evaluations for various surgeries. Expectations of postoperative pain management goals were measured by the pain levels that the patients considered "satisfactory" [21]. Overall, 41% of patients chose "no pain" as a satisfactory pain level after surgery, and the percentage of patients who chose "no pain" was not significantly different among patient scheduled for minor, moderate, or major surgery [21]. Ultimately, 36% of patients who were to undergo major surgery chose a postoperative pain goal of "no pain" [21]. However, when the administrators of the study suggested to the patients that it may not be safe to reduce the pain level to their desired satisfaction level, >80% of patients were willing to accept a higher level of pain [21].

Multivariate analysis also revealed that patients with lower education levels were more likely to choose "no pain" as their satisfactory postoperative pain level (see Fig. 6.1) [21]. Cumulatively, these data indicate the unrealistic expectations regarding postoperative pain management among many patients, thus showcasing the importance of realistic goal discussion prior to the treatment of pain. It is important that a dialog be formed between provider and patient to address the possibility that it might not be feasible or safe to substantially reduce pain in a patient below his/her baseline. Conservative pain management measures and the use of adjunct medicines should take priority to restrict opioid use. Finally, the provider and patient should interact clearly and regularly [22]. See Fig. 6.1.

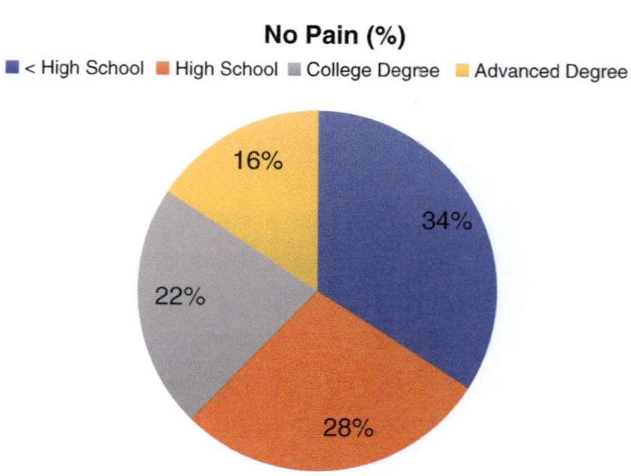

Fig. 6.1 Comparison of patients' original selection of satisfactory pain levels regardless of minor, moderate, or severe surgery [21]

Intraoperative Setting

Multimodal analgesic interventions offer an effective method of achieving optimum pain relief. Such interventions should be customized based on the nature of pain, type of surgery, and comorbid medical conditions. It is also necessary to recognize the costs of such treatments and ensure that the treatment services provided are long-term sustainable while providing patients with high-quality care.

Multimodal Analgesic Interventions

Medications used as a part of multimodal analgesic interventions include opioids and multiple opioid-sparing medications such as ketamine, alpha-2 receptor agonists, lidocaine, acetaminophen, magnesium, and dexamethasone, and their mechanisms of action have been summarized in Table 6.1. Different modes of drug delivery include regional anesthesia techniques, peripheral nerve block catheters, and local wound infiltration by analgesics.

Opioids Despite their side effects and the recent emergence of the opioid crisis, opioids remain one of the most commonly used drug classes used to treat pain during surgical procedures. Short-acting opioids are very effective in addressing short-lasting pain inflicted by surgical stimulation. However, patients with chronic opioid therapy should be given long-acting opioids along with short-acting analgesics, to prevent potential withdrawal from chronic opioid therapy [23].

Patients with a prolonged history of opioid use for chronic pain can develop opioid-induced hyperalgesia [24], experience a greater level of postoperative pain, and have an increased duration of postoperative pain before it is resolved. The total amount of opioids needed during the procedure should include the preoperative daily dose of opioids and the amount needed to address the pain elicited by surgical stimulation. Among patients with chronic opioid therapy, administration of partial opioid agonists such as nalbuphine or buprenorphine can cause sudden opioid withdrawal. The rising evidence suggestive of opioid-induced hyperalgesia further encourages pain management to begin with minimal, short-acting opioids or non-opioid combinations.

Ketamine Ketamine is an antagonist at the *N*-methyl-D-aspartate (NMDA) receptor, and multiple studies demonstrate ketamine as associated with significant reductions in postoperative pain, opioid requirements, and postoperative nausea and vomiting (PONV), including in patients who are on chronic opioid therapy [25–27]. The intraoperative boluses of ketamine vary from 0.15 to 1 mg/kg; perioperative infusions range from 1 to 5 mcg/kg/min, with a postoperative infusion rate of 2 mcg/kg/min [28].

Table 6.1 Opioid-sparing analgesic medications used during the ambulatory surgical procedures and their mechanisms of action

Opioid-sparing analgesic	Mechanism of action
Ketamine	Prevent central sensitization
Clonidine, dexmedetomidine	Prevent central sensitization
Acetaminophen	Prevent peripheral sensitization
Lidocaine	Membrane stabilizer
Magnesium	Prevent central sensitization
Glucocorticoids	Prevent peripheral sensitization

Clonidine and Dexmedetomidine Alpha-2 adrenergic receptor agonists and opioids have different mechanisms of action, and their combined use can lead to synergistic analgesic effect without a significant increase in respiratory depression, along with a reduction in side effects such as nausea and vomiting [29]. Clonidine and dexmedetomidine are alpha-2 adrenergic receptor agonists and have synergistic analgesic effect due to their different affinities for the three alpha-2 adrenergic receptor subtypes [30]. Dexmedetomidine has a more favorable pharmacokinetic profile compared to clonidine.

Intraoperative dexmedetomidine has been associated with a significant reduction in intraoperative and postoperative analgesic requirements, and such analgesic-sparing effects have been found to last up to 24 hours [31].

Acetaminophen Intraoperative IV acetaminophen can be used as an adjunct analgesic to decrease postoperative opioid requirements. Cao et al. demonstrated that intraoperative use of IV acetaminophen is associated with significantly reduced 24-hour average pain scores, decreased 24-hour opioid consumption, reduced intraoperative opioid requirements, and shorter length of hospital stay [32].

Lidocaine Lidocaine can reduce postoperative pain and improve outcomes. Lidocaine is dispensed as a bolus (100–150 mg or 1.5–2.0 mg/kg) followed by an infusion of 1–3 mg/kg/h through the end of surgery. McCarthy et al. demonstrated that patients undergoing abdominal surgery who received an intravenous lidocaine infusion during the perioperative period had lower pain scores, reduced postoperative analgesic requirements, decreased intraoperative anesthetic requirements, faster recovery of bowel function, and shortened length of hospital stay [33].

Magnesium Perioperative infusions of magnesium can reduce postoperative pain and opioid consumption [34]. Boluses are 30–50 mg/kg and the infusion rates range from 4 to 15 mg/kg/h.

Glucocorticoids Glucocorticoids reduce inflammation and tissue damage. Waldron et al. demonstrated that a single-dose perioperative dexamethasone has a small but statistically significant analgesic benefit. The use of dexamethasone was associated with reduction in postoperative pain, postoperative opioid consumption, need for rescue analgesia, length of PACU stay, and a longer time to first analgesic dose. The antiemetic effect of dexamethasone could also contribute to less postoperative nausea and vomiting [35].

Other agents used in multimodal analgesia include anticonvulsants, such as gabapentin and pregabalin, and NSAIDs, although these drugs are often used in the preoperative and postoperative periods. The use of NSAIDs is associated with opioid-sparing analgesic effects, and combined IV acetaminophen and NSAIDs have synergistic effects and offer increased analgesia [36].

Modes of Drug Delivery

Regional Anesthesia Opioid-sparing effect has been demonstrated with the use of paravertebral, femoral, lumbar plexus, and sciatic nerve blocks in lower limb surgeries and supraclavicular, interscalene, and axillary nerve blocks in upper limb surgeries; local anesthetics such as lidocaine, bupivacaine, and ropivacaine are commonly used. Regional anesthesia techniques are effective in suppressing postoperative pain and opioid consumption, and the use of adjuvant agents such as epinephrine, clonidine, dexmedetomidine, and magnesium augments effects of peripheral nerve block while reducing opioid consumption [37].

Peripheral Nerve Block Catheters Although single-bolus methods are traditionally used for peripheral nerve blocks, the use of catheters for continuous nerve blocks is becoming more popular [38, 39]. A large prospective study assessing postoperative analgesia for total hip arthroplasty found patients receiving continuous three-in-one block to have the best satisfaction compared to patient-controlled opioid analgesia and patient-controlled epidural analgesia [39].

Local Wound Infiltration Direct delivery of drugs at the surgical wound site can improve postoperative pain and decrease opioid requirements. Goldstein et al. observed that patients undergoing laparoscopic gynecological procedures were given local anesthetics to their intraperitoneal wound site followed by wound lavage, and patients had significantly decreased postoperative opioid consumption [40]. Liposomal bupivacaine (Exparel) has been studied for local wound infiltration in many types of surgeries and has showed lower cumulative pain scores, reduced opioid consumption, and shorter length of stay [41]. Exparel is administered through a proprietary foam-based delivery system and costs about $300 per dose, whereas the cost of generic bupivacaine is $3 a dose. Although expensive compared to generic bupivacaine, liposomal bupivacaine can reduce overall costs and improve quality-adjusted life-year [42].

Postoperative Setting

Postoperative pain is the major cause of delayed discharge from the post-anesthesia care unit (PACU) and unexpected hospital admission [43]. It is associated with an increase in cardiovascular and pulmonary complications which delay recovery after surgery [44]. Recently the frequency of ambulatory surgeries has increased as a result of advances in noninvasive surgical techniques, regional anesthesia, and newer anesthetic agents with decreased side effects, thus allowing patients with complex medical conditions to undergo ambulatory procedures [45]. There is a growing need for optimal management of acute postoperative pain in the PACU setting so that recovery can be enhanced and safe, expedient discharge from PACU can be achieved. While most medical centers have an established inpatient acute pain service, a regional or block service, and a chronic pain service to address the acute postoperative pain issues and prevent postoperative acute pain, flare-ups, and withdrawal syndromes, these types of specialized pain management services are often lacking or limited in ambulatory surgery centers (ASC). The first step in optimizing postoperative pain control and prevention of severe pain in PACU is identification of factors which pose higher than baseline risk of postoperative pain. Type of surgery, duration of anesthesia, preexisting chronic pain, chronic opioid dependence [46], substance abuse disorder, and higher body mass index [47] are known risk factors predisposing patients to increased risk of postoperative pain [48]. Patients with chronic opioid consumption pose a special challenge in terms of postoperative pain management in ambulatory setting.

In the ambulatory center, it is crucial to establish cost-effective, multimodal analgesia protocols for postoperative pain management. Such protocols should begin preoperatively with administration of oral non-opioid analgesics like gabapentin, acetaminophen, diclofenac, or celecoxib. Patients with chronic opioid use should take their regular oral dose of opioid medication on the day of surgery to prevent withdrawal. Intraoperative injection or infiltration of the surgical wound site with local anesthetics can also be an effective measure in managing postoperative pain. Anesthesia personnel in the PACU should be prepared for early intervention upon detection of pain issues and plan for rescue analgesia, preferably with opioid-sparing techniques to reduce unwanted side effects. Availability and utilization of regional anesthesia techniques to reduce postoperative pain with single-shot peripheral nerve blocks for upper and lower extremities and truncal blocks for abdominal surgeries and peripheral nerve catheters with homegoing catheter care programs are another effective way to deal with postoperative pain. It is important to avoid administration of partial opioid agonists nalbuphine and buprenorphine in postoperative settings to prevent the risk of acute opioid withdrawal [23].

Prescription opioid abuse has been a growing national public health concern. Potential solutions to the problem of making opioids less amenable to abuse are : (1) utilize risk evaluation and mitigation strategies for extended-release and long-acting (ER/LA) opioids and transmucosal immediate-release fentanyl products; (2) abuse-deterrent opioids designed to make manipulation of select opioids more difficult; (3) physical/chemical barriers to prevent mechanical manipulation and resist the extraction of the active ingredient when mixing the tablet with solvents; (4) addition of antagonists to agonists can interfere

Table 6.2 Summary of current strategies to reduce the abuse potential of opioid analgesics prescribed in the postoperative setting

Opioid abuse mitigation strategies	
Abuse-deterrent modality	Overview of method
Strategy/ planning	Risk mitigation and evaluation of extended-release and long-acting opioids
Physical barrier	Prevent chewing, crushing, cutting, grating, or grinding of dosage form
Chemical barrier	Complex formulation or molecular structure to resist chemical extraction
Antagonist/ agonist combination	Antagonistic compounds combined with agonists to minimize the euphoria associated with opioid abuse/misuse or attempts to manipulate the opioid
Aversive agents	Aversion substances which produce unpleasant adverse effects when opioids are consumed in large quantities or manipulated
Delivery system	Abuse-resistant opioid delivery modalities
New molecular entities and prodrugs	Novel molecular structures with decreased CNS penetrance, requirement of enzymatic activation, or unique receptor binding profiles
Combination	Combining multiple of the above strategies to further enhance the abuse-deterring properties

with or reduce the opioid-induced euphoria associated with opioid abuse, thus rendering abuse of the product less desirable; (5) aversion substances can be added to produce an unpleasant effect during abuse or when taken at higher doses than instructed; (6) unique delivery mechanisms designed to be resistant to abuse, including depot injectable formulations and subcutaneous implants; and (7) new molecular entities or prodrugs with abuse-deterring properties designed to exhibit lower and/or slower penetration into the central nervous system [49, 50]. See Table 6.2.

An ambulatory pain specialist should be available to develop structured procedures for pain management in the PACU through consults, surgeons, and anesthesiologists who practice specialized pain management. These providers should ensure safe execution of multimodal analgesic plans, including drugs, suitable regional anesthesia techniques, and safe, prompt discharge of patients from the PACU with appropriate follow-up with patients' primary care providers.

Workflow Improvements

Having a regional block team on staff at ASCs may improve patient satisfaction, increase the efficiency of surgical procedures, and reduce time spent in recovery due to postoperative pain. This team would consist of skilled anesthesiologists or nurse anesthetists, regional block nurses, and post-anesthesia care unit (PACU) nurses. A smaller, dedicated group of providers who are experienced in performing regional blocks could reduce time spent in the operating room (OR), lower the risk of misplaced blocks, and reduce opioid consumption postoperatively. Additionally, subjective factors such as team morale and rapport might also see an improvement. However, there are limitations, such as the availability of trained individuals and the need for a high volume of patients to offset the added cost of specialized personnel.

Two factors of surgery play particularly important roles in efficiency: time spent in the OR and time spent in recovery. Unlike general anesthesia, regional anesthesia is usually administered in a separate "block room," allowing more time spent in the OR to be devoted to surgery. Furthermore, regional anesthesia allows for less reliance on general anesthesia, reducing the amount of time spent in anesthesia emergence [51]. A study published in 2012 found that forming a specialized anesthesia team significantly reduced the amount of time patients spent recovering in the post-anesthesia care unit or PACU [52]. However, when comparing the ASC anesthesia group to the non-ambulatory anesthesia group, they also found significantly more postoperative nausea and vomiting (PONV). Although the research team admitted this could be attributed to center-specific policy changes in antiemetic therapy, this issue is often a large factor in patient satisfaction and timely discharge [53].

Since the advent of the US opioid crisis it is increasingly important to reduce opioid use. In anesthesia this can be seen when comparing regional blocks to general anesthetics [54]. According to a comparison of anesthesia techniques in total knee and hip replacements, regional anesthesia was associated with reduced amounts of opioids administered postoperatively. A practiced team of specialized anesthesiologists and nurses could increase the number of safe, effective nerve blocks. This could then theoretically reduce reliance on opioids in postoperative pain control [55].

Regional block nurses represent a relatively new field of nursing, although the practice of placing regional blocks itself has existed for decades. Therefore, there is a lack of standardized training among nurses that focuses specifically on block management [53]. Block nurses thus may be trained as an extension of either preoperative or PACU nurse training. This can consist of a one- or two-day course to become familiar with additional care duties. The care they offer encompasses the entire procedure, from preoperative assessment to postoperative safety monitoring [56]. Block nurses also facilitate communication between other anesthesiologists, nurse anesthetists, and surgeons, which can increase efficiency in the operating room and lead to fewer gaps in patient care. In 2010, Duke University Hospital implemented a block nurse team and subsequently reviewed its performance in 2011 [57]. This review found that the team had the greatest impact on its orthopedic surgery service: the team increased perioperative efficiency by 26%, improved on-time starts by 7%, and had no incidence of misplaced blocks. Perioperative efficiency was defined as the number of times procedure turnover met the 45-minute goal. Although the study was limited in size and duration, these findings indicate the potential for a designated block team to increase efficiency.

The goal for implementing a specialized block team would be to create a quicker, more reliable method of performing regional blocks, thereby leading to more number of surgeries of consistently high quality. Despite the potential benefits, the implementation of new programs or teams is always limited by cost-effectiveness. Cost-effectiveness encompasses a wide range of factors: patient volume, staff pay, length of recovery, and more; multiple factors must work synergistically to reduce cost. In theory, a block team could save money by allowing for more surgeries to be scheduled in one day. However, several studies have shown that decreasing time spent in anesthesia induction and emergence does not produce significant increases in overall productivity [58]. A study published in 2007 determined that while surgeons perceived greater efficiency when working with a specialized block team, there was no clear difference in the amount of surgeries performed [59]. While this does not support the use of regional block teams in ASCs, other studies have shown that increasing staffing can positively impact turnover time. An analysis published in 2002 showed that increasing the staff by even one physician and one nurse allowed for more surgeries to be performed per day and therefore achieved greater efficiency [60]. This contradiction represents a gap which could be filled with further research, perhaps focusing on the balance between higher patient volume and increased staff.

Staffing Improvements

Currently, there is no ambulatory pain physician specialty; however, there is growing evidence for their need in ambulatory care centers around the country. Ambulatory surgery is on the rise, and with this growth, there is a need for ambulatory pain management physicians to adequately achieve optimum pain control in these patients. They would also be beneficial in employing a multimodal approach to ambulatory surgeries in which they could provide safe anesthesia during procedures, conduct early intervention if problematic pain-related issues arise, and supervise readmissions for uncontrolled pain [1]. Along with the rise in ambulatory surgeries, there is a growth in patients with chronic pain, opioid use, and substance use who will undergo ambulatory surgery and will need a pain specialist who can devote the time to appropriately and ethically treat their pain pre- and postoperatively [2]. There are also some instances where specific surgeries may be associated with progression of acute pain to chronic pain, and an ambulatory pain specialist can provide the detailed plan and tailored focus to these patients [2]. A multimodal and balanced approach to anesthesia is crucial in an ambulatory care setting, and the key to successful pain management before, during, and after these surgeries is tailored treatment plans and education for patients and family/caregivers, all of which can be conducted by ambulatory pain specialists [3].

When it comes to ambulatory pain specialists and their services being covered by insurance, two studies were reviewed with one involving the use of steroid injections and NSAIDs in patients undergoing carpal tunnel surgery in an ambulatory setting and the other involving the use of nerve blocks for ambulatory orthopedic surgery. These studies outlined which type of insurance was most likely to cover the expenses incurred relating to pain management. When it comes to steroid injections and the use of NSAIDs, which could be done by an ambulatory pain specialist, it was shown that patients who were on private insurance had the highest coverage for the use of steroid injections and NSAIDs [4]. Patients who were on workers' compensation insurance (WCI) received more NSAIDs than those on Medicaid, while those on Medicaid received more steroid injections [4]. In a study reviewing the use of nerve blocks for ambulatory orthopedic surgery, patients were more likely to receive a nerve block if payment for their surgery was supported by government programs or was covered by private insurance versus those which were self-paid or paid through charity care [5]. Furthermore, an article outlining health insurance's role in pain management and cost reduction approaches to pain management are criticized for their cheaper, but less effective, means of treating pain [6]. This could pose a problem for ambulatory pain specialists and their role outside of the operating room. Part of the proposed responsibilities of an ambulatory pain specialist would be managing chronic pain in patients who undergo ambulatory surgery so these services may or may not be covered by insurance companies in the future.

Summary

Postoperative pain can often be difficult to treat. Pain is a subjective experience that varies and is often heavily influenced by factors unrelated to the specific surgery performed. Optimizing the use of all available resources can lead to decreased healthcare costs, higher patient satisfaction, and better long-term outcomes [4, 5, 61].

Ambulatory surgery accounts for a large proportion of surgeries performed in the world. It is especially important to be sensitive to the specific requirements for managing pain in these patients in the perioperative period. Poorly managed post-op pain frequently results in unscheduled early contact with healthcare providers, often leading to additional in-person visits and new prescriptions [3]. In some cases, post-op pain can result in emergency room visits or unplanned hospital admission. Ultimately, these prove to be very costly to patients and to hospitals [4].

Assessment of current readmission and post-op contact rates can be a help analyze postoperative pain control regimen quality [1, 3, 10]. Herbst et al. analyzed billing data and managed to identify five common, facility-specific factors correlated to poor postoperative pain control [10]. Although this did not ultimately eliminate preventable readmissions after ambulatory surgeries, the hospital did see a substantial decrease in pain-related admissions.

Ideal management begins with the preoperative evaluation. Information obtained through careful history taking can be help identify patients at high risk for having poorly managed pain following surgery. Several risk factors are associated with increased postoperative pain, including preoperative chronic pain and catastrophizing [1, 3, 5]. Certain surgical procedures are often associated with a higher incidence of postoperative pain than others [3, 8]. Discussion of past medical history, previous experiences, and current expectations can assist in identifying these risk factors before surgery and allow staff to prophylactically manage these patients.

Decisions concerning intraoperative management have also been shown to impact pain in the postoperative period. For example, general anesthesia is associated with a higher risk of perioperative pain than monitored anesthesia care [8]. Similarly, longer procedures are associated with a higher risk of pain after surgery than short procedures [8]. These are important considerations for pre-surgical planning as they allow for medical teams to adjust as needed before scheduling ambulatory surgeries, counsel patients on postoperative expectations, and reduce unplanned admissions.

Opioids remain the mainstay of postoperative pain management as no single medication has been shown to provide superior pain relief in the postoperative period. Many providers are hesitant to prescribe opioids due to the high abuse potential and unfavorable side effect profile. Some studies have found that opioid-sparing multimodal regimens can provide adequate postoperative analgesia with a superior safety profile [62, 63]. The use of peripheral nerve blocks is associated with faster recovery and lower total costs for treatment [64]. Such treatment regimens can be useful adjuncts in crafting a multimodal regimen for the treatment of postoperative pain.

In conclusion, the treatment of postoperative pain can be complex, but resources available for management are plentiful. Coordinated use of these resources can help decrease the burden of pain after ambulatory surgeries and prevent long-term effects. Each surgery center has access to different resources. It is recommended that careful analysis of facility-specific resources be used to determine how to best apply these recommendations for optimizing patient care.

References

1. Gramke HF, De Rijke JM, Van Kleef M, Kessels AGH, Peters ML, Sommer M, et al. Predictive factors of postoperative pain after day-case surgery. Clin J Pain. 2009;25(6):455–60.
2. Woldehaimanot TE, Eshetie TC, Kerie MW. Postoperative pain management among surgically treated patients in an Ethiopian hospital. PLoS One. 2014;9(7):e102835.
3. Brix LD, Bjørnholdt KT, Thillemann TM, Nikolajsen L. Pain-related unscheduled contact with healthcare services after outpatient surgery. Anaesthesia. 2017;72(7):870–8.
4. Coley KC, Williams BA, DaPos SV, Chen C, Smith RB. Retrospective evaluation of unanticipated admissions and readmissions after same day surgery and associated costs. J Clin Anesth [Internet]. 2002 [cited 2019 Aug 9];14(5):349–53. Available from: http://www.ncbi.nlm.nih.gov/pubmed/12208439.
5. Fletcher D, Stamer UM, Pogatzki-Zahn E, Zaslansky R, Tanase NV, Perruchoud C, et al. Chronic postsurgical pain in Europe. Eur J Anaesthesiol. 2015;32(10):725–34.
6. Roth B, Boateng A, Berken A, Carlyle D, Vadivelu N. Post-operative weaning of opioids after ambulatory surgery: the importance of physician stewardship. Vol. 22, current pain and headache reports. Current Medicine Group LLC 1; 2018. p. 1–6.
7. Tennant F. The physiologic effects of pain on the endocrine system. Pain Ther. 2013;2(2):75–86.
8. Koyyalamudi V, Sen S, Patil S, Creel JB, Cornett EM, Fox CJ, et al. Adjuvant agents in regional anesthesia in the ambulatory setting. Curr Pain Headache Rep [Internet]. 2017 [cited 2018 Jun 7];21(1):6. Available from: http://www.ncbi.nlm.nih.gov/pubmed/28210917.
9. Li J, Lam D, King H, Credaroli E, Harmon E, Vadivelu N. Novel regional anesthesia for outpatient surgery. Vol. 23, current pain and headache reports. Current Medicine Group LLC 1; 2019. p. 1–16.
10. Herbst MO, Price MD, Soto RG. Pain related readmissions/revisits following same-day surgery: have they decreased over a decade? J Clin Anesth. 2017;42:15.
11. Chung F, Ritchie E, Su J. Postoperative pain in ambulatory surgery. Anesth Analg [Internet]. 1997 [cited 2020 Jul 30];85(4):808–16. Available from: https://pubmed.ncbi.nlm.nih.gov/9322460/.
12. Vadivelu N, Kai AM, Kodumudi V, Berger JM. Challenges of pain control and the role of the ambulatory pain specialist in the outpatient surgery setting [Internet]. J Pain Res. Dove Medical Press Ltd. 2016 [cited 2020 Jul 30];9:425–35. Available from: https://pubmed.ncbi.nlm.nih.gov/27382329/.
13. Carroll IR, Angst MS, Clark JD. Management of perioperative pain in patients chronically consuming opioids [Internet]. Reg Anesth Pain Med. 2004 [cited 2020 Jul 30];29:576–91. Available from: https://pubmed.ncbi.nlm.nih.gov/15635517/.
14. Rapp SE, Ready LB, Nessly ML. Acute pain management in patients with prior opioid consumption: a case-controlled retrospective review. Pain [Internet]. 1995 [cited 2020 Jul 30];61(2):195–201. Available from: https://pubmed.ncbi.nlm.nih.gov/7659429/.

15. Osman A, Barrios FX, Kopper BA, Hauptmann W, Jones J, O'Neill E. Factor structure, reliability, and validity of the pain catastrophizing scale. J Behav Med [Internet]. 1997 [cited 2020 Jul 30];20(6):589–605. Available from: https://pubmed.ncbi.nlm.nih.gov/9429990/.
16. Sullivan MJL, Bishop SR, Pivik J. The pain catastrophizing scale: development and validation. Psychol Assess [Internet]. 1995 [cited 2020 Jul 30];7(4):524–32. Available from: /record/1996-10094-001.
17. McCracken LM, Zayfert C, Gross RT. The pain anxiety symptoms scale: development and validation of a scale to measure fear of pain. Pain [Internet]. 1992 [cited 2020 Jul 30];50(1):67–73. Available from: / record/1993-04072-001.
18. Brede E, Mayer TG, Neblett R, Williams M, Gatchel RJ. The pain anxiety symptoms scale fails to discriminate pain or anxiety in a chronic disabling occupational musculoskeletal disorder population. Pain Pract [Internet]. 2011 [cited 2020 Jul 30];11(5):430–8. Available from: /record/2011-21438-002.
19. Neblett R, Mayer TG, Hartzell MM, Williams MJ, Gatchel RJ. The fear-avoidance components scale (FACS): development and psychometric evaluation of a new measure of pain-related fear avoidance. Pain Pract [Internet]. 2016 [cited 2020 Jul 30];16(4):435–50. Available from: https://pubmed.ncbi.nlm.nih.gov/26228238/.
20. Svensson ISBHH. Influence of expectations and actual pain experiences on satisfaction with postoperative pain management. Eur J Pain. 2001;5(2):125–33.
21. Schutte SS, Le-Wendling LT. When expectations outpace reality: a survey of patient knowledge gaps in postoperative pain management. J Clin Anesth. Elsevier Inc. 2020;66:109942.
22. Stiles P, Hilliard P. Perioperative pain management: setting appropriate expectations, published in 2012, can be found here: https://anes-conf.med.umich.edu/opioidtaper/docs/setting_expectations.pdf.
23. Vadivelu N, Kai AM, Kodumudi V, Berger JM. Challenges of pain control and the role of the ambulatory pain specialist in the outpatient surgery setting. J Pain Res. 2016;9:425.
24. Laulin JP, Célèrier E, Larcher A, Le Moal M, Simonnet G. Opiate tolerance to daily heroin administration: an apparent phenomenon associated with enhanced pain sensitivity. Neuroscience. 1999;89(3):631–6.
25. Zakine J, Samarcq D, Lorne E, Moubarak M, Montravers P, Beloucif S, et al. Postoperative ketamine administration decreases morphine consumption in major abdominal surgery: a prospective, randomized, double-blind, controlled study. Anesth Analg. 2008;106(6):1856–61.
26. Laskowski K, Stirling A, McKay WP, Lim HJ. A systematic review of intravenous ketamine for postoperative analgesia. Can J Anesth. 2011;58:911–23.
27. Mebazaa MS, Mestiri T, Kaabi B, Ben Ammar MS. Clinical benefits related to the combination of ketamine with morphine for patient controlled analgesia after major abdominal surgery. Tunis Med. 2008;86(5):435–40.
28. Scott MJ, McEvoy MD, Gordon DB, Grant SA, Thacker JKM, Wu CL, et al. American Society for Enhanced Recovery (ASER) and perioperative quality initiative (POQI) joint consensus statement on optimal analgesia within an enhanced recovery pathway for colorectal surgery: part 2—from PACU to the transition home. Perioper Med. 2017;6(1):7.
29. Grosu I, Lavand'homme P. Use of dexmedetomidine for pain control. F1000 Med Rep. 2010;2:90.
30. Fairbanks CA, Stone LS, Wilcox GL. Pharmacological profiles of alpha 2 adrenergic receptor agonists identified using genetically altered mice and isobolographic analysis. Pharmacol Ther. 2009;123(2):224–38.
31. Massad IM, Mohsen WA, Basha AS, Al-Zaben KR, Al-Mustafa MM, Alghanem SM. A balanced anesthesia with dexmedetomidine decreases postoperative nausea and vomiting after laparoscopic surgery. Saudi Med J. 2009;30(12):1537–41.
32. Cao X, Yumul R, Lazo OL, Stuart J, Asatrian A, Louy C, Zhang X, Tang J, Shamloo B, Rosner H. Effect of intraoperative or postoperative intravenous acetaminophen on postoperative pain scores and opioid requirements in abdominal and spinal surgery patients. Int J Clin Exp Med. 2018;11(4):4120–5.
33. McCarthy GC, Megalla SA, Habib AS. Impact of intravenous lidocaine infusion on postoperative analgesia and recovery from surgery: a systematic review of randomized controlled trials. Drugs. 2010;70(9):1149–63.
34. De Oliveira GS, Castro-Alves LJ, Khan JH, McCarthy RJ. Perioperative systemic magnesium to minimize postoperative pain meta-analysis of randomized controlled trials. Anesthesiology. 2013;119(1):178–90.
35. Waldron NH, Jones CA, Gan TJ, Allen TK, Habib AS. Impact of perioperative dexamethasone on postoperative analgesia and side-effects: systematic review and meta-analysis. Br J Anaesth. 2013;110(2):191–200.
36. Kraglund F. Acetaminophen plus a nonsteroidal anti-inflammatory drug decreases acute postoperative pain more than either drug alone. J Am Dent Assoc. 2014;145(9):966–8.
37. Kaye A, Urman R, Rappaport Y, Siddaiah H, Cornett E, Belani K, et al. Multimodal analgesia as an essential part of enhanced recovery protocols in the ambulatory settings. J Anaesthesiol Clin Pharmacol. 2019;35(Suppl 1):S40.
38. Tetzlaff JE, Andrish J, O'Hara J, Dilger J, Yoon HJ. Effectiveness of bupivacaine administered via femoral nerve catheter for pain control after anterior cruciate ligament repair. J Clin Anesth. 1997;9(7):542–5.
39. Singelyn FJ, Gouverneur JMA. Postoperative analgesia after total hip arthroplasty: IV PCA with morphine, patient-controlled epidural analgesia, or continuous "3-in-1" block?: a prospective evaluation

by our acute pain service in more than 1,300 patients. J Clin Anesth. 1999;11(7):550–4.
40. Goldstein A, Grimault P, Henique A, Keller M, Fortin A, Darai E. Preventing postoperative pain by local anesthetic instillation after laparoscopic gynecologic surgery: a placebo-controlled comparison of bupivacaine. Anesth Analg. 2000;91(2):403–7.
41. Malik O, Kaye AD, Kaye A, Belani K, Urman RD. Emerging roles of liposomal bupivacaine in anesthesia practice. J Anaesthesiol Clin Pharmacol [Internet]. [cited 2019 Aug 9];33(2):151–6. Available from: http://www.ncbi.nlm.nih.gov/pubmed/28781438.
42. Colonna AL, Bellows BK, Enniss TM, Young JB, McCrum M, Nunez JM, et al. Reducing the pain: a cost-effectiveness analysis of transversus abdominis plane block using liposomal bupivacaine for outpatient laparoscopic ventral hernia repair. Surg Open Sci. 2020;2(2):75–80.
43. Messahel FM, Tomlin PJ. Narcotic withdrawal syndrome after intrathecal administration of morphine. Br Med J (Clin Res Ed). 1981;283(6289):471–2.
44. Shea RA, Brooks JA, Dayhoff NE, Keck J. Pain intensity and postoperative pulmonary complications among the elderly after abdominal surgery. Hear Lung J Acute Crit Care. 2002;31(6):440–9.
45. American Hospital Association. Utilization and volume, can be found here: https://www.aha.org/data-insights/utilization-and-volume.
46. Mao J. Opioid-induced abnormal pain sensitivity: implications in clinical opioid therapy. Pain. 2002;100(3):213–7.
47. Whippey A, Kostandoff G, Paul J, Ma J, Thabane L, Ma HK. Predictors of unanticipated admission following ambulatory surgery: a retrospective case-control study. Can J Anesth. 2013;60(7):675–83.
48. Chapman CR, Davis J, Donaldson GW, Naylor J, Winchester D. Postoperative pain trajectories in chronic pain patients undergoing surgery: the effects of chronic opioid pharmacotherapy on acute pain. J Pain. 2011;12(12):1240–6.
49. Vadivelu N, Chang D, Lumermann L, Suchy T, Burg MM, Fontes ML. Management of patients on abuse-deterrent opioids in the ambulatory surgery setting. Curr Pain Headache Rep. 2017;21:10.
50. Vadivelu N, Kai AM, Kodumudi V, Zhu R, Hines R. Pain management of patients with substance abuse in the ambulatory setting. Curr Pain Headache Rep. 2017;21:9.
51. Salinas FV, Joseph RS. Peripheral nerve blocks for ambulatory surgery. Anesthesiol Clin. 2014;32(2):341–55.
52. Sarin P, Philip BK, Mitani A, Eappen S, Urman RD. Specialized ambulatory anesthesia teams contribute to decreased ambulatory surgery recovery room length of stay. Ochsner J. 2012;12(2):94–100.
53. Naqib D, Purvin M, Prasad R, Hanna IM, Dimitri S, Llufrio A, et al. Quality improvement initiative to improve postoperative pain with a clinical pathway and nursing education program. Pain Manag Nurs. 2018;19(5):447–55.
54. Donauer K, Bomberg H, Wagenpfeil S, Volk T, Meissner W, Wolf A. Regional vs. general anesthesia for total knee and hip replacement: an analysis of postoperative pain perception from the International PAIN OUT Registry. Pain Pract. 2018;18(8):1036–47.
55. Caruso TJ, Lawrence K, Tsui BCH. Regional anesthesia for cardiac surgery. Curr Opin Anaesthesiol. 2019;32(5):674–82.
56. Stein RH. The perioperative nurse's role in anesthesia management. AORN J. 1995;62(5):794–804.
57. Russell RA, Burke K, Gattis K. Implementing a regional anesthesia block nurse team in the perianesthesia care unit increases patient safety and perioperative efficiency. J Perianesth Nurs. 2013;28(1):3–10.
58. Dexter F, Abouleish AE, Epstein RH, Whitten CW, Lubarsky DA. Use of operating room information system data to predict the impact of reducing turnover times on staffing costs. Anesth Analg. 2003;97(4):1119–26.
59. Eappen S, Flanagan H, Lithman R, Bhattacharyya N. The addition of a regional block team to the orthopedic operating rooms does not improve anesthesia-controlled times and turnover time in the setting of long turnover times. J Clin Anesth. 2007;19(2):85–91.
60. Sokolovic E, Biro P, Wyss P, Werthemann C, Haller U, Spahn D, et al. Impact of the reduction of anaesthesia turnover time on operating room efficiency. Eur J Anaesthesiol. 2002;19(08):560.
61. Bryan S, Goldsmith LJ, Davis JC, Hejazi S, MacDonald V, McAllister P, et al. Revisiting patient satisfaction following total knee arthroplasty: a longitudinal observational study. BMC Musculoskelet Disord. 2018;19(1):423.
62. Rafiq S, Steinbrüchel DA, Jaeger Wanscher M, Andersen LW, Navne A, Lilleoer NB, et al. Multimodal analgesia versus traditional opiate based analgesia after cardiac surgery, a randomized controlled trial. J Cardiothorac Surg. 2014;9(1):52.
63. Suner Z, Kalayci D, Sen O, Kaya M, Unver S, Oguz G. Postoperative analgesia after total abdominal hysterectomy: is the transversus abdominis plane block effective? Niger J Clin Pract. 2019;22(4):478.
64. Tighe PJ, Brennan M, Moser M, Boezaart AP, Bihorac A. Primary payer status is associated with the use of nerve block placement for ambulatory orthopedic surgery. Reg Anesth Pain Med. 2012;37(3):254–61.

7 Benefits of Optimum Pain Control in the Ambulatory Surgery Centers

Newaj Abdullah, Melissa Annette Nikolaidis, and Yi Deng

Abstract

Ambulatory surgeries are procedures that are elective and scheduled in advance and do not require overnight stays. In the United States, over 70% of surgeries are categorized as ambulatory surgery and are performed in ambulatory surgery centers (ASCs). Optimal pain control is paramount for these surgeries to ensure timely discharge and comfort at home. Data from recent studies suggest that a large portion of patients suffer from moderate to severe pain after discharge with many unintended consequences such as altered physiology, poor health-related quality of life, avoidable readmissions, and development of chronic pain. It is important for providers taking care of these patients to be knowledgeable about analgesic options after surgeries in ASC setting. Presently, options include acetaminophen, both selective and non-selective non-steroidal anti-inflammatory agents, weak opioids, and various regional techniques. With advancement in catheter and pump technology, continuous infusion is becoming another option for pain control at home.

N. Abdullah · M. A. Nikolaidis · Y. Deng (✉)
Department of Anesthesiology, Baylor College of Medicine, Houston, TX, USA
e-mail: Newaj.Abdullah@bcm.edu; Melissa.Nikolaidis@bcm.edu; yd1@bcm.edu

Scope of Ambulatory Surgery

Ambulatory surgery is defined as surgical procedure that is elective in nature and scheduled in advance and does not require overnight stays [1]. Ambulatory surgeries are performed both in acute care hospitals and in freestanding facilities called ambulatory surgery centers (ASC) [1]. The focus of this chapter will be on ambulatory surgeries performed in ASC setting. While the term ASC is coined in the recent past, the concept of it was entertained as far back as the 1930s [2]. In 1937, Hertzfeld reported on 1000 cases of pediatric hernia repair in an ambulatory setting [3]. In 1947, Ferguson published a textbook dedicated to performing surgeries outside of the traditional hospital setting [4]. With advancement in anesthesia, monitoring, and noninvasive surgical techniques, ambulatory surgeries in ASC have begun to gain momentum in the 1990s [2]. Based on the National Hospital Ambulatory Medical Care Survey from 2010, the United States performs a total of 48.3 million ambulatory surgeries each year, and 22.5 million of these surgeries are performed in ASC [1]. Today, the number of surgeries performed in ASC setting accounts for more than 70% of the surgeries done in the United States [5]. One of the paramount goals in ambulatory surgery is for same-day discharge of patients undergoing the procedure; as such, appropriate analgesic control both immediately after the surgery and post discharge is important.

K. Rajput et al. (eds.), *Pain Control in Ambulatory Surgery Centers*,
https://doi.org/10.1007/978-3-030-55262-6_7

The aim of this chapter is to evaluate our current efforts at controlling postoperative pain after ambulatory surgeries. Additionally, we will discuss the short-term and long-term consequences of inadequate postoperative pain control for surgeries performed in the ASC setting.

Pain Management After Ambulatory Surgery: How Well Are We Doing?

One of the tenets of ambulatory surgeries is optimum pain control. This includes both immediate postoperative pain control and pain control in the days after discharge. A handful of studies have explored adequacy of pain management after ambulatory surgeries. Chung and colleagues studied 10,008 consecutive patients undergoing ambulatory surgery and surveyed their pain level in the post-anesthesia care unit (PACU), ambulatory surgical unit (ASU) prior to discharge, and 24 hours after discharge [6]. Their study found that the incidence of severe pain was 5.5% in the PACU, 1.7% in the ASU prior to discharge, and 5.3% 24 hours post-surgery after oral analgesic medication. In another study, Beauregard and colleagues assessed pain control in 89 patients after undergoing ambulatory surgery [7]. Over 40% of the patients reported moderate to severe pain in the PACU. While the study does not look at the prevalence of moderate to severe pain prior to discharge, it does assess pain control at various time points after discharge. Based on telephone survey, the prevalence of moderate to severe pain was 40% at 24 hours, 24% at 48 hours, and 13% at 7 days after surgery. Rawal and colleagues looked at 1035 consecutive patients undergoing ambulatory surgery and found that approximately 10% of the patients have moderate to severe pain 48 hours after discharge [8]. Additionally, this study found that certain surgeries were particularly prone to a higher incidence of moderate to severe pain. For example, moderate to severe pain was experienced by 62% of patients undergoing inguinal hernia repair, 41% of orthopedic surgery, and 36% varicose vein surgery after discharge. Combining the findings from these studies suggests approximately 5–40% of patients continue to suffer moderate to severe pain after discharge. Recent research has implicated postoperative acute pain to poor quality of life, immune dysregulation, and development of chronic pain [7, 9]. Given the large number of surgeries performed in ASC setting, and the health implication of poor pain control, more effort needs to be placed on optimizing pain management in these settings.

Consequences of Inadequate Pain Management

Physiologic Changes

Unrelieved postoperative pain has a number of physiologic and metabolic consequences mediated primarily by the sympathetic nervous system [10]. Excessive pain can increase myocardial oxygen demand by increasing heart rate and cardiac work while decreasing myocardial oxygen supply by coronary vasoconstriction [11]. This mismatch of myocardial oxygen demand and supply can lead to myocardial ischemia and necrosis in a vulnerable individual [11]. Uncontrolled pain can also cause pulmonary complications [12, 13]. With excessive pain and muscle spasm, patients often take shallow breaths. Shallow breathing, in combination with inability to cough, can lead to atelectasis, ventilation-to-perfusion mismatch, hypoxemia, hypercarbia, and increased postoperative pulmonary infection [12, 13]. Increased sympathetic drive from untreated pain can also lead to decreased gastrointestinal motility leading to postoperative ileus [14]. Similarly, high sympathetic drive can increase urinary sphincter tone and decrease bladder muscle contractility and, thereby, contribute to postoperative urinary retention [10]. Surgical stress stimulates various factors that place a patient in hypercoagulable state. In addition to this existing hypercoagulable state, immobility from uncontrolled surgical pain can further lead to complications involving venous thromboembolism [10]. Inadequate pain control after surgery has impact on the body's immune system [15]. Excessive pain, in addition to underlying surgical stress, causes the release of glucocorticoid and beta-endorphin [15, 16]. Both of these substances have shown to impair immune cell in vitro [15, 16]. In studies involving humans, patients who received adequate pain control via multimodal or epidural analgesia had lower levels of epinephrine and cortisol and higher levels of lymphocytes and T helper cell [15, 17]. As one can appreciate, uncontrolled pain has far-reaching effects on virtually every organ system; and therefore, postoperative pain management after ambulatory surgeries in ASC setting is paramount for subsequent recovery.

Health-Related Quality of Life

Inadequate control of postoperative pain has ripple effects beyond patient satisfaction. Postoperative pain can negatively impact health-related quality of life (HRQL) which encompasses domains such as physical functioning, mental health, cognitive functioning, role and social functioning, general perception of health, sleep, and energy [18]. Admittingly there is a paucity of research assessing the effect of postoperative pain on HRQL for ambulatory surgeries done in the ASC. However, numerous studies have looked at the relationship between acute postoperative pain and HRQL for various short-stay surgeries performed in the hospital setting. In a prospective observational study, Wu and colleagues assessed the impact of postoperative pain on HRQL in 39 patients undergoing total knee replacement surgery [19]. Using visual analog scale and Short Form-12, the authors assess pain intensity and HRQL, respectively, on postoperative days 1–5, 7, and 14. In this study, the authors found a strong association between higher postoperative pain score and decreased HRQL.

In another prospective observational study, Strassels and colleagues evaluated the impact of postoperative pain on various HRQL domains as well as sexual functioning 1 month after hospital discharge in 30 patients undergoing open prostatectomy, total knee replace surgery, and total hip replacement surgery [20]. The authors used a combination of Short Form-36 and Treatment Outcomes of Pain Survey (TOPS) to assess various domains of HRQL and sexual functioning. Based on their survey, 64% of open prostatectomy, 71.4% of total hip replacement surgery, and 50% of total knee replacement surgery patients reported moderate to severe pain within the first month after discharge. In this cohort, 50% of open prostatectomy patients and 62.5% of total knee replacement surgery patient reported that their pain moderately impacted their physical activity. Likewise, 42.8% of patient who had total hip replacement surgery reported moderate, while 28.6% reported severe limitations of their physical activities due to postoperative pain. Additionally, all study participants rated their HRLQ to be lower than the average US norms in physical function, physical role, bodily pain, vitality, and social functioning domains. Furthermore, 50% of open proctectomy, 28.6% of total hip replacement surgery, and 25% of total knee replacement surgery patients reported decreased sexual functioning due to postoperative pain.

Sleep is important for healing and recovery. Numerous studies have shown that resolved postoperative pain can lead to disturbed sleep [9, 21, 22]. Pavlin and colleagues studied 171 patients with moderate to severe pain after discharge from ambulatory surgery [21]. Of these, 46% of patients reported disturbed sleep or inability to fall asleep during the first 24 hours due to pain. In another study by Diehl and colleagues, pain intensity was correlated with sleep disturbance on postoperative day 3 in 71 patients who had undergone knee replacement surgery [22]. According to this study, sleep was most affected in patient with severe pain compared to moderate or mild pain.

As mentioned earlier, vast majority of the studies that look the relationship between postoperative pain and HRQL are performed on patients undergoing non-ambulatory surgeries. One can extrapolate from these studies and extend the findings to application on ambulatory surgeries in ASC settings. Nevertheless, further studies are needed to validate this extrapolation.

Transition to Chronic Pain

Chronic postsurgical pain can develop after any surgery. Table 7.1 shows incidence of chronic postsurgical pain after various surgeries [23, 24]. The definition for chronic postsurgical pain is controversial. However, most sources agree that it is defined as persistent pain that lasts for 2–3 months after surgical healing is complete [23, 24]. Additionally, all other etiologies must be excluded prior to giving someone this diagnosis [23, 24]. There are multiple risk factors for developing chronic postsurgical pain including presence of pain conditions prior to surgery, presence of psychological conditions including pain catastrophizing nature, type of surgery, and uncontrolled postoperative pain [25]. The mechanism underlying the development of postsurgical chronic pelvic pain is complex and poorly understood. Almost all form of postsurgical chronic pain has attributes of both neuropathic and non-neuropathic pain [26, 27]. In animal studies, it has been shown that damage to nerves results in the release of cascade to inflammatory mediators [28]. These inflammatory mediators alter gene expression and produce a state of continuous noxious signal transmission to the higher brain; in turn this results in long-term neuroplastic changes giving rise to chronic neuropathic pain [28]. Alteration of these chemical cascades with adequate postoperative analgesia is therefore one strategy to avoid the development of chronic postsurgical pain. The non-neuropathic component is thought to be caused by pulling, tugging, or distortion of nearby structures by postsurgical fibrotic tissues or adhesions [29–33]. Development of non-neuropathic pain can be minimized by using careful surgical techniques and tissue handling to prevent significant postsurgical inflammation and fibrosis.

Table 7.1 Incidence of chronic postoperative pain after various ambulatory surgeries

Surgery	Incidence in percentage
Inguinal hernia	0–63%
Amputation	30–85%
Mastectomy	11–57%
Breast augmentation	13–38%
Cholecystectomy	3–56%
Hysterectomy	25%
Varicose vein stripping	27%

Economic Burden

There are economic implications for appropriate pain control after ambulatory surgeries performed in ASCs. Pavlin and colleagues studied 171 patients undergoing ambulatory surgeries in ASC setting to identify contributing factors for prolonged PACU stay and delayed recovery [34]. According to their study, uncontrolled pain control was identified as the most common cause and an independent risk factor for prolonged PACU stay and delayed discharge from ASCs [34]. While adequate pain control immediate after surgery is important, home pain management after discharge is equally important. Numerous studies have shown that pain control at home tends to be poor. This inadequate pain control at home is one common cause of readmission after outpatient surgery. For example, Gold and colleagues looked at 9616 ambulatory surgeries from 1984 to 1986 and identified pain as the most common reason for readmissions [35]. In a system review of 31 studies, Wu and colleagues identified pain as the most common cause readmission after ambulatory surgeries both in hospital and ASC setting [36]. In addition to unanticipated hospital readmissions, poor pain management can lead to delirium and cognitive dysfunction, and this can result in increased visit to general practitioners [10]. Therefore, inadequate pain control not only causes personal burden with physical limitations and suffering, but it can also cause economic burden by avoidable length of stay in PACU, readmissions, and visit to general practitioners.

Strategies for Postoperative Pain Control

Surgical and Anesthetic Consideration

Optimal pain control for ambulatory surgeries is a shared responsibility of a surgeon and an anesthesiologist. Numerous surgical factors have been identified that can influence the extent of pain in PACU and, eventually, at home. Low-pressure CO_2 pneumoperitoneum and rigorous decompression of the abdomen after laparoscopic surgeries have shown to decrease postoperative pain and should be accomplished by surgical team [37, 38]. From an anesthetic standpoint, use of succinylcholine has been linked to myalgia in ambulatory setting despite the use of defasciculating dose of nondepolarizing neuromuscular blocking agents [39]. Avoidance of succinylcholine should be practiced as much as possible. Additionally, use of endotracheal tube is associated with throat pain. Therefore, supraglottic airway device can be used to minimize such discomfort [37].

Pain Management in PACU

Postoperative pain management should begin intraoperatively. Patient should be treated during surgery with agents such acetaminophen, non-steroidal anti-inflammatory agents, and short-acting opioids such as fentanyl or hydromorphone [37]. Morphine can provide pain control for a longer duration than fentanyl and hydromorphone; however, due to longer half-life of morphine, this agent tends to delay discharge [37]. Additionally, after ambulatory surgeries, use of morphine has been linked to increased incidence of nausea and vomiting after discharge [40].

Analgesic options in the PACU include acetaminophen, NSAIDs, and short-acting opioids such as fentanyl or hydromorphone [37, 41]. Acetaminophen should be used as a first-line agent for mild postoperative pain unless otherwise contraindicated [37, 41]. The mechanism of its actions is poorly understood but postulated to work centrally by inhibiting cyclooxygenase-2 enzymes (COX-2) [42–44]. Recent evidence also suggests that acetaminophen exerts its antinociceptive activity by modulating inhibitory serotonergic pathways [42]. For individuals >50 kg, 1000 mg of oral acetaminophen can be used every 4 hours with maximum dose of 4000 mg per day [41, 45]. It has a favorable side effect profile but must be used cautiously or avoided in individuals with compromised liver function [37, 41, 45]. Non-steroidal anti-inflammatory agents are the drug of choice for moderate pain in the PACU settings [37]. Ketorolac is commonly used in PACU as it is intravenously available. The current recommended dose of ketorolac is 0.5 mg/kg up to 30 mg every 6 hours with maximum daily dose of 120 mg [41]. Its mechanism involves inhibition of both COX-1 and COX-2 enzymes [37]. The analgesia is achieved through inhibition of COX-2 enzyme, whereas inhibition of COX-1 is responsible for mediating the side effect profile of NSAIDs [37, 41]. Adverse effects include gastric ulcer formation, deterioration of platelet function, and decreased renal function; therefore, ketorolac should be avoided in individuals with underlying ulcerative conditions, platelet dysfunction or proclivity to bleeding, and poor renal function [37]. For severe pain in PACU, short-acting intravenous opioids such as fentanyl or hydromorphone are usually the agents of choice. Side effects include nausea, respiratory depression, pruritus, and ileus, which correlate with cumulative dosing. It has been reported in literature that a combination of NSAIDs such as ketorolac and weak opioid such as tramadol can be effective for severe pain; however, given tramadol's slow time of onset, it may not be feasible as a rescue medication in the PACU [37]. Lastly, ketamine as an analgesic has gained popularity in the recent years. Ketamine is an N-methyl-D-aspartate receptor inhibitor [46]. Administration of 20–40 mg of ketamine intraoperatively has been shown to decrease both postoperative pain and opioid consumption [41, 46]. It can be a great choice in the PACU as rescue medication for severe pain, as its side effect profile differs from that of opioids. One must be wary however that ketamine can induce severe hallucinations and should not be used in individuals with underlying psychiatric conditions such as schizophrenia [41, 46]. As an analgesic, it can be given in increments of 20 mg up to 1 mg/kg dose [41]. Table 7.2 summarizes the mechanism of action and side effect profile of various agents used for surgeries performed in ASC setting.

Table 7.2 Mechanism of action and side effect profile of drugs used for postoperative pain control in ASCs

Drug name	Mechanism of action	Major concerns and contraindications
Acetaminophen	Inhibition of COX-2 enzymes in the central nervous system; modulation of inhibitory serotonergic pathway	Contraindicated in patient with hypersensitivity to acetaminophen, severe hepatic impairment, or active liver disease
Non-steroidal anti-inflammatory agents *Ibuprofen* *Naproxen* *Ketorolac*	Inhibition of COX-1 and COX-2 enzymes	Increased risk of bleeding, gastrointestinal ulcer, and renal failure in susceptible patients Contraindicated during 3rd trimester pregnancy and should be avoided during 1st and 2nd trimester pregnancy Contraindicated for treatment of perioperative pain in the setting of coronary artery bypass graft surgery
Celecoxib	Selective inhibition of COX-2 enzymes	Contraindicated during 3rd trimester pregnancy and should be avoided during 1st and 2nd trimester pregnancy Contraindicated for treatment of perioperative pain in the setting of coronary artery bypass graft surgery
Codeine	Agonist of opioid receptor	Can cause respiratory and CNS depression in elderly Contraindicated in children after tonsillectomy due to concern for ultra-metabolizer Contraindicated in the setting of paralytic ileus Ten percent Caucasians are non-responder
Tramadol	Weak agonist of opioid receptor; inhibition of serotonin/noradrenaline uptake	Risk of serotonin syndrome in patients taking SSRI, MAO inhibitor, TCA Contraindicated in patient who are suicidal or addition-prone
Intravenous opioids Fentanyl Hydromorphone	Agonist of opioid receptor	Increased risk of respiratory failure
Ketamine	N-methyl D-aspartate receptor antagonism	Ketamine may cause vivid dream or hallucination, increases intraocular pressure, increases blood pressure

Pain Management After Discharge

Oral analgesics are the mainstay of pain control after discharge from ambulatory surgery. Commonly used agents for pain management after ambulatory surgery include acetaminophen, NSAIDs, and weak opioids [37]. Table 7.3 shows the common dosage for medications used for pain control after surgeries performed in ASCs. Use of acetaminophen has been discussed earlier. Acetaminophen can be used for mild pain at home. The dose for oral acetaminophen is 650 mg every 4 hours or 1000 mg every 6 hours with a maximum daily dose of 4000 mg [41, 45]. The maximum daily dose should not exceed 2500 mg when the duration of treatment is greater than 10 days [41, 45]. Non-steroidal anti-inflammatory agents alone or in combination with weak opioids are highly effective for moderate to severe pain [37, 41]. Choice of NSAIDs includes ibuprofen, naproxen, and, rarely, oral ketorolac. In adults the daily maximum dose of ibuprofen should not exceed 2400 mg divided into 3–6 doses [41, 47]. A reasonable regimen can be 600 mg of ibuprofen every 6 hours. The recommended dose for naproxen is 550 mg every 8 hours [41, 48]. Oral ketorolac should not be used for longer than 5 days [41, 49]. The recommended dose is 20 mg for first dose and then 10 mg every 6 hours [41, 49]. The side effect profile of oral NSAIDs is like that of intravenous counterpart. It is noteworthy that ibuprofen is contraindicated during third trimester of pregnancy and should be avoided during first and

Table 7.3 Commonly used medications and dose regimen used for surgeries performed in ambulatory surgery centers

Medications	Dosage regiment
Acetaminophen	650 mg every 4 hours *OR* 1000 mg every 6 hours Maximum daily dose is 4000 mg Maximum daily dose is 2500 mg after 10 days of treatment
Ibuprofen	600 mg every 6 hours *OR* 800 mg every 8 hours Maximum daily dose is 2400 mg
Naproxen	500 mg every 12 hours Maximum daily dose is 1000 mg
Toradol	20 mg for first dose followed by 10 mg every 6 hours Maximum daily dose is 40 mg Do not continue for more than 5 days
Codeine	15 mg every 4 hours *OR* 30 mg every 6 hours Maximum daily dose is 360 mg
Tramadol	50 mg every 4 hours *OR* 100 mg every 6 hours Maximum daily dose is 400 mg
Celecoxib	100 mg every 12 hours *OR* 200 mg once daily Maximum daily dose is 200 mg

second trimester pregnancy as well [41, 50]. Selective non-steroidal anti-inflammatory agents are a subcategory of NSAIDs that works by inhibiting COX-2 enzymes only and, thereby, avoid the side effects of non-selective NSAIDs [37, 41]. Celecoxib is one of the commonly used non-selective NSAIDs. The daily maximum dose of celecoxib is 200 mg and can be given in 1–2 doses [41]. It is contraindicated during pregnancy and in lactating mother [41, 51].

Weak opioids include codeine and tramadol. Codeine is a prodrug which is metabolized to morphine and is responsible for its analgesic efficacy [37]. Only about 5–10% of codeine is metabolized to morphine, and the rest is metabolized to other metabolic end products with no analgesic effects [52]. The daily maximum dose of codeine is 360 mg, and it can be prescribed as 15 mg every 6 hours or 30 mg every 4 hours depending on the anticipated pain from the surgery [53]. It is important to note that the enzyme responsible for the conversion of codeine to morphine is lacking in approximately 10% of the Caucasian population; and therefore, these individuals will not receive any benefit from codeine [52, 53]. Tramadol is another oral agent for management of severe pain at home. Tramadol exerts its analgesic effect by acting both as a weak opioid agonist and a serotonin/noradrenaline reuptake inhibitor [54]. The daily maximum dose of tramadol is 400 mg [55]. It can be prescribed as 50 mg every 4 hours or 100 mg every 6 hours depending on the surgery and the anticipated postoperative pain [55]. Unlike strong opioid agonist, tramadol lacks the risk of respiratory depression, constipation, and nausea and vomiting [37, 51].

Regional Anesthesia for Postoperative Pain

Regional anesthesia is emerging as a new tool for postoperative pain control in ASC setting. Depending on the surgery performed, there are a wide variety of peripheral nerve blocks that can be utilized. The type and technical details of peripheral nerve block are beyond the scope of this chapter and will not be discussed here. Traditionally, single-shot peripheral nerve blocks have been most commonly utilized in ASC setting for postoperative pain control [37]. However, with advancement in catheter and disposable pump technologies, it is possible to discharge patients on peripheral nerve block infusions. There are reports in literature of patients being managed with perineural, intra-articular, and perosseous local anesthetic infusions in ambulatory setting [37]. Furthermore, numerous studies in the recent year have demonstrated the efficacy and safety of ambulatory continuous interscalene blocks, infraclavicular blocks, sciatic nerve blocks, femoral nerve blocks, psoas compartment block, and paravertebral blocks [56–61]. Continuous regional anesthesia techniques are beneficial because they provide continuous pain relief which results in better quality of sleep and engagement of activities. They additionally reduce the need for opioid consumption and side effects of these medications. The pumps are programmed at a variety of preset infusion rates, and there are often additional options for patient-controlled bolus administration. With appropriate education, it is very facile to use. When the infusion is complete (usually 1–3 days after initiation), the catheter can then be removed by the patient or caregiver.

Intra-articular Opioids and Local Anesthetics

Many orthopedics surgeries are performed in ASC setting. Intra-articular analgesia is a unique opportunity for pain management for this particular patient population. Intra-articular local anesthetics have been used in ambulatory setting with mixed results [62–65]. In a systemic review of 20 studies, Nagasaka and colleagues found evidence of improved pain relief in nine of these studies [66]. In addition to intra-articular local anesthetics, intra-articular opioid is another approach to postoperative pain control after joint surgeries. For example, intra-articular morphine has been shown to provide mild analgesic effect for 24 hours in a systemic review by Gupta and colleagues [67]. Despite their role as analgesic options, intra-articular local anesthetic and opioids have shown mixed results and are not recommended to be used as a solo pain management option.

Future Direction

Percutaneous peripheral nerve stimulation (pPNS) is a novel technique that is gaining popularity for management of postoperative acute pain [68]. The technology involves implantation of very thin electrical lead adjacent to a target nerve using ultrasound [69]. The lead is then stimulated using an external electrical stimulator. The mechanism of pPNS is based on gate control theory, where electrical stimulation of large-diameter myelinated afferent peripheral nerve inhibits transmission of pain signal by small-diameter pain fibers to the central nervous system [70]. Percutaneous peripheral nerve stimulation is new and has demonstrated positive outcomes in total knee arthroplasty, rotator cuff repair, and anterior cruciate ligament repair [68, 71–73]. Complications of pPNS include infection, lead migration, and lead fracture [68]. The infection rate is lower for pPNS compared to perineural catheter [68]. In the event of lead fracture, the fracture piece can be left in place and does not interfere with magnetic resonance imaging [68]. While pPNS has been mostly used in orthopedic surgery, its utility in other surgeries is currently being explored.

Patient Education

Finally, patient education and setting realistic expectation are key to optimal pain management after discharge following ambulatory surgery. It should be conveyed to patients that 20–40% of patients will have moderate to severe pain that home that can last for 2–4 days [37]. Patients should be provided with clear written instruction on which medications to take for appropriate level of pain. Many patients do not take pain medication until they begin to experience pain. Patients should be advised to take pain medication in a timely fashion around the clock to prevent unnecessary suffering, particularly during the first 2–4 days after surgery when the pain level is heightened [59]. Finally, patients should be given proper contact information should they have problem managing their pain. This not only helps to alleviate anxiety for them but also prevents unnecessary emergency room visits.

References

1. Hall MJ, Schwartzman A, Zhang J, Liu X. Ambulatory surgery data from hospitals and ambulatory surgery centers: United States, 2010. Natl Health Stat Rep. 2017;102:1–15.
2. Pregler JL, Kapur PA. The development of ambulatory anesthesia and future challenges. Anesthesiol Clin N Am. 2003;21(2):207–28. https://doi.org/10.1016/s0889-8537(02)00073-1.
3. Henderson J. Ambulatory surgery: past, present, and future. In: Wetchler B, editor. Anesthesia for ambulatory surgery. 2nd ed. Philadelphia: Lippincott; 1991. p. 1–27.
4. Ferguson L. A survey of the field of ambulatory surgery. In: Surgery of the ambulatory patient. 3rd ed. Philadelphia: Lippincott; 1955. p. 1–3.

5. Kamming D, Chung F, Williams D, McGrath BM, Curti B. Pain management in ambulatory surgery. J Perianesth Nurs. 2004;19(3):174–82. https://doi.org/10.1016/j.jopan.2004.03.001.
6. Chung F, Ritchie E, Su J. Postoperative pain in ambulatory surgery. Anesth Analg. 1997;85(4):808–16. https://doi.org/10.1097/00000539-199710000-00017.
7. Beauregard L, Pomp A, Choinière M. Severity and impact of pain after day-surgery. Can J Anaesth. 1998;45(4):304–11. https://doi.org/10.1007/BF03012019.
8. Rawal N, Hylander J, Nydahl PA, Olofsson I, Gupta A. Survey of postoperative analgesia following ambulatory surgery. Acta Anaesthesiol Scand. 1997;41(8):1017–22. https://doi.org/10.1111/j.1399-6576.1997.tb04829.x.
9. Sinatra R. Causes and consequences of inadequate management of acute pain. Pain Med Malden Mass. 2010;11(12):1859–71. https://doi.org/10.1111/j.1526-4637.2010.00983.x.
10. Joshi GP, Ogunnaike BO. Consequences of inadequate postoperative pain relief and chronic persistent postoperative pain. Anesthesiol Clin N Am. 2005;23(1):21–36. https://doi.org/10.1016/j.atc.2004.11.013.
11. Liu SS, Block BM, Wu CL. Effects of perioperative central neuraxial analgesia on outcome after coronary artery bypass surgery: a meta-analysis. Anesthesiology. 2004;101(1):153–61. https://doi.org/10.1097/00000542-200407000-00024.
12. Ballantyne JC, Carr DB, deFerranti S, et al. The comparative effects of postoperative analgesic therapies on pulmonary outcome: cumulative meta-analyses of randomized, controlled trials. Anesth Analg. 1998;86(3):598–612. https://doi.org/10.1097/00000539-199803000-00032.
13. Desai PM. Pain management and pulmonary dysfunction. Crit Care Clin. 1999;15(1):151–66, vii. https://doi.org/10.1016/s0749-0704(05)70045-2.
14. Fotiadis RJ, Badvie S, Weston MD, Allen-Mersh TG. Epidural analgesia in gastrointestinal surgery. Br J Surg. 2004;91(7):828–41. https://doi.org/10.1002/bjs.4607.
15. Baratta JL, Schwenk ES, Viscusi ER. Clinical consequences of inadequate pain relief: barriers to optimal pain management. Plast Reconstr Surg. 2014;134(4 Suppl 2):15S–21S. https://doi.org/10.1097/PRS.0000000000000681.
16. Weissman C. The metabolic response to stress: an overview and update. Anesthesiology. 1990;73(2):308–27. https://doi.org/10.1097/00000542-199008000-00020.
17. Ahlers O, Nachtigall I, Lenze J, et al. Intraoperative thoracic epidural anaesthesia attenuates stress-induced immunosuppression in patients undergoing major abdominal surgery. Br J Anaesth. 2008;101(6):781–7. https://doi.org/10.1093/bja/aen287.
18. Guyatt GH, Feeny DH, Patrick DL. Measuring health-related quality of life. Ann Intern Med. 1993;118(8):622–9. https://doi.org/10.7326/0003-4819-118-8-199304150-00009.
19. Wu CL, Naqibuddin M, Rowlingson AJ, Lietman SA, Jermyn RM, Fleisher LA. The effect of pain on health-related quality of life in the immediate postoperative period. Anesth Analg. 2003;97(4):1078–85, table of contents. https://doi.org/10.1213/01.ane.0000081722.09164.d5.
20. Strassels SA, McNicol E, Wagner AK, Rogers WH, Gouveia WA, Carr DB. Persistent postoperative pain, health-related quality of life, and functioning 1 month after hospital discharge. Acute Pain. 2004;6(3):95–104. https://doi.org/10.1016/j.acpain.2004.08.002.
21. Pavlin DJ, Chen C, Penaloza DA, Buckley FP. A survey of pain and other symptoms that affect the recovery process after discharge from an ambulatory surgery unit. J Clin Anesth. 2004;16(3):200–6. https://doi.org/10.1016/j.jclinane.2003.08.004.
22. Dihle A, Helseth S, Paul SM, Miaskowski C. The exploration of the establishment of cutpoints to categorize the severity of acute postoperative pain. Clin J Pain. 2006;22(7):617–24. https://doi.org/10.1097/01.ajp.0000210905.57546.c1.
23. Macrae W, Devies H. Chronic post-surgical pain. In: Crombie IK, Croft PR, Linton SJ, Leresche L, Korff MV, editors. Epidemiology of pain: a report of the Task Force on Epidemiology of the International Association for the Study of Pain. 1st ed. Seattle: IASP Press; 1999.
24. Macrae WA. Chronic post-surgical pain: 10 years on. Br J Anaesth. 2008;101(1):77–86. https://doi.org/10.1093/bja/aen099.
25. Perkins FM, Kehlet H. Chronic pain as an outcome of surgery. A review of predictive factors. Anesthesiology. 2000;93(4):1123–33. https://doi.org/10.1097/00000542-200010000-00038.
26. Bjurstrom MF, Nicol AL, Amid PK, Chen DC. Pain control following inguinal herniorrhaphy: current perspectives. J Pain Res. 2014;7:277–90. https://doi.org/10.2147/JPR.S47005.
27. Hakeem A, Shanmugam V. Current trends in the diagnosis and management of post-herniorrhaphy chronic groin pain. World J Gastrointest Surg. 2011;3(6):73–81. https://doi.org/10.4240/wjgs.v3.i6.73.
28. Richebé P, Capdevila X, Rivat C. Persistent postsurgical pain: pathophysiology and preventative pharmacologic considerations. Anesthesiology. 2018;129(3):590–607. https://doi.org/10.1097/ALN.0000000000002238.
29. Aasvang E, Kehlet H. Chronic postoperative pain: the case of inguinal herniorrhaphy. Br J Anaesth. 2005;95(1):69–76. https://doi.org/10.1093/bja/aei019.
30. Poobalan AS, Bruce J, Smith WCS, King PM, Krukowski ZH, Chambers WA. A review of chronic pain after inguinal herniorrhaphy. Clin J Pain. 2003;19(1):48–54. https://doi.org/10.1097/00002508-200301000-00006.
31. Nienhuijs S, Staal E, Strobbe L, Rosman C, Groenewoud H, Bleichrodt R. Chronic pain after mesh repair of inguinal hernia: a systematic review.

Am J Surg. 2007;194(3):394–400. https://doi.org/10.1016/j.amjsurg.2007.02.012.
32. Tan WP, Levine LA. What can we do for chronic scrotal content pain? World J Mens Health. 2017;35(3):146–55. https://doi.org/10.5534/wjmh.17047.
33. Calixte N, Brahmbhatt J, Parekattil S. Chronic testicular and groin pain: pathway to relief. Curr Urol Rep. 2017;18(10):83. https://doi.org/10.1007/s11934-017-0722-7.
34. Pavlin DJ, Chen C, Penaloza DA, Polissar NL, Buckley FP. Pain as a factor complicating recovery and discharge after ambulatory surgery. Anesth Analg. 2002;95(3):627–34, table of contents. https://doi.org/10.1097/00000539-200209000-00025.
35. Gold BS, Kitz DS, Lecky JH, Neuhaus JM. Unanticipated admission to the hospital following ambulatory surgery. JAMA. 1989;262(21):3008–10.
36. Wu CL, Berenholtz SM, Pronovost PJ, Fleisher LA. Systematic review and analysis of post-discharge symptoms after outpatient surgery. Anesthesiology. 2002;96(4):994–1003. https://doi.org/10.1097/00000542-200204000-00030.
37. Rawal N. Postoperative pain treatment for ambulatory surgery. Best Pract Res Clin Anaesthesiol. 2007;21(1):129–48. https://doi.org/10.1016/j.bpa.2006.11.005.
38. Cuschieri A. Day-case (ambulatory) laparoscopic surgery. Let us sing from the same hymn sheet. Surg Endosc. 1997;11(12):1143–4. https://doi.org/10.1007/s004649900555.
39. Mikat-Stevens M, Sukhani R, Pappas AL, Fluder E, Kleinman B, Stevens RA. Is succinylcholine after pretreatment with d-tubocurarine and lidocaine contraindicated for outpatient anesthesia? Anesth Analg. 2000;91(2):312–6. https://doi.org/10.1097/00000539-200008000-00015.
40. Andersen R, Krohg K. Pain as a major cause of postoperative nausea. Can Anaesth Soc J. 1976;23(4):366–9. https://doi.org/10.1007/BF03005916.
41. Malek J, Sevcik P. Postoperative pain management. https://www.wfsahq.org/components/com_virtual_library/media/125136f77e1b7daf7565bd66530 26c35-Postoperative-Pain-Management-170518.pdf. Accessed 8 June 2020.
42. Bonnefont J, Courade J-P, Alloui A, Eschalier A. Antinociceptive mechanism of action of paracetamol. Drugs. 2003;63(Spec No 2):1–4.
43. Warner TD, Mitchell JA. Cyclooxygenase-3 (COX-3): filling in the gaps toward a COX continuum? Proc Natl Acad Sci U S A. 2002;99(21):13371–3. https://doi.org/10.1073/pnas.222543099.
44. Botting JH. Nonsteroidal antiinflammatory agents. Drugs Today. 1999;35(4–5):225. https://doi.org/10.1358/dot.1999.35.4-5.552199.
45. FDA Package Insert for Acetaminophen. https://www.accessdata.fda.gov/drugsatfda_docs/label/2015/204767s000lbl.pdf. Accessed 8 June 2020.
46. Bell RF, Dahl JB, Moore RA, Kalso E. Perioperative ketamine for acute postoperative pain. Cochrane Database Syst Rev. 2006;(1):CD004603. https://doi.org/10.1002/14651858.CD004603.pub2.
47. FDA Package Insert for Ibuprofen. https://www.accessdata.fda.gov/drugsatfda_docs/label/2011/018989Orig1s079lbl.pdf. Accessed 8 June 2020.
48. FDA Package Insert for Naproxen. https://www.accessdata.fda.gov/drugsatfda_docs/label/2007/017581s108,18164s58,18965s16,20067s14lbl.pdf. Accessed 8 June 2020.
49. FDA Package Insert for Toradol. https://www.accessdata.fda.gov/drugsatfda_docs/label/2013/019645s019lbl.pdf. Accessed 8 June 2020.
50. Research C for DE and. FDA Drug Safety Communication: FDA has reviewed possible risks of pain medicine use during pregnancy. FDA. Published February 9, 2019. https://www.fda.gov/drugs/drug-safety-and-availability/fda-drug-safety-communication-fda-has-reviewed-possible-risks-pain-medicine-use-during-pregnancy. Accessed 8 June 2020.
51. FDA Package Insert for Celebrex. https://www.accessdata.fda.gov/drugsatfda_docs/label/2018/020998s050lbl.pdf. Accessed 8 June 2020.
52. Caraco Y, Sheller J, Wood AJ. Pharmacogenetic determination of the effects of codeine and prediction of drug interactions. J Pharmacol Exp Ther. 1996;278(3):1165–74.
53. FDA Package Insert for Codeine. https://www.accessdata.fda.gov/drugsatfda_docs/label/2013/022402s006lbl.pdf. Accessed 8 June 2020.
54. Raffa RB, Friderichs E, Reimann W, Shank RP, Codd EE, Vaught JL. Opioid and nonopioid components independently contribute to the mechanism of action of tramadol, an "atypical" opioid analgesic. J Pharmacol Exp Ther. 1992;260(1):275–85.
55. FDA Package Insert for Tramadol. https://www.accessdata.fda.gov/drugsatfda_docs/label/2010/022370s000lbl.pdf. Accessed 8 June 2020.
56. Klein SM, Grant SA, Greengrass RA, et al. Interscalene brachial plexus block with a continuous catheter insertion system and a disposable infusion pump. Anesth Analg. 2000;91(6):1473–8. https://doi.org/10.1097/00000539-200012000-00033.
57. Ilfeld BM, Morey TE, Wright TW, Chidgey LK, Enneking FK. Continuous interscalene brachial plexus block for postoperative pain control at home: a randomized, double-blinded, placebo-controlled study. Anesth Analg. 2003;96(4):1089–95, table of contents. https://doi.org/10.1213/01.ane.0000049824.51036.ef.
58. Ilfeld BM, Morey TE, Enneking FK. Continuous infraclavicular brachial plexus block for postoperative pain control at home: a randomized, double-blinded, placebo-controlled study. Anesthesiology. 2002;96(6):1297–304. https://doi.org/10.1097/00000542-200206000-00006.
59. Rawal N, Allvin R, Axelsson K, et al. Patient-controlled regional analgesia (PCRA) at home: controlled comparison between bupivacaine and ropivacaine brachial

plexus analgesia. Anesthesiology. 2002;96(6):1290–6. https://doi.org/10.1097/00000542-200206000-00005.

60. Ilfeld BM, Morey TE, Wang RD, Enneking FK. Continuous popliteal sciatic nerve block for postoperative pain control at home: a randomized, double-blinded, placebo-controlled study. Anesthesiology. 2002;97(4):959–65. https://doi.org/10.1097/00000542-200210000-00031.
61. Buckenmaier CC, Kwon KH, Howard RS, et al. Double-blinded, placebo-controlled, prospective randomized trial evaluating the efficacy of paravertebral block with and without continuous paravertebral block analgesia in outpatient breast cancer surgery. Pain Med Malden Mass. 2010;11(5):790–9. https://doi.org/10.1111/j.1526-4637.2010.00842.x.
62. Smith I, Van Hemelrijck J, White PF, Shively R. Effects of local anesthesia on recovery after outpatient arthroscopy. Anesth Analg. 1991;73(5):536–9.
63. Henderson RC, Campion ER, DeMasi RA, Taft TN. Postarthroscopy analgesia with bupivacaine. A prospective, randomized, blinded evaluation. Am J Sports Med. 1990;18(6):614–7. https://doi.org/10.1177/036354659001800610.
64. Milligan KA, Mowbray MJ, Mulrooney L, Standen PJ. Intra-articular bupivacaine for pain relief after arthroscopic surgery of the knee joint in day case patients. Anaesthesia. 1988;43(7):563–4. https://doi.org/10.1111/j.1365-2044.1988.tb06688.x.
65. Reuben SS, Sklar J. Pain management in patients who undergo outpatient arthroscopic surgery of the knee. J Bone Joint Surg Am. 2000;82(12):1754–66. https://doi.org/10.2106/00004623-200012000-00010.
66. Nagasaka H, Awad H, Yaksh TL. Peripheral and spinal actions of opioids in the blockade of the autonomic response evoked by compression of the inflamed knee joint. Anesthesiology. 1996;85(4):808–16. https://doi.org/10.1097/00000542-199610000-00016.
67. Gupta A, Bodin L, Holmström B, Berggren L. A systematic review of the peripheral analgesic effects of intraarticular morphine. Anesth Analg. 2001;93(3):761–70. https://doi.org/10.1097/00000539-200109000-00042.
68. Gabriel RA, Ilfeld BM. Percutaneous peripheral nerve stimulation and other alternatives for perineural catheters for postoperative analgesia. Best Pract Res Clin Anaesthesiol. 2019;33(1):37–46. https://doi.org/10.1016/j.bpa.2019.02.002.
69. Deer TR, Levy RM, Rosenfeld EL. Prospective clinical study of a new implantable peripheral nerve stimulation device to treat chronic pain. Clin J Pain. 2010;26(5):359–72. https://doi.org/10.1097/AJP.0b013e3181d4d646.
70. Melzack R, Wall PD. Pain mechanisms: a new theory. Science. 1965;150(3699):971–9. https://doi.org/10.1126/science.150.3699.971.
71. Ilfeld BM, Gilmore CA, Grant SA, et al. Ultrasound-guided percutaneous peripheral nerve stimulation for analgesia following total knee arthroplasty: a prospective feasibility study. J Orthop Surg. 2017;12(1):4. https://doi.org/10.1186/s13018-016-0506-7.
72. Ilfeld BM, Said ET, Finneran JJ, et al. Ultrasound-guided percutaneous peripheral nerve stimulation: neuromodulation of the femoral nerve for postoperative analgesia following ambulatory anterior cruciate ligament reconstruction: a proof of concept study. Neuromodulation J Int Neuromodulation Soc. 2019;22(5):621–9. https://doi.org/10.1111/ner.12851.
73. Ilfeld BM, Finneran JJ, Gabriel RA, et al. Ultrasound-guided percutaneous peripheral nerve stimulation: neuromodulation of the suprascapular nerve and brachial plexus for postoperative analgesia following ambulatory rotator cuff repair. A proof-of-concept study. Reg Anesth Pain Med. Published online February 15, 2019. https://doi.org/10.1136/rapm-2018-100121.

8 Analgesic Strategies in Ambulatory Surgery Centers

Olabisi Lane

Abstract

The use of ambulatory surgery centers continues to increase with more than 48.3 million surgical and nonsurgical procedures performed in 2010. Postoperative pain continues to be a challenging problem with inadequate pain control impeding recovery, reducing patient satisfaction, quality of life, delaying discharge and leading to unanticipated hospital admissions. Opioids are the mainstay treatment of postoperative pain. However, a multimodal approach has proved beneficial and utilizes various therapeutic options including adjuvant medications such as acetaminophen, antineuropathic agents, peripheral nerve blocks, nonsteroidal anti-inflammatory drugs (NSAIDs), antagonist of the N-methyl-D-aspartate (NMDA) receptors, and parenteral analgesics to name a few. The long-term consequences of uncontrolled acute postoperative pain may be the progression to persistent pain.

O. Lane (✉)
Department of Anesthesiology/Pain Medicine, Emory University Hospital, Atlanta, GA, USA
e-mail: olabisi.lane@emory.edu

Introduction

Since the 1980s, the use of ambulatory surgery centers continues to increase with more than 48.3 million surgical and nonsurgical procedures performed in 2010 during 28.6 million ambulatory surgery visits to hospitals and ASCs combined [1]. Advances in perioperative care, surgical and anesthetic techniques have facilitated the growth of this number [2]. The appeal of performing operations in ambulatory care centers is seen in all surgical specialties, as is evident by the rise in the number of surgery centers in the United States.

Postoperative pain continues to be a challenging problem with inadequate pain control impeding recovery, patient satisfaction, quality of life, and discharge after outpatient surgery. It may also lead to an unanticipated hospital admission as determined by Coley et al., where more than one third of all readmissions were as a result of inadequate pain control [3]. Unanticipated hospital admissions lead to a substantial increase in cost. The exact cause of uncontrolled pain remains undetermined, but it is thought that several factors play a role in the amount of pain a patient experiences after surgery. Patient-specific factors such as opioid tolerance, response to pain, surgical procedure, and choice of anesthetic may play a role [2]. The long-term consequences of uncontrolled acute postoperative pain may be the progression to persistent pain. Chronic postsurgical pain, that is, pain that persists greater than

K. Rajput et al. (eds.), *Pain Control in Ambulatory Surgery Centers*,
https://doi.org/10.1007/978-3-030-55262-6_8

3 months after surgery, is underdiagnosed. Over 10% of patients who have had surgery continue to complain of moderate to severe pain [4]. Risk factors for developing persistent postsurgical pain include the intensity and type of surgery, genetics, preexisting psychological and social factors, younger age, and female gender [5].

It is thought that the key to improving a patient's recovery after surgery involves the use of a multimodal or a balanced analgesia technique. This requires the use of more than one analgesic compound or modality of pain control to achieve an opioid-sparing effect, obtain additive and synergistic pain relief while minimizing adverse effects. This approach has become the gold standard for postoperative pain management [6]. It is important to know that multimodal analgesia translates to an individualized pain management regimen.

Preventative analgesia involves the administration of various analgesic medications prior to, during, and after surgery to prevent central and peripheral sensitization that can result after a noxious insult. This approach is more comprehensive and proactive than preemptive analgesia but similarly employs a multimodal treatment approach to attain this goal.

While opioids are the most commonly used treatment for pain control, a multimodal approach utilizes various therapeutic options including adjuvant medications such as acetaminophen, antineuropathic agents, peripheral nerve blocks, nonsteroidal anti-inflammatory drugs (NSAIDs), antagonist of the N-methyl-D-aspartate (NMDA) receptors, and regional and parenteral analgesics to name a few.

Preoperative Analgesia

A diverse class of medications and regional anesthesia may be utilized in the preoperative period.

Regional Anesthesia

Regional anesthesia has many advantages as it can be used as part of conscious sedation and provides superior analgesia while minimizing adverse effects of opioid medications and general anesthesia. Regional anesthesia may consist of neuraxial (spinal and epidural) anesthesia; local anesthesia infiltration (intra- and peri-articular); peripheral nerve block of the upper and lower extremity, head, and neck; facial blocks; truncal blocks; and intravenous regional anesthesia. Liposomal bupivacaine and adjuvants (clonidine, dexmedetomidine, etc.) can be used in combination with a local anesthetic agent to prolong the duration of effect. Perineural catheters can be placed in preparation for discharge to provide continued postoperative pain relief for a period longer than a single shot with or without adjuvant medication. Table 8.1 illustrates commonly used regional nerve blocks in the ambulatory surgery.

Patients should be given clear written instructions before a peripheral nerve block is performed and prior to discharge from the ambulatory surgery center. Depending on the block performed, the patient should be advised to reposition the limb frequently. If an upper extremity block is performed, the patient should be provided with a sling/brace and educated on proper use. Crutches or an assist device should be provided if a lower extremity block is performed. The patient should be instructed on signs and symptoms of neurologic deficits. The patient should be educated on starting prescribed oral pain medications once the effects of the block start to wear off. The contact information of a pain team member, anesthesiologist, or ASC staff member should be provided in the event that the patient has questions.

See below for CPNB.

Adjuvants to Regional Anesthesia

Perineural adjuvant medications can improve onset of blockade and/or increase duration and analgesic properties. The benefits of these agents may be secondary to their ability to allow lower volume of local anesthetic be used while achieving longer duration and improved analgesic effects. There has been no reported incidence of long-term deleterious effects or neurotoxicity.

Table 8.1 Commonly used regional nerve blocks in ambulatory surgery

Peripheral nerve block	Indication/surgery	Target	Complications
Interscalene + [7]	Shoulder Proximal humerus Clavicle	Interscalene groove C5–C7 nerve roots of brachial plexus	Ipsilateral phrenic nerve paralysis Horner's syndrome
Supraclavicular + [8]	Mid-humeral to hand	Trunk and divisions of brachial plexus	Phrenic nerve block (~50%) Horner's syndrome Pneumothorax
Infraclavicular + [8]	Surgery distal to elbow	Divisions and cord of the brachial plexus	Pneumothorax Hemothorax Chylothorax (left) vascular injection
Axillary + [8]	Surgery distal to elbow	Terminal branches of medial, lateral, and posterior cord Median, ulnar, radial nerve within axillary sheath Musculocutaneous Blocked separately	Hematoma Ecchymosis and pain at injection site
Individual blocks at elbow [9]	Hand surgery Wrist surgery	Radial nerve Median nerve Ulnar nerve	Ecchymosis and pain at injection site Nerve injury
Digital blocks [10]	Minor surgery or procedure of the digits	Digital nerves arise from median and ulnar nerves	Ecchymosis and pain at injection site Nerve injury Compromise of blood flow to digit
PEC I/II + [11]	Breast surgery Device implantation Ex:pacemaker	I-lateral and medial pectoral nerves II-long thoracic nerve, intercostobrachial and the lateral branch of intercostal nerves T2–T5	Pneumothorax LAST Vascular injury Infection
Serratus plane block + [12]	Breast surgery Chest wall surgery	Thoracic intercostal Nerves (lateral branch) Deep and superficial block. Superficial with better pain control	Pneumothorax Intravascular injection Vascular injury
Erector spinae + [13, 14]	Abdominal surgery Breast surgery Chest wall surgery	Ventral and dorsal rami of spinal nerves	Pneumothorax Unintended motor block if injection in lower thoracic or lumbar
Paravertebral + [15]	Breast surgery Chest wall surgery Abdominal surgery	Thoracic: Paravertebral space Somatic and sympathetic nerves Spread to intercostal and epidural space Lumbar: spinal nerves with spread into epidural space	Thoracic: Pleural puncture Pneumothorax Vascular injection Hypotension Intrathecal, epidural administration Lumbar: Motor weakness Injection into vasculature, epidural, intrathecal space Intraperitoneal injection Visceral injury
Subcostal TAP+ [16]	Abdominal surgery (above umbilicus)	Intercostal nerves T6-T9	Infection Peritoneal injection Hematoma Vascular injection LAST

(continued)

Table 8.1 (continued)

Peripheral nerve block	Indication/surgery	Target	Complications
Rectus sheath + [17]	Umbilical surgery Umbilical hernia surgery Midline incisions	Anterior cutaneous nerves 9–11 intercostal nerve	Infection Peritoneal injection Hematoma Vascular injection LAST
TAP*+ [18]	Abdominal surgery	Anterior rami of T7–L1 reliably blocks T10–L1	Infection Peritoneal injection Hematoma Vascular injection LAST
Ilioinguinal and iliohypogastric + [19]	Groin surgery Hernia repair	Ilioinguinal and iliohypogastric nerve which arise from L1 Contribution of fibers from T12 in 25% of patient	Uncommon Injection in vasculature
Femoral nerve + [20]	Anterior thigh surgery Surgery of medial leg below knee Hip surgery	Anterior rami of L2–L4 forms the femoral nerve	Infection Hematoma Nerve injury Vascular injection LAST
Adductor canal block + [21]	Knee surgery Vein harvesting/ stripping Ankle surgery (combine with popliteal nerve block)	Saphenous nerve within adductor canal	Infection Hematoma Nerve injury Vascular injection LAST
Infiltration between popliteal artery and capsule of knee (iPACK) [22]	Posterior knee capsule after knee surgery	Articular branches of tibial and obturator nerves (interspace between popliteal artery and posterior knee cap)	Infection Hematoma Vascular injection LAST
Popliteal sciatic nerve block + [23]	Lower leg surgery Ankle/foot surgery	Sciatic splits into tibial and common peroneal nerve	Infection Hematoma Nerve injury Vascular injection LAST
Sciatic nerve block (anterior or transgluteal approach)	Lower leg surgery Ankle/foot surgery Knee surgery (posterior)	Sciatic nerve	Infection Hematoma Nerve injury Vascular injection LAST
Lateral femoral cutaneous Nerve block [24]	Surgery on lateral thigh Hip surgery (combination with other block)	Lateral femoral cutaneous nerve	Infection Hematoma Nerve injury Vascular injection LAST
Obturator nerve block [25]	TURBT (prevent thigh adduction) Procedure on medial thigh Knee surgery	Primary rami of L2–L4 forms the obturator nerve (anterior and posterior branch)	Infection Pain at injection site
Ankle block [26]	Foot surgery	Saphenous nerve Sural nerve Posterior tibial nerve Deep peroneal nerve Superficial peroneal nerve	Infection Vascular injection LAST

TAP tranversus abdominis plane, *LAST* local anesthetic systemic toxicity; abdominal surgery: laparotomy, laparoscopy, laparotomy; + continuous peripheral nerve block (CPNB) is possible

Buprenorphine

Buprenorphine is a lipophilic analgesic with strong agonist properties at the mu receptor. It also has antagonist properties at the kappa receptor owing to its antihyperalgesic effects. It binds to opioid receptors on axons in the periphery and is able to block sodium channels, thus exerting effects similar to a local anesthetic agent. Buprenorphine is able to prolong the duration of analgesia when administered with a local anesthetic agent for a peripheral nerve block. However, similar to systemic administered doses, perineural administration is associated with an increased incidence of postoperative nausea and vomiting (PONV) which may impede discharge from the ambulatory surgery center [27]. 300 mcg of buprenorphine has been shown to cause opioid related side effects, while 150–200 mcg is thought to reduce the incidence of PONV and itching. Buprenorphine should be avoided in patients with a history of PONV [28].

Magnesium

Magnesium is an N-methyl-D-aspartate (NMDA) receptor antagonist. It augments the excitation threshold in peripheral nerves, and its effects on peripheral nerve are thought to be due to its positive divalent charge on the neuronal membrane or its role as a calcium antagonist. Perineural magnesium is said to prolong duration of analgesia and sensory and motor block [28]. Most studies do not report side effects or toxicity with the use of this agent, but Lee et al. saw an increase in nausea when 200 mg but not 150 mg of magnesium was used as an adjuvant [30].

Dexmedetomidine

Dexmedetomidine is a selective α2-adrenoceptor agonist. It has sedative, analgesic, and opioid-sparing effects. In the periphery, nerve fiber action potentials are inhibited as well as the release of norepinephrine. The blockade of the hyperpolarization-activated cation current (I_h current) has been proven to prolong the duration of analgesia, by as much as a 75% increase in duration. When compared to clonidine, it is eight times more selective at the α2-adrenoceptor receptor making it a valuable sedative and analgesic agent. It is used to extend the duration of peripheral nerve blocks, improves the quality of neuraxial (intrathecal and epidural) anesthesia, and allows a lower volume of local anesthetic agent [31, 32]. Dexmedetomidine at doses of 50 mcg and 75 mcg is beneficial, although transient bradycardia was seen, as well as hypotension with the higher dose [33].

Clonidine

Clonidine is also an α2-adrenergic agonist. Its mechanism of action in the periphery is not as apparent but is thought to be work via four proposed mechanisms, including direct effects on the peripheral nerve resulting in slowing or blockade of conduction [34]. This effect is thought to occur when clonidine is injected perineurally with or without local anesthetic, although not consistently demonstrated. It is able to extend analgesia of all local anesthetics with onset and duration of motor and sensory block varying depending on local anesthetic. It is worth mentioning the motor blockade when administered with bupivacaine is twice as long when compared with ropivacaine. This needs to be taken into consideration if postoperative discharge is dependent on resolution of blockade [35, 36]. Absorption into the systemic circulation is thought to be behind commonly seen adverse effects such as sedation, hypotension, and bradycardia. Clonidine at doses of 150 mcg appears to provide benefit without significant adverse effects [37].

Dexamethasone

Dexamethasone is a potent, long-acting glucocorticoid with anti-inflammatory and analgesic effects. It has been proven to prolong peripheral nerve blockade when combined with a local anesthetic agent. The exact mechanism of action is unknown but thought to be due to glucocorticoid receptors leading to inhibition of potassium channel-mediated discharge in excitable cells and attenuation of inflammatory mediators or via vasoconstrictive effects. Dexamethasone is able to prolong the duration of analgesia without affecting the sensory and motor blockade. In fact, it is also believed to aid in the healing process as it may have positive effects on sleep such as improving the quality with fewer disruptions [38, 39]. Neurological complications associated with its use are rare and typically due to direct injury to the nerve although hyperglycemia and infection may be a cause of concern. Choi et al. believe that dexamethasone may be the best medication to prolong analgesia and may be superior to other additives [40]. Interestingly, intravenous administration of dexamethasone also extends the duration and quality of analgesia similarly to perineural administration; however, perineural dexamethasone results in a quicker onset of motor and sensory blockade [41, 42]. There is conflicting information about the optimal dose to use, but doses of 1–2 mg of perineural dexamethasone appear to prolong the block. While Deshpande et al. described the benefits of 4 mg of dexamethasone in a patient who received bilateral TAP blocks [43], Sharnouby et al. observed that 4 mg was equipotent to 8 mg when used for TAP block [44].

Epinephrine

When used as an additive to local anesthetic agents, epinephrine acts as a vasoconstrictor and reduces systemic toxicity by limiting local anesthetic absorption into the bloodstream. It can prolong the duration and intensity of the block. However, unintentional absorption can lead to sympathomimetic effects such as hypertension and tachycardia. Caution should be employed when using epinephrine in patients in whom sympathetic stimulation could be detrimental, such as those with history of uncontrolled hyperthyroidism, arrhythmias, or cardiovascular disease. It is beneficial when a large volume of a long-acting agent (bupivacaine or ropivacaine) is used as epinephrine reduces the peak concentration. It does not affect the duration of long-acting local anesthetic agent as it will outlast the effect of the epinephrine. Local anesthetic agents have differing effects in a dose-dependent manner on peripheral nerve blood flow. Bupivacaine enhances blood flow, while lidocaine reduces blood flow. This reduction in blood flow is made worse when epinephrine is also administered. Fortunately, epinephrine is deemed safe, and the potential to cause peripheral nerve injury in normal patients is low, as these patients can tolerate reduced perineural blood flow. However, one must be careful in patients with preexisting nerve damage or injury [45]. Brummet et al. advise against the use of epinephrine except for as a marker of intravascular injection or when ultrasound is not utilized [31].

Liposomal Bupivacaine

This injectable suspension is approved by the US Food and Drug Administration (FDA) for single-dose infiltration into the surgical site, transversus abdominis plane (TAP) blocks, and interscalene brachial plexus blocks to produce postsurgical analgesia. It is said to improve pain over a 72-hour period via encapsulated bupivacaine in multivesicular liposomal particles that are slowly released over that time period [46]. It is marketed as providing long-lasting pain without the burden, toxicity, and cost associated with catheters and pumps. Several randomized controlled trials have revealed that the first 24 hours is where the most analgesic control is seen with no significant reduction in pain after the first 24 hours [47, 48]. More recently, Patel et al. determined it is safe and provides improved analgesia with a decrease in opioid use in the first 72 hours after shoulder surgery [49]. In pediatrics, Cohen et al. saw no cases of local anesthetic systemic toxicity when used for surgical wound infiltration [50]. Overall there are not enough high-quality studies for surgical infiltration suggesting a change in practice from unencapsulated to liposomal bupivacaine. However, its use in epidural and perineural nerve shows more promise [51]. Most commonly reported adverse effects of liposomal bupivacaine include headache, constipation, nausea, vomiting, and dizziness [52, 53]. It has been noted to have a favorable cardiac safety profile [54].

Continuous Perineural Nerve Block (CPNB)

Management of postoperative pain with continuous peripheral nerve block (CPNB) has now become widely popular in the ambulatory surgery center (ASC). Benefits of this analgesic modality include adequate pain control, reduced need for supplemental opioids, decreased opioid-related side effects, improved patient satisfaction, same-day discharge, and reduced incidence of unanticipated readmissions.

CPNB can be used to target pain after shoulder surgery via a catheter positioned in the posterior interscalene groove or for surgery distal to the proximal humerus via a supraclavicular block. Patients can be discharged after surgery with an adductor canal catheter in place after knee surgery. The use of CPNB has expanded beyond orthopedic surgeries and may now be used for breast, pelvic, urologic, and abdominal surgeries. The catheter may also be tunneled to prevent dislodgement [55]. Despite many benefits there are concerns about catheter site leakage, migration, obstruction, and inadvertent removal of the catheter.

Short-acting agents and local anesthetic agents have been used, but typically a longer-acting medication such as 0.2% ropivacaine or 0.125% bupivacaine may be instilled in the delivery device.

The economic impact of this analgesic technique is apparent as surgeries that previously required hospitalization can be performed. Those with preexisting conditions, such as COPD, can be discharged with a multimodal treatment regimen that removes opioids from the forefront . The cost of the delivery system has to be taken into consideration especially when comparing pumps with set infusion rates versus a pump capable of providing patient-initiated boluses [56].

Patient education is an integral part and must be completed prior to discharge. Patients should be properly educated and provided written instructions on the signs and symptoms of neurologic complications, infections, and local anesthetic toxicity. Instructions should be provided reinforcing care of the catheter site and proper techniques to remove and discard the device. If an extremity is involved, the patient should be given proper equipment (splint, cast, crutches) to safeguard the limb from injury and should be educated on falls. The contact information of a pain team member, anesthesiologist, or ASC staff member should be provided in the event that the patient has questions.

The use of peripheral nerve blocks has grown significantly with adjuvants frequently being added to local anesthetics to shorten the duration of action, increase the intensity, and prolong analgesia following the procedure. Various opioids (such as buprenorphine), dexamethasone, and dexmedetomidine to name a few have been added with beneficial effects, but caution should be used as this indication with the exception of liposomal bupivacaine for shoulder surgery is not approved by the FDA [28]. Although results have been demonstrated with agents such as ketamine, neostigmine, and magnesium for both neuraxial and perineural uses, widespread acceptance hasn't occurred, and some studies revealed neurotoxicity [57, 58].

Neuraxial Techniques in Ambulatory Surgery Center

The use of neuraxial anesthesia (spinal and epidural) is popular in ambulatory surgery. They are used for various surgery types including urologic, orthopedic, and abdominal surgeries. While sufficient as primary anesthesia for the operation, they are often not enough for providing postoperative pain control after the patient has recovered and is discharged from the ambulatory surgery center. Capdevila et al. conducted a study that showed in ambulatory surgery centers, spinal anesthesia with a short-acting local anesthetic was chosen over general anesthesia and conferred higher patient satisfaction [59]. However, Naghibi et al. demonstrated that spinal anesthesia conferred lower pain scales in the first 6 hours after surgery but then the pain score was no different than that of a patient who had general anesthesia [60]. When used in the ambulatory surgery center, epidural anesthesia has several advantages including shorter time to void when compared to spinal anesthesia, room turnover time shorter if epidural placed at holding area, and better hemodynamic stability. Despite the many advantages of both techniques, neither result in adequate postoperative pain control necessitating a plan for a multimodal treatment regimen prior to and after discharge.

Midazolam for Preoperative Anxiolysis

Stress and anxiety have been shown to negatively impact postoperative recovery and pain control. White et al., demonstrated that midazolam is able to modify the threshold for perception of tactile and painful stimulation and thus may have analgesic, specifically antinociceptive, properties. The exact mechanism of this phenomenon is unclear, but researchers are correct in saying anxiety and pain are intimately connected and uncontrolled anxiety will lead to worsening pain. These authors concluded that midazolam is effective in reducing pain after third molar surgery [61]. Contrary to their finding, Kim et al. discovered that midazolam does not improve quality of recovery after surgery but did allow for less propofol to be used during induction [62].

Midazolam is a potent anxiolytic agent and the most commonly administered anxiolytic in the perioperative period. It also has sedative and amnesic properties. It works via GABA-A receptor resulting in neuronal inhibition via a chloride channel. Advantages of this medication include rapid onset and short half-life; it has major metabolites with no pharmacologic action that are renally eliminated. 2 mg of midazolam is often used as an anxiolytic agent while procedures are performed or prior to transferring the patient to the operating room.

Oral Preoperative Analgesia

Selective Nonsteroidal Anti-inflammatory Agents

Celecoxib

Celecoxib is an inhibitor of the cyclooxygenase (COX) pathway, specifically the COX-2 isoform. It has antipyretic, analgesic, and anti-inflammatory properties with an added advantage of reduced gastrointestinal adverse effects (gastrointestinal bleeding, ulceration, or perforation) that is typically seen with nonselective anti-inflammatory agents. Patients are often advised to discontinue all nonsteroidal anti-inflammatory drugs (NSAIDs) due to concerns of platelet dysfunction leading to clinically significant bleeding. It has since been determined by Teerawattananon et al. that celecoxib, currently the only FDA-approved COX-2 selective agent, does not cause platelet dysfunction, nor does it increase the risk of bleeding or blood loss in the perioperative period [63]. Khan et al. determined that celecoxib conveys a small decrease in postoperative morphine use, nausea, vomiting, and pain in the postoperative period. In addition, no differences were noted between doses of 200 mg and 400 mg, given as a single preoperative dose or continued in the postoperative period [64]. Maund et al. also reported a modest but unlikely clinically significant difference when acetaminophen, NSAIDs, and COX-2 inhibitors were compared with each other as it pertains to a reduction in morphine consumption. The reduction in morphine-related adverse effects also does not favor one drug class [65]. Clinical studies have shown an increased risk of cardiovascular (CV) thrombotic events such as myocardial infarction (MI) and stroke but unsure if it is similar in all NSAIDs. This risk is seen in those with and without a predisposition or baseline cardiovascular disease. However, those with increased risk factors have a higher frequency of events typically early in treatment and with higher doses [66]. Finally, after gastrointestinal surgery there is the concern of anastomotic leak, but Peng et al. demonstrated that selective NSAIDs had no major impact on the numbers of anastomotic leak, while nonselective NSAIDs perhaps appreciably increase the frequency of anastomotic leak [67]. Celecoxib continues to be used as part of a multimodal treatment regimen. Each patient should be assessed and benefits must be carefully weighed against associated risks.

Acetaminophen

Acetaminophen is a well-known non-opioid analgesic with potent antipyretic effects but weak anti-inflammatory properties. The exact mechanism of acetaminophen remains poorly understood but is thought to work via the cyclooxygenase (COX) pathway with central and peripheral properties. An advantage of this medication is multiple dosage forms exist, with intravenous (IV) acetaminophen approved by the US

Food and Drug Administration in 2010. Benefits of the IV formulation over oral include faster onset of action, higher plasma levels, predictable pharmacokinetics and pharmacodynamics properties, and potentially reduced hepatotoxicity [68, 69]. The increased medication cost, time of administration (~15 minutes) and associated risks, infection, and phlebitis must be considered [70]. Evidence does suggest that oral doses between 600 and 1000 mg confer a 50% reduction in pain relief based over 4–6 hours [71]. Higher doses, such as 1000 mg, by mouth do have better bioavailability, and Jibril et al. determined that oral acetaminophen may not be inferior to the IV formulation [72]. The use of the IV formulation continues to increase given a demonstrable opioid-sparing effect when compared to placebo, although there is a lack of consistent reduction in adverse effects secondary to opioids [70].

Gabapentinoids (Gabapentin and Pregabalin)

Gabapentinoids are now seen as a desirable option for use in prevention of acute postoperative pain. Gabapentinoids inhibit the alpha 2-delta subunit of the voltage-gated calcium channels. Hu et al. showed a decrease in 24 hours perioperative opioid use with increasing doses of gabapentinoids. This study discovered that doses of ≥150 mg of pregabalin and ≥900 mg of gabapentin resulted in a decrease in pain score and opioid consumption when compared with lower doses [73]. Most studies recommend preoperative administration at least 1–2 hours before surgery and may be considered postoperatively if appropriate. This drug class has also been found to be effective in increasing patient satisfaction and reducing postoperative nausea, vomiting, itching, and anxiety but is noted to increase somnolence and dizziness [74].

In December 2019, the FDA issued a warning involving the use alone, in elderly or those with comorbid pulmonary conditions, as well as the coadministration of gabapentinoids with opioid or sedative medications. Serious consequences including but not limited to respiratory depression and death were reported [75]. The benefits of this treatment option in terms of pain control must be carefully weighed against the likelihood of delayed discharged due to adverse effects.

Intraoperative Analgesia

Ketamine

Ketamine is a N-methyl-D-aspartate (NMDA) receptor antagonist with analgesic, antihyperalgesic, and opioid-sparing effects when given at subanesthetic doses. Ketamine exerts effects on other receptors including μ-opioid receptors, γ-aminobutyric acid receptors, and muscarinic receptor to name a few [76]. The blockade of the NMDA receptor reduces pain by modulating centrally mediated pain, and this effect lasts even after the infusion is terminated [77] Ketamine used for acute pain either alone or in combination with an opioid has been shown to be beneficial [78]. Significant reduction in postoperative pain scores and opioid consumption was seen with a bolus of 0.1–0.3 mg/kg followed by an infusion rate of 0.1–0.3 mg/kg/min [79] Ketamine may cause hallucination and a “dissociated state”; however at subanesthetic doses consciousness and arousal are not substantially affected. At anesthetic doses ketamine can increase blood pressure and heart rate. It can also cause a small increase in intracranial pressure and CO_2 levels. The psychomimetic and sympathomimetic effects are greatly reduced at lower doses. Caution should be employed in patients with renal and hepatic dysfunction, active psychosis, or schizophrenia. There is no consensus on the effects of ketamine in patients with seizures [80].

Magnesium

Magnesium is the second most common intracellular ion and important in neurotransmission [81]. Its exact mechanism of analgesia isn’t fully understood but thought to be due to regulation of calcium influx into the cell, as well as antagonism of N-methyl-D-aspartate (NMDA) receptor in the central nervous system [82, 83]. During general anesthesia, it can be used to reduce the intraoperative use of opioid [84]. Albrecht et al. determined that in all types of surgery studied, the use of magnesium in the perioperative period can result in a reduction in opioid consumption and pain score within the first 24 hours [85]. De Oliveira et al. demonstrated an overall reduction in postoperative opioid use even when lower limits of magnesium were used. These effects were even more pronounced when magnesium was infused in the operating room and in the postoperative period versus intraoperative infusion only. Furthermore, this study reported that intravenous magnesium is a valuable addition and can minimize rest pain in the early and late postoperative period, as well as pain with movement in the late postoperative period. Magnesium was also beneficial in reducing the incidence of postoperative shivering. No systemic adverse effects were noted in this study [81]. A 30–50 mg/kg loading dose given 10–15 minutes either before or right after induction followed by an infusion at a rate of 8–15 mg/kg/h resulted in a reduction in fentanyl use, especially in surgeries associated with significant pain. Doses higher than 10 mg/kg/h did not yield more benefit and resulted in hemodynamic instability [86]. Patients with certain comorbidities may not be ideal candidates for magnesium, including those with prior history of renal failure, heart block, and neuromuscular disease [87].

Lidocaine

Lidocaine is an amide local anesthetic agent with antihyperalgesic, analgesic, and anti-inflammatory properties. There is literature to suggest that lidocaine also has anti-metastatic effects in cancer patients [88]. Its mechanism of action is via blockade of sodium channels in nerves disrupting neuronal transmission and best seen when administered perineurally. However how it exerts analgesic effects systemically is not completely understood [89]. It has a relatively safe background; therapeutic and toxic levels of the drug have been well established, given that it has also been used as an antiarrhythmic agent for many years.

Lidocaine use in the perioperative period is said to reduce pain scores and opioid consumption in the first 24 hours in patients undergoing ambulatory surgery, but its effects may differ depending on the specific type of surgery. The exact reason for this difference is unknown, but it may be due to variables in each study conducted [90]. It can hasten the recovery of bowel function, reduce the length of hospital stay, and allow patients to participate in rehabilitation [91]. The use of this medication, particularly as an infusion, must be discussed with the surgeon or regional team as one must be cautious when combining intravenous lidocaine infusion or single dose with injection of liposomal bupivacaine [92]. Although rare, signs of toxicity may include arrhythmias, perioral numbness, and tinnitus. A typical loading dose is 1–2 mg/kg followed by an infusion of 1–2 mg/kg/h. Monoethylglycinexylidide (MEGX) and glycinexylidide (GX) are two major active metabolites of lidocaine [93]. Patients with history of heart block (any degree), heart failure, or seizures may not be a candidate for lidocaine infusion. Hepatic and renal dysfunction, as well as drug interactions, may impair its clearance [89].

Opioid Analgesics (Fentanyl and Hydromorphone)

Opioids are a class of medications derived from opium. The natural alkaloids are termed opiates and include morphine and codeine. There are many synthetic derivatives including fentanyl, hydromorphone, methadone, and buprenorphine to name a few. The primary mechanism of opioids is via mu receptor agonism but some are able to bind other receptors including the kappa and delta opiate receptors. Opioid receptors are found in different locations throughout the body including the brain, spinal cord, gut, lungs, and vasculature. Receptor binding leads to intracellular processes that ultimately result in a decrease in neurotransmission via a reduction in cell excitability [94].

In the perioperative period, there are many reasons to utilize intravenous opioid medications including ensuring patient compliance and comfort with the performance of a procedure such as neuraxial or peripheral nerve block, as part of balanced anesthetic plan when inducing general anesthesia, a component of monitored anesthesia care (MAC) and postoperative pain control. In the operating room, opioids are also able to ensure analgesia, act in a synergistic manner with other agents including inhalation agents, blunt autonomic responses to laryngoscopy and intubation, as well as reduce pain during surgery. There are associated side effects with this drug class including respiratory depression, hypoventilation, bradycardia, postoperative nausea and vomiting, decreased gastrointestinal motility, chest wall rigidity, and pruritus. Fentanyl and hydromorphone are two of the most commonly used opioid medications in the perioperative period.

IV Dexamethasone

As previously discussed, dexamethasone is a potent, long-acting glucocorticoid with anti-inflammatory and analgesic effects. It can be used to prolong nerve blocks and is often used to prevent and treat nausea. Intravenously administered dexamethasone also plays a role in postoperative pain control and has been shown to decrease pain scores and opioid consumption postoperatively [95, 96]. A one-time dose of greater than or equal to 0.1 mg/kg or a range of 8–10 mg seems to confer the greatest benefit. This dose is more than what is usually administered for the prevention of postoperative nausea and vomiting. There are concerns that this medication at higher doses can lead to hyperglycemia, infection, and poor wound healing. In a study done by Waldron et al., no differences were seen in wound healing and infection, but a modest increase in blood glucose level was noted 24 hours after surgery [97]. This increase was higher in patients who were diabetic [98]. These patients should be advised to monitor their blood glucose levels carefully upon discharge.

Intravenous (IV) Acetaminophen (Ofirmev)

See above. As discussed, IV acetaminophen results in higher plasma concentration than oral administration and peaks within 15 minutes. The question of preemptive or preventative analgesia was answered by Khalili et al., who determined both preemptive and preventive acetaminophen used similarly resulted in lower pain scores and a longer duration of time to first opioid use when compared to placebo [99]. It might be worth it to administer intravenous acetaminophen toward the end of the case to allow for its analgesic benefits to peak as the case is completed. The cost of the medication must also be considered.

IV Nonsteroidal Anti-inflammatory Agents (Ketorolac)

Ketorolac is a nonsteroidal anti-inflammatory drug (NSAID). Its mechanism of action is via inhibition of the cyclooxygenase (COX) enzymes. It has analgesic and anti-inflammatory properties. It can be administered intravenously, intramuscularly, and per oral. Its use in the perioperative period may be limited by concerns of adverse effects, particularly postoperative bleeding. Ketorolac has been shown to cause a slight but significant increase in bleeding time. However, this increase was noted to the same magnitude as a patient using aspirin, and overall it was not found to cause significant bleeding. A decrease in platelet was also seen although not clinically significant [100]. Stephen et al. discovered there were no significant association between the use of ketorolac and the development of postoperative hematoma [101]. Perioperative use of ketorolac in ankle fracture surgery revealed no substantial differences in fracture patterns, healing, and complications. It was also linked with a high rate of union [102]. McClain showed there was not an increased risk of bleeding in patients undergoing tonsillectomy with or without adenoidectomy or UPPP [103]. The review of both colorectal and non-colorectal gastrointestinal surgeries (appendectomies and colon resections) revealed an undesirable association with the use of ketorolac. The results show an increased risk of emergency room visits, readmissions, and reintervention in patients who receive perioperative ketorolac; as such it may not be ideal in this population type [104]. Lyon et al. demonstrated that 10 mg of ketorolac was just as effective as higher doses including 15 mg, 30 mg, and 60 mg. 10 mg of ketorolac is not commercially available and would have to be specially formulated. As such, the authors recommend the use of the lowest possible effective dose [105].

Caution should be exercised when administering these medications to patients with congestive heart failure or underlying renal and hepatic dysfunction.

Dexmedetomidine Infusion

Dexmedetomidine is a selective α2-adrenoceptor agonist. As was previously discussed, it has sedative, analgesic, and opioid-sparing effects and is beneficial when administered as an adjuvant in peripheral nerve blocks. Adverse effects associated with the use of this medication include hypotension, bradycardia, and postoperative nausea and vomiting. Lundorf et al. performed a Cochrane review of abdominal surgeries and determined the perioperative use of this medication results in decreased opioid use, although there was no significant decrease in postoperative pain scores [106]. Ge et al. exhibited that the addition of dexmedetomidine resulted in less morphine consumption via PCA, lower pain scores, and higher recovery in patients who underwent abdominal hysterectomy [107]. Dexmedetomidine was shown to substantially reduce the consumption of morphine in the first 24 hours after knee arthroplasty [98]. Similarly Shin et al. found that the intraoperative addition of dexmedetomidine leads to a modest but clinically significant reduction in opioid consumption [108]. Finally, Kundra et al. demonstrated that patients undergoing one- to two-level laminectomy who received dexmedetomidine infusion at 0.3 mcg/kg/h remained hemodynamically stable, had lower intraoperative blood loss, required less anesthetic agents, and were extubated sooner when compared to patients who received saline [109].

Wound Infiltration

Intraoperative wound infiltration with a local anesthetic agent can easily be accomplished by the surgeon and has been shown to help with postoperative pain control. It is thought that the local anesthetic binds to fast sodium channels at the surface of the wound and directly blocks the transmission of pain from nociceptive afferents. It is also thought to reduce inflammation, thereby lessening pain and hyperalgesia [110]. Several methods of administration have been trialed including intraoperative infiltration with or without additives, continuous catheters, slow-release liposomal bupivacaine, and via tumescent analgesia. There is the concern for infection, local anesthetic systemic toxicity, and appropriate location of the catheter when used.

Philippi et al. investigated extracapsular local infiltration analgesia in hip arthroscopy patients and showed that this technique did not result in a significant reduction in pain [111]. Greimel et al. showed that the use of local infiltration anesthesia (LIA) in total knee arthroplasty did not reduce the need for opioid medications despite increasing patient satisfaction [112].

Postoperative Analgesia

Acute postoperative pain that is inadequately managed can lead to delayed recovery time, delayed discharge, impaired function and quality of recovery and life, increased morbidity, prolonged duration of opioid use, patient dissatisfaction, unanticipated admissions and has an economic impact. Poorly controlled postoperative pain can lead to persistent postsurgical pain [113]. The approach to the treatment of postoperative pain should follow the multimodal treatment approach, maximizing non-opioid

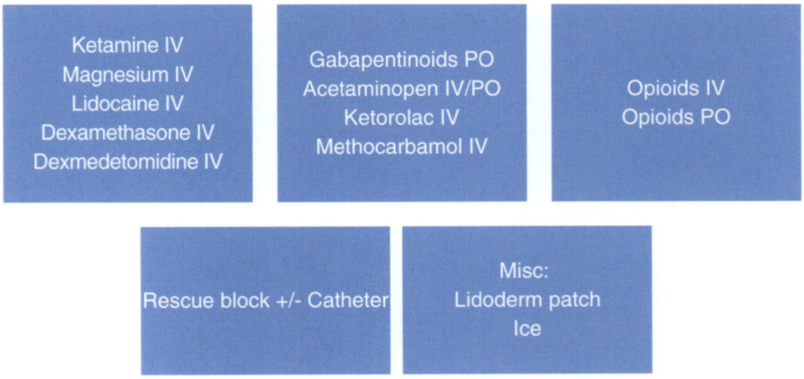

Fig. 8.1 Various treatment options for management of postoperative pain control

medications while minimizing opioids and its associated side effects. However, control of pain can be very difficult to acheive in the post-anesthesia care unit (PACU). Some patients may initially require opioid medications such as short-acting fentanyl and then benefit from the addition of other medications. Figure 8.1 demonstrates various treatment options that can be used to improve pain control in the post-anesthesia care unit (PACU).

Methocarbamol

Methocarbamol is one of the oldest muscle relaxants available. Its mechanism of action is not clear but is thought to target the spinal cord and inhibit muscle spasms. It has been used in the treatment of acute postoperative pain and after orthopedic procedures. Hidalgo et al. investigated the use of this medication in the treatment of postoperative pain and found that preoperative administration of methocarbamol improved early pain in breast augmentation surgery when compared to intercostal nerve blocks plus methocarbamol, intercostal blocks alone, and the use of neither [114]. Its benefit in perioperative hip and knee replacement was investigated by Looke et al., via a new pain protocol, and revealed improvement in patient care that was in part attributed to the use of intravenous methocarbamol and acetaminophen [115]. In contrary to the previously mentioned favorable findings, Aljuhani et al. investigated the use of this medication in the treatment of acute traumatic injury and found that methocarbamol did not improve pain [116].

Lidocaine 5% Transdermal Patch

Lidocaine 5% is an amide local anesthetic manufactured as a topical transdermal agent and approved for the relief of pain secondary to postherpetic neuralgia. It contains 700 mg of lidocaine (50 mg/gram adhesive). Its mechanism of action is believed to inhibit ion fluxes needed for initiation and conduction of impulses, thereby stabilizing neuronal membranes [117]. It is applied to intact skin close to the site of incision or pain and continuously penetrates the area of application. Lau et al. showed that lidocaine 5% patch was effective at decreasing pain intensity at rest without any adverse effects after gynecological surgery [118]. Similarly, results were favorable when Kwon et al. investigated the benefits of topical lidocaine at laparoscopic port sites in wound pain after gynecological laparoscopic surgery [119]. Its efficacy with treating postsurgical knee pain is mixed, with one report noting no significant improvement in postsurgical knee pain and another detailing improvement in tourniquet-induced pain. Smoker et al. performed a systemic review and revealed that in certain surgery types, it may lessen short-term pain and is fairly well tolerated. Its utility is yet to be determined, as it does not reliably reduce opioid use and does not improve patient function [120].

Sample Combination of Medications

	Abdominal surgery
Preoperative	Midazolam 2 mg Gabapentin 600–900 mg Acetaminophen 975–1000 mg ± Celecoxib 200–400 mg (if no contraindications) Midazolam (anxiolysis) Preoperative TAP block with liposomal bupivacaine
Intraoperative	Magnesium 2 gm IV Ketorolac 15 mg IV PRN fentanyl and hydromorphone IV Decadron 8–10 mg IV
Postoperative	Robaxin 1 g IV Consider repeating acetaminophen 1 g IV Dexmedetomidine 0.5 mg/kg IV Ice Lidocaine 5% topical patch IV opioids PRN
	Breast surgery (reconstruction)
Preoperative	Midazolam 2 mg Gabapentin 600–900 mg Acetaminophen 975–1000 mg Ketorolac 15 mg IV Preoperative erector spinae plane block with catheters – 0.2% ropivacaine with dexmedetomidine and dexamethasone at 8 ml/h
Intraoperative	Lidocaine PRN fentanyl and hydromorphone IV Decadron 8–10 mg IV
Postoperative	Robaxin 1 g IV Magnesium 2 gm IV Consider repeating acetaminophen 1 g IV Consider bolus of catheter in PACU IV opioids PRN
	Knee surgery
Preoperative	Midazolam 2 mg Gabapentin 600–900 mg Acetaminophen 975–1000 mg Ketorolac 15 mg IV Preoperative adductor canal block with catheter – 0.2% ropivacaine at 8 ml/h
Intraoperative	Intraoperative spinal anesthesia MAC + propofol + dexmedetomidine Decadron 8–10 mg ± Fentanyl or hydromorphone PRN
Postoperative	Ketamine 0.1–0.3 mg/kg IV Magnesium 2 gm IV Consider iPACK IV opioids for posterior knee pain

References

1. Hall MJ. Ambulatory surgery data from hospitals and ambulatory surgery centers: United States, 2010. Natl Health Stat Rep. 2017;(102):15.
2. Pavlin DJ, Chen C, Penaloza DA, Polissar NL, Buckley FP. Pain as a factor complicating recovery and discharge after ambulatory surgery. Anesth Analg. 2002;95(3):627–34.
3. Coley KC, Williams BA, DaPos SV, Chen C, Smith RB. Retrospective evaluation of unanticipated admissions and readmissions after same day surgery and associated costs. J Clin Anesth. 2002;14(5):349–53.
4. Fletcher D, Stamer UM, Pogatzki-Zahn E, Zaslansky R, Tanase NV, Perruchoud C, et al. Chronic postsurgical pain in Europe: an observational study. Eur J Anaesthesiol. 2015;32(10):725–34.
5. Cintron L, MD, MS. Persistent postsurgical pain [Internet]. Practical pain management. [cited 2020 Jun 6]. Available from: https://www.practicalpainmanagement.com/persistent-postsurgical-pain.
6. White PF. Multimodal pain management--the future is now! Curr Opin Investig Drugs. 2007;8(7):517–8.
7. Vaid VN, Shukla A. Inter scalene block: revisiting old technique. Anesth Essays Res. 2018;12(2):344–8.
8. Dhir S, Brown B, Mack P, Bureau Y, Yu J, Ross D. Infraclavicular and supraclavicular approaches to brachial plexus for ambulatory elbow surgery: a randomized controlled observer-blinded trial. J Clin Anesth. 2018;48:67–72.
9. McCahon RA, Bedforth NM. Peripheral nerve block at the elbow and wrist. Contin Educ Anaesth Crit Care Pain. 2007;7(2):42–4.
10. Digital Nerve Block Periprocedural Care: Equipment, Anesthesia, Positioning [Internet]. [cited 2020 Jun 24]. Available from: https://emedicine.medscape.com/article/80887-periprocedure#b7.
11. Battista C, Krishnan S. Pectoralis nerve block. In: StatPearls [Internet]. Treasure Island: StatPearls Publishing; 2020 [cited 2020 Jun 22]. Available from: http://www.ncbi.nlm.nih.gov/books/NBK547691/.
12. Blanco R, Parras T, McDonnell JG, Prats-Galino A. Serratus plane block: a novel ultrasound-guided thoracic wall nerve block. Anaesthesia. 2013;68(11):1107–13.
13. Krishnan S, Cascella M. Erector spinae plane block. In: StatPearls [Internet]. Treasure Island: StatPearls Publishing; 2020 [cited 2020 Jun 22]. Available from: http://www.ncbi.nlm.nih.gov/books/NBK545305/.
14. Tulgar S, Selvi O, Senturk O, Serifsoy TE, Thomas DT. Ultrasound-guided erector spinae plane block: indications, complications, and effects on acute and chronic pain based on a single-center experience. Cureus [Internet]. [cited 2020 Jun 22];11(1). Available from: https://www.ncbi.nlm.nih.gov/pmc/articles/PMC6402723/.
15. Župčić M, Dedić D, Graf Župčić S, Đuzel V, Šimurina T, Šakić L, et al. The role of paravertebral blocks in ambulatory surgery: review of the literature. Acta Clin Croat. 2019;58(Suppl 1):43–7.
16. Soliz JM, Lipski I, Hancher-Hodges S, Speer BB, Popat K. Subcostal transverse abdominis plane block for acute pain management: a review. Anesth Pain Med [Internet]. 2017 [cited 2020 Jun 23];7(5). Available from: https://www.ncbi.nlm.nih.gov/pmc/articles/PMC5903215/.
17. Quek KHY, Phua DSK. Bilateral rectus sheath block as the single anaesthetic technique for an open infraumbilical hernia repair. Singap Med J. 2014;55(3):e39–41.
18. Tsai H-C, Yoshida T, Chuang T-Y, Yang S-F, Chang C-C, Yao H-Y, et al. Transversus abdominis plane block: an updated review of anatomy and techniques. Biomed Res Int [Internet]. 2017 [cited 2020 Jun 24];2017. Available from: https://www.ncbi.nlm.nih.gov/pmc/articles/PMC5684553/.
19. Zhou Y, Chen M, Zhang Y, Zhou H, Yu X, Chen G. Ilioinguinal/iliohypogastric nerve block versus transversus abdominis plane block for pain management following inguinal hernia repair surgery: a systematic review and meta-analysis of randomized controlled trials. Medicine (Baltimore). 2019;98(42):e17545.
20. Sykes Z, Pak A. Femoral nerve block. In: StatPearls [Internet]. Treasure Island: StatPearls Publishing; 2020 [cited 2020 Jun 23]. Available from: http://www.ncbi.nlm.nih.gov/books/NBK546704/.
21. Sun C, Zhang X, Song F, Zhao Z, Du R, Wu S, et al. Is continuous catheter adductor canal block better than single-shot canal adductor canal block in primary total knee arthroplasty? Medicine (Baltimore) [Internet]. 2020 [cited 2020 Jun 24];99(20). Available from: https://www.ncbi.nlm.nih.gov/pmc/articles/PMC7254479/.
22. Kandarian B, Indelli PF, Sinha S, Hunter OO, Wang RR, Kim TE, et al. Implementation of the IPACK (Infiltration between the Popliteal Artery and Capsule of the Knee) block into a multimodal analgesic pathway for total knee replacement. Korean J Anesthesiol. 2019;72(3):238–44.
23. Ma H-H, Chou T-FA, Tsai S-W, Chen C-F, Wu P-K, Chen W-M. The efficacy and safety of continuous versus single-injection popliteal sciatic nerve block in outpatient foot and ankle surgery: a systematic review and meta-analysis. BMC Musculoskelet Disord [Internet]. 2019 [cited 2020 Jun 24];20. Available from: https://www.ncbi.nlm.nih.gov/pmc/articles/PMC6788034/.
24. Coraci D, Giovannini S, Loreti C, Ruggeri F, Padua L. The lateral femoral cutaneous nerve: ultrasound support in nerve assessing. Reg Anesth Pain Med. 2018;43(6):650–1.
25. Yoshida T, Nakamoto T, Kamibayashi T. Ultrasound-guided obturator nerve block: a focused review on anatomy and updated techniques. Biomed Res Int. 2017;2017:7023750.
26. Girón-Arango L, Vásquez-Sadder MI, González-Obregón MP, Gamero-Fajardo CE. Ultrasound-guided ankle block: an attractive anaesthetic technique for foot surgery. Colombian J Anesthesiol. 2015;43(4):283–9.

27. Schnabel A, Reichl SU, Zahn PK, Pogatzki-Zahn EM, Meyer-Frießem CH. Efficacy and safety of buprenorphine in peripheral nerve blocks: a meta-analysis of randomised controlled trials. Eur J Anaesthesiol (EJA). 2017;34(9):576–86.
28. YaDeau JT, Gordon MA, Goytizolo EA, Lin Y, Fields KG, Goon AK, et al. Buprenorphine, Clonidine, Dexamethasone, and Ropivacaine for Interscalene Nerve Blockade: A Prospective, Randomized, Blinded, Ropivacaine Dose-Response Study. Pain Med. 2015;14;pnv010.
29. Kirksey MA, Haskins SC, Cheng J, Liu SS. Local anesthetic peripheral nerve block adjuvants for prolongation of analgesia: a systematic qualitative review. PLoS One [Internet]. 2015 [cited 2020 Jun 20];10(9). Available from: https://www.ncbi.nlm.nih.gov/pmc/articles/PMC4565585/.
30. Lee AR, Yi H, Chung IS, Ko JS, Ahn HJ, Gwak MS, et al. Magnesium added to bupivacaine prolongs the duration of analgesia after interscalene nerve block. Can J Anaesth. 2012;59(1):21–7.
31. Brummett CM, Williams BA. Additives to local anesthetics for peripheral nerve blockade. Int Anesthesiol Clin. 2011;49(4):104–16.
32. Swain A, Nag DS, Sahu S, Samaddar DP. Adjuvants to local anesthetics: current understanding and future trends. World J Clin Cases. 2017;5(8):307–23.
33. Abdulatif M, Fawzy M, Nassar H, Hasanin A, Ollaek M, Mohamed H. The effects of perineural dexmedetomidine on the pharmacodynamic profile of femoral nerve block: a dose-finding randomised, controlled, double-blind study. Anaesthesia. 2016;71(10):1177–85.
34. Dalle C, Schneider M, Clergue F, Bretton C, Jirounek P. Inhibition of the I(h) current in isolated peripheral nerve: a novel mode of peripheral antinociception? Muscle Nerve 2001;24:254–261. https://doi.org/10.1002/1097-4598(200102)24:2<254::aid mus110>3.0.co;2-#.
35. Pöpping DM, Elia N, Marret E, Wenk M, Tramèr MR. Clonidine as an adjuvant to local anesthetics For peripheral nerve and plexus blocks a meta-analysis of randomized trials. Anesthesiology. 2009;111(2):406–15.
36. Erlacher W, Schuschnig C, Koinig H, Marhofer P, Melischek M, Mayer N, et al. Clonidine as adjuvant for mepivacaine, ropivacaine and bupivacaine in axillary, perivascular brachial plexus block. Can J Anaesth. 2001;48(6):522–5.
37. Murphy DB, McCartney CJL, Chan VWS. Novel analgesic adjuncts for brachial plexus block: a systematic review. Anesth Analg. 2000;90(5):1122–8.
38. Alarasan AK, Agrawal J, Choudhary B, Melhotra A, Uike S, Mukherji A. Effect of dexamethasone in low volume supraclavicular brachial plexus block: a double-blinded randomized clinical study. J Anaesthesiol Clin Pharmacol. 2016;32(2):234.
39. Marks R, Barlow JW, Funder JW. Steroid-induced vasoconstriction: glucocorticoid antagonist studies. J Clin Endocrinol Metab. 1982;54(5):1075–7.
40. Choi S, Rodseth R, McCartney CJL. Effects of dexamethasone as a local anaesthetic adjuvant for brachial plexus block: a systematic review and meta-analysis of randomized trials. Br J Anaesth. 2014;112(3):427–39.
41. Desmet M, Braems H, Reynvoet M, Plasschaert S, Van Cauwelaert J, Pottel H, et al. I.V. and perineural dexamethasone are equivalent in increasing the analgesic duration of a single-shot interscalene block with ropivacaine for shoulder surgery: a prospective, randomized, placebo-controlled study. Br J Anaesth. 2013;111(3):445–52.
42. Mathew R, Radha KR, Hema VR. Effect of perineural and intravenous dexamethasone on duration of analgesia in supraclavicular brachial plexus block with bupivacaine: a comparative study. Anesth Essays Res. 2019;13(2):280–3.
43. Deshpande JP, Ghodki PS, Sardesai SP. The analgesic efficacy of dexamethasone added to ropivacaine in transversus abdominis plane block for transabdominal hysterectomy under subarachnoid block. Anesth Essays Res. 2017;11(2):499–502.
44. Sharnouby NME, Gendy HAAE. Ultrasound-guided single injection transversus abdominis plane block of isobaric bupivacaine with or without dexamethasone for bariatric patients undergoing laparoscopic vertical banded gastroplasty: a comparative study of different doses. Ain-Shams J Anaesthesiol. 2015;8(2):194.
45. Neal J. Effects of epinephrine in local anesthetics on the central and peripheral nervous systems: neurotoxicity and neural blood flow. Reg Anesth Pain Med. 2003;28(2):124–34.
46. Mont MA, Beaver WB, Dysart SH, Barrington JW, Del Gaizo DJ. Local infiltration analgesia with liposomal bupivacaine improves pain scores and reduces opioid use after total knee arthroplasty: results of a randomized controlled trial. J Arthroplast. 2018;33(1):90–6.
47. Gorfine SR, Onel E, Patou G, Krivokapic ZV. Bupivacaine extended-release liposome injection for prolonged postsurgical analgesia in patients undergoing hemorrhoidectomy: a multicenter, randomized, double-blind, placebo-controlled trial. Dis Colon Rectum. 2011;54(12):1552–9.
48. Lonner J. Role of liposomal bupivacaine in pain management after total joint arthroplasty. J Surg Orthop Adv. 2014;23(1):37–41.
49. Patel MA, Gadsden JC, Nedeljkovic SS, Bao X, Zeballos JL, Yu V, et al. Brachial plexus block with liposomal bupivacaine for shoulder surgery improves analgesia and reduces opioid consumption: results from a multicenter, randomized, double-blind, controlled trial. Pain Med. 2020;21(2):387–400.
50. Cohen B, Glosser L, Saab R, Walters M, Salih A, Zafeer-Khan M, et al. Incidence of adverse events attributable to bupivacaine liposome injectable suspension or plain bupivacaine for postoperative pain in pediatric surgical patients: a retrospec-

tive matched cohort analysis. Paediatr Anaesth. 2019;29(2):169–74.

51. Shafer SL. Letter to the editor on "Local infiltration analgesia with liposomal bupivacaine improves pain scores and reduces opioid use after total knee arthroplasty: results of a randomized controlled trial". J Arthroplast. 2018;33(8):2694.
52. Bramlett K, Onel E, Viscusi ER, Jones K. A randomized, double-blind, dose-ranging study comparing wound infiltration of DepoFoam bupivacaine, an extended-release liposomal bupivacaine, to bupivacaine HCl for postsurgical analgesia in total knee arthroplasty. Knee. 2012;19(5):530–6.
53. Golf M, Daniels SE, Onel E. A phase 3, randomized, placebo-controlled trial of DepoFoam® bupivacaine (extended-release bupivacaine local analgesic) in bunionectomy. Adv Ther. 2011;28(9):776–88.
54. Bergese SD, Onel E, Morren M, Morganroth J. Bupivacaine extended-release liposome injection exhibits a favorable cardiac safety profile. Reg Anesth Pain Med. 2012;37(2):145–51.
55. Chelly JE, Ghisi D, Fanelli A. Continuous peripheral nerve blocks in acute pain management. Br J Anaesth. 2010;105(suppl_1):i86–96.
56. Swenson JD, Cheng GS, Axelrod DA, Davis JJ. Ambulatory anesthesia and regional catheters: when and how. Anesthesiol Clin. 2010;28(2):267–80.
57. Swami SS, Keniya VM, Ladi SD, Rao R. Comparison of dexmedetomidine and clonidine (α2 agonist drugs) as an adjuvant to local anaesthesia in supraclavicular brachial plexus block: a randomised double-blind prospective study. Indian J Anaesth. 2012;56(3):243–9.
58. Hemmings HC, Egan TD. Pharmacology and physiology for anesthesia e-book: foundations and clinical application: Elsevier Health Sciences; Elsevier Philadelphia PA. 2018. 986 p.
59. Capdevila X, Aveline C, Delaunay L, Bouaziz H, Zetlaoui P, Choquet O, et al. Factors determining the choice of spinal versus general anesthesia in patients undergoing ambulatory surgery: results of a multicenter observational study. Adv Ther. 2020;37(1):527–40.
60. Naghibi K, Saryazdi H, Kashefi P, Rohani F. The comparison of spinal anesthesia with general anesthesia on the postoperative pain scores and analgesic requirements after elective lower abdominal surgery: a randomized, double-blinded study. J Res Med Sci. 2013;18(7):543–8.
61. White PF. Multimodal analgesia: its role in preventing postoperative pain. Curr Opin Investig Drugs. 2008;9(1):76–82.
62. Kim MH, Kim MS, Lee JH, Seo JH, Lee J-R. Can quality of recovery be enhanced by premedication with midazolam? Medicine (Baltimore) [Internet]. 2017 [cited 2020 Jun 24];96(7). Available from: https://www.ncbi.nlm.nih.gov/pmc/articles/PMC5319519/.
63. Teerawattananon C, Tantayakom P, Suwanawiboon B, Katchamart W. Risk of perioperative bleeding related to highly selective cyclooxygenase-2 inhibitors: a systematic review and meta-analysis. Semin Arthritis Rheum. 2017;46(4):520–8.
64. Khan JS, Margarido C, Devereaux PJ, Clarke H, McLellan A, Choi S. Preoperative celecoxib in noncardiac surgery: a systematic review and meta-analysis of randomised controlled trials. Eur J Anaesthesiol (EJA). 2016;33(3):204–14.
65. Maund E, McDaid C, Rice S, Wright K, Jenkins B, Woolacott N. Paracetamol and selective and non-selective non-steroidal anti-inflammatory drugs for the reduction in morphine-related side-effects after major surgery: a systematic review. Br J Anaesth. 2011;106(3):292–7.
66. DailyMed – CELECOXIB- celecoxib capsule [Internet]. [cited 2020 Jun 16]. Available from: https://dailymed.nlm.nih.gov/dailymed/drugInfo.cfm?setid=27d813ea-7798-09cb-734b-b970d7248f1f.
67. Peng F, Liu S, Hu Y, Yu M, Chen J, Liu C. Influence of perioperative nonsteroidal anti-inflammatory drugs on complications after gastrointestinal surgery: a meta-analysis. Acta Anaesthesiol Taiwanica. 2016;54(4):121–8.
68. Jaeschke H. Acetaminophen – dose-dependent drug hepatotoxicity and acute liver failure in patients. Dig Dis. 2015;33(4):464–71.
69. O'Neal JB. The utility of intravenous acetaminophen in the perioperative period. Front Public Health [Internet]. 2013 [cited 2020 Jun 15];1. Available from: https://www.ncbi.nlm.nih.gov/pmc/articles/PMC3854978/.
70. Yeh Y-C, Reddy P. Clinical and economic evidence for intravenous acetaminophen. Pharmacotherapy. 2012;32(6):559–79.
71. Toms L, McQuay HJ, Derry S, Moore RA. Single dose oral paracetamol (acetaminophen) for postoperative pain in adults. Cochrane Database Syst Rev [Internet]. 2008 [cited 2020 Jun 15];2008(4). Available from: https://www.ncbi.nlm.nih.gov/pmc/articles/PMC4163965/.
72. Jibril F, Sharaby S, Mohamed A, Wilby KJ. Intravenous versus oral acetaminophen for pain: systematic review of current evidence to support clinical decision-making. Can J Hosp Pharm. 2015;68(3):238–47.
73. Hu J, Huang D, Li M, Wu C, Zhang J. Effects of a single dose of preoperative pregabalin and gabapentin for acute postoperative pain: a network meta-analysis of randomized controlled trials. J Pain Res. 2018;11:2633–43.
74. Doleman B, Heinink TP, Read DJ, Faleiro RJ, Lund JN, Williams JP. A systematic review and meta-regression analysis of prophylactic gabapentin for postoperative pain. Anaesthesia. 2015;70(10):1186–204.
75. Commissioner O of the. FDA In Brief: FDA requires new warnings for gabapentinoids about risk of respiratory depression. FDA [Internet]. 2019 [cited 2020 Jun 14]. Available from: https://www.fda.gov/

news-events/fda-brief/fda-brief-fda-requires-new-warnings-gabapentinoids-about-risk-respiratory-depression.
76. Maher DP, Chen L, Mao J. Intravenous ketamine infusions for neuropathic pain management: a promising therapy in need of optimization. Anesth Analg. 2017;124(2):661–74.
77. Goswami D, Nisa N, Sharma A, Dadhwal V, Baidya DK, Arora M. Low-dose ketamine for outpatient hysteroscopy: a prospective, randomised, double-blind study. Turk J Anaesthesiol Reanim. 2020;48(2):134–41.
78. Schwenk ES, Viscusi ER, Buvanendran A, Hurley RW, Wasan AD, Narouze S, et al. Consensus guidelines on the use of intravenous ketamine infusions for acute pain management from the American Society of Regional Anesthesia and Pain Medicine, the American Academy of Pain Medicine, and the American Society of Anesthesiologists. Reg Anesth Pain Med. 2018;43(5):456–66.
79. Kaur S, Saroa R, Aggarwal S. Effect of intraoperative infusion of low-dose ketamine on management of postoperative analgesia. J Nat Sci Biol Med. 2015;6(2):378–82.
80. Gorlin AW, Rosenfeld DM, Ramakrishna H. Intravenous sub-anesthetic ketamine for perioperative analgesia. J Anaesthesiol Clin Pharmacol. 2016;32(2):160–7.
81. De Oliveira GS, Castro-Alves LJ, Khan JH, McCarthy RJ. Perioperative systemic magnesium to minimize postoperative pain: a meta-analysis of randomized controlled trials. Anesthesiology. 2013;119(1):178–90.
82. Iseri LT, French JH. Magnesium: nature's physiologic calcium blocker. Am Heart J. 1984;108(1):188–93.
83. Woolf CJ, Thompson SW. The induction and maintenance of central sensitization is dependent on N-methyl-D-aspartic acid receptor activation; implications for the treatment of post-injury pain hypersensitivity states. Pain. 1991;44(3):293–9.
84. Cavalcanti IL, de Lima FLT, da Silva MJS, da Cruz Filho RA, Braga ELC, Verçosa N. Use profile of magnesium sulfate in anesthesia in Brazil. Front Pharmacol [Internet]. 2019 26 [cited 2020 Jun 20];10. Available from: https://www.ncbi.nlm.nih.gov/pmc/articles/PMC6499034/.
85. Albrecht E, Kirkham KR, Liu SS, Brull R. Peri-operative intravenous administration of magnesium sulphate and postoperative pain: a meta-analysis: Peri-operative intravenous magnesium and postoperative pain. Anaesthesia. 2013;68(1):79–90.
86. Rodríguez-Rubio L, Nava E, Del Pozo JSG, Jordán J. Influence of the perioperative administration of magnesium sulfate on the total dose of anesthetics during general anesthesia. A systematic review and meta-analysis. J Clin Anesth. 2017;39:129–38.
87. ASRA News – "Oh Mg!" Magnesium: A Powerful Tool in the Perioperative Setting – American Society of Regional Anesthesia and Pain Medicine [Internet]. [cited 2020 Jun 20]. Available from: https://www.asra.com/asra-news/article/105/oh-mg-magnesium-a-powerful-tool-in-the.
88. Chamaraux-Tran T-N, Piegeler T. The amide local anesthetic lidocaine in cancer surgery-potential anti-metastatic effects and preservation of immune cell function? A narrative review. Front Med (Lausanne). 2017;4:235.
89. Eipe N, Gupta S, Penning J. Intravenous lidocaine for acute pain: an evidence-based clinical update. BJA Educ. 2016;16(9):292–8.
90. Dunn LK, Durieux ME. Perioperative use of intravenous lidocaine. Anesthesiology. 2017;126(4):729–37.
91. Groudine SB, Fisher HA, Kaufman RP, Patel MK, Wilkins LJ, Mehta SA, et al. Intravenous lidocaine speeds the return of bowel function, decreases postoperative pain, and shortens hospital stay in patients undergoing radical retropubic prostatectomy. Anesth Analg. 1998;86(2):235–9.
92. Butterworth JF, Strichartz GR. Molecular mechanisms of local anesthesia: a review. Anesthesiology. 1990;72(4):711–34.
93. Boysen PG, Pappas MM, Evans B. An evidence-based opioid-free anesthetic technique to manage perioperative and periprocedural pain. Ochsner J. 2018;18(2):121–5.
94. Opioids. In: LiverTox: clinical and research information on drug-induced liver injury [Internet]. Bethesda: National Institute of Diabetes and Digestive and Kidney Diseases; 2012 [cited 2020 Jun 25]. Available from: http://www.ncbi.nlm.nih.gov/books/NBK547864/.
95. De Oliveira GS, Castro-Alves LJS, Ahmad S, Kendall MC, McCarthy RJ. Dexamethasone to prevent postoperative nausea and vomiting: an updated meta-analysis of randomized controlled trials. Anesth Analg. 2013;116(1):58–74.
96. Oliveira GSD, Almeida MD, Benzon HT, McCarthy RJ. Perioperative single dose systemic dexamethasone for postoperative pain a meta-analysis of randomized controlled trials. Anesthesiology. 2011;115(3):575–88.
97. Waldron NH, Jones CA, Gan TJ, Allen TK, Habib AS. Impact of perioperative dexamethasone on postoperative analgesia and side-effects: systematic review and meta-analysis. Br J Anaesth. 2013;110(2):191–200.
98. Hans P, Vanthuyne A, Dewandre PY, Brichant JF, Bonhomme V. Blood glucose concentration profile after 10 mg dexamethasone in non-diabetic and type 2 diabetic patients undergoing abdominal surgery. Br J Anaesth. 2006;97(2):164–70.
99. Khalili G, Janghorbani M, Saryazdi H, Emaminejad A. Effect of preemptive and preventive acetaminophen on postoperative pain score: a randomized, double-blind trial of patients undergoing lower extremity surgery. J Clin Anesth. 2013;25(3):188–92.
100. Conrad KA, Fagan TC, Mackie MJ, Mayshar PV. Effects of ketorolac tromethamine on hemostasis in volunteers. Clin Pharmacol Ther. 1988;43(5):542–6.

101. Stephens DM, Richards BG, Schleicher WF, Zins JE, Langstein HN. Is ketorolac safe to use in plastic surgery? A critical review. Aesthet Surg J. 2015;35(4):462–6.
102. McDonald E, Winters B, Nicholson K, Shakked R, Raikin S, Pedowitz DI, et al. Effect of postoperative ketorolac administration on bone healing in ankle fracture surgery. Foot Ankle Int. 2018;39(10):1135–40.
103. McClain K, Williams AM, Yaremchuk K. Ketorolac usage in tonsillectomy and uvulopalatopharyngoplasty patients. Laryngoscope. 2020;130(4):876–9.
104. Kotagal M, Hakkarainen TW, Simianu VV, Beck SJ, Alfonso-Cristancho R, Flum DR. Ketorolac use and postoperative complications in gastrointestinal surgery. Ann Surg. 2016;263(1):71–5.
105. PURLs: less is more when it comes to ketorolac for pain [Internet]. [cited 2020 Jun 25]. Available from: https://www.ncbi.nlm.nih.gov/pmc/articles/PMC6484969/.
106. Jessen Lundorf L, Korvenius Nedergaard H, Møller AM. Perioperative dexmedetomidine for acute pain after abdominal surgery in adults. Cochrane Database Syst Rev. 2016;2:CD010358.
107. Ge D-J, Qi B, Tang G, Li J-Y. Intraoperative dexmedetomidine promotes postoperative analgesia and recovery in patients after abdominal hysterectomy: a double-blind, randomized clinical trial. Sci Rep. 2016;6:21514.
108. Shin H-J, Do S-H, Lee J-S, Kim T-K, Na H-S. Comparison of intraoperative sedation with dexmedetomidine versus propofol on acute postoperative pain in total knee arthroplasty under spinal anesthesia: a randomized trial. Anesth Analg. 2019;129(6):1512–8.
109. Kundra S, Taneja S, Choudhary AK, Katyal S, Garg I, Roy R. Effect of a low-dose dexmedetomidine infusion on intraoperative hemodynamics, anesthetic requirements and recovery profile in patients undergoing lumbar spine surgery. J Anaesthesiol Clin Pharmacol. 2019;35(2):248–53.
110. Whiteman A, Bajaj S, Hasan M. Novel techniques of local anaesthetic infiltration. Contin Educ Anaesth Crit Care Pain. 2011;11(5):167–71.
111. Philippi MT, Kahn TL, Adeyemi TF, Maak TG, Aoki SK. Extracapsular local infiltration analgesia in hip arthroscopy patients: a randomized, prospective study. J Hip Preserv Surg. 2018;5(3):226–32.
112. Greimel F, Maderbacher G, Baier C, Schwarz T, Zeman F, Meissner W, et al. Matched-pair analysis of local infiltration analgesia in total knee arthroplasty: patient satisfaction and perioperative pain management in 846 cases. J Knee Surg. 2019;32(10):953–9.
113. Gan TJ. Poorly controlled postoperative pain: prevalence, consequences, and prevention. J Pain Res. 2017;10:2287–98.
114. Hidalgo DA, Pusic AL. The role of methocarbamol and intercostal nerve blocks for pain management in breast augmentation. Aesthet Surg J. 2005;25(6):571–5.
115. Looke TD, Kluth CT. Effect of preoperative intravenous methocarbamol and intravenous acetaminophen on opioid use after primary total hip and knee replacement. Orthopedics. 2013;36(2):25–32.
116. Aljuhani O, Kopp BJ, Patanwala AE. Effect of methocarbamol on acute pain after traumatic injury. Am J Ther. 2017;24(2):e202–6.
117. DailyMed – LIDODERM- lidocaine patch [Internet]. [cited 2020 Jun 26]. Available from: https://dailymed.nlm.nih.gov/dailymed/drugInfo.cfm?setid=f1c40164-4626-4290-9012-c00e33420a33.
118. Lau LL, Li CY, Lee A, Chan SK. The use of 5% lidocaine medicated plaster for acute postoperative pain after gynecological surgery. Medicine (Baltimore) [Internet]. 2018 [cited 2020 Jun 26];97(39). Available from: https://www.ncbi.nlm.nih.gov/pmc/articles/PMC6181576/.
119. Kwon Y-S, Kim JB, Jung HJ, Koo Y-J, Lee I-H, Im K-T, et al. Treatment for postoperative wound pain in gynecologic laparoscopic surgery: topical lidocaine patches. J Laparoendosc Adv Surg Tech A. 2012;22(7):668–73.
120. Smoker J, Cohen A, Rasouli MR, Schwenk ES. Transdermal lidocaine for perioperative pain: a systematic review of the literature. Curr Pain Headache Rep. 2019;23(12):89.

9 Preoperative Planning of Acute Pain Management in an Academic Ambulatory Surgical Center

Suwarna Anand and Anand M. Prem

Abstract

Optimal pain management is integral to enhanced recovery of patients undergoing ambulatory surgery. Medicare and Medicaid reimbursements which are based on pain management scores and the Hospital Consumer Assessment of Healthcare Providers and Systems (HCAHPS) survey which evaluates performance of US hospitals and used by patients to compare healthcare facilities for their elective surgery have been an added incentive to improve postoperative pain. As a result, understanding the incidence and severity of postsurgical pain is more important now than ever before. The key components that influence the pain management strategies are patient's comorbid conditions, the type of surgery and expected severity of pain, patient's pain tolerance and preferences, the available resources, and the risk-benefit ratio of the technique. This review highlights the significance of preoperative planning in the management of acute pain in an academic ambulatory surgical center.

S. Anand (✉) · A. M. Prem
Department of Anesthesiology, University of Mississippi Medical Center, Jackson, MS, USA
e-mail: sanand2@umc.edu; aprem@umc.edu

Introduction

Ambulatory surgery is coming to the hospital for surgery and leaving within 23 h of surgery. According to the National Center for Health Statistics (NCHS) data in 2010, 48.3 million surgical and nonsurgical procedures were performed [1]. This was made possible in part due to the medical and technological advancements in anesthesia and analgesia.

Multimodal Analgesia as an Essential Part of Enhanced Recovery After Surgery (ERAS) Protocol (2019)

Strategies implemented in ambulatory surgery are intended to increase the cost-effectiveness of surgical procedures, reduce surgical morbidity, decrease length of stay, and prevent readmission. This can lead to reduced risks of hospital-acquired infections, cognitive defects resulting from an unfamiliar environment, thromboembolism associated with immobilization, and the financial burden associated with hospitalization.

Adequate pain control plays a pivotal role in ambulatory surgery. Postoperative pain is a key factor leading to hospital admission or delaying discharge from a day surgery center. It can also cause persisting pain leading to chronic physical disability, delayed functional recovery and psychosocial

K. Rajput et al. (eds.), *Pain Control in Ambulatory Surgery Centers*,
https://doi.org/10.1007/978-3-030-55262-6_9

distress, and metabolic complications. 30–60% of patients still have moderate to severe pain after surgery [2–4]. Challenges associated with good postoperative analgesia are that patients must control their pain by themselves at home and it must be effective, easy, and safe.

Factors predictive of postoperative pain in an ambulatory center are the following:

1. Presence of preoperative pain
2. Patients with low pain threshold
3. Preoperative anxiety and psychological profile
4. Previous experiences with surgery
5. Type of surgery

Preoperative Evaluation

The important aspect of perioperative pain control is preoperative patient evaluation. This involves pain history, physical examination, and an interdisciplinary approach involving surgeon, anesthesiologist, and physical therapy. Patient factors to consider in formulating a plan include the type of surgery, expected severity of postoperative pain, underlying medical conditions (e.g., presence of respiratory or cardiac disease, allergies), the risk-benefit ratio for the available techniques, and patient's preferences or experience with pain.

Pain experience is multifactorial and is based on previous pain experience, patient's tolerance, culture, and behavioral responses. It is essential for the surgeons and anesthesiologist to have a discussion with the patient about what to expect with regard to postoperative pain and the options available.

Communication and patient education plays an essential role in establishing realistic expectations regarding perioperative pain management as well as helping to reduce stress and anxiety, known risk factors for increased pain.

Pain Management in an Ambulatory Setting

Opioids were the commonly used analgesics for perioperative pain control. The perioperative period may be a patient's first exposure to these medications, and indiscriminate prescription can lead to addiction, overdose, and death from the prescribed opioids. With the recognition of the opioid crisis, there has been a paradigm shift in healthcare. It had led to a surge in the multimodal pain control approaches that minimize the need for powerful opioids.

Multimodal analgesia is the use of multiple analgesic techniques simultaneously targeting various pain pathways for the effective management of intraoperative and postoperative pain while reducing drug-related adverse events. This includes the use of analgesics drugs with a different modes of action and side effect profile leading to synergistic effects and minimal side effects.

Multimodal analgesia commences in the preoperative phase. It plays a pivotal role in minimizing the stress response following surgery and avoiding delayed discharge, unplanned hospital admission, or readmission. Optimizing the perioperative use of opioids while minimizing the risk of overdose or relapse is challenging in opioid-tolerant patients. But this can be achieved with multimodal analgesia which can have a positive impact on their recovery [5].

Anesthesiologists have been at the forefront of research addressing the above challenges by developing, exploring, and refining primary therapies, adjuvant medications, regional anesthesia and analgesia techniques, local anesthetic additives, acupuncture, and other alternative therapies, and various combinations of the above.

Premedication

Premedication is a vital component of ambulatory anesthesia. Medication given in the preoperative period can serve various roles including, but not limited to, anxiolysis, preemptive analgesia, and prophylaxis for PONV.

Preemptive analgesia is defined as an antinociceptive treatment that prevents central sensitization of a painful stimulus by blunting the afferent input associated with tissue injury and inflammation [6].

Nonopioid Analgesics: Commonly Used Premedications

The rationale behind combining opioids and nonopioid adjuvants is based on the ability to synergistically modulate pain pathways at central and peripheral sites, thereby enhancing analgesia and decreasing the opioid requirement as well as opioid-related side effects. Though preemptive analgesia with nonopioid analgesics may reduce the opioid requirement, they cannot by themselves provide adequate pain relief. This is particularly relevant in ambulatory surgery where immediate postoperative mobilization is essential.

Acetaminophen

Acetaminophen is the most commonly used analgesic in the perioperative period due to its low incidence of adverse events and few contraindications [8, 9]. The primary analgesic effect of acetaminophen is central through modulation of the central activity of CB1/TRPV1 supraspinal receptors and reinforces the activity of the descending bulbo spinal inhibitory sensory pathway [7] and much less from a peripheral COX inhibition. Several studies have reported that the plasma concentrations of acetaminophen needed to offer a clinical analgesic effect to 50% of the patients (EC_{50} for analgesic effect) were 15–16 mcg/ml, and this was achieved in only 28% of patients who took oral acetaminophen 1 g versus 100% of those who received the same dose intravenously. It was reported that opioids significantly impacted the analgesic effect of the oral acetaminophen by reducing or delaying its absorption and bioavailability [7]. Intravenous administration was shown to be effective in controlling postoperative pain [8, 9].

Nonsteroidal Anti-inflammatory Drugs (NSAIDs)

NSAIDs in perioperative analgesia regimens reduce opioid requirements by 20–30% [10]. In the absence of contraindication, NSAIDs, and COX-2 inhibitors can be used for preemptive analgesia. COX-2 inhibitors have fewer side effects than NSAIDs such as gastric ulceration, renal dysfunction, and perioperative bleeding [11–13].

Dexmedetomidine

Dexmedetomidine is an α2-adrenoreceptor agonist that possesses sedative and anxiolytic properties. Its central antinociceptive activity (mediated by the stimulation of α2-adrenoreceptors located in the dorsal horns of the spinal cord and the locus coeruleus) makes it appealing to use as an analgesic adjuvant [14]. Dexmedetomidine has been reported to delay discharge from PACU because of prolonged sedation [15].

Ketamine

Ketamine is an N-methyl-D-aspartate (NMDA) receptor antagonist that decreases nociceptive and inflammatory pain transmission [16]. It plays a vital role in the control of chronic, cancer, neuropathic, and postsurgical pain. Evidence suggests that ketamine can also exert its analgesic effect by interacting with μ-opioid and δ-opioid receptors [17, 18]. A review article that analyzed the data from 39 RCTs concluded that a subanesthetic dose of intravenous ketamine provides a 40% opioid-sparing effect after a variety of surgical interventions [16].

To make it an effective analgesic, ketamine needs to be used throughout the operation and into the postoperative phase, to reduce sensitization of central and peripheral pathways. Ketamine also reduces postoperative nausea and vomiting. Psychomimetic events (hallucinations, dreams, and diplopia) associated with ketamine has deterred some from administering the drug in the perioperative setting.

Gabapentinoids (Gabapentin and Pregabalin)

Gabapentin is an antiepileptic drug that is commonly used for the treatment of chronic neuropathic pain [19]. Its analgesic properties are mediated by its interaction with α2δ subunits of voltage-gated calcium channels in the central nervous system, decreasing the release of excitatory neurotransmitters. Gabapentinoids are effective in reducing postoperative pain, opioid consumption, and opioid-related adverse effects after surgery [20–23].

Compared with gabapentin, pregabalin has greater potency, better bioavailability, and fewer side effects [24].

A meta-analysis of 55 RCTs concluded that all dosing regimens of pregabalin provided a significant reduction in pain scores and opioid consumption at 2 and 24 h compared to placebo [25]. With 300 mg pregabalin, a statistically significant increase in dizziness and blurred vision was seen [26].

Recent publications have shown that preoperative pregabalin has been effective in reducing anxiety and improving sleep quality [27], in preventing succinylcholine-induced fasciculations and myalgia [28], and in prolonging the duration of spinal anesthesia [14] and peripheral nerve blocks [29].

Dexamethasone

De Oliveira et al. [30] in their meta-analysis of randomized controlled trials of 2500 patients showed that a perioperative single dose of 8–10 mg systemic dexamethasone effectively reduced postoperative pain and opioid consumption. Single-dose glucocorticoid was not associated with increased infection rates or delayed wound healing, and the hyperglycemic response was modest at most [31].

Intermediate doses of dexamethasone (0.11–0.2 mg/kg) have beneficial effects on postoperative pain and a reduction in opioid consumption in addition to decreased nausea and vomiting [32]. The time to peak effect of dexamethasone is 45 min to 1 h. A potential limitation to the preoperative administration of dexamethasone is that it can frequently (50–70%) produce extreme perineal pain when given rapidly in low volumes [33]. This effect can be avoided if the dexamethasone dose is diluted in 50 ml saline solution and infused over 10 min or the dose is given after induction [34].

Lidocaine

Lidocaine possesses adjuvant analgesic properties when administered intravenously. Mechanisms of action include decreased release of proinflammatory cytokines (e.g., interleukin-6, interleukin-8), nuclear factor-kB-modulated downregulation at the mRNA level, and inhibition of NMDA receptors [35].

A 2015 Cochrane review [36] pooled the results of 43 RCTs (1700 patients) comparing intravenous lidocaine to placebo/treatment and concluded that a bolus of lidocaine (100 mg or 1–3 mg/kg) followed by an infusion (1–5 mg/kg/h or 2–4 mg/min) significantly lowers pain scores at 1–4 h and 24 h (but not at 48 h) and decreases perioperative opioid requirements, which was more pronounced in patients undergoing laparoscopic and open abdominal surgery [36]. Lidocaine significantly decreases postoperative nausea and vomiting (PONV) as well as ileus and, as a result, may shorten the length of hospital stay by approximately 8 h [36].

Regional Anesthesia: Component of Multimodal Analgesia

Regional anesthesia is a robust tool in an anesthesiologist's armamentarium to enhance perioperative analgesia and improve patient satisfaction. This has been primarily driven by advancements in technology, improved patient satisfaction, quicker recovery, increased clinician awareness, and enhanced patient safety.

The development and improvement of ultrasound technology has increased safety and efficacy of administration of an enlarging repertoire of medications [37–39] in peripheral nerve blocks. Evidence of improvements in the types of drugs administered and nerve blocking techniques has led to a reduction in the number of complications including nerve and vascular injury, failure of the block, and systemic toxicity.

Regional anesthesia, an important part of multimodal analgesia, has been incorporated in the enhanced recovery after surgery (ERAS) protocols. This has shown to decrease the healthcare cost and enhance patient safety and experience.

Depot Delivery Systems: Intended for Slow and Sustained Release of Local Anesthetic over an Extended Duration

They include liposomal bupivacaine (depobupivacaine), SABER-bupivacaine, bupivacaine collagen matrix, and HTX-011, a combination product of bupivacaine and meloxicam.

Liposomal bupivacaine has a liposomal bilayer that encapsulates bupivacaine and allows its sustained release for up to 72 h after a single use leading to prolonged analgesia. SABER-bupivacaine is another depot formulation of bupivacaine encapsulated in a biodegradable sucrose acetate isobutyrate biolayer.

Bupivacaine is presently the only local anesthetic commercially available using multivesicular encapsulation [40]. Bimodal peaks in concentration have been reported, with initial peaks occurring 1–8 h after drug administration and the second peak occurring 12–36 h later. It can elicit an anesthetic effect lasting for up to 96 h after a single injection. The most common adverse events were considered mild to moderate in severity and included gastrointestinal upset, pyrexia, headache, and pain at the injection site [41–43].

Liposomal bupivacaine is available in vials of 10 and 20 ml with a 13.3 mg/mL formulation for a total of 133 mg and 266 mg per vial, respectively [44]. Currently, the maximum dose per the manufacturer is 266 mg or 20 ml. Liposomal bupivacaine can be used in its undiluted state, or it can be diluted with normal saline or lactated ringers. Drawbacks include high cost, and some encapsulated drugs have been reported to leak secondary to oxidation, hydrolysis, and destabilization of the liposome.

Peripheral nerve blockade can decrease the risk of postoperative nausea/vomiting, altered mental status, and pruritus by reducing the opioid requirement and thus expediting the ambulatory surgical center discharge [45–47].

In a randomized, controlled trial by Apfel and colleagues [48], regional anesthesia in an ambulatory surgery setting has been associated with a relative risk reduction of 77% in postoperative nausea and vomiting, comparable with using quadruple antiemetic therapies.

Regional anesthesia has beneficial effects on perioperative morbidity due to its lower incidence of cardiac dysrhythmias, venous thromboembolic events (VTE), and pulmonary complications postoperatively [49–51].

Orthopedic surgery is one of the most painful and commonly performed surgeries in an ambulatory setting. Hence postoperative pain prevention and treatment are key to the success of an ambulatory procedure.

As per the orthopedic surgery literature, in pediatrics and adults, regional anesthesia was associated with significantly less blood loss, with fewer venous thromboembolisms and respiratory complications [52].

Peripheral nerve block when used as an adjunct to general anesthesia has shown to reduce postoperative hospital admission after ambulatory surgery.

In a randomized, controlled trial of 133 patients undergoing laparoscopic colorectal surgery, spinal anesthesia was associated with reduced early neuroendocrine response (interleukin-6, cortisol, glucose) and morphine requirements when compared with opioid patient-controlled analgesia.

Globally an estimated 10% of the population undergoing procedures and surgery are aged 75 years or older [53]. Elderly population has continued to grow over time with improvement in lifestyle. Regional anesthesia in elderly patients reduces the systemic effects of anesthetic drugs and their potential toxicities.

Adjuvant Drugs

Regional anesthesia has become a cornerstone in modern clinical practice. Adjuvants are medications that work synergistically with local anesthetics to help quicken the onset of action, increase the duration of analgesia, improve the quality of analgesia, and limit potential medication-related adverse effects.

Adjuvants for regional techniques include dexamethasone, alpha-2 agonists such as clonidine and dexmedetomidine, buprenorphine, tramadol, midazolam, neostigmine, epinephrine, sodium bicarbonate, nonsteroidal anti-inflammatory drugs, and NMDA antagonists such as ketamine and magnesium. Opioids are not used as adjuvants for peripheral nerve blocks as there is no evidence of any opioid receptor along the peripheral nerve. Epinephrine, clonidine, and dexmedetomidine are recommended for single-shot block [54, 55]. As the use of adjuvants is currently off-label indication with peripheral nerve blocks, studies are underway to evaluate their safety and efficacy.

Anticoagulation

Despite the benefits of regional anesthesia, it is not safe in patients with comorbidities that lead to chronic use of anticoagulants.

Regional anesthesia in patients on anticoagulants has been evolving. Due to insufficient evidence in the literature regarding peripheral nerve blocks, the American Society of Regional Anesthesia and Pain Medicine (ASRA) recommends similar anticoagulation management for patients undergoing peripheral blocks to those undergoing neuraxial blockade. ASRA recommends using block site compressibility, vascularity, and ramifications of hemorrhage to help guide management of other peripheral blockades [56].

Anticoagulant management is agent-specific, and concomitant use of herbal and over-the-counter products can result in synergistic effects increasing the risk of bleeding. Variability in renal function, advanced age, female gender, inherent coagulopathy, and difficult needle placement can influence the response to anticoagulant and independently increase the risk of hemorrhage. The risk vs benefit profile for altering the anticoagulation regimen for the underlying conditions should be assessed in order to optimize anesthetic management.

Perioperative Pain Management in Patients on Chronic Pain Medications

Acute pain management in patients on medications such as methadone or buprenorphine for chronic pain can be challenging. Methadone and buprenorphine have been used in patients with long-standing pain states and/or substance abuse history. The first step in obtaining a comprehensive history is to establish good communication and trust with these patients. It is also important to be professional, nonjudgmental, and focus on the history of drug dosage, frequency, time of last dose, and any possible illicit drug use.

Methadone is a long-acting opioid, used to treat heroin and other opioid abuse disorders. It is a mu-opioid receptor agonist that reduces craving for opioids, prevents withdrawal symptoms for a very significant period and, by maintaining high levels of opioid tolerance, reduces the euphoric effects of subsequent illicit opioid use [57, 58]. Its half-life is 1 day, and it takes five half-lives for most of the drug to be eliminated. Therefore, it would take 4–5 days for withdrawal symptoms to become evident.

The daily methadone dose should be continued until the day of surgery and in the perioperative period [59]. The correct dose of methadone should be verified with the patient and by the methadone-prescribing clinic. Further, the clinic should be informed of the patient's perioperative requirements of opioids. The most common ratio used to convert methadone from oral to IV form is 2:1, but some may require dose escalation to ratios of 1:1.

Buprenorphine is an opioid with partial agonist at mu-opioid receptors but is a kappa-opioid receptor antagonist with a half-life of 37 h. It is used for both chronic pain and opioid use disorder management and may have an analgesic ceiling. This could be problematic in management of acute pain.

Suboxone is a combination of buprenorphine and naloxone, a mu-opioid antagonist. Naloxone reverses the effects of opioids when the drug is inappropriately crushed for intravenous or intranasal use, which either may result in overdose with respiratory failure [60].

Lembke and colleagues most recently supported continuation of perioperative buprenorphine with evidence from case reports and series [61]. They recommend continuation of buprenorphine in the preoperative period in order to avoid disruption of the existing regimen and exacerbation of the underlying disorder in an unmonitored setting. The recommendations in this section apply to all doses, formulations (not including newly introduced extended-release formulations), surgery types, patient risk levels, and indications for buprenorphine therapy like chronic pain or opioid use disorder.

Percutaneous Peripheral Nerve Stimulation for Acute Postoperative Pain

Peripheral nerve stimulation (PNS) or peripheral neuromodulation has been used for decades to manage chronic pain. The analgesia provided by single and continuous peripheral nerve blocks has fallen short in terms of duration for postoperative pain for different types of surgeries. To overcome this shortcoming, PNS has received FDA approval for management of postoperative pain. Studies include one randomized controlled trial in postamputation pain [62] and multiple case series in axial low back pain [63, 64], acute postoperative pain after rotator cuff surgery [65], total knee arthroplasty [66], and foot surgery [67]. Analgesic benefits up to 12 months [62] and 4 months [63, 64] after extraction of the PNS were noted in postamputation and low back pain patients, respectively.

Ultrasound-guided percutaneous peripheral nerve stimulation has overcome some of the constraints associated with peripheral nerve blocks like limited duration of action (i.e., 3–7 days), a risk of infection, dislodgement of catheter, local anesthetic toxicity, and dense motor/sensory blockade (which may be associated with higher risk of falls or inability to participate in physical therapy maneuvers) [37].

Peripheral neuromodulation systems can be used in both acute and chronic pain management. Some systems have received FDA clearance for the symptomatic relief of acute post-traumatic and postoperative pain and/or chronic, intractable pain involving the back and/or extremities. These systems generally have several components. Several percutaneous lead designs are available. The one indicated for short-term acute pain is insulated, helically coiled, monopolar, and made of stainless steel. The systems designed for long-term use in chronic pain are linear, multipolar, and made of platinum/iridium contacts. These are deployed under ultrasound or nerve stimulation with an introducer needle. They are then stimulated via a battery-powered external pulse generator. Some systems require a small internal programmable generator, but the systems indicated for acute pain do not. These latter systems are approved for up to 60 days of use. An electrical stimulus is delivered to the percutaneous lead. The intensity of the electrical stimulus can be controlled with a handheld remote to elicit distal motor or sensory responses until a comfortable sensation over the region of pain is achieved without producing muscle contractions. The non-IPG lead systems are left in place for up to 60 days and can be removed by gentle external traction. "Gate control" is the proposed theory for PNS analgesia, in which large-diameter myelinated peripheral nerve fibers are electrically activated causing the inhibition of pain signals from the smaller-diameter pain fibers to the central nervous system [68].

Summary

Most of the factors predictive of postoperative pain can be assessed in the preoperative phase with effective and complete evaluation.

Multimodal analgesics less centered on opioids play a vital role in improving postoperative pain and reducing perioperative opioid analgesic use.

Specific analgesic strategy catered to the patient facilitates the smooth intraoperative and postoperative course leading to improved quality of care and shortening time to discharge.

References

1. Hall MJ, Schwartzman A, Zhang J, Liu X. Ambulatory surgery data from hospitals and ambulatory surgery centers: United States, 2010. Natl Health Stat Rep. 2017;102:1–5.
2. McGrath B, Elgendy H, Chung F, et al. Thirty percent of patients have moderate to severe pain 24 hours after ambulatory surgery: a survey of 5,703 patients. Can J Anaesth. 2004;51:886–91.
3. McHugh GA, Thoms GMM. The management of pain following day-case surgery. Anaesthesia. 2002;57:270–5.
4. Sommer M, de Rijke JM, van Kleef M, et al. The prevalence of postoperative pain in a sample of 1490 surgical inpatients. Eur J Anaesthesiol. 2008;25:267–74.
5. Kumar K, Kirksey MA, Duong S, Wu CL. A review of opioid-sparing modalities in perioperative pain management: methods to decrease opioid use postoperatively. Anesth Analg. 2017;125(5):1749–60.
6. Devin CJ, McGirt MJ. Best evidence in multimodal pain management in spine surgery and means of assessing postoperative pain and functional outcomes. J Clin Neurosci. 2015;22(6):930–8.
7. Raffa RB, Pawasauskas J, Pergolizzi JV Jr, et al. Pharmacokinetics of oral and intravenous paracetamol (acetaminophen) when co-administered with intravenous morphine in healthy adult subjects. Clin Drug Investig. 2018;38:259–68.
8. De Oliveira GS Jr, Castro-Alves LJ, McCarthy RJ. Single-dose systemic acetaminophen to prevent postoperative pain: a meta-analysis of randomized controlled trials. Clin J Pain. 2015;31:86–93.
9. McNicol ED, Ferguson MC, Haroutounian S, et al. Single dose intravenous paracetamol or intravenous propacetamol for postoperative pain. Cochrane Database Syst Rev. 2016;(5):CD007126.
10. Dahl V, Raeder JC. Non-opioid postoperative analgesia. Acta Anaesthesiol Scand. 2000;44(10):1191–203.
11. Hegi TR, Bombeli T, Seifert B, et al. Effect of rofecoxib on platelet aggregation and blood loss in gynaecological and breast surgery compared with diclofenac. Br J Anaesth. 2004;92:523–31.
12. Lee A, Cooper MG, Craig JC, et al. Effects of nonsteroidal anti-inflammatory drugs on postoperative renal function in adults with normal renal function. Cochrane Database Syst Rev. 2007;(2):CD002765.
13. Schug SA. The role of COX-2 inhibitors in the treatment of postoperative pain. J Cardiovasc Pharmacol. 2006;47(Suppl 1):S82–6.
14. Chan AK, Cheung CW, Chong YK. Alpha-2 agonists in acute pain management. Expert Opin Pharmacother. 2010;11:2849–68.
15. St-Pierre P, Tanoubi I, Verdonck O, et al. Dexmedetomidine versus remifentanil for monitored anesthesia care during endobronchial ultrasound-guided transbronchial needle aspiration: a randomized controlled trial. Anesth Analg. 2019;128:98–106.
16. Jouguelet-Lacoste J, La Colla L, Schilling D, Chelly JE. The use of intravenous infusion or single dose of low-dose ketamine for postoperative analgesia: a review of the current literature. Pain Med. 2015;16:383–403.
17. Smith DJ, Bouchal RL, deSanctis CA, et al. Properties of the interaction between ketamine and opiate binding sites in vivo and in vitro. Neuropharmacology. 1987;26:1253–60.
18. Pacheco Dda F, Romero TR, Duarte ID. Central antinociception induced by ketamine is mediated by endogenous opioids and μ- and δ-opioid receptors. Brain Res. 2014;1562:69–75.
19. Vorobeychik Y, Gordin V, Mao J, Chen L. Combination therapy for neuropathic pain: a review of current evidence. CNS Drugs. 2011;25:1023–34.
20. Peng PW, Wijeysundera DN, Li CC. Use of gabapentin for perioperative pain control – a meta-analysis. Pain Res Manag. 2007;12:85–92.
21. Alayed N, Alghanaim N, Tan X, Tulandi T. Preemptive use of gabapentin in abdominal hysterectomy: a systematic review and meta-analysis. Obstet Gynecol. 2014;123:1221–9.
22. Zhai L, Song Z, Liu K. The effect of gabapentin on acute postoperative pain in patients undergoing total knee arthroplasty: a meta-analysis. Medicine (Baltimore). 2016;95:e3673.
23. Han C, Li XD, Jiang HQ, Ma JX, Ma XL. The use of gabapentin in the management of postoperative pain after total hip arthroplasty: a meta-analysis of randomised controlled trials. J Orthop Surg Res. 2016;11:79.
24. Dauri M, Faria S, Gatti A, Celidonio L, Carpenedo R, Sabato AF. Gabapentin and pregabalin for the acute post-operative pain management. A systematic-narrative review of the recent clinical evidences. Curr Drug Targets. 2009;10:716–33.
25. Mishriky BM, Waldron NH, Habib AS. Impact of pregabalin on acute and persistent postoperative pain: a systematic review and meta-analysis. Br J Anaesth. 2015;114:10–31.
26. Hetta DF, Mohamed MA, Mohammad MF. Analgesic efficacy of pregabalin in acute postmastectomy pain: placebo-controlled dose ranging study. J Clin Anesth. 2016;34:303–9.
27. Shimony N, Amit U, Minz B, et al. Perioperative pregabalin for reducing pain, analgesic consumption, and anxiety and enhancing sleep quality in elective neurosurgical patients: a prospective, randomized, double-blind, and controlled clinical study. J Neurosurg. 2016;125:1513–22.

28. Srivastava VK, Agrawal S, Nimbhorkar VK, et al. Prophylactic use of pregabalin for prevention of succinylcholine-induced fasciculation and myalgia: a randomized, double-blinded, placebo-controlled study. Braz J Anesthesiol. 2016;66:165–70.
29. Cegin MB, Soyoral L, Yuzkat N, et al. Pregabalin administered as an anxiolytic agent in ultrasound-guided infraclavicular block: a controlled, double-blind, dose-ranging trial. Eur Rev Med Pharmacol Sci. 2016;20:568–74.
30. De Oliveira GS, Almeida MD, Benzon HT, McCarthy RJ. Perioperative single dose systemic dexamethasone for postoperative pain. A meta-analysis of randomized controlled trials. Anesthesiology. 2011;115:575–88.
31. Mathiesen O, Wetterslev J, Kontinen VK, et al. Adverse effects of perioperative paracetamol, NSAIDs, glucocorticoids, gabapentinoids and their combinations: a topical review. Acta Anaesthesiol Scand. 2014;58:1182–98.
32. Karanicolas PJ, Smith SE, Kanbur B, Davies E, Guyatt GH. The impact of prophylactic dexamethasone on nausea and vomiting after laparoscopic cholecystectomy: a systematic review and meta-analysis. Ann Surg. 2008;248:751–62.
33. Neff SP, Stapelberg F, Warmington A. Excruciating perineal pain after intravenous dexamethasone. Anaesth Intensive Care. 2002;30:370–1.
34. Bell A. Preventing perineal burning from i.v. dexamethasone. Oncol Nurs Forum. 1988;15:199.
35. Brinkrolf P, Hahnenkamp K. Systemic lidocaine in surgical procedures: effects beyond sodium channel blockade. Curr Opin Anaesthesiol. 2014;27:420–5.
36. Kranke P, Jokinen J, Pace NL, et al. Continuous intravenous perioperative lidocaine infusion for postoperative pain and recovery. Cochrane Database Syst Rev. 2015;(7):CD009642.
37. Ilfeld BM. Continuous peripheral nerve blocks: an update of the published evidence and comparison with novel, alternative analgesic modalities. Anesth Analg. 2017;124(1):308–35.
38. Ilfeld BM, Grant SA. Ultrasound-guided percutaneous peripheral nerve stimulation for postoperative analgesia: could neurostimulation replace continuous peripheral nerve blocks? Reg Anesth Pain Med. 2016;41:720–2.
39. Ilfeld BM, Meunier MJ, Macario A. Ambulatory continuous peripheral nerve blocks and the perioperative surgical home. Anesthesiology. 2015;123:1224–6.
40. Santamaria CM, Woodruff A, Yang R, et al. Drug delivery systems for prolonged duration local anesthesia. Mater Today. 2017;20:22. https://doi.org/10.1016/j.mattod.2016.11.019.
41. Viscusi ER, Candiotti KA, Onel E, et al. The pharmacokinetics and pharmacodynamics of liposome bupivacaine administered via a single epidural injection to healthy volunteers. Reg Anesth Pain Med. 2012;37:616. https://doi.org/10.1097/AAP.0b013e318269d29e.
42. Hu D, Onel E, Singla N, et al. Pharmacokinetic profile of liposome bupivacaine injection following a single administration at the surgical site. Clin Drug Investig. 2013;33:109. https://doi.org/10.1007/s40261-012-0043-z.
43. Rice D, Heil JW, Biernat L. Pharmacokinetic profile and tolerability of liposomal bupivacaine following a repeated dose via local subcutaneous infiltration in healthy volunteers. Clin Drug Investig. 2017;37:249. https://doi.org/10.1007/s40261-017-0495-2.
44. Pacira Pharmaceuticals, IncExparel (bupivacaine liposomal injection suspension) Pacira Pharmaceuticals, Inc., San Diego; 2018 [Web 5 April 2018]. Available from: www.exparel.com/hcp/prescriptioninformation.pdf.
45. Chou R, Gordon DB, de Leon-Casasola OA, et al. Management of postoperative pain: a clinical practice guideline from the American Pain Society, the American Society of Regional Anesthesia and Pain Medicine, and the American Society of Anesthesiologists' Committee on Regional Anesthesia, Executive Committee, and Administrative Council. J Pain. 2016;17(2):131–57.
46. Hadzic A, Williams BA, Karaca PE, et al. For outpatient rotator cuff surgery, nerve block anesthesia provides superior same-day recovery over general anesthesia. Anesthesiology. 2005;102:1001–7.
47. Brummett CM, Williams BA. Additives to local anesthetics for peripheral nerve blockade. Int Anesthesiol Clin. 2011;49(4):104–16.
48. Apfel CC, Korttila K, Abdalla M, et al. A factorial trial of six interventions for the prevention of postoperative nausea and vomiting. N Engl J Med. 2004;350:2441–51.
49. Chery J, Semaan E, Darji S, et al. Impact of regional versus general anesthesia on the clinical outcomes of patients undergoing major lower extremity amputation. Ann Vasc Surg. 2014;28(5):1149–56.
50. Hausman MS Jr, Jewell ES, Engoren M. Regional versus general anesthesia in surgical patients with chronic obstructive pulmonary disease: does avoiding general anesthesia reduce the risk of postoperative complications? Anesth Analg. 2015;120(6):1405–12.
51. Vadivelu N, Gesquire M, Mitra S, et al. Safety of local anesthesia combined with monitored intravenous sedation for American Society of Anesthesiologists 3 and 4 patients undergoing lower limb-preservation procedures. J Foot Ankle Surg. 2010;49(2):152–4.
52. Stevens RD, Van Gessel E, Flory N, et al. Lumbar plexus block reduces pain and blood loss associated with total hip arthroplasty. Anesthesiology. 2000;93:115–21.
53. He W, Goodkind D, Kowal P. An aging world: 2015. International population reports. Washington, DC: U.S. Government Publishing Office; 2016.
54. Bailard NS, Ortiz J, Flores RA. Additives to local anesthetics for peripheral nerve blocks: evidence, limitations, and recommendations. Am J Health Pharm. 2014;71:373–85.
55. Kirksey MA, Haskins SC, Cheng J, Liu SS. Local anesthetic peripheral nerve block adjuvants for pro-

longation of analgesia: a systematic qualitative review. PLoS One. 2015;10:e0137312.
56. Horlocker TT, Vandermeulen E, Kopp SL, Gogarten W, Leffert LR, Benzon HT. Regional anesthesia in the patient receiving antithrombotic or thrombolytic therapy: American Society of Regional Anesthesia and Pain Medicine evidence-based guidelines (fourth edition). Reg Anesth Pain Med. 2018;43:263–309.
57. Donnadieu S. Use of methadone as analgesic. Ann Med Interne. 2000;151(1):A40–3.
58. Mattick RP, Breen C, Kimber J, Davoli M. Methadone maintenance therapy versus no opioid replacement therapy for opioid dependence. Cochrane Database Syst Rev. 2009;(3):CD002209.
59. Sen S, Arulkumar S, Cornett EM, et al. New pain management options for the surgical patient on methadone and buprenorphine. Curr Pain Headache Rep. 2016;20:16.
60. Olofsen E, van Dorp E, Teppema L, Aarts L, Smith TW, Dahan A, et al. Naloxone reversal of morphine- and morphine-6-glucuronide-induced respiratory depression in healthy volunteers: a mechanism-based pharmacokinetic-pharmacodynamic modeling study. Anesthesiology. 2010;112(6):1417–27.
61. Lembke A, Ottestad E, Schmiesing C. Patients maintained on buprenorphine for opioid use disorder should continue buprenorphine through the perioperative period. Pain Med. 2019;20:425–8.
62. Gilmore C, Ilfeld B, Rosenow J, et al. Percutaneous peripheral nerve stimulation for the treatment of chronic neuropathic postamputation pain: a multicenter, randomized, placebo-controlled trial. Reg Anesth Pain Med. 2019;44:637–45.
63. Gilmore C, Kapural L, McGee M, Boggs J. Percutaneous peripheral nerve stimulation (PNS) for the treatment of chronic low Back pain provides sustained relief. Neuromodulation. 2018;22:615–20.
64. Kapural L, Gilmore C, Chae J, et al. Percutaneous peripheral nerve stimulation for the treatment of chronic low Back pain: two clinical case reports of sustained pain relief. Pain Pract. 2017;18:94–103.
65. Ilfeld B, Finneran J, Gabriel R, et al. Ultrasound-guided percutaneous peripheral nerve stimulation: neuromodulation of the suprascapular nerve and brachial plexus for postoperative analgesia following ambulatory rotator cuff repair. A proof-of-concept. Reg Anesth Pain Med. 2019;44:310.
66. Ilfeld B, Ball S, Gabriel R, et al. A feasibility study of percutaneous peripheral nerve stimulation for the treatment of postoperative pain following total knee arthroplasty. Neuromodulation. 2018;22:653–60.
67. Ilfeld B, Gabriel R, Said E, et al. Ultrasound-guided percutaneous peripheral nerve stimulation. Reg Anesth Pain Med. 2018;43:580–9.
68. Melzack R, Wall PD. Pain mechanisms: a new theory. Science. 1965;150(3699):971.

Part II

Multimodal Analgesia

Comprehensive Pain Management: Opioid-Naïve Versus Opioid-Tolerant Patients

10

Alexander Bautista, Robert Liu, and Jianguo Cheng

Abstract

Management of acute postoperative pain is essential to decrease the risk of developing chronic pain. Inadequate pain control may lead to poor patient outcomes, increased readmission rate, increased healthcare costs, and patient dissatisfaction. The use of opioids has been the mainstay for perioperative pain management. However, there exists a difference on how to approach patients who are opioid naïve and those who are opioid tolerant from prolonged opioid use. It is imperative to identify both of these patients presenting for surgery to be able to appropriately provide adequate analgesia. With the current opioid crisis, it is a challenge in itself to balance and weigh the benefits and risks for continuous opioid use. This chapter aims to provide a narrative review of multimodal approach to perioperative management of opioid-naïve and opioid-tolerant patients.

A. Bautista · R. Liu
Department of Anesthesiology and Perioperative Medicine, University of Louisville, Louisville, KY, USA
e-mail: alexander.bautista@louisville.edu; Robert.liu@louisville.edu

J. Cheng (✉)
Department of Pain Management, Cleveland Clinic Foundation, Cleveland, OH, USA
e-mail: CHENGJ@ccf.org

Introduction

Pain is defined as "an unpleasant sensory and emotional experience associated with actual or potential damage, or described in terms of such damage" [1]. This definition tells us that apart from the sensation of pain, it involves an emotional experience that is unique to an individual. Taking the experiential component of pain as a given, the difference between nociception and pain should be delineated especially in the acute setting, in particular as a result of a surgical procedure. There has been a growing interest in optimizing pain control to facilitate recovery; shorten hospital stays after surgery, trauma, or illness; and reduce complications [2]. However, previous studies have shown that more than 50% of patients undergoing surgery report inadequate pain relief postoperatively [3]. The difficulties in managing these patients may be attributed to challenging clinical scenarios such as chronic pain patients with high tolerance to opioids on top of the metabolic or physical challenges that limit the dosing of pain medications [4]. Hence, identification of an ideal analgesic that is devoid of undesired side effects may prove to be difficult. Even though the progression of acute to chronic pain does not always happen, acute pain should be aggressively treated to minimize the risk of the development of chronic pain.

Managing pain-tolerant patients can be challenging in a healthcare facility such as an

K. Rajput et al. (eds.), *Pain Control in Ambulatory Surgery Centers*,
https://doi.org/10.1007/978-3-030-55262-6_10

Ambulatory Surgery Center (ASC) that offers elective surgical and non-surgical procedures that typically do not require overnight hospital stay. It is important to know that the success of the ASC is dependent on preventing postoperative complications as well as appropriately managing pain.

The goal for managing pain is to establish an appropriate and individualized plan of care. This also entails proper assessment of the patient in pain with accurate monitoring of response to treatment. Recognition of any social, psychiatric, and behavioral issues that may hinder effective pain management should be determined. It is also important to prevent adverse events related to possible opioid withdrawal.

Pathophysiology of Pain and Opioid Tolerance

The pain pathway mediates the transmission of pain signals from nociceptors to somatosensory cortex and the limbic system (Fig. 10.1). Noxious stimuli induce the release of chemicals such as inflammatory cytokines and prostaglandins (PG) from the site of injury [5]. These chemicals activate nociceptors and generate action potentials. These impulses are transmitted via first-order neuron to the dorsal horn of the spinal cord where the first-order neuron synapses with the second-order neuron to relay the signals upon release of glutamate and neuropeptides such as substance P, calcitonin gene-related peptide, cholecystokinin, and brain-derived neurotrophic factor [5]. The second-order neuron crosses over to the contralateral side of the spinal cord via anterior white commissure and ascends to the brainstem and the thalamus of the brain. In the thalamus, the second-order neuron synapses with the third-order neuron. The third-order neuron carries the input to the somatosensory cortex where it is interpreted as pain sensation in terms of spatial distribution, intensity, and characteristics. In the brainstem, collaterals of the spinothalamic projection make synaptic connections in the brachial nucleus which relay the pain information to specific areas of the brain such as the amygdala, the cingulate cortex, and the insular cortex. These brain structures are related to the emotional aspect of pain. Also in the brainstem, collaterals of the spinothalamic projection make synaptic connections with the periaqueductal gray and the

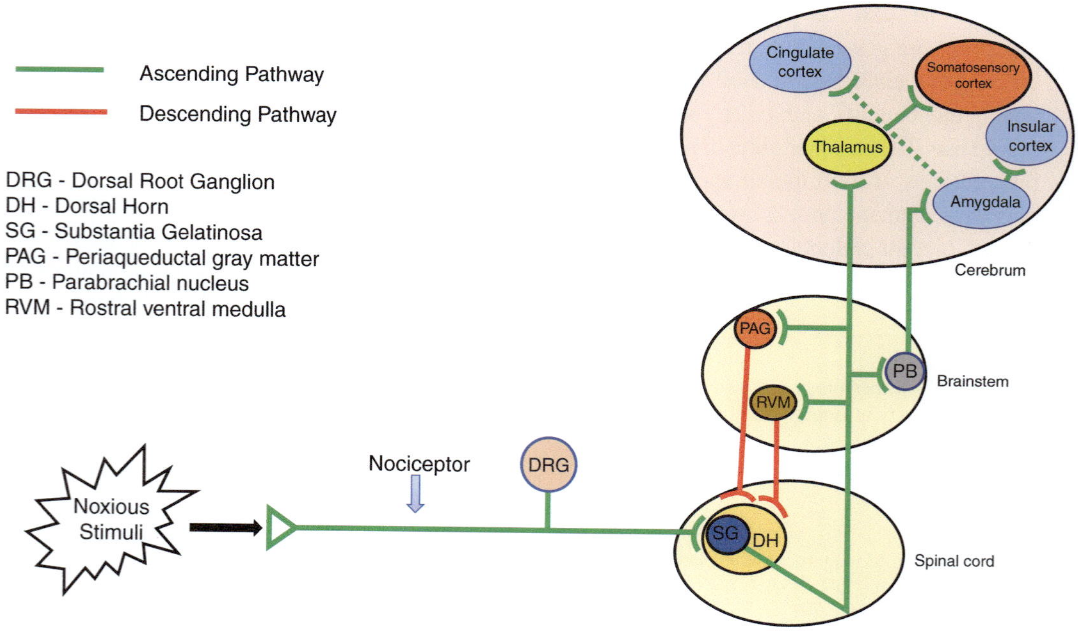

Fig. 10.1 Pain pathway

rostral ventral medulla to regulate descending pathways that can profoundly modulate nociceptive transmission in the dorsal horn of the spinal cord [5]. The periaqueductal gray matter of the midbrain and the nucleus raphe magnus of the medulla are crucial areas of the descending pathway. Neurons stemming from these two areas synapse with serotonergic/noradrenergic neurons and descend to the substantia gelatinosa located within the dorsal horn of the spinal cord. Here, the transmission of pain signal is inhibited by the release of serotonin and noradrenaline which subsequently prevents the release of substance P and stimulates the release of endogenous opioids such as enkephalins, dynorphins, and endorphins [5]. Ultimately, these endogenous opioids inhibit the ascending pain pathway.

Opioids have been found to be effective analgesics to address pain; however, the development of tolerance limits their effectiveness. Opioid tolerance is defined as a decrease in analgesic response with increasing dose or frequency of administration. It is a result of progressive loss of active receptor sites from prolonged agonist exposure. There are two hypotheses on how opioid tolerance develops. One hypothesis is due to the homeostatic upregulation during opioid exposure of non-opioid-dependent ascending pain pathways. The second hypothesis is that adjuvant non-opioid therapies may inhibit ascending non-opioid-dependent pathways and support the clinical observations that monotherapy with opioids often fails [6]. It is also thought that tolerance develops from desensitization and internalization of opioid receptors would result in higher requirements [7].

N-methyl-D-aspartate (NMDA) receptor and the second-messenger protein kinase C (PKC) have both been implicated in the development of opioid tolerance. PKC has been shown to increase opioid regulation of NMDA receptor. This has been supported by animal studies using competitive and non-competitive NMDA receptor antagonists and reversing opioid tolerance [8].

Morphologic changes in the receptive field zone of the spinal cord occur with heightened response in opioid-tolerant patients, relating to both higher requirements of opioids postoperatively and uncontrolled pain [9]. It is therefore imperative that blockade of afferent pain signals before visceral stimulus starts is more beneficial with opioid-tolerant than in opioid-naïve patients [10, 11].

Overview on Multimodal Analgesia

Multimodal analgesia refers to analgesia techniques combining pharmacological (drugs acting on different therapeutic targets), non-pharmacological (cognitive and behavioral therapy, e.g.), and interventional (nerve blocks and nerve catheters) approaches to maximize analgesic effects and minimize adverse/side effects. Acetaminophen, also known as paracetamol in other parts of the world, is a commonly used analgesic. It can be administered preoperatively via oral route or intraoperatively via intravenous route. However, a double-blinded randomized controlled trial by Pearson et al. demonstrated that postoperative plasma levels of acetaminophen were higher if given intravenously during the surgery [12]. Additionally, intravenous acetaminophen has shown to result in higher cerebrospinal fluid levels than oral dosing [13]. The side effects of acetaminophen are rare in recommended dosage of 4000 mg/day, and it has opioid-sparing effects, making it an attractive analgesic option. However, its routine use for opioid sparing and pain care has not been supported by clinical outcomes research [14].

Non-steroidal anti-inflammatory drugs (NSAIDs) are effective analgesics. It can be administered to all patients provided there are no contraindications. The combination of NSAIDs and acetaminophen has demonstrated enhanced pain relief in 17 out of 20 randomized controlled trials [15]. In addition, NSAID use has been shown to reduce opioid consumption and speed up the postoperative recovery compared with opioid-based analgesia after laparoscopic procedures [16].

Gabapentinoids include gabapentin and pregabalin. They can be used as part of the multimodal analgesic approach as well. Preoperative administration of gabapentinoids has demonstrated improved postoperative pain control. In addition, patients on gabapentinoids postoperatively had decreased morphine consumption [17]. Hence, continuation of gabapentinoids for 2 weeks postoperatively has been suggested [17]. However, healthcare providers must consider the side effects (i.e., dizziness and sedation) and the patient risk factors (i.e., renal dysfunction) prior to prescribing gabapentinoids. A recent systematic review concluded that preoperative use of gabapentinoids was able to reduce postoperative pain, total morphine consumption, and morphine-related complications following spine surgery [18].

Dexamethasone, a glucocorticoid, has multiple positive effects such as anti-inflammation, pain management, and antiemetic [19, 20]. It is frequently used intraoperatively due to its antiemetic and analgesic effects [21]. It has shown to reduce "postoperative pain and time to discharge readiness" [22]. Given the known benefits, it is an important part of multimodal analgesic regimen.

Ketamine, an NMDA antagonist, at subanesthetic doses provides pain relief [21]. Administration of ketamine has shown to decrease early (~4 h) and late (24–72 h) pain scores by 37.5% and 25%, respectively [20]. Moreover, it decreases opioid requirements, opioid-induced hyperalgesia, and the incidence of postsurgical pain [23]. These benefits are especially helpful in patients who are opioid tolerant. However, the side effects (i.e., nystagmus, hallucinations, unpleasant dreams, and psychiatric disturbances) are a limiting factor. Therefore, patient selection and procedure-specific administration of ketamine are vital [23]. A systematic review of a large number of studies concluded that perioperative intravenous ketamine probably reduces postoperative analgesic consumption and pain intensity. Results were consistent in different operation types or timing of ketamine administration and by higher and lower pain intensity. In addition, perioperative intravenous ketamine probably reduces postoperative nausea and vomiting by a small extent of arguable clinical relevance. Central nervous system (CNS) adverse events were little different with ketamine or control [24].

Central-acting alpha-2 agonist like dexmedetomidine is a promising non-opioid analgesic option. It has been shown to reduce intra- and postoperative opioid requirement coupled with a decrease in general anesthetic use [25, 26]. Dexmedetomidine can be administered intravenously, intramuscularly, and orally. Its various routes of administration make it an attractive option in children and patients without intravenous access. Despite all the benefits, dexmedetomidine has potential side effects such as bradycardia and hypotension which must be taken into consideration prior to administration.

In addition to the analgesics discussed above, regional anesthetic techniques are a crucial part of the analgesic armamentarium. Regional anesthesia offers significant intra- and postoperative pain relief. It also reduces opioid consumption and associated side effects. Regional anesthesia consists of administering local anesthetics via single-shot perineural injections and/or continuous perineural catheter infusions. Ideally, regional anesthetic procedures are performed preoperatively and with ultrasound guidance to decrease the opioid requirements and provide prolonged duration of pain relief. However, both the patient and the caretaker must be educated about the potential self-harm that can result with an insensate limb before getting discharged.

Upper Extremity Surgery

Shoulder surgery pain can be managed with an interscalene (IS) nerve block. This peripheral nerve block almost always results in ipsilateral phrenic nerve paralysis. Hence, caution must be taken in patient selection. Patients with chronic obstructive pulmonary disease, obstructive sleep apnea, and other diseases that impair the respiratory function are advised to avoid IS nerve block. Alternatively, the combination of supraclavicular (SC) and axillary nerve block can provide equal analgesic efficacy with less risk of hemidiaphragmatic paresis.

Peripheral nerve block targeting the axillary and musculocutaneous nerve provides excellent analgesia for forearm and hand surgeries without general anesthesia. Bier block is an alternate option. However, it has been associated with rare but severe side effects such as local anesthetic systemic toxicity, seizures, and cardiac arrest.

Lower Extremity Surgery

The sciatic nerve block provides analgesia to the hamstring muscles, posterior aspect of the knee, and down to the toes except the medial aspect of the leg and foot. The femoral nerve block provides analgesia of the anteromedial aspect of the thigh down to the medial aspect of the ankle. It is often performed to supplement sciatic nerve block to provide complete anesthesia of the lower leg and ankle. The fascia iliaca compartment block also provides magnificent analgesia for procedures involving the hip, knee, and foot. The popliteal fossa block is performed to anesthetize the lower limb below the knee except the medial aspect of the leg and foot. All the above blocks provide both sensory and motor blockade. Alternatively, adductor canal block of the saphenous nerve provides anesthesia to the medial leg and foot with minimal motor blockade. One of the concerns with lower limb blocks is delayed mobility or impaired proprioception possibly resulting in falls. This dilemma can be mitigated by reducing the concentration of the local anesthetic or selecting peripheral nerve blocks that have minimal motor blockade effects.

Trunk Surgery

Pain related to surgeries involving the chest wall can be managed with epidural or paravertebral block. However, these treatment options are sometimes contraindicated or are limited by coagulopathy. Erector spinae plane block is an alternative option. The advantages of this procedure include no contraindication with coagulopathy, improved analgesic efficacy, and low complication risk [27]. Lower abdominal postoperative pain can be treated with transversus abdominis plane (TAP) block. However, injecting local anesthetic within the correct plane with ultrasound guidance is key to achieving optimal pain control.

Perineural Catheters

Single-shot peripheral nerve blocks have limited duration of localized pain relief. In order to lengthen the duration of analgesia, a continuous infusion of local anesthetic via catheters can be implemented. The prolonged pain control can promote postoperative mobilization and increase patient satisfaction [28, 29]. Patients may need rescue opioid prescriptions with written instructions about catheter removal and healthcare provider contact information should they have any questions.

Opioid-Naïve Versus Opioid-Tolerant Patients

There are two subsets of patients presenting for surgery, the opioid-naïve and the opioid-tolerant patients. Opioid-naïve patients are those who have not previously taken an opioid medication or has not been taking opioid medication on a regular basis. Patients who are already taking chronic opioid prescription who may or may not have tolerance to the analgesic properties of opioids are labeled as opioid tolerant. Both of these patients who present for surgery have differences in their analgesic requirements.

Opioid-tolerant patients seeking elective operations may require significant dose escalations after surgery. These patients may confer tolerance to usual analgesics leading to inadequate pain control and disproportionate reports of pain. Opioid-tolerant patients should not be wrongly labeled as drug-seeking. Still, opioids remain the mainstay for perioperative pain management due to their efficacy, familiarity, accessibility, and wide range of available formulations to providers [30]. A growing body of literature supports that chronic opioid use also predisposes to immediate postoperative complications such as infection and impaired wound healing [31].

Table 10.1 Summary of perioperative consideration for opioid-tolerant and opioid-naïve patients

Preoperative considerations
Documentation of drug abuse history with underlying psychological comorbidities
Recognizing signs and symptoms of opioid misuse and opioid withdrawal
Discussion of expectations and anticipation of post-procedure level of pain
Discussion of multimodal analgesia regimen including regional anesthetic techniques for pain control
Discussion of opioid-tapering plan
Discussion of potential post-procedure hospital admission for uncontrolled pain
Continue chronic opioid medications including the morning dose prior to procedure
Consider continuing buprenorphine in patients with OUD in the perioperative period
Intraoperative considerations
Select opioids specific to procedure for short-term and long-term pain control
Titrate opioid dose to patient's requirement to achieve adequate pain control
Target different mechanisms using multimodal analgesic approach (i.e., dexmedetomidine, lidocaine, ketamine, and magnesium sulfate, clonidine, etc.)
Include wound infiltration with local anesthetic as adjunct pain management
Postoperative considerations
Increased opioid requirement and duration of treatment in opioid-tolerant patients
Utilization of patient-controlled analgesia (PCA) for breakthrough pain and opioid withdrawal in patients with oral restrictions
Regional anesthesia as adjunct pain management if not performed preoperatively
Rescue opioid prescriptions with written instructions about peripheral nerve catheter removal and healthcare provider contact information
Pharmacokinetics, pharmacodynamics, drug-drug interactions, and potential risks for cardiorespiratory depression in patients on methadone or buprenorphine
Follow-up with addiction specialist for patients on maintenance therapy (i.e., buprenorphine, methadone) for addiction

More than the opioid-naïve patients, opioid-tolerant patients who have acute pain postoperatively are prone to under treatment of pain due to stigma or bias. Hence, it is necessary to have a strategy on how to approach these patients before surgery at the ASC (Table 10.1).

Preoperative Evaluation and Identification of Risk

The goal of preoperative evaluation is to identify risk factors and reduce the patient's surgical and anesthetic perioperative morbidity and mortality [32]. During this time, the physician's responsibility is to take them through the surgical continuum, also trying to facilitate referrals to providers who can help in the optimization of these patients. Germane to the visit is to identify patients who are on medically directed opioid therapy and patients with substance use disorders, including opioid use disorder (OUD). Preoperative considerations should include education in weaning off opioids, use of multimodal regimen, and identifying patients with OUD history and those who have underlying psychological comorbidities [33]. It is important to recognize signs and symptoms for OUD and opioid withdrawal at this time. It is imperative to obtain a comprehensive assessment including history and physical examination and review diagnostic studies. Preoperative opioid misuse and opioid-tolerant patients are associated with prolonged hospital length of stay and increased resource utilization [34]. A perioperative plan on managing pain for both patients should be underway. A review of effective pain management strategies from previous procedures should be documented. Discussion on analgesic strategies, especially the use of multimodal anesthesia, should be explained to patient that include regional techniques when suitable, patient-controlled analgesia and the use of opioid-sparing medications such as acetaminophen, NSAIDs, or COX-2 inhibitors as preoperative medication. There should be a documentation of the treatment plan with a written opioid pain care agreement with patients [34, 35]. More importantly, patients should be reassured that despite a previous or an ongoing history of opioid dependency, effective pain control is an achievable goal and assurance that relapses and withdrawals will be minimized [34]. During the preoperative assessment, discussion should be made of expectations and anticipated level of pain associated with the procedure including perceptions from past surgical experiences.

There is no consensus about whether patients with OUD should discontinue buprenorphine therapy before elective surgery. Adequate pain control was reported in five patients maintained on buprenorphine perioperatively and given supplemental opioids as needed for breakthrough pain [36]. A retrospective cohort study of 22 patients presenting for surgery and taking buprenorphine did not show significant difference in outcomes [37]. Half of the patients were maintained on buprenorphine, and the remainder had their buprenorphine doses held postoperatively. Pain control was similar between groups on postoperative day 1. It was concluded that buprenorphine can be continued perioperatively and co-administered opioid agonists can effectively treat acute pain. We recommend a team approach to this complex and challenging population of patients, by including surgeons, anesthesiologist, pain physician, addiction specialists, and behavioral health professionals in the decision-making process.

Intraoperative Considerations

There is a paucity of data regarding the ideal opioid for intraoperative use. Opioid-naïve patients usually would require a smaller dose of opioids in comparison to opioid-tolerant patients in achieving adequate pain control. The anesthesia provider's responsibility is to select the opioid and titrate the doses per demand. The dosage and requirements vary in different clinical settings and are usually guided by heart rate, pupil dilation, blood pressure, and patient movement and most recently by analgesia nociception index monitoring [34, 38]. Regional anesthesia, local anesthetics, wound infiltration, and subanesthetic doses of ketamine have been shown to be helpful in reducing intraoperative opioid requirements and improved pain scores [34, 39].

The analgesic regimen should be tailored to each opioid-naïve or opioid-tolerant patient. Patients who are on chronic opioid regimen should be allowed to continue taking their medications up until the time of surgery, including their morning dose. Multimodal analgesia as discussed above should be employed while taking into account and understanding the type of pain and the need to target multiple mechanisms along the pain pathway to achieve synergistic effects with the different classes of analgesics.

Postoperative Considerations

The duration of postoperative treatment has been found to be three times longer in opioid-tolerant patients compared with opioid-naïve patients [40]. Opioid-tolerant patients have fourfold increase in requirements in comparison with opioid-naïve patients [34]. If regional anesthesia was not performed preoperatively, it may have some utility in reducing opioid consumption after surgery. However, in opioid-tolerant patient, the baseline opioid requirement should be taken into consideration to avoid withdrawal symptoms. The use of patient-controlled analgesia (PCA) may be helpful to address breakthrough pain and opioid withdrawal especially if they cannot take oral medications. Although opioid withdrawal may not be life-threatening, it can be unpleasant. But as soon as their condition improves, transition to oral opioids should be continued upon discharge from ASC. For some patients who are on maintenance therapy for addiction with either methadone or buprenorphine, it is important to be aware of their complex pharmacokinetics and pharmacodynamics, its drug-drug interaction, and potential risk for cardiorespiratory depression [41]. It is oftentimes necessary to seek recommendations on discharge regimens from physicians who are experienced in pain management since doses may exceed many surgeons' comfort levels.

Summary

It could not be overemphasized that uncontrolled postoperative pain can result in significant morbidity and mortality. Opioid-tolerant patients presenting for a procedure at an ASC may result in unanticipated admission if their pain is poorly controlled. With advances in surgical procedures, improvements in analgesia specific to procedure are evolving to meet the demands of optimal postoperative pain control. There is no single medication or technique that provides ideal pain relief; instead, a combination of systemic, local, and regional techniques utilizing non-opioids, opioids, and local anesthetics will result in the best patient outcome.

References

1. International Association for the Study of Pain. 2012. Available from: http://www.iasp-pain.org/Taxonomy#Pain
2. Tighe P, Buckenmaier CC 3rd, Boezaart AP, Carr DB, Clark LL, Herring AA, et al. Acute pain medicine in the United States: a status report. Pain Med. 2015;16(9):1806–26.
3. Joshi GP, Ogunnaike BO. Consequences of inadequate postoperative pain relief and chronic persistent postoperative pain. Anesthesiol Clin North Am. 2005;23(1):21–36.
4. Gandhi K, Heitz JW, Viscusi ER. Challenges in acute pain management. Anesthesiol Clin. 2011;29(2):291–309.
5. Schaible HG, Richter F. Pathophysiology of pain. Langenbeck's Arch Surg. 2004;389(4):237–43.
6. Goldberg JS. Chronic opioid therapy and opioid tolerance: a new hypothesis. Pain Res Treat. 2013;2013:407504.
7. Mehta V, Langford RM. Acute pain management for opioid dependent patients. Anaesthesia. 2006;61(3):269–76.
8. Herman BH, Vocci F, Bridge P. The effects of NMDA receptor antagonists and nitric oxide synthase inhibitors on opioid tolerance and withdrawal. Medication development issues for opiate addiction. Neuropsychopharmacology. 1995;13(4):269–93.
9. Dubner R. Pain and hyperalgesia following tissue injury: new mechanisms and new treatments. Pain. 1991;44(3):213–4.
10. Woolf CJ. Recent advances in the pathophysiology of acute pain. Br J Anaesth. 1989;63(2):139–46.
11. de Leon-Casasola O, Yarussi A. Pathophysiology of opioid tolerance and clinical approach to the opioid-tolerant patient. Curr Rev Pain. 2000;4(3):203–5.
12. Brett CN, Barnett SG, Pearson J. Postoperative plasma paracetamol levels following oral or intravenous paracetamol administration: a double-blind randomised controlled trial. Anaesth Intensive Care. 2012;40(1):166–71.
13. Lachiewicz PF. The role of intravenous acetaminophen in multimodal pain protocols for perioperative orthopedic patients. Orthopedics. 2013;36(2 Suppl):15–9.
14. Wasserman I, Poeran J, Zubizarreta N, Babby J, Serban S, Goldberg AT, et al. Impact of intravenous acetaminophen on perioperative opioid utilization and outcomes in open colectomies: a claims database analysis. Anesthesiology. 2018;129(1):77–88.
15. Ong CK, Seymour RA, Lirk P, Merry AF. Combining paracetamol (acetaminophen) with nonsteroidal anti-inflammatory drugs: a qualitative systematic review of analgesic efficacy for acute postoperative pain. Anesth Analg. 2010;110(4):1170–9.
16. White PF, Sacan O, Tufanogullari B, Eng M, Nuangchamnong N, Ogunnaike B. Effect of short-term postoperative celecoxib administration on patient outcome after outpatient laparoscopic surgery. Can J Anaesth. 2007;54(5):342–8.
17. Schmidt PC, Ruchelli G, Mackey SC, Carroll IR. Perioperative gabapentinoids: choice of agent, dose, timing, and effects on chronic postsurgical pain. Anesthesiology. 2013;119(5):1215–21.
18. Liu B, Liu R, Wang L. A meta-analysis of the preoperative use of gabapentinoids for the treatment of acute postoperative pain following spinal surgery. Medicine (Baltimore). 2017;96(37):e8031.
19. Helander EM, Menard BL, Harmon CM, Homra BK, Allain AV, Bordelon GJ, et al. Multimodal analgesia, current concepts, and acute pain considerations. Curr Pain Headache Rep. 2017;21(1):3.
20. Kaye AD, Cornett EM, Helander E, Menard B, Hsu E, Hart B, et al. An update on nonopioids: intravenous or oral analgesics for perioperative pain management. Anesthesiol Clin. 2017;35(2):e55–71.
21. Colin B, Gan TJ. Cancer recurrence and hyperglycemia with dexamethasone for postoperative nausea and vomiting prophylaxis: more moot points? Anesth Analg. 2014;118(6):1154–6.
22. De Oliveira GS Jr, Almeida MD, Benzon HT, McCarthy RJ. Perioperative single dose systemic dexamethasone for postoperative pain: a meta-analysis of randomized controlled trials. Anesthesiology. 2011;115(3):575–88.
23. Laskowski K, Stirling A, McKay WP, Lim HJ. A systematic review of intravenous ketamine for postoperative analgesia. Can J Anaesth. 2011;58(10):911–23.
24. Brinck EC, Tiippana E, Heesen M, Bell RF, Straube S, Moore RA, et al. Perioperative intravenous ketamine for acute postoperative pain in adults. Cochrane Database Syst Rev. 2018;12:CD012033.
25. Unlugenc H, Gunduz M, Guler T, Yagmur O, Isik G. The effect of pre-anaesthetic administration of intravenous dexmedetomidine on postoperative pain in patients receiving patient-controlled morphine. Eur J Anaesthesiol. 2005;22(5):386–91.
26. Tufanogullari B, White PF, Peixoto MP, Kianpour D, Lacour T, Griffin J, et al. Dexmedetomidine infusion during laparoscopic bariatric surgery: the effect on recovery outcome variables. Anesth Analg. 2008;106(6):1741–8.
27. Kot P, Rodriguez P, Granell M, Cano B, Rovira L, Morales J, et al. The erector spinae plane

block: a narrative review. Korean J Anesthesiol. 2019;72(3):209–20.
28. Mulroy MF, McDonald SB. Regional anesthesia for outpatient surgery. Anesthesiol Clin North Am. 2003;21(2):289–303.
29. Little K, Pillai A, Fazzi U, Storey N. Local anaesthetic infusion with elastomeric pump after arthroscopic subacromial decompression. Ann R Coll Surg Engl. 2007;89(4):410–3.
30. Maremmani I, Gerra G, Ripamonti IC, Mugelli A, Allegri M, Vigano R, et al. The prevention of analgesic opioids abuse: expert opinion. Eur Rev Med Pharmacol Sci. 2015;19(21):4203–6.
31. Gulur P, Nelli AH. The opioid-tolerant patient: opioid optimization. J Arthroplast. 2020;35:S50.
32. Apfelbaum JL, Connis RT, Nickinovich DG, Committee on Standards and Practice Parameters; American Society of Anesthesiologists Task Force on Preanesthesia Evaluation, et al. Practice advisory for preanesthesia evaluation: an updated report by the American Society of Anesthesiologists Task Force on Preanesthesia Evaluation. Anesthesiology. 2012;116(3):522–38.
33. Vetter TR, Kain ZN. Role of the perioperative surgical home in optimizing the perioperative use of opioids. Anesth Analg. 2017;125(5):1653–7.
34. Coluzzi F, Bifulco F, Cuomo A, Dauri M, Leonardi C, Melotti RM, et al. The challenge of perioperative pain management in opioid-tolerant patients. Ther Clin Risk Manag. 2017;13:1163–73.
35. Devin CJ, Lee DS, Armaghani SJ, Bible J, Shau DN, Martin PR, et al. Approach to pain management in chronic opioid users undergoing orthopaedic surgery. J Am Acad Orthop Surg. 2014;22(10):614–22.
36. Kornfeld H, Manfredi L. Effectiveness of full agonist opioids in patients stabilized on buprenorphine undergoing major surgery: a case series. Am J Ther. 2010;17(5):523–8.
37. Macintyre PE, Russell RA, Usher KA, Gaughwin M, Huxtable CA. Pain relief and opioid requirements in the first 24 hours after surgery in patients taking buprenorphine and methadone opioid substitution therapy. Anaesth Intensive Care. 2013;41(2):222–30.
38. Daccache G, Jeanne M, Fletcher D. The analgesia nociception index: tailoring opioid administration. Anesth Analg. 2017;125(1):15–7.
39. Mitra S, Sinatra RS. Perioperative management of acute pain in the opioid-dependent patient. Anesthesiology. 2004;101(1):212–27.
40. de Leon-Casasola OA, Myers DP, Donaparthi S, Bacon DR, Peppriell J, Rempel J, et al. A comparison of postoperative epidural analgesia between patients with chronic cancer taking high doses of oral opioids versus opioid-naive patients. Anesth Analg. 1993;76(2):302–7.
41. Cornett EM, Kline RJ, Robichaux SL, Green JB, Anyama BC, Gennuso SA, et al. Comprehensive perioperative management considerations in patients taking methadone. Curr Pain Headache Rep. 2019;23(7):49.

Opioid Use in the Treatment of Pain States

11

Ethan Williamson, Kelley L. Sharp, and Steven D. Waldman

Abstract

Opioid medications are used ubiquitously in the treatment of moderate and severe pain. They are a safe, convenient, and reliable method used to alleviate pain related to cancer and should be considered first-line therapies. This chapter will discuss safe prescribing guidelines, practical applications of opioid medications, common medications used, strategies for the management of adverse effects, and methods of effectively achieving optimal analgesia in patients suffering from pain related to cancer. It will also offer more nuanced recommendations of treatment as they may relate to specific subpopulations of patients and specific medications used in their treatment.

Introduction

Every year millions of people are diagnosed with cancer. Of those diagnosed with cancer, 66% will survive for at least 5 years, and 40% will live more than 10 years after their initial diagnoses [1, 2]. Pain is the most common symptom of cancer [3], reported in 59% of patients undergoing cancer treatment, in 64% of patients with advanced disease, and in 33% of patients after treatment concludes [4–6]. Additionally, pain is one of the symptoms that patients fear most.

More than three decades have passed since the WHO guidelines for cancer pain relief were published, but significant inadequacies remain in the relief of cancer-related pain. It is reported that more than one third of cancer patients suffering from pain are undertreated likely due to inadequate attention to pain during treatment and delayed access to opioid medications [7, 8]. Uncontrolled pain can lead to significant morbidity for cancer patients, resulting in physical disabilities, emotional distress, and a reduced quality of life.

As such, improving the patient experience with cancer-related pain is of significant importance. Proper attention must be given to the patient's expressed needs, goals of care, and physical condition so that appropriate measures are taken to ensure optimal pain control while minimizing adverse effects experienced by the patient [9].

Opioid analgesics have been, and continue to be, a safe and effective tool to manage chronic cancer pain. They are broadly used for the reduction of cancer-related pain due to their known safety, ease of dose titration, multiple routes of

E. Williamson · S. D. Waldman (✉)
University of Missouri – Kansas City School of Medicine, Kansas City, MO, USA
e-mail: waldmans@umkc.edu

K. L. Sharp
Frank H. Netter School of Medicine – Quinnipiac University, North Haven, CT, USA

K. Rajput et al. (eds.), *Pain Control in Ambulatory Surgery Centers*,
https://doi.org/10.1007/978-3-030-55262-6_11

administration, reliability, and effectiveness for various types of pain. However, it is important to note that opioids are potential drugs of abuse with significant public health consequences when prescribed irresponsibly.

This chapter will cover the use of opioids in the treatment of pain related to cancer to provide optimal analgesia as well as discuss safe prescribing strategies and methods to minimize adverse effects from medications prescribed.

Opioid Drugs Commonly Used for Management of Cancer Pain

Opioids bind mu-, kappa-, and delta-opioid receptors which elicit their systemic and local effects. These receptors are present in varying concentrations throughout the body, leading to different effects based on their locations.

Opioids are classically divided by their effect on the mu-opioid receptor which can be pure agonism, agonist-antagonist (mixed action), or pure antagonism (Table 11.1). While agonist and mixed action drugs provide analgesia when given in appropriate doses, mu receptor antagonists reverse this process, have no intrinsic analgesic effect, and are instead used to treat opioid overdoses.

Table 11.1 Classification of opioids

Type of opioid	Medications	Notes
Pure agonists	Codeine Hydrocodone Dihydrocodeine Morphine Hydromorphone Fentanyl Oxycodone Oxymorphone Levorphanol Methadone Meperidine	Cornerstone of treatment for moderate to severe cancer pain No analgesic ceiling effect; as dose is increased, analgesic effect will increase until proper analgesia is achieved or dose escalation is limited by adverse effects Methadone must be used with caution and only by those experienced in its use and knowledgeable of its variable half-life, unpredictable potency, and QTc-prolonging effect
Mixed agonist-antagonists	Buprenorphine Butorphanol Nalbuphine Dezocine Pentazocine	Include partial agonists and drugs with agonist effects on one receptor and antagonist effects on another receptor May induce acute abstinence syndrome in patients with physical dependence to pure opioid agonists Most have ceiling effect for analgesia
Mixed-mechanism drugs	Tramadol Tapentadol	Have agonist actions at the mu receptor and block monoamine re-uptake

Morphine

Morphine is considered to be the standard for comparison in the treatment of moderate to severe cancer pain; however, the superiority of morphine when compared to other commonly used mu receptor agonists (such as oxycodone, oxymorphone, or fentanyl) in terms of both efficacy and tolerability has not been demonstrated [10–13]. As such, it should not be considered the drug of choice, but rather one of many reasonable choices that may be used to treat cancer pain.

Morphine is both a mu-opioid receptor agonist and a weak agonist of the kappa receptor and is known for its relatively short half-life of 1.5–4 hours and a duration of analgesia of between 3 and 7 hours. It is available in a wide array of formulations including instant- and extended-release varieties with varying routes of administration including parenteral, oral, and rectal [14].

All formulations of morphine are hepatically metabolized and renally excreted. Morphine yields two active metabolites after hepatic processing, morphine-3-glucuronide (M3G) and morphine-6-glucuronide (M6G) [15]. There is some data from limited human studies to suggest that the M6G metabolite may contribute to the drug's overall analgesic effect [16].

Special dosing considerations should be taken for patients who accumulate idiosyncratically high levels of morphine metabolites. The presence of excessive metabolite collection may occur in patients with renal disease or in patients with largely unknown genetic variations. If metabolites accumulate, the drug can exhibit unexpected and potentially harmful potency, as well as significant adverse effects. Morphine should be administered with caution in the setting of renal insufficiency and may not be the preferred opioid if kidney function is anticipated to decline [17].

Morphine's various routes of administration and modified-release formulations allow for convenient once- or twice-daily dosing in most patients. Oral administration is the preferred route for most patients who are able tolerate PO intake out of convenience. In opioid-naïve patients, a starting dose of 5–15 mg of short-acting morphine sulfate given orally is recommended. Patients who present with severe pain requiring urgent analgesia should receive parenteral opioids, generally through intravenous or subcutaneous delivery mechanisms. The equianalgesic dose of parenteral morphine is one third that of the oral dose. When using parenteral routes of administration, an initial dose of 2–5 mg of morphine sulfate or equivalent is recommended in the opioid-naïve patient.

Oxycodone, Hydrocodone, Hydromorphone, and Oxymorphone

Similar to morphine, oxycodone, hydrocodone, hydromorphone, and oxymorphone all have short half-lives and are available in numerous formulations, including modified-release variants, allowing for more convenient dosing.

Oxycodone produces agonistic effects on the mu-, delta-, and kappa-opioid receptors [18]. This interaction with several receptors may suggest a theoretical advantage, but clinical studies have failed to identify differences in efficacy or tolerability when oxycodone is compared to morphine or other pure mu receptor agonists. Oxycodone provides overall similar levels of analgesia with comparable adverse effects when compared to morphine and other pure mu agonists and can be viewed as interchangeable when considering which opioid to initiate [19].

Hydromorphone is primarily a mu-opioid receptor agonist, but it also exhibits weak delta-opioid receptor agonism. It is available in several dosage forms including an oral liquid formulation, immediate- and modified-release tablets, as a suppository, and as a solution for intravenous or subcutaneous use. The extended modified-release variant of hydromorphone is available in strengths of 8, 12, and 16 mg and is dosed once daily [4, 18]. A hydromorphone solution of 10 mg/ml is commercially available and facilitates administration of high doses when necessary for adequate pain control.

Hydromorphone is a preferred agent for use in patients with renal insufficiency as its active metabolites maintain lower concentrations than the active metabolites of morphine which may lead to a reduction in adverse effects in this population (see Section "Drugs for Use in Patients with Known Renal Disease" for further discussion).

Oxymorphone is comparable to other opioids in analgesic efficacy [20]. Of note, this drug has a relatively low likelihood of releasing histamine which may reduce the risk of opioid-associated pruritus or urticaria. Although this factor may improve patient experience, there is no evidence to suggest that the difference is clinically useful in pain management.

Immediate-release hydrocodone is available in the United States only in combination with acetaminophen, limiting the use of this relatively short-acting combination to opioid-naïve patients with mild to moderate pain due to the risk of acetaminophen toxicity with higher doses.

A modified-release formulation of hydrocodone is available as a single drug entity that does not include acetaminophen (Zohydro ER). It is approved for use in patients with severe pain requiring constant long-term pain management, but this formulation should only be used when alternative treatments have proven to be inadequate [21].

Fentanyl

Fentanyl is a highly lipophilic opioid that is indicated for patients with moderate to severe pain. Because of its high lipid solubility, it is not recommended for rapid analgesic titration and rather should be utilized after pain is sufficiently controlled with other medications in opioid-tolerant patients [4].

Fentanyl can be given through parenteral, transdermal, or transmucosal routes of administration. The transdermal formulation may be particularly useful for patients with chronic pain as it requires infrequent dosing (every 2–3 days) and does not require oral intake. Caution should be exercised when using the transdermal patch as exposing the patch to excess heat may increase systemic fentanyl absorption leading to respiratory depression and even death. Since heating blankets and other warming devices are commonly utilized in the operating room, many best practice recommendations include taking a fentanyl patch off in the preoperative period. Also, fentanyl patches are not recommended for acute pain. Each patch also contains small amounts of metal and must be removed before undergoing MRI procedures. Failure to remove the patch may result in localized burns.

There is some data to suggest that fentanyl may exhibit a reduced risk of opioid-induced constipation than modified-release formulations of oral morphine [22, 23]. It is therefore reasonable to use fentanyl for pain management in patients with constipation refractory to treatment.

Rapid-acting formulations of fentanyl do exist but are limited to the management of breakthrough pain. These unique formulations will be discussed further in section "Management of Breakthrough Pain."

Methadone

Although commonly used in pain control, methadone is the most difficult opioid to use effectively and requires experience in application. It is a mu-opioid agonist as well as an antagonist of the NMDA receptor. Challengingly, methadone is known to have a widely variable half-life between individuals due to enzymatic polymorphisms, with some half-lives extending beyond 100 hours [24]. Methadone is metabolized primarily by the CYP3A4 and CYP2B6 isoenzymes. Drugs that interfere with this metabolic pathway may prolong the half-life of methadone and should be used concurrently with caution (Table 11.4).

The dramatic variation in half-lives between patients can present difficulty in dose titration, and clinicians lacking experience with methadone use should consult a pain and/or palliative care specialist with experience in methadone therapy when initiating treatment. Additionally, due to the difficulty of dose titration, it is necessary to provide the patient with an adequate rescue medication in the event of significant breakthrough pain. This will be discussed further in section "Management of Breakthrough Pain." Close monitoring of the patient is required when initiating treatment as true steady-state conditions may not be met for up to 2 weeks.

Generally, RCT data have shown that methadone, when appropriately titrated, is similar in effectiveness and tolerability to morphine when treating cancer pain [25]. There is some evidence to suggest that doses of methadone exceeding 120 mg may lead to a prolonged QT interval and may precipitate *torsades de pointes* [26]; however, further studies have shown that cancer patients with baseline QT interval prolongation do not experience further QT interval change with the addition of methadone. Currently, the use of methadone in cancer patients is supported, but due to a lack of conclusive evidence related to cardiac impact, baseline and follow-up electrocardiograms are necessary in patients with known heart disease or who are on other drugs known to elongate the QT interval [4]. It is recommended that alternative opioid medications should be considered in patients with QTc of 450–500 ms and that methadone should not be used in patients with QTc greater than 500 ms [27].

Levorphanol

Levorphanol is an agonist to the mu-, delta-, and kappa-opioid receptors. Like methadone, it is also an antagonist to the NDMA receptor. It is distinguished from methadone by its shorter half-life (12–16 hours), lack of QT interval prolongation, and more predictable metabolism with no known drug-drug interactions involving hepatic cytochrome P450 enzymes [28, 29].

Levorphanol may be viewed as an alternative to methadone with similar benefits and decreased complexity of management. It may be used for moderate to severe pain when other treatment options have proven to be inadequate or are contraindicated [29].

Mu Agonists Rarely Used for Cancer Pain

Codeine

Codeine was once considered a first-line agent for mild to moderate pain in opioid-naïve patients, but as a weak agonist of the mu- and delta-opioid receptors, it has little direct analgesic effect. When metabolized in the liver via the CYP2D6 enzyme, it produces codeine-6-glucuronide, norcodeine, morphine, morphine-3-glucuronide, and normorphine which collectively exhibit a much larger analgesic effect. The CYP2D6 enzyme, however, exhibits marked polymorphisms within different ethnic groups and individuals leading to significant differences in metabolism. Some polymorphisms lead to greatly reduced conversion of codeine into its active metabolites which leads to pronounced reductions in analgesic effect, while other polymorphisms cause extremely rapid metabolism of codeine leading to the possibility of toxicity at seemingly reasonable doses [30]. As codeine is metabolized into several active metabolites including morphine, it is prudent to exercise the same caution when using this medication in patients with renal disease as the risk for toxicity is increased, and it should be avoided in the setting of renal failure [31].

Due to its weak analgesic effect as a parent drug, its numerous active metabolites that rely on a highly polymorphic enzyme for activation, and its increased risk of toxicity in patients with renal insufficiency, codeine is not a preferred drug in the treatment of cancer pain.

Meperidine

Meperidine is not a preferred drug for use in the treatment of pain associated with cancer as it is metabolized into normeperidine, which is relatively toxic and can cause seizure activity, delirium, and arrhythmias. An increase in metabolite level is most likely to occur with repeated administration, with dose escalation, or in patients with renal insufficiency [32]. For these reasons, it is recommended that an alternative mu receptor agonist be selected for the management of chronic cancer pain.

Mixed-Mechanism Drugs Used in the Treatment of Cancer Pain

Tramadol

Tramadol is an atypical opioid (codeine analog) that exhibits weak activity on mu-opioid receptors and inhibits the re-uptake of norepinephrine and serotonin. Tramadol is considered to be generally less potent than other opioids and is approximately one tenth as potent as morphine. It is widely used outside the United States and may be used in patients with moderate to severe pain as an alternative to more traditional opioids if they are not tolerated well. Its dose is limited by its neuromodulating effects, and it should be used with caution in patients who are concomitantly taking other neuromodulating drugs such as serotonergic drugs and monoaminoxidase inhibitors [33].

In adults with normal hepatic and renal function, a maximum daily dose should not exceed 400 mg of IR formulation, or 300 mg of ER formulation is recommended. Special dosing considerations should be taken for the elderly (patients over the age of 75) as well as in patients with hepatic or renal dysfunction due to an increased risk of seizure. Tramadol is associated with more adverse effects including dizziness, weakness, nausea, and vomiting when compared to hydrocodone and codeine [34], and there is little evidence supporting its use in the treatment of cancer pain as it is likely not as effective as morphine while exhibiting increased adverse effects [33].

Tapentadol

Like tramadol, tapentadol exhibits weak mu-opioid receptor agonism as well as a neuromodulatory effect by inhibiting the re-uptake of norepinephrine [35]. It is available in instant- and modified extended-release formulations and may be used in the treatment of moderate to severe pain including neuropathic pain. Typical doses range from 50 to 100 mg orally every 4 hours as needed, and a maximum daily dose should not exceed 500 mg of modified extended release or 600 mg of instant release as the effects of higher doses have not been studied to date. Tapentadol should be used at lower doses in patients with moderate hepatic impairment and should be avoided in all patients with severe hepatic or renal impairment [4].

Agonist-Antagonist Drugs Used in the Treatment of Cancer Pain

Buprenorphine

Buprenorphine is a partial mu-opioid receptor agonist with high receptor affinity that has been approved for used in patients with chronic pain who are opioid naïve or opioid tolerant [4]. Because it is only a partial agonist of the mu-opioid receptor, it may also be used in the treatment of opioid addiction. There is limited evidence suggesting that it is effective in treating pain related to cancer and it may be used in the short-term management of severe cancer-related pain. Buprenorphine may hold special status in the treatment of cancer patients with significant renal impairment as it is cleared primarily in fecal matter [36].

As it is a partial agonist, buprenorphine does exhibit an analgesic ceiling limiting its use in severe cancer-related pain. Partial agonism may also elicit withdrawal in patients already on other opioids that exhibit lower receptor affinity [37]. Buprenorphine has been shown to prolong the QT interval, although not to the degree seen with methadone treatment. FDA guidelines recommend that doses not exceed 20 mcg/hour for this reason. Due to the difficulty in dose conversion between buprenorphine and other opioids, it is suggested that physicians who lack experience in its use consider a consultation with a pain specialist before initiating therapy in complex cases.

Considerations in the Practical Use of Opioids

Selecting the Opioid

Although efforts have been made to standardize the process of initiating opioid therapy, many recommendations continue to be based mostly on clinical experience. Conventionally, opioid-naïve patients exhibiting pain necessitating opioid-level pain management are offered an opioid-nonopioid combination drug or a pure mu agonist at a low dose. If an opioid-nonopioid medication is preferred, acetaminophen-oxycodone (5 mg/tablet standard dosing, 2.5 mg/tablet in older or very frail patients) or acetaminophen-hydrocodone (5–7.5 mg/tablet) may be used. The dosing of these medications is typically 1–2 tablets every 2–3 hours as needed. If a low-dose pure mu agonist drug is preferred, an opioid-naïve patient with moderate to severe pain may be trialed on several oral options including morphine (5–10 mg every 3–4 hours), oxycodone (2.5–5 mg every 3–4 hours), or hydromorphone (2–4 mg every 3–4 hours). In some cases, transdermal fentanyl (12 mcg/hour every 72 hours) may be used, but this is typically reserved for use once a daily opioid requirement has been established.

In patients requiring several doses per day of short-acting pain medication or in patients who awaken at night due to pain, a transition to a modified extended-release formulation may be beneficial. There is no evidence to suggest that any one of the commonly used long-acting opioid medications available in the United States such as morphine, oxycodone, oxymorphone, or fentanyl is likely to be more effective than another; therefore, drug selection may be dictated by the patient's prior experiences and comorbidities, the clinicians' experience, cost, and availability. The convenience of administration and the side effect profile associated with the drug are also important considerations when selecting the medication of use.

Methadone, while less costly and equally as effective as other drugs typically used for the long-term management of cancer pain, carries significant challenges to safe prescribing as previously noted. Due to its variable half-life and difficulty of titration, it should only be considered a first-line agent for the management of chronic pain by prescribers experienced in its use. For all others, it should remain a second-line agent and may be trialed if other drugs fail to provide adequate analgesia with manageable side effects.

Opioid Use in Patients with Renal Failure

Drugs to Use with Caution

Meperidine

Meperidine is contraindicated for use in patients with renal insufficiency as its active metabolite, normeperidine, has been shown to accumulate. Normeperidine has a long half-life and is known to cause seizure activity, delirium, and cardiac arrhythmias. For these reasons, meperidine is not a preferred medication for the treatment of cancer-related pain [38].

Morphine

Although morphine is a standard drug used to treat cancer-related pain, it should be used cautiously in the setting of renal insufficiency. It is hepatically metabolized into morphine-6-glucuronide which exhibits potent analgesic effects and morphine-3-glucuronide which is associated with neurotoxic side effects. Both metabolites are renally excreted and may accumulate in patients with renal insufficiency [39]. The effects of toxicity related to these metabolites are not fully understood at this point in time. Regardless, in the setting of stable renal insufficiency, morphine should be administered with caution and close follow-up monitoring for neurotoxicity; in patients with changing kidney function or those with renal failure, it is prudent to select a different first-line opioid medication for pain management.

Codeine and Tramadol

The metabolites of codeine and tramadol may accumulate in patients with renal failure, extending their effects and leading to possible toxicity.

Drugs for Use in Patients with Known Renal Disease

These recommendations are based primarily on pharmacokinetics and physician experience as there is little evidence available to guide the choice of opioid in patients with renal impairment.

Hydromorphone

Hydromorphone produces active metabolites at a relatively low concentration when compared to morphine and may be less likely to precipitate toxicity in patients with renal insufficiency. Toxicity may still occur with its use, but it will require relatively high doses to manifest [40]. Hydromorphone may be considered a preferred agent in treating pain related to cancer in patients with renal insufficiency.

Fentanyl and Methadone

Both fentanyl and methadone lack active metabolites and, therefore, should be considered for pain management in patients with renal insufficiency. The aforementioned challenges associated with methadone use may preclude it from being used in treatment by physicians who are not experienced with its use. Additionally, methadone should be avoided in patients who are metabolically unstable. Both fentanyl and methadone may be considered secondary agents for treating pain related to cancer in patients with renal insufficiency.

Buprenorphine

Buprenorphine is another viable option for pain control in the setting of renal insufficiency for opioid-naïve patients, but as a partial agonist, it has an associated analgesic ceiling and may not provide significant relief for moderate to severe pain [36].

Opioid Use in Patients with Liver Failure

Most opioids are metabolized to some degree in the liver which complicates their use in patients with hepatic disease [41]. Safe prescribing of analgesics for these patients can be achieved with the application of two general principles:

1. A lower starting dose of most opioids should be used in patients with liver disease.
2. Caution should be exercised with prescribing at conventional dosing intervals until tolerance has been demonstrated. Dosing intervals may have to be increased as the patient's liver disease progresses.

Codeine and meperidine should not be used in the setting of liver failure. Codeine relies on hepatic metabolism to form morphine, and other active compounds with analgesic effects and pain control may be inadequate if hepatic function is diminished. Meperidine clearance is diminished in patients with liver failure, and the half-life may be increased, leading to increased likelihood of toxicity.

Management of Breakthrough Pain

Breakthrough pain is pain that occurs transiently in the setting of chronic pain that is otherwise adequately controlled by the patient's opioid regimen. This type of pain is very common in cancer as the disease is continually changing. Breakthrough pain may lead to negative clinical consequences; as such, patients should be provided with rescue dosing to relieve this burden and facilitate adequate pain control. Rescue doses typically consist of a supplemental short-acting opioid medication available on an as-needed basis to treat breakthrough pain in concurrence with the patient's fixed-schedule long-acting drug. It may consist of an opioid-nonopioid combination drug or an immediate-release single-entity drug such as morphine, oxycodone, hydromorphone, or oxymorphone. The choice of rescue medication will vary based on patient-specific needs such as the dose required, among other factors. The typical rescue dose is typically 5–15% of the patient's daily opioid requirement [42].

Breakthrough pain may also be treated with transmucosal fentanyl formulations. These formulations are specifically indicated for cancer-related breakthrough pain, and six options are now available in the United States. These include an oral transmucosal lozenge (Actiq), an immediate-release tablet (Abstral), a buccal tablet (Fentora), a nasal spray (Lazanda), and a sublingual spray (Subsys). These drugs exhibit an onset of effect that is faster than that expected from oral formulations [43–46]. Unfortunately, these medications are often cost prohibitive and as such are typically considered for use only after a patient exhibits a poor response to other rescue medications. To prescribe these medications in the United States, physicians must complete online education related to their use, and each patient treated must be registered along with the prescribing physician and dispensing pharmacist.

Selecting a Route of Administration

Oral

Typically, the oral route of administration is preferred for the treatment of chronic cancer pain because of its convenience. Most patients experience peak analgesia 1–1.5 hours after ingestion of immediate-release compounds and between 3 and 5 hours after ingestion of modified-release formulations. For patients with odynophagia or dysphagia when swallowing solid tablets, as well as patients who are feeding tube dependent, liquid formulations of several drugs are available.

Modified-release formulations of drugs should never be crushed and administered to patients as this may negate part of the modified-release mechanism and creates an increased risk for overdose and toxicity. Some modified-release formulations of opioids may also lead to an effective dose increase when taken with alcohol as it may dissolve the matrix that the drug is embedded in. Patients should be counseled to avoid coadministration of alcohol with their opioid medications.

The oral route of administration may not be feasible to use in certain patients including those with oral mucositis, dysphagia, bowel obstruction, or severe nausea. In these instances, it is advisable to trial alternative routes of administration which may be more readily available. Should other routes not be available, and the patient require modified extended-release opioid therapy, certain modified-release formulations of morphine (Kadian) are prepared as caplets which may be opened, and the contents thereof spread over food or in drinks that the patient is able to ingest. This does not change the delivery characteristics of the drug and permits the mediation to be administered through a large feeding tube if necessary.

Transdermal

Transdermally delivered fentanyl is used widely in the treatment of chronic pain, including chronic cancer-related pain. In most cases, each patch provides 48–72 hours of drug delivery. This route of administration may be preferred over the oral route in patients with poor gastrointestinal tract absorption or dysphagia. It may also be indicated if the patient is experiencing significant constipation, if the patient is distressed by the number of tablets required to maintain adequate analgesia, or if there is an issue with adherence to a medication regimen.

Transdermal fentanyl may not be effective in cachectic patients or other patients lacking the adipose tissue necessary to maintain an adequate subcutaneous drug reservoir. Without adequate subcutaneous fat reservoirs, serum levels of fentanyl may never reach therapeutic levels due to poor delivery of the drug into the bloodstream and rapid hepatic metabolization. Patients with low albumin levels or who have frequent infections are at increased risk of developing fentanyl toxicity due to sudden increases in the free fraction of fentanyl as well as increased absorption of the drug if the patient's temperature exceeds 102 °F.

Transdermal formulations of buprenorphine also exist, but as discussed earlier, its uses are limited to short-term treatment of opioid-naïve patients with moderate to severe pain.

Rectal

In rare instances, patients may be treated with rectal administration of opioids [47]. Several short-acting rectal formulations are available in the United States including morphine (5, 10, 20, and 30 mg), hydromorphone (3 mg), and oxymorphone (5 mg). There is only limited anecdotal experience in the use of long-acting modified-release drugs for this application.

Rectally delivered opioids exhibit a potency approximately equivalent to their oral formulations, but absorption can be variable; therefore, the relative potency may be higher or lower than predicted [48]. Because of this variation, switching from an oral to rectal dose should be accompanied by a reduction in equivalent dose with close follow-up monitoring.

Subcutaneous and Intravenous

It is common for patients with pain related to cancer who are started and maintained on an oral medication regimen to eventually be transitioned, at least temporarily, to a continuous intravenous (IV) or subcutaneous (SC) analgesic infusion. While the intramuscular route is available, it is generally not preferred as it is significantly more painful and does not provide a pharmacological advantage.

If the transition from oral medications to SC infusion occurs, it may be easily facilitated through the use of a butterfly catheter placed under the skin of the chest or abdomen which may be left in place for more than a week. Placement of this catheter allows for use of any drug with an injectable formulation, with the exception of methadone, and precise titration of analgesic dose [49]. Methadone is not a preferred medication for use via the SC route as it may lead to significant localized irritation of the skin.

When delivering medications via the SC route, the rate of infusion should not exceed 5 mL/hour in order to maintain patient comfort. If higher volumes are required, hyaluronidase may be added to the infusion to facilitate faster dispersion of the drug depot. Special consideration should be given to hydromorphone when selecting a medication to be given via SC infusion as it exhibits a greater water solubility than other frequently used drugs such as fentanyl or morphine [50]. Hydromorphone is available for use in a concentrated 10 mg/mL solution for use with injection which may be useful in this application [51].

Patients who are utilizing either the IV or SC routes of administration may still find benefit from access to a short-acting rescue medication in the event of breakthrough pain. In these patients, it is advisable to utilize parenteral versus oral opioids as the onset of action will be shorter. When administered as an IV bolus, some drugs, such as fentanyl, exhibit analgesic effect almost immediately, while others, such as morphine, take longer to penetrate the blood-brain barrier resulting in a slightly delayed but still quite rapid analgesic effect.

Patient-Controlled Analgesia

Patient-controlled analgesia (PCA) utilizes a pump to administer IV or SC medication on a controlled as-needed basis. This facilitates both a basal drug level and the possibility of rescue dosing. PCA devices are programmed with a dose size, interval between doses, and cumulative dose allowed in 1 or 4 hours to maintain safety and effectiveness.

PCA settings that are safe and efficacious for morphine, hydromorphone, and fentanyl are widely used and accepted in the setting of acute post-operative pain relief, but these settings must be adapted when PCA is used for the treatment of cancer pain. In these cases, patients with an established opioid regimen should have their daily oral requirement converted to an equianalgesic continuous infusion. These patients should also be provided with a rescue dose to be programmed into the PCA pump which allows for 5–15% of their daily requirement in a single bolus for the treatment of breakthrough pain.

Intrathecal and Intraspinal Opioid Administration

Select patients whose pain is refractory to routine systematic methods of opioid administration may find benefit from intrathecal or intraspinal opioid use. This type of pain control is more sophisticated, and a referral to a pain management physician specializing in interventional pain management should be sought.

Dose Titration

Once a starting dose has been selected, adjustment is nearly always required to maintain proper analgesia over time. When pain is continuous or frequently occurring, it is most effectively managed using a fixed schedule of around-the-clock opioid dosing combined with an as-needed rescue dose for breakthrough pain. If the patient is requiring several doses of short-acting medication per day or is unable to obtain uninterrupted sleep due to pain, switching to a long-acting formulation for more continuous analgesia is recommended. Proper titration of fixed-schedule opioid medication and adequate rescue dosing is able to achieve adequate pain relief in most cases.

Dose titration by convention has been achieved in one of two ways for patients with sub-optimal analgesia. The initial fixed-scheduled dose may be increased by 30–100% of the total dose received in the previous 24 hours. The percent of increase should be dictated by the severity of pain remaining, frailty of the patient, comorbidities putting the patient at risk of opioid toxicity or adverse effects, and the formulations of medication available to them. Caution should be exercised in any case when adding greater than 50% of the total dose of opioid taken previously to the patient's regimen. Alternatively, the initial fixed-scheduled dose may be increased by a value determined by averaging the amount of rescue medication required over several days. Following these methods of escalation ensures the safety of the patient during a drug's dosage increase while providing the patient with relatively quick and effective pain relief.

When titrating a patient's pain medication, the absolute dose of drug delivered to a patient is relatively inconsequential with regard to opioids as long as a desirable balance between analgesia and tolerance of side effects is found. To accomplish this, it is important to reassess pain and adverse effects experienced by the patient at every office visit and with special care at every dose change.

The interval between dose escalations should be long enough for the patient to approach a new steady state. This typically requires time equal to 5 or 6 half-lives of the drug of choice regardless of the route of administration. This equates approximately to less than 24 hours when using most instant-release formulations, 2–3 days when using modified-release formulations, and 3 to 6 days for transdermal patches. In the special case of methadone, 5 days may be sufficient to determine the effect of change, but this will not always hold true as the metabolism of methadone is widely variable.

In patients with severe pain that requires rapid dose titration who are unable to wait 5–6 half-lives between dose escalation, there is a risk of "overshooting" with rapid dose increases. In these patients, a dose that initially appears beneficial and successfully treats the patient's pain may reach toxic levels once a new steady state has been achieved. The risk of overshooting should always be assessed in patients requiring rapid dose titration, patients taking medications with long half-lives (the medication of greatest concern being methadone), and those who are medically frail. For any at-risk patient, inpatient hospitalization should be considered to facilitate safe and effective rapid dose titration.

Pain That Responds Poorly to Opioids

If a patient's pain is unresponsive to opioids, it may be related to the type of pain that the patient is experiencing. Neuropathic pain often does not respond as expected to standard opioid therapy and may be better treated through the use of adjuvant analgesics. Pain is also denoted to be resistant to opioids when the dose of medication required elicits significant side effects in the patient, overwhelming the analgesic effect. Physicians should observe their patients for pain that is resistant to opioids and be prepared to promptly address any potential contributors, as well as offer alternative avenues of pain management.

To accomplish this, the physician should initially conduct a pain assessment, which should include questions regarding the patient's psychological and spiritual concerns in addition to their pain. In patients with history or suspicion of substance abuse, a detailed history relevant to nonadherence, addiction, and diversion should be obtained. The physician must also complete a detailed and targeted physical exam to assess changing causes and severity of pain as well as order any diagnostic studies that may be indicated to investigate new or evolving pain. If a treatable etiology of poorly responsive pain is not discovered and the patient is not deriving additional analgesic benefit with dose escalation, a new plan should be developed.

There are several options to consider in this case. First, a more effective opioid can be sought out using an opioid rotation strategy [52]. Each drug trialed should be dosed to achieve initial equianalgesia as the drug that was discontinued. This is essential to prevent precipitation of withdrawal or unintentional overdose. Equianalgesic tables have been developed to aid in these conversions (Tables 11.2 and 11.3). While it is important to know and understand the equianalgesic dose conversion between two drugs, there are other things to consider before switching

Table 11.2 Commonly used long-acting pure mu-opioid agonists

Drug	Brand name (US)	Initial dose in opioid-tolerant adults	Serum half-life (hours)	Duration of analgesia (hours)	Notes
Morphine	MS Contin	15 mg PO every 12 hours	Unspecified	8–12	Active metabolite clearance dependent on kidney function; avoid use or reduce dose with renal dysfunction. Accumulation may lead to neurotoxicity
	Kadian	30 mg PO daily in 1 or 2 divided doses	11–13	12–24	
	Arymo ER	15 mg PO every 8–12 hours	Unspecified	8–12	
Oxycodone	OxyContin	10 mg PO every 12 hours	4.5	8–12	Possess abuse deterrents
	Xtampza ER	10 mg PO every 12 hours	5.6	<12	
Hydromorphone	Exalgo	8 mg PO daily	11	24	Reduce dose in renal and/or hepatic impairment Exalgo possesses abuse deterrents
Hydrocodone	Hysingla ER	20 mg PO daily	7–9	24	May interact with drugs utilizing the CYP3A4 and CYP2D6 enzyme pathways Converted into active metabolite by CYP2D6 a highly polymorphic enzyme leading to variable metabolism Possess abuse deterrents
	Zohydro ER	10 mg PO every 12 hours	13	<12 in patients with non-cancer back pain	
Transdermal fentanyl	Duragesic	12 or 25 mcg per hour, new patch applied every 72 hours	17 after patch removal	48–72, some effect may exist up to 12 hours after patch removal	

Data from:

1. Lexicomp Online. Copyright 1978–2020 Lexicomp, Inc. All Rights Reserved
2. National Comprehensive Cancer Network. Adult Cancer Pain, Version 2.2016

medications such as individual patient variation, variants in metabolic enzymes, patient tolerance, and variations in drug absorption. Given the propensity for variation, clinical guidelines have been developed that incorporate the appropriate reductions in the calculated equianalgesic dose to ensure patient safety when opioid rotation is performed [53].

Second, through aggressive management of side effects, it is possible to open the therapeutic window of a given opioid and supply higher doses to the patient. This will be discussed later in section "Management of Opioid-Induced Side Effects."

Third, a systemic NSAID, adjuvant analgesic, or a trial of intrathecal or intraspinal analgesics may be added to the patient's drug regimen.

Fourth, a non-pharmacological approach may be added with the goal of reducing the patient's opioid requirement. This may include neural blockade, neurostimulation, and psychological or rehabilitative therapy.

Switching to Methadone for Pain Control

Transitioning from a pure mu agonist opioid to methadone is the most difficult aspect of opioid rotation, and the optimal way to do so is still largely debated. The ratios that have been developed for standard equianalgesic dose tables may be radically different from the dose of methadone required to achieve favorable outcomes. Studies suggest that patients receiving >1200 mg/day of morphine or morphine equivalent drugs require a fixed maximum daily dose of less than 30 mg/day of methadone [54]. These findings support an

Table 11.3 Commonly used immediate-release and parenteral opioids with approximately equivalent dosing

Drug (US)	Approx. equivalent dose	Initial dose in opioid-naïve patients	Serum half-life	Duration of analgesia	Notes
Oral immediate-release formulations					
Morphine	30 mg	15–30 mg PO every 4 hours	2–3	3–6	Active metabolite clearance dependent on kidney function; avoid use or reduce dose with renal dysfunction. Accumulation may lead to neurotoxicity
Hydromorphone	7.5 mg	2–4 mg PO every 3–4 hours	2–3	3–6	Reduce dose in renal and/or hepatic impairment
Methadone	20 mg*	2.5–10 mg orally every 4–8 hours	12–150	3–4 initially; increases with repeated use	Not a first-line analgesic due to inherent difficulty of use Guidelines must be used to reduce risk of accidental overdose
Oxycodone	20 mg	5–15 mg PO every 4–6 hours	2–3	3–6	Available only in combination with acetaminophen, ASA, or ibuprofen which limits the dose
Oxymorphone	10–15 mg	5–10 mg orally every 4–6 hours	7–9	3–6	Should be taken on an empty stomach
Parenteral formulations					
Morphine	10 mg IV/SC	2–5 mg IV every 2–4 hours 2–5 mg every 3–4 hours SC	2–3	3–4	Active metabolite clearance dependent on kidney function; avoid use or reduce dose with renal dysfunction. Accumulation may lead to neurotoxicity
Fentanyl	0.1 mg	25–50 mcg IV or SC every 1–2 hours	7–12	0.5–1 (IV) 1–2 (SC)	
Hydromorphone	1.5 mg IV/SC	0.3–1 mg IV every 2–4 hours 0.3–1 mg SC every 3–4 hours	2–3	3–4	High potency useful for SC administration
Methadone	10 mg IV/SC*	1.25–5 mg IV/SC every 4–8 hours	12–150	3–4	Duration of effect increases with repeated use Refer to text for further discussion of the safe administration of methadone
Oxymorphone	1 mg IV/SC	0.5 mg IV every 4–6 hours 0.5–1.5 mg SC every 4–6 hours	7–9	3–6	

*Not a first-line analgesic due to inherent difficulty of use. Guidelines must be used to reduce risk of accidental overdose

*Duration of effect increases with repeated use. Refer to text for further discussion of the safe administration of methadone

Data from:

1. Lexicomp Online. Copyright 1978–2020 Lexicomp, Inc. All Rights Reserved
2. National Comprehensive Cancer Network. Adult Cancer Pain, Version 2.2016

Table 11.4 Cytochrome P450 3A inhibitors and inducers

Strong inducers	Moderate inducers	Moderate inhibitors	Strong inhibitors
Apalutamide	Bexarotene	Amiodarone	Atazanavir
Carbamazepine	Bosentan	Aprepitant	Ceritinib
Enzalutamide	Cenobamate	Cimetidine	Clarithromycin
Fosphenytoin	Dabrafenib	Conivaptan	Cobicistat
Lumacaftor	Dexamethasone	Crizotinib	Darunavir
Mitotane	Efavirenz	Cyclosporine	Idelalisib
Phenobarbital	Eslicarbazepine	Diltiazem	Indinavir
Phenytoin	Etravirine	Duvelisib	Itraconazole
Primidone	Lorlatinib	Dronedarone	Ketoconazole
Rifampin	Modafinil	Erythromycin	Lopinavir
	Nafcillin	Fedratinib	Mifepristone
	Pexidartinib	Fluconazole	Nefazodone
	Rifabutin	Fosamprenavir	Nelfinavir
	Rifapentine	Fosaprepitant	Ombitasvir
	St. John's wort	Grapefruit juice	Posaconazole
		Imatinib	Ritonavir
		Isavuconazole	Saquinavir
		Lefamulin	Telithromycin
		Letermovir	Tucatinib
		Netupitant	Voriconazole
		Nilotinib	
		Ribociclib	
		Schisandra	
		Verapamil	

Data from: Lexicomp Online (Lexi-Interact). Copyright © 1978–2020 Lexicomp, Inc. All Rights Reserved

References:

1. Clinical Drug Interaction Studies — Cytochrome P450 Enzyme- and Transporter-Mediated Drug Interactions Guidance for Industry (January 2020) available at: https://www.fda.gov/regulatory-information/search-fda-guidance-documents/clinical-drug-interaction-studies-cytochrome-p450-enzyme-and-transporter-mediated-drug-interactions
2. US Food & Drug Administration. Drug Development and Drug Interactions: Table of Substrates, Inhibitors and Inducers. Available at: FDA.gov website

emphasis on safety when converting from other opioids to methadone and outline several steps to accomplish this:

1. Calculate the dose of methadone that is equianalgesic to the dose of the starting opioid by using a standard equianalgesic dose table (Table 11.3).
2. Reduce the calculated dose by 75–90% and do not exceed a starting dose of 30 mg/day.
3. Methadone should be initiated in one of the two dominant strategies: the "stop and go" method in which the previous opioid is immediately replaced with methadone or the 3-day switch method in which the previous opioid is decreased in amount by one third each day and substituted with one third of the initial methadone dose over the course of 3 days. Sufficient data does not exist at this time to recommend one course over the other [55], but switching to methadone over a 3-day period may reduce the risk of accumulation and toxicity. This method is especially beneficial for patients already on high doses of opioids [56–61] (Table 11.4).

Management of Opioid-Induced Side Effects

Opioid-Induced Constipation

The most commonly reported side effect of opioid use is constipation. Opioid therapy leads to decreased gut motility, secretions, and blood flow leading to hard and dry feces. Patients who exhibit significant constipation usually do not develop a tolerance to it, and prophylactic measures should be initiated consisting of a contact or osmotic cathartic to mitigate this adverse effect. Patients should be treated utilizing one of the strategies outlined below until they have one bowel movement either every or every other day [62].

In patients who develop opioid-induced constipation (OIC) despite an adequate prophylactic regimen, conventional laxatives are recommended as first-line agents. A transition from the patient's prophylactic laxative, whether it be a contact cathartic or an osmotic cathartic, to a member of the other family and to escalate the dose as tolerated by the patient is recommended. Stool softeners should be used only in patients who describe hard, dry stools and are not part of the initial therapy in many patients.

If a patient has passed no stool in several days but has no evidence of bowel obstruction or ileus, it is likely that they have become impacted. This impaction can often be cleared with a mineral oil enema followed by an irritant enema if located in the rectal vault or lower sigmoid colon, but it is also possible that manual disimpaction may be required. Once an impaction is ruled out or cleared, the patient may resume or start a new laxative therapy.

Select patients find that they are also able to improve their bowel function with dietary modifications including increased fluid and fiber intake, as well as with increased physical exercise. In the event that the patient is debilitated and may have a bowel obstruction or if hydration has been difficult to maintain, fiber intake should not be increased. Regular ingestion of a probiotic has shown potential to improve chronic constipation, and given the safety of this therapy, it is a reasonable addition to the treatment regimen for OIC.

Patients exhibiting OIC that is refractory to other therapies who do not have bowel obstruction are recommended to trial a peripherally acting mu-opioid receptor antagonist (PAMORA). Several agents are available for use, but subcutaneous methylnaltrexone is suggested for most patients. In the event that an oral agent is preferred, several options exist including the opioid antagonist naloxegol, oral methylnaltrexone, and naldemedine [63].

Table 11.5 Strategies for the management of opioid-induced constipation

1. Nonpharmacologic approaches for all patients without contraindication
Increase fluid intake
Increase dietary fiber (ensure adequate liquid intake)
Encourage mobility
2. Pharmacologic strategies
Intermittent suppository or enema use
Intermittent osmotic laxative use (every 2–3 days)
Stool softener trial
Intermittent use of contact cathartic
Daily use of contact cathartic
Daily lactulose or sorbitol use
Daily polyethylene glycol use
3. Adjust dose and schedule of selected therapy for optimal effect
4. Switch or combine approaches to achieve results if initial therapy is inadequate
5. Consider adding a peripheral opioid antagonist or lubiprostone if constipation remains refractory

Linaclotide, a guanylyl cyclase C agonist approved for the treatment of irritable bowel syndrome and chronic idiopathic constipation, is an alternative option (Table 11.5).

Opioid-Induced Sedation and Mental Clouding

Opioid therapy, especially at initiation of therapy or increase in dosage, may lead to sedation. This effect typically diminishes over days to weeks but may be persistent in some patients. A stepwise approach to treatment should be initiated and should include the following. If obvious contributing factors can be identified, they should be removed if it is feasible to do so and aligns with the patient's goals of care. Use of centrally acting medications such as central nervous system depressants should be reduced or eliminated if at all possible. If the patient is experiencing adequate analgesia, a trial of opioid dose reduction is a reasonable first step. Should this result in unsatisfactory levels of analgesia, opioid rotation may be considered, or a coanalgesic may be initiated to lower the dose of opioid required. If a dose reduction is not an option for a patient, empiric trials of psychostimulants such as methylphenidate or modafinil are viable options.

Nausea

Nausea is a common side effect and is reported in roughly 25% of patient initiated on opioids, but tolerance typically appears quickly, and persistent nausea is not a frequent issue. If significant nausea does occur, opioid rotation and a change in route of administration are both reasonable approaches to mitigate the issue. For patients who do not respond to these changes, pharmacologic therapy with anti-nausea medications such as metoclopramide or prochlorperazine is reasonable. In patients with nausea that is refractory to this therapy, atypical antipsychotics such as olanzapine or risperidone may be used to alleviate symptoms [64].

Respiratory Depression

Respiratory depression is commonly considered to be the most serious adverse effect of opioid use, but it is rarely a problem if therapy follows accepted guidelines. In the event that severe respiratory depression occurs, patients should be treated with opioid antagonists such as naloxone.

Pruritis

Opioid-induced pruritis affects up to 10% of patients taking opioids. Management options include antihistamines, paroxetine, and opioid rotation.

Summary and Recommendations

Choice of Initial Drug

1. Oral and transdermal routes are preferred for the treatment of chronic pain in the outpatient setting.
2. In opioid-naïve patients, short-acting mu-opioid receptor agonists such as morphine, oxycodone, or hydromorphone are preferred agents to treat moderate to severe cancer pain. There is no evidence to support one over the other in the general population. Regardless of drug choice, the dose should be the lowest effective in providing analgesia. Genetic variation in metabolism of codeine and the inability to predict its effects suggest against its use in this setting. Due to concerns for toxicity, meperidine is also not suggested for use in this setting. Combination products containing short-acting formulations of hydrocodone or oxycodone plus acetaminophen are commonly used in this setting. Other less common but viable options for moderate to severe pain in opioid-naïve patients include mixed-mechanism drugs such as tramadol or tapentadol and the partial agonist buprenorphine.
3. Hydromorphone may be a preferred agent of use in patients with renal insufficiency. In the event that high doses are required, a concentrated solution is available and may be administered via SC or IV routes. Should hydromorphone not be tolerated well by the patient, fentanyl is the preferred alternative.

Titration and Switching to Modified-Release Formulations

1. Titration of dose is almost always required after initiation of opioid therapy. If pain is continuous or frequent, a fixed medication schedule is most effective. The absolute dose of opioid is inconsequential as long as an optimum balance between analgesia and side effects remains tolerable for the patient. Titration should always be accompanied by re-evaluation of the patient and their pain.
2. Switching to a modified-release long-acting formulation is suggested if a patient is requiring several short-acting doses per day or is awakened at night because of pain.
3. Morphine by convention is the standard of comparison across opioid drug classes. When selecting a drug, any single-entity medication can be selected (Tables 11.2 and 11.3). There is no evidence to support superior efficacy or tolerability of any single agent. However:

(a) In patients with poor gastrointestinal tract absorption, dysphagia, or constipation that has proved difficult to manage, transdermal fentanyl is suggested over an oral opioid.
(b) In patients with renal insufficiency, hydromorphone is suggested as the preferred agent. If hydromorphone proves to be intolerable, fentanyl should be considered.
(c) Because of the difficulties surrounding the safe prescribing of methadone, this drug is considered a second-line agent. It should only be tried in the event that other more commonly used drugs have been shown to be ineffective. If the prescriber is inexperienced with the use of methadone, it is recommended to consult a pain management specialist before starting therapy.

Breakthrough Pain Management

1. Patients experiencing breakthrough pain should be offered a supplemental short-acting opioid to be taken on an as-needed basis along with their fixed-schedule medication. The rescue drug may consist of a single-entity formulation such as immediate-release morphine, oxycodone, or hydromorphone, or it may be a combination product. The typical rescue dose should be between 5% and 15% of the patient's daily opioid requirement.
2. Breakthrough pain may also be treated with one of the rapid onset transmucosal fentanyl preparations. These are specifically indicated for use in cancer-related breakthrough pain. These medications are often cost prohibitive and are not commonly used leading to lack of physician experience with them. These should be considered in patients who have demonstrated poor responses to other oral rescue medications.
3. Patients with severe pain requiring rapid titration may be trialed on patient-controlled analgesia pumps. These will administer continuous opioid infusions via the intravenous or subcutaneous routes with intermittent rescue blouses. The intravenous route will provide the fastest onset of action when rapid titration is required.

Management of Pain That Is Poorly Responsive to Opioids

1. Several options exist for patients who develop significant side effects during titration. These include opioid rotation, aggressive side effect management, NSAID or adjuvant analgesic use, neuraxial analgesia, as well as non-pharmacological interventions.
2. When using opioid rotation, equianalgesic tables (Tables 11.2, 11.3, and 11.6) allow for correct dosing of the new opioid based on the patient requirement for the old opioid. These guidelines are not exact, and individual patients may vary due to multiple factors discussed earlier in this chapter. Clinical guidelines exist with reductions incorporated to the suggested doses to ensure patient safety.
3. Special care is required when converting a patient to methadone from a different opioid. As there is great variability in the metabolism of methadone, initially the equianalgesic dose should be reduced by 75–90%. Methadone should never be initiated at doses higher than 30 mg/day.

Table 11.6 Dose conversions for commonly used opioids

Hydromorphone		Morphine		Oxycodone	Fentanyl
IV (mg/day)	Oral (mg/day)	IV (mg/day)	Oral (mg/day)	Oral (mg/day)	Transdermal patch (mcg/hour)
1.25	6.25	8.5	25	15	12
2.5	12.5	17	50	30	25
5	25	33	100	65	50
7.5	37.5	50	150	100	75
10	50	67	200	130	100
12.5	62.5	83	250	165	125
15	75	100	300	200	150
17.5	87.5	117	350	230	175
20	100	133	400	265	200
22.5	112.5	150	450	300	225
25	125	167	500	330	250
27.5	137.5	183	550	360	275
30	150	200	600	400	300
Equianalgesic doses and ratios for determining daily morphine equivalent dose in commonly used opioids					
Drug	Equivalent oral dose	Equivalent IV or SC dose	Morphine: Alternate opioid		
Fentanyl	Not available	0.1 mg	100:1		
Hydrocodone	30 mg	Not available	1:1 (oral)		
Hydromorphone	7.5 mg	1.5 mg	4:1 (oral); 6.7:1 (parenteral		
Morphine	30 mg	10 mg	Standard of reference		
Oxycodone	20 mg	Not available	1.5:1 (oral)		
Oxymorphone	10 to 15 mg	1 mg	3:1 or 2:1 (oral); 10:1 (parenteral)		

Data from:

1. Lexicomp Online. Copyright 1978–2020 Lexicomp, Inc. All Rights Reserved
2. National Comprehensive Cancer Network. Adult Cancer Pain, Version 2.2016

References

1. Ferlay J, Steliarova-Foucher E, Lortet-Tieulent J, Rosso S, Coebergh JWW, Comber H, et al. Cancer incidence and mortality patterns in Europe: estimates for 40 countries in 2012. Eur J Cancer. 2013;49(6):1374–403. https://doi.org/10.1016/j.ejca.2012.12.027.
2. Glare PA, Davies PS, Finlay E, Gulati A, Lemanne D, Moryl N, et al. Pain in cancer survivors. J Clin Oncol. 2014;32(16):1739–47. https://doi.org/10.1200/jco.2013.52.4629.
3. Breivik H, Cherny N, Collett B, deConno F, Filbet M, Foubert AJ, et al. Cancer-related pain: a pan-European survey of prevalence, treatment, and patient attitudes. Ann Oncol. 2009;20:1420–33. https://doi.org/10.1093/annonc/mdp001.
4. Swarm RA, Paice JA, Anghelescu DL, Are M, Bruce J, Buga S, Chwistek M, Cleeland C, Craig D, Gafford E. Adult Cancer pain, version 3.2019, NCCN clinical practice guidelines in oncology. J Natl Compr Cancer Netw. 2019;17(8):977–1007. Retrieved Apr 19, 2020, from https://jnccn.org/view/journals/jnccn/17/8/article-p977.xml.
5. van den Beuken-van Everdingen MH, Hochstenbach LM, Joosten EA, Tjan-Heijnen VC, Janssen DJ. Update on prevalence of pain in patients with cancer: Systematic review and meta-analysis. J Pain Symptom Manage. 2016;51:1070–90.
6. Boland EG, Ahmedzai SH. Persistent pain in cancer survivors. Curr Opin Support Palliat Care. 2017;11(3):181–190.
7. Gagnon B, Scott S, Nadeau L, Lawlor PG. Patterns of community-based opioid prescriptions in people dying of cancer. J Pain Symptom Manage. 2015;49(1):36–44.e1. https://doi.org/10.1016/j.jpainsymman.2014.05.015.
8. Ziegler L, Mulvey M, Blenkinsopp A, Petty D, Bennett MI. Opioid prescribing for patients with cancer in the last year of life: a longitudinal population cohort study. Pain. 2016;157(11):2445–51.
9. Bennett MI, Eisenberg E, Ahmedzai SH, et al. Standards for the management of cancer-related pain across Europe-A position paper from the EFIC Task Force on Cancer Pain. Eur J Pain. 2019;23(4):660–8. https://doi.org/10.1002/ejp.1346.
10. Quigley C. Opioids in people with cancer-related pain. BMJ Clin Evid. 2008;2008.

11. Mercadante S, Tirelli W, David F, et al. Morphine versus oxycodone in pancreatic cancer pain: a randomized controlled study. Clin J Pain. 2010;26:794.
12. Pigni A, Brunelli C, Caraceni A. The role of hydromorphone in cancer pain treatment: a systematic review. Palliat Med. 2011;25:471.
13. Riley J, Branford R, Droney J, et al. Morphine or oxycodone for cancer-related pain? A randomized, open-label, controlled trial. J Pain Symptom Manag. 2015;49:161.
14. MS Contin (morphine sulfate extended-release tablets) package insert. Stamford: Purdue Pharma L.P.; 2019.
15. Sjögren P. Clinical implications of morphine metabolites. In: Portenoy RK, Bruera EB, editors. Topics in palliative care, vol. 1. New York: Oxford University Press; 1997. p. 163.
16. Penson RT, Joel SP, Gloyne A, et al. Morphine analgesia in cancer pain: role of the glucuronides. J Opioid Manag. 2005;1:83.
17. Vieira CM, Fragoso RM, Pereira D, Medeiros R. Pain polymorphisms and opioids: an evidence based review. Mol Med Rep. 2019;19(3):1423–34.
18. Trescott AM, Datta S, Kee M, et al. Opioid pharmacology. Pain Physician. 2008;11(2 Suppl):S133–53.
19. Schmidt-Hansen M, Bennett MI, Arnold S, et al. Oxycodone for cancer related pain. Cochrane Database Syst Rev. 2017;8:CD003870.
20. Mayyas F, Fayers P, Kaasa S, Dale O. A systematic review of oxymorphone in the management of chronic pain. J Pain Symptom Manag. 2010;39:296.
21. Baek SK, Shin HW, Choi YJ, et al. Noninterventional observational study using high-dose controlled-release oxycodone (CR oxycodone) for cancer pain management in outpatient clinics. Pain Med. 2013;14:1866.
22. Tassinari D, Sartori S, Tamburini E, et al. Adverse effects of transdermal opiates treating moderate-severe cancer pain in comparison to long-acting morphine: a meta-analysis and systematic review of the literature. J Palliat Med. 2008;11:492.
23. Tassinari D, Sartori S, Tamburini E, et al. Transdermal fentanyl as a front-line approach to moderate-severe pain: a meta-analysis of randomized clinical trials. J Palliat Care. 2009;25:172.
24. Davis MP, Homsi J. The importance of cytochrome P450 mono-oxygenase CYP2D6 in palliative medicine. Support Care Cancer. 2001;9:442–51.
25. Nicholson AB, Watson GR, Derry S, et al. Methadone for cancer pain. Cochrane Database Syst Rev. 2017;2:CD003971.
26. Krantz MJ, Lewkowiez L, Hays H, et al. Torsade de pointes associated with very-high dose methadone. Ann Intern Med. 2002;137:501–4.
27. Chou R, Cruciani RA, Fiellin DA, et al. Heart Rhythm Society. Methadone safety: a clinical practice guideline from the American Pain Society and College on Problems of Drug Dependence, in collaboration with the Heart Rhythm Society. J Pain. 2014;15:321–37.
28. McNulty JP. Can Levorphanol be used like methadone for intractable refractory pain? J Palliat Med. 2007;10:293–6.
29. Gudin J, Fudin J, Nalamachu S. Levorphanol use: past, present and future. Postgrad Med. 2016;128(1):46–53. https://doi.org/10.1080/00325481.2016.1128308.
30. Kirchheiner J, Schmidt H, Tzvetkov M, Keulen JT, Lötsch J, Roots I, Brockmöller J. Pharmacokinetics of codeine and its metabolite morphine in ultra-rapid metabolizers due to CYP2D6 duplication. Pharmacogenomics J. 2007 Aug;7(4):257–65.
31. Murtagh FE, Chai MO, Donohoe P, Edmonds PM, Higginson IJ. The use of opioid analgesia in end-stage renal disease patients managed without dialysis: recommendations for practice. J Pain Palliat Care Pharmacother. 2007;21(2):5–16.
32. Sjöstrom S, Hartvig P, Persson MP, Tamsen A. Pharmacokinetics of epidural morphine and meperidine in humans. Anesthesiology. 1987;67(6):877–88.
33. Wiffen PJ, Derry S, Moore RA. Tramadol with or without paracetamol (acetaminophen) for cancer pain. Cochrane Database Syst Rev. 2017;5:CD012508.
34. Rodriguez RF, Bravo LE, Castro F, et al. Incidence of weak opioids adverse events in the management of cancer pain: a double-blind comparative trial. J Palliat Med. 2007;10:56–60.
35. Hartrick CT, Rozek RJ. Tapentadol in pain management. CNS Drugs. 2011;25(5):359–70.
36. Melilli G, Samolsky Dekel BG, Frenquelli C, et al. Transdermal opioids for cancer pain control in patients with renal impairment. J Opioid Manag. 2014;10:85–93.
37. Johnson RE, Fudala PJ, Payne R. Buprenorphine: considerations for pain management. J Pain Symptom Manag. 2005;29:297–326.
38. Sande TA, Laird BJ, Fallon MT. The use of opioids in cancer patients with renal impairment-a systematic review. Support Care Cancer. 2017;25:661.
39. Kurita GP, Lundström S, Sjøgren P, et al. Renal function and symptoms/adverse effects in opioid-treated patients with cancer. Acta Anaesthesiol Scand. 2015;59:1049.
40. Kullgren J, Le V, Wheeler W. Incidence of hydromorphone-induced neuroexcitation in hospice patients. J Palliat Med. 2013;16:1205.
41. Oliverio C, Malone N, Rosielle DA. Opioid use in liver failure #260. J Palliat Med. 2012;15:1389.
42. Azhar A, Kim YJ, Haider A, et al. Response to oral immediate-release opioids for breakthrough pain in patients with advanced cancer with adequately controlled background pain. Oncologist. 2019;24:125.
43. Rauck R, North J, Gever LN, et al. Fentanyl buccal soluble film (FBSF) for breakthrough pain in patients with cancer: a randomized, double-blind, placebo-controlled study. Ann Oncol. 2010;21:1308.
44. Fallon M, Reale C, Davies A, et al. Efficacy and safety of fentanyl pectin nasal spray compared with immediate-release morphine sulfate tablets in the treatment of breakthrough cancer pain: a multicenter, randomized, controlled, double-blind, double

dummy multiple-crossover study. J Support Oncol. 2011;9:224.
45. Rauck R, Reynolds L, Geach J, et al. Efficacy and safety of fentanyl sublingual spray for the treatment of breakthrough cancer pain: a randomized, double-blind, placebo controlled study. Curr Med Res Opin. 2012;28:859.
46. Jandhyala R, Fullarton JR, Bennett MI. Efficacy of rapid-onset oral fentanyl formulations vs. oral morphine for cancer-related breakthrough pain: a meta-analysis of comparative trials. J Pain Symptom Manag. 2013;46:573.
47. Bruera E, Fainsinger R, Spachynski K, et al. Clinical efficacy and safety of a novel controlled-release morphine suppository and subcutaneous morphine in cancer pain: a randomized evaluation. J Clin Oncol. 1995;13:1520.
48. Wilkinson TJ, Robinson BA, Begg EJ, et al. Pharmacokinetics and efficacy of rectal versus oral sustained-release morphine in cancer patients. Cancer Chemother Pharmacol. 1992;31:251.
49. Wilcock A, Jacob JK, Charlesworth S, et al. Drugs given by a syringe driver: a prospective multicentre survey of palliative care services in the UK. Palliat Med. 2006;20:661.
50. McNeill JA, Sherwood GD, Starck PL. The hidden error of mismanaged pain: a systems approach. J Pain Symptom Manag. 2004;28:47.
51. Dilaudid (hydromorphone) injection package insert. Lake Zurich: Fresenius Kabi; 2019.
52. Reddy A, Yennurajalingam S, Pulivarthi K, et al. Frequency, outcome, and predictors of success within 6 weeks of an opioid rotation among outpatients with cancer receiving strong opioids. Oncologist. 2013;18:212.
53. Fine PG, Portenoy RK. Ad hoc expert panel on evidence review and guidelines for opioid rotation. Establishing "best practices" for opioid rotation: conclusions of an expert panel. J Pain Symptom Manag. 2009;38:418.
54. Bruera E, Palmer JL, Bosnjak S, et al. Methadone versus morphine as a first-line strong opioid for cancer pain: a randomized, double-blind study. J Clin Oncol. 2004;22:185.
55. McLean S, Twomey F. Methods of rotation from another strong opioid to methadone for the management of cancer pain: a systematic review of the available evidence. J Pain Symptom Manag. 2015;50:248.
56. Lawlor PG, Turner KS, Hanson J, Bruera ED. Dose ratio between morphine and methadone in patients with cancer pain: a retrospective study. Cancer. 1998;82:1167.
57. Ripamonti C, De Conno F, Groff L, et al. Equianalgesic dose/ratio between methadone and other opioid agonists in cancer pain: comparison of two clinical experiences. Ann Oncol. 1998;9:79.
58. Benítez-Rosario MA, Salinas-Martín A, Aguirre-Jaime A, et al. Morphine-methadone opioid rotation in cancer patients: analysis of dose ratio predicting factors. J Pain Symptom Manag. 2009;37:1061.
59. Mercadante S, Casuccio A, Calderone L. Rapid switching from morphine to methadone in cancer patients with poor response to morphine. J Clin Oncol. 1999;17:3307.
60. Mercadante S, Casuccio A, Fulfaro F, et al. Switching from morphine to methadone to improve analgesia and tolerability in cancer patients: a prospective study. J Clin Oncol. 2001;19:2898.
61. Parsons HA, de la Cruz M, El Osta B, et al. Methadone initiation and rotation in the outpatient setting for patients with cancer pain. Cancer. 2010;116:520.
62. Poulsen JL, Brock C, Olesen AE, et al. Evolving paradigms in the treatment of opioid induced bowel dysfunction. Ther Adv Gastroenterol. 2015;8:360.
63. Candy B, Jones L, Vickerstaff V, et al. Mu-opioid antagonists for opioid-induced bowel dysfunction in people with cancer and people receiving palliative care. Cochrane Database Syst Rev. 2018;6:CD006332.
64. Coluzzi F, Rocco A, Mandatori I, Mattia C. Non-analgesic effects of opioids: opioid-induced nausea and vomiting: mechanisms and strategies for their limitation. Curr Pharm Des. 2012;18:6043.

12 Maximization of Non-opioid Multimodal Therapy in Ambulatory Surgery Centers

Mitchell C. Fuller, Harley J. Bordelon, Raquel E. Candal, Sam Carlson, Elyse M. Cornett, and Alan David Kaye

Abstract

After nearly two decades of evolution, enhanced recovery after anesthesia has become a best practice pathway for most types of surgeries. A key feature includes multimodal analgesia from which many evidence-based studies have demonstrated reduced opioid consumption and quicker discharge after surgery. In the present chapter, we summarize the key components of these recipes that currently represent mainstream thinking, in particular in ambulatory surgical centers. Although there is continuous refinement to the details of best practice enhanced recovery protocols, the present chapter highlights important concepts and components in the setting of ambulatory surgery.

M. C. Fuller · S. Carlson
Medical College of Wisconsin, Wauwatosa, WI, USA

H. J. Bordelon
Louisiana State University Health Sciences Center Shreveport, Shreveport, LA, USA

R. E. Candal
Department of Surgery, Louisiana State University Health Sciences Center Shreveport, Shreveport, LA, USA

E. M. Cornett
Department of Anesthesiology, Louisiana State University Health Shreveport, Shreveport, LA, USA

A. D. Kaye (✉)
Departments of Anesthesiology and Pharmacology, Toxicology, and Neurosciences, Louisiana State University Health Shreveport, Shreveport, LA, USA
e-mail: akaye@lsuhsc.edu

Introduction

Surgery in the ambulatory setting has rapidly gained popularity over the last several decades, with 28.6 million operations conducted at over 5400 ambulatory surgery centers (ASCs) being performed each year [1]. Moreover, advances in medical technology have shifted higher-risk patients and a wider range of procedures to the ASC hemisphere [2]. The trend toward ambulatory surgery has underscored attention toward quality and infection control, while postoperative pain remains the number one patient complaint in outpatient and inpatient care [3]. The significance of poorly controlled pain is complex, wherein pain directly correlates with patient discomfort, suffering, and physiologic as well as psychologic maladaptation. In a phenomenon called central sensitization, heightened activity of the neuroendocrine system drives adverse perioperative outcomes (i.e., deep vein thrombosis, pulmonary embolism, hypertension, etc.). Chronically, uncontrolled pain can lead to long-term emotional and psychological distress, both of which propagate a cost to the patient and health system as a whole [4].

K. Rajput et al. (eds.), *Pain Control in Ambulatory Surgery Centers*,
https://doi.org/10.1007/978-3-030-55262-6_12

Opioids are a class of potent analgesic drugs, which act on one or more of three distinct receptors (mu, kappa, delta) at the supraspinal and spinal levels. Opioids directly bind to G protein-coupled receptors at the supraspinal level, working to increase potassium conduction and hyperpolarize neurons. At the spinal level, opioids inhibit the release of pain pathway mediators (glutamate, substance p, nitric oxide) to abolish nociception [5]. Related to a resounding potency, opioids were once the favored postoperative pain management agent. However, in the wake of serious and persistent concern over the US opioid epidemic, as well as the growing number of ambulatory operations performed each year, a more judicious opioid prescription practice has developed. As an alternative, the non-opioid multimodal approach to anesthesia care was borne. Multimodal analgesia incorporates agents such as NSAIDs, acetaminophen, glucocorticoids, alpha-2 agonists, benzodiazepines, liposomal bupivacaine, ketamine, and patient-controlled analgesia pumps in addition to intraoperative analgesia modalities such as regional nerve blocks. Interestingly, augmentation of more traditional analgesia with homeopathic remedies such as transcutaneous nerve stimulation (TENS), acupuncture, music therapy, and virtual reality are also becoming mainstream alternatives for comprehensive pain control [6, 7].

Enhanced Recovery After Surgery Guidelines

Over the last two decades, enhanced recovery after surgery (ERAS) pathways have emerged as a mainstay of quality patient care. ERAS protocols were originally conceptualized in 2001 for colorectal operations but have since expanded to include everything from neurosurgical operations to ambulatory orthopedic operations. The intent of ERAS is to minimize surgical stress response in the perioperative setting by standardizing procedure-specific guidelines, providing interconnecting services, and reducing the time to return to physiologic homeostasis (i.e., bladder function, cardiovascular stability) [8]. Included in ERAS are eight overarching goals based on common surgical and anesthesiology items: evaluation of preoperative risk, prevention of postoperative nausea and vomiting, minimizing invasive surgical approach, avoiding intraoperative hypothermia, providing adequate opioid-sparing pain treatment, individualized fluid administration, early mobilization, and quick oral intake restart [7]. These eight items are incorporated into the preoperative, intraoperative, and postoperative course. Randomized control trials have validated the effectiveness of ERAS when adhered to, demonstrating a 2.5-day reduced length of stay (LOS) in the hospital on average [9]. Despite the surgical efficacy, recent literature has pointed to poor anesthesia adherence to ERAS guidelines [10]. It is paramount to the improvement of patient pain control that enhanced surgical pathways be followed, and as they evolve based on clinical studies and other evidence-based medicine, our practices continue to evolve.

Enhanced surgical pathways, which are referred to as fast track guidelines, incorporate a robust multimodal analgesic approach. Particular to the ambulatory setting, pain remains the most common cause of discharge delay. Opioids do have an important place in the postoperative pain management protocol, but their utilization is minimal related to their concern of long-term dependence in the outpatient setting, hence opioid sparing [11]. Alternatively, agents such as IV acetaminophen, nonsteroidal anti-inflammatory drugs, magnesium, ketamine, liposomal bupivacaine (Exparel), dexmedetomidine, and the more modern advent of neuraxial as well as peripheral regional techniques have all taken their place in the anesthesiologist's toolkit [12]. Of particular interest, gabapentinoids have grown as a popular antinociceptive modality although more recent meta-analyses have mounted concern over the efficacy of their routine use [13]. Of note, several large meta-analyses have reviewed patient-controlled analgesia (PCA) in comparison to conventional opioid analgesia, collectively finding that PCAs demonstrated lower visual pain scores and superior satisfaction with anesthesia care [14, 15]. As a result of reduced hospital length of stay, frequency of adverse effects, and improved patient satisfaction, PCA-administered opioids remain an attractive option for low-risk patients. A major advantage of ERAS standardization in the perioperative antinociceptive course is special attention to the importance of pain relief for postoperative care on a procedure-specific basis. The consequences of inadequate analgesia for specific procedures at high risk of developing chronic pain such as knee arthroplasty are more severe in nature [16]. In these special cases, more invasive analgesic modalities such adductor canal or neuraxial block are validated tools for minimizing morbidity. On the contrary, less risk adverse procedures such as laparoscopic operations may not warrant the added risk of neuraxial or regional technique. The fast track pathways give careful consideration to the individual risks in each ambulatory situation in order to minimize morbidity while expediting full patient return to function.

Preemptive Analgesia

Woolf originally published a 1983 article which provided support for analgesic administration prior to surgical incision for their antinociceptive effect compared to postoperative pain control [17]. This method has evolved into a quintessential component of anesthesiology called preemptive analgesia. Preemptive analgesia, in theory, augments postoperative pain control via prevention of central sensitization [18]. Enhancement in neuron membrane excitability and decreased inhibition in nociceptive circuits within the spinal cord underlies the process of central sensitization. This process, in addition to synaptic plasticity and recruitment, results in central amplification of noxious inputs which enhances the response to painful stimuli [19]. These noxious stimuli released by damaged tissues from thermal or mechanical injury include many common inflammatory mediators including prostaglandins, bradykinin, 5-hydroxytryptamine (5-HT), and histamine. Unfortunately, the patient perceives these changes as worsened pain with reduced pain thresholds. In sum, the goal of analgesia in the preoperative period is to decrease nociceptive pathway activation before going under the knife.

With the intent of optimizing postoperative pain control, a multimodal analgesic model is often implemented which utilizes various adjuncts possessing different mechanisms of action. Numerous non-opioid medications including acetaminophen, nonsteroidal anti-inflammatory drugs (NSAID), dexamethasone, gabapentin, alpha-2 agonist, NMDA receptor antagonist, and benzodiazepines are some of the many adjuncts used in multimodal analgesia. These same adjuncts are currently being utilized and researched to provide preemptive analgesia as well.

Acetaminophen

Acetaminophen, also known as paracetamol, possesses both analgesic and antipyretic effects; however, despite being used clinically since 1887, little is fully understood about its mechanism of action [20]. Possible functions include activation of the descending serotonergic inhibitory pathways, decreased prostaglandin production, and inhibitory effects on hypothalamic thermoregulatory neurons [20]. Adverse acetaminophen effects are relatively rare under recommended dosing and include skin rash, nephrotoxicity with chronic overdose, and pancytopenia [21]. Metabolism to NAPQI (N-acetyl-p-benzoquinone imine) can result in serious adverse effects including hepatotoxicity and potential hepatic failure, renal tubular acidosis, and hypoglycemia [20]. Intravenous acetaminophen given preemptively reduced both postoperative pain scores and total analgesic consumption in 24 hours in patients undergoing lower extremity surgeries compared to placebo, in one study [22]. Interestingly enough, one study looked at IV versus oral acetaminophen for preemptive analgesia in women undergoing total laparoscopic hysterectomy and found no difference in pain quality which further suggest oral use as a potential to save money without compromised care [23]. However, in another study, IV acetaminophen given before pelvic organ prolapse repair did not reduce pain scores or opioid consumption [24]. A current ongoing randomized control trial is comparing the postoperative analgesic effectiveness of preemptive intravenous ibuprofen and acetaminophen in laparoscopic cholecystectomy [25].

NSAIDs (Nonsteroidal Anti-inflammatory Drugs)

NSAIDs are some of the most widely recognized anti-inflammatory, antipyretic, and analgesic agents on the market. NSAIDs include both irreversible (e.g., aspirin) and reversible (e.g., diclofenac, ibuprofen, ketorolac, naproxen, etc.) agents in terms of their inhibition of cyclooxygenase (COX) enzymes 1 and 2 [26]. COX-1 is primarily responsible for metabolism of arachidonic acid into thromboxane A2 which promotes platelet aggregation and increased vascular tone and prostaglandin E2 which regulates peripheral vasodilation and gastric mucosal integrity. COX-2 also metabolizes arachidonic acid; however, its products are primarily prostaglandins which mediate pain and inflammation including prostaglandin D2 [27, 28]. COX-2 selective NSAIDs, including celecoxib and etoricoxib, provide pain relief and anti-inflammatory effects without gastrointestinal mucosal barrier inhibition [29]. Adverse effects from nonselective NSAID usage include dyspepsia, peptic ulcer disease, and increased risk of gastrointestinal bleeding due to antiplatelet effects. Additionally, acute renal failure development secondary to renal vasoconstriction and electrolyte abnormalities including hyperkalemia and hyponatremia have also been observed. Both acute and chronic NSAID use has been shown to increase risk of myocardial infarction and stroke [30]. Aspirin-exacerbated respiratory disease can present as bronchospasms in patients with underlying asthma who were recently treated with aspirin [27]. Despite these effects, surgeons have widely used NSAIDs to reduce postoperative pain. Older studies [31, 32] concluded postoperative NSAID use was more beneficial in pain control than preoperative administration in regard to molar surgeries; however, more recent randomized control trials [33] demonstrate promise over single-dose intravenous ibuprofen. Patients have greater postoperative analgesia and lower need for acetaminophen or opioids as rescue pain relief. Based on research over the past 10 years, more effective oral medications have begun to replace nonselective NSAID usage as preemptive analgesia [34]. One randomized trial found preemptive use of oral celecoxib prior to lower extremity orthopedic surgery to be better than oral acetaminophen for postoperative pain control [35]. Furthermore, COX-2 selective inhibitors have shown promise as preemptive analgesics in reducing postoperative pain and overall opioid use for a wide variety of procedures including arthroscopic knee surgeries, laparoscopic cholecystectomies, and thoracotomies [29, 34, 36].

Corticosteroids

Endogenous glucocorticoids (e.g., cortisol) provide numerous effects and regulatory functions especially during times of stress including maintaining blood glucose homeostasis via gluconeogenesis; anti-inflammatory effects via decrease phospholipase A2 activity; inhibited IL-2, cytokine, and histamine production; and adrenergic receptor upregulation which promotes alpha-1-mediated vasoconstriction [20]. Synthetic corticosteroids, like dexamethasone, are used to achieve similar effects in patients undergoing procedures. Dexamethasone has widely been used for the prevention of postoperative nausea and vomiting, to suppress inflammation, and as an adjuvant to peripheral nerve blockade to prolong regional anesthesia [37]. In the DREAMS trial study, it was found that a single dose of 8 mg dexamethasone significantly reduced the 24-hour incidence of postoperative nausea and vomiting and decreased the need for rescue anti-emetics for up to 72 hours in patients undergoing large and small bowel surgery [38]. A meta-analysis on the preemptive effects of dexamethasone in third-molar surgery, when compared to methylprednisolone and NSAIDs, found dexamethasone to be more effective in reduction of edema and trismus. However, there was insufficient evidence to conclude its role as effective preemptive analgesia [39]. Another study examined dexamethasone's effects on postoperative pain in patients undergoing abdominal surgery and concluded a small but significant reduction in pain scores 24 hours after but no difference 36 hours after procedure [40]. A randomized clinical trial comparing dexamethasone and ketorolac found a reduction in both the 24-hour incidence and severity of postoperative sore throat in patients undergoing thyroidectomy in the dexamethasone group compared to the ketorolac group [41]. Well-known long-term effects of steroids include secondary adrenal insufficiency, increased infection risk, hyperglycemia and insulin resistance, osteoporosis, and hypertension [42]. A Cochrane review article found insufficient evidence to determine whether dexamethasone usage results in delayed wound healing [42].

Gabapentinoids

Gabapentin is a structural analog of gamma aminobutyric acid (i.e., GABA) and has traditionally been used as an adjunctive therapy for seizures; however, it is often prescribed for diabetic neuropathy, neuropathic pain, postherpetic neuralgia, and restless leg syndrome [34]. Gabapentin works by binding to the $\alpha 2\delta 1$-subunit on voltage-gated calcium channels and modulating the release of excitatory neurotransmitters [43]. Serious adverse reactions include depression, anaphylaxis, Steven-Johnson syndrome, and rhabdomyolysis. Common adverse reactions include ataxia, somnolence, fatigue, dizziness, tremor, fever, peripheral edema, diplopia, headache, nausea, and vomiting. A systematic review looked at eight studies including seven randomized placebo-controlled trials and one nonrandomized retrospective cohort study [34]. These studies examined preemptive gabapentin usage for a variety of procedures including lower extremity orthopedic surgery (total knee arthroplasty), lumbar discectomy, abdominal surgeries including laparoscopic cholecystectomy, thyroid surgery, and cesarean section delivery. In these studies, patients in the preoperative gabapentin group had significantly lower pain scores within the first 24 hours and showed decreased opioid consumption postoperatively and/or decreased need for breakthrough pain control compared to the control group which used standard morphine, tramadol, or diclofenac [34]. In another meta-analysis, a single preoperative dose of gabapentin or pregabalin was associated with decreased postoperative pain and opioid consumption at 24 hours; however, there appeared to be an increase in postoperative sedation, dizziness, and visual disturbances [44].

Alpha-2 Agonists

Alpha-2 agonists bind to and activate alpha-2 receptors, which stimulates inhibitory G proteins. These proteins inhibit calcium entry which result in decreased release of norepinephrine from presynaptic neurons within the central nervous system and lead to decreased sympathetic response [45]. Furthermore, stimulation of alpha-2A and alpha-2C receptors in the locus coeruleus results in sedation [46]. Examples include dexmedetomidine and clonidine. In a randomized control trial on patients undergoing laparoscopic surgery, there was a clinically significant reduction in cumulative postoperative analgesia consumption in patients receiving dexmedetomidine preemptively compared to the placebo (normal saline) group [46]. Another meta-analysis examined the addition of dexmedetomidine to brachial plexus nerve blocks and concluded a significant increase in block duration with faster onset and improved analgesia with reduced postoperative opioid consumption [47]. However, due to risk of hypotension and sedation, dexamethasone was found to be the preferred adjunct to brachial plexus blocks compared to dexmedetomidine [48]. In another set of randomized trials, pretreatment with IV dexmedetomidine prior to propofol injection not only was safe and effective in reducing pain incidence but also showed decreased pain response compared to pretreatment with lidocaine [49, 50]. A systematic review comparing dexmedetomidine to midazolam in patients requiring procedural sedation concluded dexmedetomidine provided higher sedation efficacy, improved patient satisfaction scores, and provided greater analgesic effects [51]. In review, dexmedetomidine is a well-known selective alpha-2a receptor agonist used to control hemodynamic stress response to surgery, reduce postoperative pain, reduce anesthetic requirements, serve as an adjuvant in local anesthetic nerve blocks, and provide sedative effects [52]. Significant side effects concerning dexmedetomidine include systolic hypertension and/or hypotension, atrial fibrillation, xerostomia, bronchospasm, syncope, dizziness, and electrolyte abnormalities including hypokalemia, hyperglycemia, and hypocalcemia [52]. The high cost of dexmedetomidine will likely limit clinical use until a generic option becomes available, particularly considering historically safe and effective alternatives (midazolam, propofol, etc.).

Clonidine, another alpha-2 adrenoreceptor agonist, possesses many sedative-hypnotic, sympatholytic, and analgesic properties [53]. In a randomized control trial comparing preoperative clonidine administration with midazolam, researchers found lower postoperative pain scores, improved sedation, reduced perioperative fentanyl usage, and more stable heart rate and blood pressure in patients undergoing supraclavicular blocks for upper extremity procedures. Researchers pointed to midazolam's variable metabolism rate leading to short duration of action and labile blood levels compared to the long elimination half-life of clonidine as possible reasons [53]. Additionally, addition of clonidine to epidural analgesia improves duration of action and shortens analgesia onset. A randomized double-blind study concluded that clonidine added as an adjuvant to ropivacaine administered via epidural route provided significantly shorter onset of motor and sensory block and longer analgesic effect compared to ropivacaine alone for lower extremity orthopedic surgery [54]. Adverse effects of clonidine include drowsiness, fatigue, headache, dizziness, xerostomia, bradycardia with epidural administered routes most likely causing hypotension, bradycardia, orthostatic hypotension, dizziness, and confusion [55].

NMDA Receptor Antagonists

N-methyl-D-aspartate (NMDA) receptors located on neurons function as ionotropic glutamate (an excitatory neurotransmitter) ion channels [56]. Locations of action include three primary sites: brain and brainstem, peripheral nociceptive nerve, and dorsal root ganglion [56]. Functioning as a noncompetitive antagonist, ketamine blocks the activity of NMDA receptors, thus preventing the transmission of painful stimuli to higher processing centers [57]. In addition, it modulates development of central sensitization due to NMDA receptors' ability to alter gene expression and receptor expression [56]. Ketamine possesses dissociative properties. Ketamine's dose-dependent effects allow it to be used for induction ($\geq$1 mg/kg IV) and maintenance (0.5–2 mg/kg/minute) of anesthesia and with subtherapeutic (0.1–0.3 mg/kg q30–60 minutes) dosing provide analgesic effects and reduce postoperative opioid consumption [58]. A meta-analysis reviewing preemptive ketamine usage found a reduction in postoperative morphine consumption and prolongation of first analgesia use time [57]. In another review, ketamine was also associated with decreased incidence of postoperative nausea and vomiting, a significant complaint of many patients [59]. Significant side effects include an initial sympathomimetic effect driving increased heart rate and blood pressure, as well as clinically significant laryngospasm at high doses. The later hemodynamic profile of ketamine can include bradycardia, hypotension in addition to confusion, delirium, respiratory depression, and laryngospasm [56]. A dutiful anesthesiologist will give apt attention to the risk of delayed discharge secondary to this side effect profile, particularly in a high-risk patient.

Benzodiazepines

Benzodiazepines are a broad class of drugs used to provide sedation, anxiolytic, and anticonvulsant effects and include alprazolam, diazepam, lorazepam, midazolam, and others. Benzodiazepines are commonly given preemptively to patients as an anxiolytic to reduce procedural anxiety and increase patient's comfort during the procedure [60]. Additionally, high doses of short-acting benzodiazepine (e.g., midazolam) have shown anterograde amnesia effects [61]. Benzodiazepines bind to the GABA-A receptor and enhance inhibitory effects of GABA by increasing chloride ion influx. This results in a rise in the threshold potential and decreased firing of the subsequent neuron [62]. Several studies show that intrathecal addition of midazolam to anesthetic agents such as ropivacaine or bupivacaine shortens onset duration and prolongs duration of postoperative analgesia [63–66]. Irrespective of benzodiazepines' anxiolytic, analgesic, and amnesic effects, controversy exists on its antinociceptive properties. In a systematic review for pain control in postoperative hysterectomy patients, benzodiazepines did not show a reduction in narcotic usage or postoperative pain scores [67]. However, according to another meta-analysis on knee arthroscopy, significantly lower pain scores and rescue analgesic consumption was found in patients receiving midazolam [68]. These differences could result from the fact that benzodiazepines mediate pain perception primarily with little effect on intrinsic products eliciting pain [69]. Adverse effects of benzodiazepines included drowsiness, confusion, syncope, tremor, respiratory depression/arrest, and paradoxical worsening of anxiety [51]. These effects can be reduced by careful titration in elderly and pediatric patients.

Intraoperative Analgesia

If local anesthesia is properly applied in the perioperative period, it diminishes the inflammatory response as well as decreases the nociceptive afferent nerves to keep from sensitizing pain receptors. Because these receptors contribute to hyperalgesia, local anesthesia can successfully decrease pain in the postoperative period, decreasing the need for opioid consumption [70]. Local anesthetics have traditionally consisted of diluted bupivacaine and ropivacaine often with adjuvants such as epinephrine or ketorolac. However, liposomal bupivacaine has been approved for several procedures, and other formulations have been the subject of investigation, such as HTX-011 (combination of bupivacaine and meloxicam). These different formulations aim at increasing the duration of local anesthetics [71, 72].

Advances in regional anesthesia techniques play a critical role in the setting of ambulatory surgeries. Motor-sparing peripheral nerve blocks permit quicker recovery postoperatively, allowing surgeries such as total knee arthroplasty and total hip arthroplasty [73]. Obturator nerve blocks in conjunction with femoral and sciatic nerve blocks show decreased pain profile and need for opioids following total knee replacements [74]. Additionally, truncal peripheral nerve blocks show promise when compared to neuraxial anesthesia, limiting the need for urinary catheterization postoperatively as well as improving hemodynamic instability [73]. In ambulatory centers specifically, some nerve blocks that are seeing a rise in utility are paravertebral blocks for breast surgery and inguinal/umbilical hernia repairs; transversus abdominis plane blocks for urology and gynecologic surgery; and saphenous nerve block at the adductor canal for knee and lower limb surgery [75]. One final mainstay of regional anesthesia in the perioperative ambulatory setting is the interscalene block which provides anesthesia relief to most of the brachial plexus (C5-T1), sparing the ulnar nerve distribution (C8-T1). It is a tremendous block for the distal clavicle, shoulder, and proximal humerus procedures, particularly in orthopedics. The goal of this block is to place the needle and catheter in the tissue space between the anterior and middle scalene muscles, first injecting local anesthesia to provide comfort to the patient and ensure proper needle placement followed by injection of longer-acting antinociceptive agents such as liposomal bupivacaine. Adding to the peripheral nerve blocks in the operating room, patients can be sent home with perineural catheters supplying continuous analgesia, which decreases opioid consumption postoperatively [76].

Monitored anesthesia care (MAC) is a multimodal method requiring a combination of local or regional anesthesia as well as sedation and analgesia. It is growing in popularity due to the quicker discharge times and decrease in anesthesia-related side effects such as postoperative nausea and vomiting (PONV) and ileus [77, 78]. If the anesthesiologist is not attentive, MAC can cause oversedation and consequent respiratory depression. Usually MAC requires propofol infusions, but dexmedetomidine and ketamine are also used because these drugs alleviate adverse effects of propofol infusions [78]. Due to ketamine's analgesic properties, it can be used in combination with propofol sedation. This reduces need for postoperative opioids as well as enhanced sedation [79].

General anesthesia in the ambulatory setting is still commonly employed, related to a multitude of reasons ranging from type of procedure to surgeon preference. In ambulatory setting, it is important to use anesthetics that provide quality sedation but with minimal side effects such as PONV [78]. Volatile anesthetics have long been known to induce PONV; therefore, patients who are high risk for PONV should be preemptively treated and/or receive TIVA (total intravenous anesthesia) [80]. PONV is detrimental in the ambulatory setting since it can lead to unplanned admissions as well as problems with wound healing [81]. Additionally, if volatile agents are used for general anesthesia, they should be fast acting with quick offset, such as desflurane or sevoflurane, in order to permit same-day discharge with the quickest recovery profiles [78].

Postoperative Management and Pain Control

Postoperative urinary retention (POUR) can significantly affect patient morbidity following surgery. Not only does urinary catheterization increases risk for urinary tract infection, but it also causes psychological disturbance that may hinder a speedy recovery [82]. Awan et al. found that POUR accounted for 20% of hospital admissions following day surgery [83]. Proper identification of patients at risk for POUR before going into the operating room is necessary for prevention. Increased age and presence of lower urinary tract symptoms increase the probability of POUR; however, the use of alpha blocking agents has the potential to protect against POUR [82]. Additionally, certain measures such as avoiding spinal anesthesia can decrease the risk of POUR. Limiting oral water intake following surgery has also been shown to reduce the risk of POUR [82].

Postoperative nausea and vomiting (PONV) continues to be another major cause of hospital admission following surgery [81]. As with other complications, it is important to understand which patients are particularly at risk for PONV. Patient risk factors for PONV include those who have had prior episodes of PONV, have female gender, are less than 50 years old, and have a history of motion sickness. Because the mechanism of PONV is complex, using several anti-emetics that have different mechanisms of action prior to surgery reduces PONV [81]. Reducing anesthesia-related risk factors, such as the use of opioids, volatile agents, nitric oxide, and high doses of neostigmine, also diminishes the risk for PONV [81]. Opioids are a major source of PONV; therefore, non-opioid analgesics and a multimodal approach to pain management have become the primary focus for pain relief [84].

Pain control in the perioperative period is the primary responsibility of the anesthesiologist. Poorly controlled acute postoperative pain continues to harrow ambulatory patients despite major efforts to mitigate it. Chronic pain has been widely shown to propagate worse long-term health outcomes with functional limitations [85, 86]. Herein, correct management of pain while keeping side effects to a minimum is central to any type of ambulatory operation.

Execution of a verified multimodal pain regimen can augment therapy, both short and long term, following surgery. Multimodal pain regimens have largely replaced the use of opioids, reserving opioids for rescue pain management [87]. As explained earlier, multimodal pain management involves using a variety of pain relief regimens with different mechanisms of action involving the use of NSAIDs, acetaminophen, COX-2 inhibitors, ketamine, gabapentin, and alpha-2 adrenergic agonists [88]. NSAIDs are central to the multimodal pain regimen by blocking prostaglandins and inhibiting COX 1 and 2. This decreases inflammatory mediators and both peripheral nociception and a central response to pain [88]. Ketamine is a drug with a variety of uses, one being an analgesic drug if given in small doses. As an NMDA receptor antagonist, ketamine is used with local or regional anesthesia to control the central pain response to prevent pain memory and central sensitization. Due to the attenuated pain memory, need for postoperative narcotics is lessened [89]. Gabapentin, a GABA structural analog, has been used for chronic neuropathic pain as well as treating postoperative pain [88]. Additionally, local and regional anesthesia have also been used to amplify the effects of multimodal pain techniques. Upon application, local anesthesia causes a temporary reduction in nociception in several ways. Local anesthetics directly block the afferent nociceptive fibers that surround the wound. Additionally, local anesthetics can interrupt the inflammatory cascade by reducing the release of inflammatory mediators from neutrophils. This results in decreased edema as well as decreased hyperalgesia [70]. These drugs reduce postoperative pain and, in turn, the need for postoperative opioids. Moreover, local anesthetics can be administered as wound catheters or different formulations of injections perioperatively [70]. Interestingly, lidocaine is rapidly becoming a more popular preoperative antinociceptive modality due to its wide availability and comfortability among clinicians.

Liposomal bupivacaine, also known as Exparel, was devised to have an increased duration of action as compared to standard bupivacaine or other local anesthetics [71]. This aids in the recovery and rehabilitation process; however, Exparel's efficacy has produced conflicting results. One meta-analysis of nine randomized control trials found no significant decrease in consumption of opioids post-surgery when patients were given Exparel versus standard bupivacaine [71]. However, Dasta et al. found a lowered cumulative pain intensity score in patients postoperatively when using Exparel as opposed to standard bupivacaine HCl [90].

HTX-011, a combination of meloxicam and bupivacaine, has promising preliminary results in phase III trials when administered intraoperatively. This dual-acting extended-release local anesthetic has shown greater pain relief 72 hours post-operation and decreased opioid consumption when compared with bupivacaine hydrochloride and saline placebo [72].

Ambulatory pain specialist, an onsite anesthesiologist that specializes in acute postoperative pain, is an emerging concept [91]. Ambulatory pain specialists are in charge of pain management preoperatively, intraoperatively, and postoperatively. The role of these specialists includes establishing a standard of care at their ambulatory center, identifying patients at increased risk for pain, providing rescue techniques for pain control, and controlling PONV [92]. With the continued emergence of surgical and anesthetic techniques, the role of ambulatory surgery will continue to grow. Therefore, it is important to keep improving the postoperative recovery process to optimize patient experience and reduce hospitalizations.

Special Population: Geriatric Population

Ambulatory surgery has numerous positive implications for the geriatric population such as a decrease in risk of nosocomial infections and quicker recovery [93]. With the increase of ambulatory surgeries, a better understanding of pain control is necessary to prevent admissions after surgery. The geriatric population, especially, still continues with difficulties in proper pain control postoperatively [94]. Reasons why the geriatric population disproportionately suffers with pain are not exactly known. Possibilities include providers being more hesitant to provide analgesics to the elderly due to their increased sensitivity to drugs or perhaps the elderly are not reporting their pain accurately [94]. Already, the elderly are at increased risk for delirium and confusion after surgery; therefore, giving additional sedative drugs, such as opioids, is detrimental for the geriatric population in ambulatory centers where follow-up is nil [95]. Additionally, elderly patients have altered pharmacologic effects of anesthetic drugs due to aging. As patients age, the central nervous system depressant effects of some analgesics occur at lower blood concentration. Therefore, it is important to use caution when using analgesics in the elderly population [93]. Hepatic and renal mass declines as patients age, which affects metabolism of anesthetic and analgesic drugs. Because of this, special attention to dosing and drug interactions is crucial in the elderly population [96].

Related to the increased sensitivity of opioids on elderly patients, multimodal analgesic techniques are critical for alleviating the negative side effects of opioids. The fundamental components of multimodal pain relief include NSAIDs, which should be used mostly in the early postoperative period to avoid cardiovascular and renal damage [94]. Additional methods of pain control include acetaminophen, ketamine, clonidine, gabapentin, regional nerve blocks, and local anesthetics [87]. Local anesthetics, especially, have shown promise in assisting with recovery of total hip arthroplasty (THA) and knee arthroscopy, which can be done on an ambulatory basis [87, 97]. Peripheral nerve blocks have proven to be useful in the elderly population as nerve blocks have minimal drug interactions with anticoagulants and aspirin [94]. However, in the ambulatory setting, special attention has to be taken with dosage of these blocks to minimize altered sensation in the recovery process [98].

Other non-opioid analgesics that show some promise include adenosine, capsaicin, and beta blockers (esmolol, labetalol) [94]. These drugs require more research to truly understand their benefit; however, White et al. showed that esmolol and labetalol given perioperatively reduce pain score and need for opioids after surgery [99]. Nonpharmacologic techniques are also used to amplify the effects of pharmacologic techniques. Transcutaneous electrical nerve stimulation (TENS) is a noninvasive method shown to improve postoperative pain and decrease opioid consumption [100]. Other nonpharmacologic techniques consist of low-level laser therapy, acupuncture, hydrotherapy, mindful meditation, and stress management [94].

Ultimately, physicians should carefully assess older patients on a case-by-case basis and devise a tailored approach for pain management with shared decision-making between all parties involved [101]. By taking into account the patient's drug list, comorbidities, and aging changes, the anesthesia team can prevent excessive pain and postoperative complications in the ambulatory setting [94].

Special Population: Pediatric Population

Children have a number of factors that contribute to an increase in perioperative stress and anxiety. These include an increased vulnerability to stressors, less developed self-control, increased self-reliance, and a limited experience and knowledge of health care, including a potential inability to understand why they are undergoing surgery [102]. In addition, parents may also have similar feelings of stress and anxiety, which can translate to their children [103]. Preoperative anxiety has been shown to correlate with an increased need for anesthesia, delayed anesthesia induction, and increased anesthetic risk [104]. AL-Sagarat et al. [102] reviewed three nonpharmacologic themes which may reduce preoperative stress and anxiety in pediatric patients and their families, including information preparation, therapeutic play intervention, and clown intervention. Patient education is a critical aspect of patient care, with multiple literature reviews concluding that preoperative education and literature distribution regarding anesthesia reduced parent's anxiety [102]. Therapeutic play is a structured activity which can educate and prepare children for surgery while effectively minimizing anxiety associated with hospitalization and surgery in both patients and their parents [102]. Clown intervention has been shown in a number of studies to decrease emotional side effects of pediatric surgery [105].

Many pediatric patients experience significant postoperative pain, warranting IV opioid administration. In light of the opioid epidemic, adequate analgesia while avoiding unnecessary opioid medications remains paramount in pediatric pain management. Additionally, acute postoperative pain contributes to complication rates, prolongs post-anesthesia care unit stay time, delays ambulation, and predisposes to unplanned hospitalization [106]. One approach is to identify at-risk pediatric populations for higher postoperative pain reporting, in order to achieve proactive analgesia. Nafiu et al. [107] determined that pediatric PACU IV opioid requirements can be predicted with perioperative parameters, including female sex, decreasing age, increased duration of surgery, non-Caucasian ethnicity, pharyngeal surgery, and higher first recorded PACU pain score. When all these factors are considered during the perioperative period, a more personalized experience for the patient may be attainable, and analgesic management can be tailored to provide optimal pain control with the lowest possible opioid use rate attainable.

Ultrasound-guided regional anesthesia use has increased the utilization of peripheral nerve blocks in pediatric patients recently. However, few studies have examined pharmacodynamics of these locally acting anesthetics in the pediatric population [108]. Additionally, the current utilization of local blocks demonstrates a large difference in dosages used, ranging from five- to tenfold difference in dosage used. This poses potential detrimental effects to patients' safety and the effectiveness of the locally acting block [109]. Despite these findings, both upper and lower extremity blocks and fascial plane blocks are a successful and safe methodology for pediatric postoperative analgesia, when doses are within the recommended 0.5–1.5 mg/kg for extremity blocks and 0.25–0.75 mg/kg for fascial blocks [108].

Nonpharmacologic Pain Management

Nonpharmacologic pain management, employed in a multimodal therapeutic strategy, may be beneficial as an alternative for both acute and chronic pain. Examples include transcutaneous electrical nerve stimulation (TENS), low-level laser therapy (LLLT), physical therapies (e.g., acupuncture, massage, hot-cold treatment, and hydrotherapy), and psychological therapies (e.g., music therapy, mindfulness, guided imagery) [94]. TENS units are a small device thought to activate the endogenous descending inhibitory pain pathway, reducing pain via stimulation of large afferent nerves [101]. LLLT therapy involves a nonthermal laser which may decrease the intensity of pain [94]. In an attempt to mitigate opioid-induced side effect profiles, a combination of nonpharmacologic analgesia may have a prominent role in multimodality pain management. While inadequate alone, the utilization of nonpharmacologic modalities in conjunction with opioid and non-opioid analgesics may provide superior analgesic effects and reduce necessary medication doses, thus being safer, especially in elderly patients with other medications and comorbidities [94]. Analgesia efficacy is dependent upon a number of modifiable and non-modifiable risk factors, including the type of surgical procedure, surgical trauma, type of incision, surgery site and length, patient physical and psychological status, preoperative preparation, and prior surgical history, with surgical site contributing the most to postoperative pain [110]. While effective as combination therapy for a multimodal approach to achieve analgesia, the benefits may be smaller in extensive surgical procedures. Additionally, one should carefully consider the adverse effects and efficacy of each modality relating to the specific surgical procedure, prior to its inclusion in a multimodal patient-centered approach to postoperative analgesia [94].

Summary

Ambulatory surgery is one of the fastest growing fields of medicine, yet literature demonstrates a failure of pain control specialists to adequately treat perioperative pain. In the post-opioid era, multimodal analgesia is becoming the mainstay approach due to its superior safety and efficacy profile. Emerging agents such as Exparel and HTX-011 are showing great promise in adjuvant therapy with more traditional agents such as benzodiazepines, NMDA antagonists, and NSAIDs. Beyond pharmacotherapy, it is becoming increasingly apparent that special attention must be given to the pediatric and geriatric populations, who have unique challenges to the short-term handling of pain. Moving forward, homeopathic modalities including transcutaneous electrical nerve stimulation, low-level laser therapy, and a myriad of physical and psychological approaches may provide optimal combinatorial pain control and patient satisfaction.

References

1. Hall MJ, Schwartzman A, Zhang J, Liu X. Ambulatory surgery data from hospitals and ambulatory surgery centers: United States 2010. Natl Health Stat Report. 2017;2017(102):1–15.
2. Davis KK, Mahishi V, Singal R, et al. Quality improvement in ambulatory surgery centers: a major national effort aimed at reducing infections and other surgical complications. J Clin Med Res. 2019;11(1):7–14. https://doi.org/10.14740/jocmr3603w.
3. Roth B, Boateng A, Berken A, Carlyle D, Vadivelu N. Post-operative weaning of opioids after ambulatory surgery: the importance of physician stewardship. Curr Pain Headache Rep. 2018;22(6):1–6. https://doi.org/10.1007/s11916-018-0694-4.
4. Sherman M, Sethi S, Hindle AK, Chanza T. Multimodal pain management in the perioperative setting. Open J Anesthesiol. 2020;10(02):47–71. https://doi.org/10.4236/ojanes.2020.102005.
5. Stoeber M, Jullié D, Lobingier BT, et al. A genetically encoded biosensor reveals location bias of opioid drug action. Neuron. 2018;98(5):963–976.e5. https://doi.org/10.1016/j.neuron.2018.04.021.
6. Arruda APN, Ayala AP, Lopes LC, et al. Herbal medications for surgical patients: a systematic review protocol. BMJ Open. 2017;7(7):e014290. https://doi.org/10.1136/bmjopen-2016-014290.
7. Mitra S, Carlyle D, Kodumudi G, Kodumudi V, Vadivelu N. New advances in acute postoperative pain management. Curr Pain Headache Rep. 2018;22(5):1–11. https://doi.org/10.1007/s11916-018-0690-8.
8. Cabrini L, Redaelli MB, Turi S, Beretta L. The ERAS protocol. Cham: Springer; 2020. p. 37–42. https://doi.org/10.1007/978-3-030-17305-0_5.
9. Gustafsson UO, Scott MJ, Hubner M, et al. Guidelines for perioperative care in elective colorectal surgery: enhanced recovery after surgery (ERAS®) society recommendations: 2018. World J Surg. 2019;43(3):659–95. https://doi.org/10.1007/s00268-018-4844-y.
10. Berian JR, Ban KA, Liu JB, Ko CY, Feldman LS, Thacker JK. Adherence to enhanced recovery protocols in NSQIP and association with colectomy outcomes. Ann Surg. 2019;269(3):486–93. https://doi.org/10.1097/SLA.0000000000002566.
11. Kaye A, Urman R, Rappaport Y, et al. Multimodal analgesia as an essential part of enhanced recovery protocols in the ambulatory settings. J Anaesthesiol Clin Pharmacol. 2019;35(5):40–5. https://doi.org/10.4103/joacp.JOACP_51_18.
12. Kehlet H, Wilmore DW. Evidence-based surgical care and the evolution of fast-track surgery. Ann Surg. 2008;248(2):189–98. https://doi.org/10.1097/SLA.0b013e31817f2c1a.
13. Joshi GP, Kehlet H. Postoperative pain management in the era of ERAS: an overview. Best Pract Res Clin Anaesthesiol. 2019;33(3):259–67. https://doi.org/10.1016/j.bpa.2019.07.016.
14. Mcnicol ED, Ferguson MC, Hudcova J. Patient controlled opioid analgesia versus non-patient controlled opioid analgesia for postoperative pain. Cochrane Database Syst Rev. 2015;2015(6):CD003348. https://doi.org/10.1002/14651858.CD003348.pub3.
15. Dinges H-C, Otto S, Stay DK, et al. Side effect rates of opioids in equianalgesic doses via intravenous patient-controlled analgesia. Anesth Analg. 2019;129(4):1153–62. https://doi.org/10.1213/ANE.0000000000003887.
16. Lee B, Schug SA, Joshi GP, et al. Procedure-specific pain management (PROSPECT) – an update. Best Pract Res Clin Anaesthesiol. 2018;32(2):101–11. https://doi.org/10.1016/j.bpa.2018.06.012.
17. Woolf CJ. Evidence for a central component of post-injury pain hypersensitivity. Nature. 1983;306(5944):686–8. https://doi.org/10.1038/306686a0.
18. Rosero EB, Joshi GP. Preemptive, preventive, multimodal analgesia: what do they really mean? Plast Reconstr Surg. 2014;134(4):85S–93S. https://doi.org/10.1097/PRS.0000000000000671.
19. Woolf CJ. Central sensitization: implications for the diagnosis and treatment of pain. Pain. 2011;152(SUPPL.3):S2–S15. https://doi.org/10.1016/j.pain.2010.09.030.
20. Candido KD, Perozo OJ, Knezevic NN. Pharmacology of acetaminophen, nonsteroidal

antiinflammatory drugs, and steroid medications: implications for anesthesia or unique associated risks. Anesthesiol Clin. 2017;35(2):e145–62. https://doi.org/10.1016/j.anclin.2017.01.020.

21. Ndetan H, Evans MW, Singal AK, Brunner LJ, Calhoun K, Singh KP. Light to moderate drinking and therapeutic doses of acetaminophen: an assessment of risks for renal dysfunction. Prev Med Reports. 2018;12:253–8. https://doi.org/10.1016/j.pmedr.2018.10.013.
22. Khalili G, Janghorbani M, Saryazdi H, Emaminejad A. Effect of preemptive and preventive acetaminophen on postoperative pain score: a randomized, double-blind trial of patients undergoing lower extremity surgery. J Clin Anesth. 2013;25(3):188–92. https://doi.org/10.1016/j.jclinane.2012.09.004.
23. Atkins JR, Titch JF, Norcross WP, Thompson JA, Muckler VC. Preemptive oral acetaminophen for women undergoing total laparoscopic hysterectomy. Nurs Womens Health. 2019;23(2):105–13. https://doi.org/10.1016/j.nwh.2019.01.003.
24. Turner LC, Zyczynski HM, Shepherd JP. Intravenous acetaminophen before pelvic organ prolapse repair: A randomized controlled trial. Obstet Gynecol. 2019;133(3):492–502. https://doi.org/10.1097/AOG.0000000000003102.
25. Alanoglu Z. Comparison of the postoperative analgesia effectiveness of preemptive intravenous ibuprofen and paracetamol in patients undergoing laparoscopic cholecystectomy.
26. Xu J, Li H, Zheng C, et al. Correction to: the efficacy of pre-emptive analgesia on pain management in total knee arthroplasty: a mini-review. Arthroplasty. 2019;1(1):1–6. https://doi.org/10.1186/s42836-019-0013-5.
27. Wongrakpanich S, Wongrakpanich A, Melhado K, Rangaswami J. A comprehensive review of non-steroidal anti-inflammatory drug use in the elderly. Aging Dis. 2018;9(1):143–50. https://doi.org/10.14336/AD.2017.0306.
28. Ricciotti E, GA FG. [Eicosanoid neuroinflammation] prostaglandins and inflammation. Arter Thromb Vasc Biol. 2011;31(5):986–1000. https://doi.org/10.1161/ATVBAHA.110.207449.Prostaglandins.
29. Kaye AD, Baluch A, Kaye AJ, Ralf G, Lubarsky D. Pharmacology of cyclooxygenase-2 inhibitors and preemptive analgesia in acute pain management. Curr Opin Anesthesiol. 2008;21(4):439–45.
30. Varga Z, Sabzwari SRA, Vargova V. Cardiovascular risk of nonsteroidal anti-inflammatory drugs: an under-recognized public health issue. Cureus. 2017;9(4):e1144. https://doi.org/10.7759/cureus.1144.
31. Kaczmarzyk T, Wichlinski J, Stypulkowska J, Zaleska M, Woron J. Preemptive effect of ketoprofen on postoperative pain following third molar surgery. A prospective, randomized, double-blinded clinical trial. Int J Oral Maxillofac Surg. 2010;39(7):647–52. https://doi.org/10.1016/j.ijom.2010.02.019.
32. Jung YS, Kim MK, Um YJ, Park HS, Lee EW, Kang JW. The effects on postoperative oral surgery pain by varying NSAID administration times: comparison on effect of preemptive analgesia. Oral Surg Oral Med Oral Pathol Oral Radiol Endod. 2005;100(5):559–63. https://doi.org/10.1016/j.tripleo.2005.02.065.
33. Demirbas AE, Karakaya M, Bilge S, Canpolat DG, Kütük N, Alkan A. Does single-dose preemptive intravenous ibuprofen reduce postoperative pain after third molar surgery? A prospective, randomized, double-blind clinical study. J Oral Maxillofac Surg. 2019;77(10):1990–7. https://doi.org/10.1016/j.joms.2019.04.019.
34. Penprase B, Brunetto E, Dahmani E, Forthoffer JJ, Kapoor S. The efficacy of preemptive analgesia for postoperative pain control: a systematic review of the literature. AORN J. 2015;101(1):94–105.e8. https://doi.org/10.1016/j.aorn.2014.01.030.
35. Honarmand A, Kashefi P, Safavi M. Effects of preemptive analgesia with celecoxib or acetaminophen on postoperative pain relief following lower extremity orthopedic surgery. Adv Biomed Res. 2012;1(1):66. https://doi.org/10.4103/2277-9175.100197.
36. Rodriguez-Aldrete D, Candiotti KA, Janakiraman R, Rodriguez-Blanco YF. Trends and new evidence in the management of acute and chronic post-thoracotomy pain – an overview of the literature from 2005 to 2015. J Cardiothorac Vasc Anesth. 2016;30(3):762–72. https://doi.org/10.1053/j.jvca.2015.07.029.
37. Gupta B. Role of dexamethasone in peri-operative anesthesia management: a review of literature. Res Pract Anesthesiol. 2017;2(2):33–9. https://doi.org/10.17140/rpaoj-2-114.
38. Collaborators DT, Midlands W. Dexamethasone versus standard treatment for postoperative nausea and vomiting in gastrointestinal surgery: randomised controlled trial (DREAMS trial). BMJ. 2017;357:j1455. https://doi.org/10.1136/bmj.j1455.
39. Falci SG, Lima TC, Martins CC, Santos CR, Pinheiro ML. Preemptive effect of dexamethasone in third-molar surgery: a meta-analysis. Anesth Prog. 2017;64(3):136–43. https://doi.org/10.2344/anpr-64-05-08.
40. Valdivia-Sanchez CG, Prieto-Duarte ML. Effectiveness of dexamethasone as an adjuvant in preemptive analgesia for postoperative pain in patients undergoing abdominal surgery. Gac Med Mex. 2017;153(3):390–6.
41. Yang C, Jung SM, Bae YK, Park S. The effect of ketorolac and dexamethasone on the incidence of sore throat in women after thyroidectomy: a prospective double-blinded randomized trial. Korean J Anesthesiol. 2017;70(1):64.
42. Polderman JAW, Farhang-Razi V, Van Dieren S, et al. Adverse side effects of dexamethasone in surgical patients. Cochrane Database Syst Rev. 2018;11(11):CD011940. https://doi.org/10.1002/14651858.CD011940.pub2.

43. Arumugam S, Lau CSM, Chamberlain RS. Use of preoperative gabapentin significantly reduces postoperative opioid consumption: a meta-analysis. J Pain Res. 2016;9:631–40. https://doi.org/10.2147/JPR.S112626.
44. Mishriky BM, Waldron NH, Habib AS. Impact of pregabalin on acute and persistent postoperative pain: a systematic review and meta-analysis. Br J Anaesth. 2015;114(1):10–31. https://doi.org/10.1093/bja/aeu293.
45. Weerink MAS, Struys MMRF, Hannivoort LN, Barends CRM, Absalom AR, Colin P. Clinical pharmacokinetics and pharmacodynamics of dexmedetomidine. Clin Pharmacokinet. 2017;56(8):893–913. https://doi.org/10.1007/s40262-017-0507-7.
46. Panchgar V, Shetti AN, Sunitha HB, Dhulkhed VK, Nadkarni AV. The effectiveness of intravenous dexmedetomidine on perioperative hemodynamics, analgesic requirement, and side effects profile in patients undergoing laparoscopic surgery under general anesthesia. Anesth Essays Res. 2017;11(1):72–7.
47. Vorobeichik L, Brull RAF. Evidence basis for using perineural dexmedetomidine to enhance the quality of brachial plexus nerve blocks: a systematic review and meta-analysis of randomized controlled trials. Br J Anaesth. 2017;118(2):167–81.
48. Albrecht E, Vorobeichik L, Jacot-Guillarmod A, Fournier N, Abdallah FW. Dexamethasone is superior to dexmedetomidine as a perineural adjunct for supraclavicular brachial plexus block: systematic review and indirect meta-analysis. Anesth Analg. 2019;128(3):543–54. https://doi.org/10.1213/ANE.0000000000003860.
49. He L, Xu JM, He T, Liu L, Zhu R. Dexmedetomidine pretreatment alleviates propofol injection pain. Ups J Med Sci. 2014;119(4):338–42. https://doi.org/10.3109/03009734.2014.941049.
50. Aditya K, Krishna Simha A, Reddy MHR. Comparison of intravenous dexmedetomidine and intravenous lignocaine for the prevention of conventional propofol injection pain: a prospective randomised double_blind study. J Clin Sci Res. 2018;7(4):170.
51. Barends CRM, Absalom A, Van Minnen B, Vissink A, Visser A. Dexmedetomidine versus midazolam in procedural sedation. A systematic review of efficacy and safety. PLoS One. 2017;12(1):1–12. https://doi.org/10.1371/journal.pone.0169525.
52. Kaye AD, Chernobylsky DJ, Thakur P, et al. Dexmedetomidine in enhanced recovery after surgery (ERAS) protocols for postoperative pain. Curr Pain Headache Rep. 2020;24(5):21. https://doi.org/10.1007/s11916-020-00853-z.
53. Mosaffa F, Mohajerani SA, Aminnejad R, Solhpour A, Dabir S, Mohseni GR. Preemptive oral clonidine provides better sedation than intravenous midazolam in brachial plexus nerve blocks. Anesthesiol Pain Med. 2016;6(3):4–10. https://doi.org/10.5812/aapm.28768.
54. Singh M, Pathak A, Khan AL, Srivastava A, Negi D. Comparative study of clonidine with ropivacaine versus ropivacaine alone in epidural anesthesia for lower limb orthopedic surgery. Anesth Essays Res. 2017;11(4):1035–9. https://doi.org/10.4103/aer.aer_67_17.
55. Nigam S, Rastogi S, Tyagi A, Bhandari RA. Comparative study for the analgesic efficacy and safety profile of fentanyl versus clonidine as an adjuvant to epidural Ropivacaine 0.75% in lower abdominal surgeries. Anesth Essays Res. 2017;11(3):692–6. https://doi.org/10.4103/aer.aer_254_16.
56. Gorlin AW, Rosenfeld DM, Ramakrishna H. Intravenous sub-anesthetic ketamine for perioperative analgesia. J Anaesthesiol Clin Pharmacol. 2016;32(2):160–7. https://doi.org/10.4103/0970-9185.182085.
57. Yang L, Zhang J, Zhang Z, Zhang C, Zhao D, Li J. Preemptive analgesia effects of ketamine in patients undergoing surgery. A meta-analysis. Acta Cir Bras. 2014;29(12):819–25. https://doi.org/10.1590/S0102-86502014001900009.
58. Vadivelu N, Schermer E, Kodumudi V, Belani K, Urman RD, Kaye AD. Role of ketamine for analgesia in adults and children. J Anaesthesiol Clin Pharmacol. 2016;32(3):298–306. https://doi.org/10.4103/0970-9185.168149.
59. Visser E, Schug SA. The role of ketamine in pain management. Biomed Pharmacother. 2006;60(7):341–8. https://doi.org/10.1016/j.biopha.2006.06.021.
60. Sheen MJ, Chang FL, Ho ST. Anesthetic premedication: new horizons of an old practice. Acta Anaesthesiol Taiwanica. 2014;52(3):134–42. https://doi.org/10.1016/j.aat.2014.08.001.
61. Bulach R, Myles PS, Russnak M. Double-blind randomized controlled trial to determine extent of amnesia with midazolam given immediately before general anaesthesia. Br J Anaesth. 2005;94(3):300–5. https://doi.org/10.1093/bja/aei040.
62. Hasani A, Soljakova M, Jakupi M, Ustalar-Ozgen S. Preemptive analgesic effects of midazolam and diclofenac in rat model. Bosn J Basic Med Sci. 2011;11(2):113–8. https://doi.org/10.17305/bjbms.2011.2593.
63. Paleti S, Prasad PK, Lakshmi BS. A randomized clinical trial of intrathecal magnesium sulfate versus midazolam with epidural administration of 0.75% ropivacaine for patients with preeclampsia scheduled for elective cesarean section. J Anaesthesiol Clin Pharmacol. 2018;34(1):23–8.
64. Tucker AP, Lai C, Nadeson R, Goodchild CS. Intrathecal midazolam I: a cohort study investigating safety. Anesth Analg. 2004;98(6):1512–20.
65. Ho KMIH. Use of intrathecal midazolam to improve perioperative analgesia: a meta-analysis. Anesth Intensive Care. 2008;36(3):365–73.
66. Shirmohammadie M, Soltani AE, Arbabi S, Nasseri K. A randomized-controlled, double-blind study to evaluate the efficacy of caudal midazolam, ketamine

and neostigmine as adjuvants to bupivacaine on postoperative analgesic in children undergoing lower abdominal surgery. Acta Biomed. 2018;89(4):513–8. https://doi.org/10.23750/abm.v89i4.5775.
67. Steinberg AC, Schimpf MO, White AB, et al. Preemptive analgesia for postoperative hysterectomy pain control: systematic review and clinical practice guidelines. Am J Obstet Gynecol. 2017;217(3):303–313.e6. https://doi.org/10.1016/j.ajog.2017.03.013.
68. Chen X, Mou X, He Z, Zhu Y. The effect of midazolam on pain control after knee arthroscopy: a systematic review and meta-analysis. J Orthop Surg Res. 2017;12(1):179. https://doi.org/10.1186/s13018-017-0682-0.
69. Frölich MA, Kui Zhang TN. Effect of sedation on pain perception. Anesthesiology. 2013;118(3):611–21. https://doi.org/10.1038/jid.2014.371.
70. Liu SS, Richman JM, Thirlby RC, Wu CL. Efficacy of continuous wound catheters delivering local anesthetic for postoperative analgesia: a quantitative and qualitative systematic review of randomized controlled trials. J Am Coll Surg. 2006;203:914. https://doi.org/10.1016/j.jamcollsurg.2006.08.007.
71. Kendall MC, Castro Alves LJ, De Oliveira G. Liposome bupivacaine compared to plain local anesthetics to reduce postsurgical pain: an updated meta-analysis of randomized controlled trials. Pain Res Treat. 2018;2018:1. https://doi.org/10.1155/2018/5710169.
72. Viscusi E, Gimbel JS, Pollack RA, Hu J, Lee GC. HTX-011 reduced pain intensity and opioid consumption versus bupivacaine HCl in bunionectomy: phase III results from the randomized EPOCH 1 study. Reg Anesth Pain Med. 2019;44:700. https://doi.org/10.1136/rapm-2019-100531.
73. Li J, Lam D, King H, Credaroli E, Harmon E, Vadivelu N. Novel regional anesthesia for outpatient surgery. Curr Pain Headache Reports. 2019;23(10):69.
74. McNamee DA, Parks L, Milligan KR. Postoperative analgesia following total knee replacement: an evaluation of the addition of an obturator nerve block to combined femoral and sciatic nerve block. Acta Anaesthesiol Scand. 2002;46:95. https://doi.org/10.1034/j.1399-6576.2002.460117.x.
75. Rana MV, Desai R, Tran L, Davis D. Perioperative pain control in the ambulatory setting. Curr Pain Headache Rep. 2016;20(3):18. https://doi.org/10.1007/s11916-016-0550-3.
76. O'Donnell BD, Iohom G. Regional anesthesia techniques for ambulatory orthopedic surgery. Curr Opin Anaesthesiol. 2008;21:723. https://doi.org/10.1097/ACO.0b013e328314b665.
77. Hammond LM, Hardy J. Monitored anesthesia care. In: Essential clinical Anesthesia review: keywords, questions and answers for the boards. Cambridge: Cambridge University Press.; 2015. https://doi.org/10.1017/CBO9781139584005.051.
78. Prabhakar A, Cefalu JN, Rowe JS, Kaye AD, Urman RD. Techniques to optimize multimodal analgesia in ambulatory surgery. Curr Pain Headache Rep. 2017;21(5):24. https://doi.org/10.1007/s11916-017-0622-z.
79. Badrinath S, Avramov MN, Shadrick M, Witt TR, Ivankovich AD. The use of a ketamine-propofol combination during monitored anesthesia care. Anesth Analg. 2000;90:858. https://doi.org/10.1213/00000539-200004000-00016.
80. Apfel CC, Kranke P, Katz MH, et al. Volatile anaesthetics may be the main cause of early but not delayed postoperative vomiting: a randomized controlled trial of factorial design. Br J Anaesth. 2002;88(5):659–68. https://doi.org/10.1093/bja/88.5.659.
81. Cao X, White PF, Ma H. An update on the management of postoperative nausea and vomiting. J Anesth. 2017;31:617. https://doi.org/10.1007/s00540-017-2363-x.
82. Mason SE, Scott AJ, Mayer E, Purkayastha S. Patient-related risk factors for urinary retention following ambulatory general surgery: a systematic review and meta-analysis. Am J Surg. 2016;211:1126. https://doi.org/10.1016/j.amjsurg.2015.04.021.
83. Awan FN, Zulkifli MS, Mc Cormack O, et al. Factors involved in unplanned admissions from general surgical day-care in a modern protected facility. Ir Med J. 2013;106(5):153–4.
84. Lee JH. Anesthesia for ambulatory surgery. Korean J Anesthesiol. 2017;70:398. https://doi.org/10.4097/kjae.2017.70.4.398.
85. Peters ML, Sommer M, De Rijke JM, et al. Somatic and psychologic predictors of long-term unfavorable outcome after surgical intervention. Ann Surg. 2007;245:487. https://doi.org/10.1097/01.sla.0000245495.79781.65.
86. Gan TJ. Poorly controlled postoperative pain: prevalence, consequences, and prevention. J Pain Res. 2017;Volume 10:2287. https://doi.org/10.2147/JPR.S144066.
87. Elvir-Lazo OL, White PF. The role of multimodal analgesia in pain management after ambulatory surgery. Curr Opin Anaesthesiol. 2010;23:697. https://doi.org/10.1097/ACO.0b013e32833fad0a.
88. Jafra A, Mitra S. Pain relief after ambulatory surgery: progress over the last decade. Saudi J Anaesth. 2018;12(4):618–25. https://doi.org/10.4103/sja.SJA_232_18.
89. Kohrs R, Durieux ME. Ketamine: teaching an old drug new tricks. Anesth Analg. 1998;87:1186. https://doi.org/10.1097/00000539-199811000-00039.
90. Dasta J, Ramamoorthy S, Patou G, Sinatra R. Bupivacaine liposome injectable suspension compared with bupivacaine HCl for the reduction of opioid burden in the postsurgical setting. Curr Med Res Opin. 2012;28:1609. https://doi.org/10.1185/03007995.2012.721760.
91. Thomas DA, Chang D, Zhu R, Rayaz H, Vadivelu N. Concept of the ambulatory pain physician. Curr Pain Headache Rep. 2017;21(1):7. https://doi.org/10.1007/s11916-017-0611-2.

92. Vadivelu N, Kai AM, Kodumudi V, Berger JM. Challenges of pain control and the role of the ambulatory pain specialist in the outpatient surgery setting. J Pain Res. 2016;9:425. https://doi.org/10.2147/JPR.S86579.
93. White PF, White LM, Monk T, et al. Perioperative care for the older outpatient undergoing ambulatory surgery. Anesth Analg. 2012;114:1190. https://doi.org/10.1213/ANE.0b013e31824f19b8.
94. Cao X, Elvir-Lazo OL, White PF, Yumul R, Tang J. An update on pain management for elderly patients undergoing ambulatory surgery. Curr Opin Anaesthesiol. 2016;29(6):674–82. https://doi.org/10.1097/ACO.0000000000000396.
95. Warren KG, Froehlich M, Feldman DL. The role multimodal pain management plays with successful total knee and hip arthroplasty. Top Geriatr Rehabil. 2019;35:42. https://doi.org/10.1097/TGR.0000000000000215.
96. Schmucker DL. Age-related changes in liver structure and function: implications for disease? Exp Gerontol. 2005;40:650. https://doi.org/10.1016/j.exger.2005.06.009.
97. Nelson SJ, Webb ML, Lukasiewicz AM, Varthi AG, Samuel AM, Grauer JN. Is outpatient total hip arthroplasty safe? J Arthroplast. 2017;32:1439. https://doi.org/10.1016/j.arth.2016.11.053.
98. Ilfeld BM, Moeller LK, Mariano ER, et al. Continuous peripheral nerve blocks: Is local anesthetic dose the only factor, or do concentration and volume influence infusion effects as well? Anesthesiology. 2010;112(2):347–54. https://doi.org/10.1097/ALN.0b013e3181ca4e5d.
99. White PF, Wang B, Tang J, Wender RH, Naruse R, Sloninsky A. The effect of intraoperative use of esmolol and nicardipine on recovery after ambulatory surgery. Anesth Analg. 2003;97:1633. https://doi.org/10.1213/01.ANE.0000085296.07006.BA.
100. Wang B, Tang J, White PF, et al. Effect of the intensity of transcutaneous acupoint electrical stimulation on the postoperative analgesic requirement. Anesth Analg. 1997;85:406. https://doi.org/10.1097/00000539-199708000-00029.
101. Chou R, Gordon DB, De Leon-Casasola OA, et al. Management of postoperative pain: a clinical practice guideline from the American pain society, the American society of regional anesthesia and pain medicine, and the American society of anesthesiologists' committee on regional anesthesia, executive commi. J Pain. 2016;17(2):131–57. https://doi.org/10.1016/j.jpain.2015.12.008.
102. AL-Sagarat AY, Al-Oran HM, Obeidat H, Hamlan AM, Moxham L. Preparing the family and children for surgery. Crit Care Nurs Q. 2017;40(2):99–107. https://doi.org/10.1097/CNQ.0000000000000146.
103. Frisch AM, Johnson A, Timmons S, Weatherford C. Nurse practitioner role in preparing families for pediatric outpatient surgery. Pediatr Nurs. 2010;36(1):41–7.
104. Scrimin S, Haynes M, Altoe G, Bornstein MH, Axia G. Anxiety and stress in mothers and fathers in the 24 hours after their child's surgery. Child Care Heal Dev. 2012;35(2):227–33. https://doi.org/10.1111/j.1365-2214.2008.00920.x.Anxiety.
105. Dionigi A, Sangiorgi D, Flangini R. Clown intervention to reduce preoperative anxiety in children and parents: a randomized controlled trial. J Health Psychol. 2014;19(3):369–80. https://doi.org/10.1177/1359105312471567.
106. Beauregard L, Pomp A, Choinière M. Severity and impact of pain after day-surgery. Can J Anaesth. 1998;45(4):304–11. https://doi.org/10.1007/BF03012019.
107. Nafiu OO, Thompson A, Chiravuri SD, Cloyd B, Reynolds PI. Factors associated with recovery room intravenous opiate requirement after pediatric outpatient operations. Anesth Analg. 2019;128(6):1225–33. https://doi.org/10.1213/ANE.0000000000003701.
108. Suresh S, Ecoffey C, Bosenberg A, et al. The European society of regional anaesthesia and pain therapy/American society of regional anesthesia and pain medicine recommendations on local anesthetics and adjuvants dosage in pediatric regional anesthesia. Reg Anesth Pain Med. 2018;43(2):211–6. https://doi.org/10.1097/AAP.0000000000000702.
109. Suresh S, De Oliveira GS. Local anaesthetic dosage of peripheral nerve blocks in children: analysis of 40 121 blocks from the pediatric regional anesthesia network database. Br J Anaesth. 2018;120(2):317–22. https://doi.org/10.1016/j.bja.2017.10.019.
110. Pereira RJ, Munechika M, Sakata RK. Pain management after outpatient surgical procedure. Rev Dor. 2013;14(1):61–7.

The Role of Ultrasound in the Ambulatory Setting

13

Amit Prabhakar, Vanessa Moll, Katie Frith, Mason E. Triay, Raquel E. Candal, Levin Fairchild, Elyse M. Cornett, and Alan David Kaye

Abstract

Ultrasound use has become an integral part of modern medical practice in the past two decades. Ultrasound technology allows clinicians to quickly, easily, and safely identify patient anatomy for diagnostic and therapeutic purposes. Diagnostic ultrasound utilization includes transthoracic, abdominal, and airway assessment. Therapeutic ultrasound utilization includes securing difficult intravenous access, central hemodynamic access, and peripheral nerve blocks. The ease, quickness, and safety of ultrasound use has made it an integral component of ambulatory surgical centers' healthare. This chapter will review the wide utility of ultrasound in ambulatory surgical centers.

Introduction

The ambulatory surgical center (ASC) was first introduced in 1970, and its creation had an immediate and lasting impact on the landscape of healthcare. Not even two decades after its introduction, over half of all surgeries took place in these specialized centers. This percentage has continued to rise as the popularity and efficacy of

A. Prabhakar
Department of Anesthesiology, Division of Critical Care Medicine, Emory University School of Medicine, Atlanta, GA, USA
e-mail: Amit.prabhakar@emory.edu

V. Moll
Department of Anesthesiology, Division of Critical Care Medicine, Emory University School of Medicine, Atlanta, GA, USA

University Hospital Zurich, Zurich, Switzerland
e-mail: vanessa.moll@emory.edu

K. Frith · L. Fairchild
Louisiana State University Health Shreveport, Shreveport, LA, USA
e-mail: kfrit1@lsuhsc.edu; lfair1@lsuhsc.edu

M. E. Triay
Louisiana State University Health Shreveport, School of Medicine, Shreveport, LA, USA
e-mail: mtriay@lsuhsc.edu

R. E. Candal
Department of Surgery, Louisiana State University Health Sciences Center Shreveport, Shreveport, LA, USA
e-mail: rcanda@lsuhsc.edu

E. M. Cornett (✉)
Department of Anesthesiology, Louisiana State University Health Shreveport, Shreveport, LA, USA
e-mail: ecorne@lsuhsc.edu

A. D. Kaye
Departments of Anesthesiology and Pharmacology, Toxicology, and Neurosciences, Louisiana State University Health Shreveport, Shreveport, LA, USA
e-mail: akaye@lsuhsc.edu

K. Rajput et al. (eds.), *Pain Control in Ambulatory Surgery Centers*,
https://doi.org/10.1007/978-3-030-55262-6_13

minimally invasive surgical techniques continue to improve [1, 2]. Numerous studies have shown that procedures and surgeries performed in ambulatory surgery centers can have a decreased risk of hospital-acquired infections and other postoperative complications when compared to their inpatient counterparts [3]. Additionally, many patients find greater patient satisfaction with outpatient surgery centers, as they are more convenient and accessible. Related to lower overhead costs and high patient satisfaction, ambulatory surgery centers are integral components of the rapidly changing modern healthcare landscape.

Point-of-care ultrasound (POCUS) use has proven to be an indispensable tool in ambulatory surgery centers for both diagnostic and therapeutic interventions. Once trained and facile, clinicians can view patient anatomy in real-time with no radiation exposure or discomfort to the patient. Ultrasound use has proven clinical utility for a broad range of scenarios including but not limited to, securing intravenous access, transthoracic ultrasound, difficult airway evaluation, and regional nerve blocks.

Clinicians who work in ASCs need to be prepared to care for a wide variety of patient populations, including those who have a history of chronic pain. Members of the perioperative team are continually striving to enhance multimodal analgesic strategies and protocols to help minimize peri-procedural pain. The utilization of peripheral nerve blocks is a core component of multimodal analgesia and has been shown to decrease pain, improve patient satisfaction, speed recovery, and improve overall outcomes. Peripheral nerve blocks include upper extremity, lower extremity, neuraxial, and truncal sites. Peripheral nerve blocks can function as the sole anesthetic, as a supplement to anesthesia, or even as an outpatient approach to help mitigate chronic pain. While complications from regional anesthesia performed under ultrasound guidance can occur, severe adverse events are extremely rare. Regardless, ambulatory surgery centers need to be equipped and prepared to deal with any potential complications. This book chapter will detail the many ways ultrasound can be used in an ambulatory setting.

Pain Treatment and Ultrasound

Efficiency is the cornerstone of a successful ASC. Numerous tools and methods have been investigated to allow for optimal patient care and safety while also ensuring maximal productiveness of the ASC. Clinicians working in ASCs are faced with the unique challenge of providing numerous safe and efficient analgesic approaches that allow for appropriate patient recovery within a finite time period [1]. Optimizing pain control is important for both the patient experience and decreasing admissions to the hospital. Poorly controlled pain can result in an increased length of stay in the post-anesthesia care unit and is one of the most common reasons to admit a patient after an outpatient procedure [4]. The increased utilization of ultrasound for regional anesthetic approaches has played a pivotal role in advancing anesthesia in outpatient settings. Ultrasound guidance for peripheral nerve blocks has been shown to increase fast pass success, decrease time to block onset, improve overall analgesia, and minimize the risk for adverse events like unintended nerve injury, vascular injury, or local anesthetic systemic toxicity (LAST). Performing regional anesthetics with the administration of local anesthetics under direct ultrasound visualization can minimize the total dose given and decrease the risk of LAST.

While there are numerous advantages supporting the use of ultrasound for regional anesthetics, deciding whether or not to perform a peripheral nerve block is ultimately made collaboratively by the clinician, patient, and surgeon. This decision is also dependent on the procedure that is being performed, patient anatomy, and psychosocial factors that may affect the block's assessment (see Table 13.1) [4]. Special considerations in the ambulatory setting include limited observation in the post-anesthesia care unit with a heavy reliance on both patient and caretaker to adhere to discharge instructions. Patients who are best suited for peripheral nerve blocks include those patients in which opioids need to be used sparingly, such as chronic pain patients, patients with obstructive sleep apnea, and/or patients with a

Table 13.1 Selection criteria for ambulatory center nerve blocks

Procedure with moderate to severe postoperative pain
No contraindications to regional anesthesia
Has a working telephone and can be reliably contacted after discharge from the facility
Patient or caregiver is proficient in English and can facilitate a follow-up conversation
Lives within a reasonable distance to medical facility in the case emergent assessment is warranted

history of severe nausea and vomiting after anesthesia [5].

It is currently estimated that nearly one in five individuals suffers from some form of chronic pain [6]. Since their creation, ambulatory surgery centers have been molded to fit the needs of the healthcare community better. In 2012, it was noted that four of the ten top procedures performed in these centers were considered to be a form of interventional pain management [2]. As with peripheral nerve blocks, many of these pain management treatments – including stellate ganglion blocks, vertebral facet injections, and non-spine procedures – have blossomed with the aid of the ultrasound. The stellate ganglion block (most often used to treat complex regional pain syndrome) is considered high risk due to the target site's vascular anatomy. Ultrasound guidance has been shown to decrease the incidence of post-procedure hematoma formation. It helps to identify the correct fascial plane in which the ganglion is located, minimizing the spread of the injected anesthetic to surrounding neurovascular structures.

For similar reasons, ultrasound is now being used for cervical spinal injections. The procedure's major complication is potential damage to nearby vessels, the most important being the vertebral artery. When using ultrasound, this vasculature can be visualized, leading to fewer needle passes and decreased procedure time. The utility of ultrasound varies with traveling down the spinal column due to patient anatomy and factors such as the depth of target structures and overlying bone. For lumbar vertebral injections, the ultrasound can be used to help identify and map relevant anatomy. Non-spine pain management procedures have also started to take advantage of the ultrasound. This includes peripheral joint injections, intercostal nerve blocks, and ilioinguinal/iliohypogastric injections for chronic pain after hernia repair [7].

Peripheral Nerve Blocks and Multimodal Analgesia Using Ultrasound in Outpatient Setting

The use of ultrasound in an outpatient setting is gaining popularity for several reasons. The increased usage is attributed to its utility in visualizing soft tissues (muscles, ligaments, fascial planes) and vascular structures in real-time, ease of performance, and avoidance of ionizing radiation and contrast agents that may cause renal damage or allergic reactions [7].

When examining the efficacy of ultrasound guidance for perioperative neuraxial and peripheral nerve blocks in children, it was found that ultrasonography-assisted techniques resulted in improved pain scores 1 hour postoperatively, longer block duration, reduced number of required needle passes, and shorter time to perform the preoperative patient pre-scan [8]. Ultrasound use is still heavily operator dependent and requires substantial knowledge of the external and internal landmarks necessary for analgesic injections.

Upper Extremity Peripheral Nerve Blocks

Upper extremity peripheral nerve blocks are ideal for outpatient forearm and hand surgeries. Depending on the injury and type of surgical procedure being performed, single target nerve blocks, facilitated by real-time ultrasound imaging, are very successful within one needle entry point [9]. A distal approach to blocking the arm's peripheral nerves (radial, median, ulnar) has numerous benefits. This approach avoids vital structures, such as the subclavian vasculature, axillary artery, pleura, or phrenic nerve, while preserving the arm and hand's proximal motor function. A recent randomized controlled trial comparing ultrasound-guided supraclavicular plexus block with distal peripheral nerve blocks for ambulatory hand surgery resulted in better strength preservation, in addition to greater patient satisfaction with ultrasound-guided distal nerve blocks [9].

Lower Extremity Nerve Blocks

When considering lower extremity nerve blocks safe ambulation during the postoperative period is of paramount importance. Delayed mobility and altered proprioception from residual local anesthetic can lead to falls or other adverse events. The lumbar plexus and sciatic nerves are deeper and more difficult anatomic structures to isolate, increasing the risk of LAST. LAST will be discussed in more detail later in the chapter. Some experts recommend using both nerve stimulation and ultrasound guidance for lower extremity blocks [10].

Ultrasound-guided sciatic nerve blocks (SNB) in the gluteal region have been shown to safe alternative to treating postherpetic neuralgia (PHN) in herpes zoster patients. Some patients with acute refractory herpetic neuralgia had a rapid disappearance of pain and dysesthesia with a significant sleep quality improvement after receiving a continuous peripheral nerve block under ultrasound guidance [11]. Ultrasound guidance has also improved the quality of motor and sensory blocks, in addition to a reduction in the total dose of local anesthetic used in femoral nerve blocks. A grade A recommendation is that ultrasound guidance for lower extremity peripheral nerve blocks provides improvements in both onset and success of sensory block, a decrease in local anesthetic dosing, and decreased time to perform lower extremity procedures [12].

Truncal Blocks

Truncal nerve block targets include the paravertebral, intercostal, suprascapular, ilioinguinal, and iliohypogastric nerves. The ilioinguinal, iliohypogastric, and genitofemoral nerves are routinely blocked to help mitigate postoperative orchiectomy, appendectomy, nephrectomy, or ureteral pain [13]. Blocking the thoracic paravertebral nerve results in an ipsilateral somatic motor and sensory blockade of multiple thoracic dermatomes above and below the site of injection. Locating this space is technically challenging and can result in several needle redirections, leading to pain and increasing the risk of causing a pneumothorax [14]. The use of ultrasound offers real-time imaging and visualization of the vertebral transverse processes and parietal pleura giving a measurement of depth from skin to paravertebral space. Ultrasound-guided paravertebral blockade has also gained popularity in breast surgeries due to improved postoperative pain scores and the potential effects general anesthesia may have on cancer progression [15].

Adjuvant Medications and Multimodal Analgesia

The ability to control postoperative pain via a multimodal approach can improve pain scores while also minimizing the risk for pharmacologic adverse effects. The addition of adjuvant medications work additively and/or synergistically with local anesthetics to enhance opioid-sparing analgesia. Examples of adjuvants include gabapentinoids, nonsteroidal anti-inflammatory drugs (NSAIDs), cyclooxygenase-1, and cyclooxygenase-2 (COX-1 and COX-2) inhibitors, glucocorticoids, ketamine, clonidine, and lidocaine infusions. Studies demonstrate that the addition of these medications can reduce postoperative opioid use by 20–60% [16]. Local anesthetics can be paired with adjuvant drugs to achieve prolonged pain control, to reduce toxicity with higher local anesthetic injections, and to potentially reduce prolonged motor blockade [16]. The balance between maintaining a patient's motor strength and providing adequate postoperative analgesia has shown to be difficult with single local injections. Certain adjuvant medications can prolong the duration of single-injection peripheral nerve blocks. Dexamethasone is one of these adjuvants that can prolong or enhance the duration of pain control when injected intravenously or perineurally [16]. A systematic review found that ultrasound-guided upper and lower extremity blocks with adjuvants resulted in faster onset and longer duration of analgesia when compared to other techniques [17].

Ultrasound Complications in the Ambulatory Setting

Ultrasound is a proven reliable, and safe imaging modality. Risks associated with ultrasound use are minimal, and any complications associated with ultrasound use are generally attributable to the procedure itself. An example of this is regional anesthetics. Common risks associated with regional anesthetics include peripheral nerve injury, local anesthetic system toxicity (LAST), hemidiaphragmatic paresis, and pneumothorax [18]. This list is the same regardless of if ultrasound is utilized or not.

LAST is seen when local anesthetics inadvertently enter the systemic vasculature with eventual migration to the cardiac and central nervous system. Local anesthetic inhibition of voltage-gated Na + channels results in both inhibitory and excitatory downstream effects [19]. Symptoms are wide-ranging and can include mild systemic symptoms like metallic taste or circumoral numbness to more severe symptoms like seizures, coma, and/or cardiac arrest [20]. Thankfully, current evidence shows that ultrasound use for peripheral nerve blocks does reduce the occurrence of LAST [18, 21]. Treatment of LAST includes prompt recognition, initiation of lipid infusion, and supportive measures [22].

Peripheral nerve injuries can result from direct trauma, excessive stretching, hypoperfusion, or exposure to a neurotoxic substance [24]. While ultrasound use can help to minimize potential nerve injury, it does not completely preclude its occurrence. Peripheral nerve injuries can be challenging to classify and may not be immediately recognized, but thankfully are mostly transient [23]. Direct trauma can result from intraneural injections and high injection pressures (greater than or equal to 25 PSI) [24, 27]. Unintentional trauma to the surrounding vasculature may cause a hematoma formation resulting in compression and subsequent ischemia. A review of peripheral nerve injuries found that most patients who experience symptoms after the peripheral nerve block already had preexisting peripheral neuropathy [24]. This point emphasizes the importance for clinicians to perform and document a comprehensive physical exam before performing a peripheral nerve block.

Other potential adverse effects associated with upper extremity peripheral nerve blocks include ipsilateral phrenic nerve paralysis, pneumothorax, and Horner's syndrome. As mentioned previously, brachial plexus nerve blocks are used for upper extremity analgesia. Ipsilateral phrenic nerve paralysis can result from the spread of local anesthetic to the phrenic nerve roots and result in hemidiaphragmatic paralysis [29]. Partial paralysis of the diaphragm can significantly impact a patient's respiratory mechanics, resulting in a 25% reduction in pulmonary function [29]. Thus, upper extremity peripheral nerve blocks, such as an interscalene approach, need to be either avoided entirely or done with extreme caution in patients who have a preexisting pulmonary compromise. Iatrogenic pneumothorax is another potential complication that can occur and is most commonly associated with the supraclavicular approach. Patients may present with shortness of breath and/or tracheal deviation. If suspicious, clinicians should order a chest x-ray and auscultate for the presence or absence of breath sounds. Treatment includes expeditious decompression with chest tube placement. Horner's syndrome is a less severe and transient complication that may occur with either a supraclavicular or interscalene nerve block approach. This complication occurs when local anesthetic unintentionally migrates to the stellate ganglion resulting in ipsilateral pupillary miosis, blurry vision, ptosis, and anhidrosis.

PACU Discharge Criteria

Postoperative pain is the most commonly reported complication of ambulatory surgery [25]. Uncontrolled pain can result in a cascade of detrimental downstream effects resulting in delayed discharge or even in-patient admission. A multimodal approach to analgesia that starts in the preoperative phase and continues through the intra- and postoperative phase of care can ensure adequate analgesia while also minimizing the risk of adverse medication reactions such as nausea and emesis [32].

One of the most important components in ambulatory surgical center patient care is the post-anesthesia care unit or PACU. The PACU consists of two phases. The first phase involves close monitoring and frequent assessments with nurse staffing equivalent to the ICU. The second phase is a transitional period before the patient is either sent home or admitted to the hospital. Patients who have undergone regional anesthetics should not leave phase 1 until motor, and sensory function is restored [25]. As analgesic approaches have continued to evolve and improve, there are a certain subset of patients that can bypass phase 1 and proceed directly to phase 2, also known as being "fast-tracked." This can help to decrease healthcare costs by expediting discharge home. Fast-tracking patients can also increase patient comfort and satisfaction because in phase 2, patients can recover while having their loved ones present at the bedside [25].

Historically, Aldrete's score has been used to determine when a patient can be discharged from the PACU [29]. This scoring system considers a patient's activity, respiratory status, hemodynamics, consciousness, and oxygen saturation (see Table 13.2). Patients with a score of 9 or greater can be safely discharged from the PACU to progress with their other phases of care [25].

There are additional criteria to help clinicians ascertain which patients are appropriate candidates to skip phase 1. These criteria include scoring pain and emesis as seen in Table 13.3. Patients who score a combined minimum score of 12 are deemed appropriate to fast-track to phase 2 [33].

Table 13.2 Aldrete scoring system

Criteria		Points
Activity	Able to move four extremities on command	2
	Able to move two extremities on command	1
	Able to move zero extremities on command	0
Breathing	Breathe deeply and cough freely	2
	Tachypnea with good cough	1
	Dyspnea with weak cough	0
Circulation	Systemic B.P. ± 20% of pre-anesthetic level	2
	Systemic B.P. ± 20–40% of pre-anesthetic level	1
	Systemic B.P. >40% of pre-anesthetic level	0
Consciousness	Fully awake	2
	Arousable	1
	Not arousable	0
Oxygen saturation	While breathing room air: 92%	2
	Needs supplemental oxygen to maintain >90%	1
	<90% even with supplemental oxygen	0

As ambulatory surgery centers continue to grow in popularity due to the advancement of surgical and anesthesia techniques, it is important to address complications promptly to prevent hospital admissions following day surgeries. A multimodal approach to anesthesia is a central component to minimize the severity of potential complications associated with anesthesia in the ambulatory setting. While ultrasound use has profoundly decreased the amount of complications associated with regional anesthesia, complications can still occur, and it is important for clinicians to recognize and treat such adverse effects.

Important Clinical Findings

Emerging literature continues to investigate the various aspects of ultrasound use and its effects on different metrics. Here, we discuss the most recent literature and clinical findings for POCUS. POCUS use has proven utility in a

Table 13.3 Scoring system with additional criteria of pain and nausea and vomiting

Additional criteria		
Pain	Controllable with oral analgesics	2
	Moderate to severe pain controlled with IV analgesics	1
	Persistent severe pain	0
Nausea and vomiting	Minimal nausea with no emesis	2
	Transient vomiting or retching	1
	Persistent moderate to severe nausea and vomiting	0

variety of different clinical scenarios (see Table 13.4). While there have been numerous publications showing the benefits of ultrasound utilization, most have been retrospective reviews, leaving a lack of randomized controlled trial methodology [26, 28]. A recent prospective and controlled study of 80 patients investigated the impact of POCUS on resource utilization, diagnostic accuracy, and clinical management in medical and surgical (ICUs) [30]. Patients in the ultrasound-driven protocol had fewer chest radiographs, ultrasound studies, and computed tomography scans ordered compared to those who received a conventional standard of care [30]. This same study also found that the ultrasound cohort had reduced time from admission to first ultrasound study, better characterization of ICU admitting diagnosis with pertinent changes to clinical management, less duration on mechanical ventilation, and more precise fluid management [30]. Despite the relatively small sample size, this study applied a controlled trial methodology to demonstrate the utility of bedside ultrasound and the positive outcomes associated with its increased use in ICU patients. While more prospective studies in other clinical settings need to be done, the findings of this study should also translate to the ambulatory setting. POCUS has the potential to decrease healthcare costs and improve patient mortality by ordering fewer diagnostic imaging studies, decreasing time spent on ventilators, and allowing for more precise fluid management.

Table 13.4 Major advantages and disadvantages of POCUS (please note that there are other potential advantages and disadvantages; this is not an exhaustive list)

Potential advantages of POCUS	Potential disadvantages of POCUS
Fewer chest radiographs, CT	Need ultrasound available
Better admission diagnosis	No standardized methods/training
Duration of time mechanically ventilated	Need physician trained in using/reading
Fluid management	Time needed to perform procedure
Predictive difficult laryngoscopy	Physician perception of traditional methods
Predictive adverse cardiac events	No unanimous protocols for specific findings
Regional/neuraxial anesthesia Accurate epidural depth Appropriate tool selection Improved success of first needle insertion Identifying midline and interlaminar landmarks	
Vascular access Peripheral IV Midline catheters Peripherally inserted central catheter	

Airway Assessment

Ultrasound has also been a useful adjunct for airway assessment and predicting potentially difficult airway management. A recent prospective, observational study evaluated the use of POCUS for airway evaluation and correlation with traditional clinical indicators of potential difficult airway management. The study included 200 operative patients and was relevant for finding a strong positive correlation with ultrasound airway measurements compared to conventional predictors to difficult intubation, such as the Cormack-Lehane grades [39]. Examples of ultrasound soft tissue measurements include the depth of the peri-epiglottic space and thyrohyoid membrane. It is important to recognize other cofactors such as obesity, pregnancy, operator experience, and patient positioning play a key role in potential difficult airway management. The increased utilization of ultrasound for airway assessment can be a powerful clinical adjunct when used in addition to traditional airway assessment tools.

Transthoracic Echocardiography

Transthoracic echocardiography (TTE) has emerged as one of the most useful clinical adjuncts to quickly assess cardiovascular function [39]. In general, there should be minimal need to assess the adequacy of cardiac function in the ambulatory surgical setting. However, as the patient selection for ambulatory surgery continues to expand to include sicker patients, all perioperative clinicians should be cognizant of the utility of TTE. A prospective and observational study looked at TTE feasibility and effects in the perioperative setting [41].

Anesthesiologists with TTE training were able to obtain diagnostic-quality images in 98% of patients. More importantly, these findings had a direct impact on the acute management of patients [41]. A recent prospective interventional study compared TTE-guided management to conventional non-TTE-guided management in hemodynamically unstable patients [43]. Findings showed that TTE use in situations of hemodynamic instability resulted in improved outcomes by changing clinical management 66% of the time [43]. TTE is a potentially lifesaving clinical adjunct, and all perioperative clinicians should be facile in basic TTE principles.

Neuraxial Anesthesia

As mentioned previously, ultrasound can be a valuable tool for neuraxial anesthetics. A 2019 prospective randomized controlled study compared using preprocedural ultrasound exams to conventional blind techniques for lumbar epidural blocks [31, 34]. This study found that ultrasound use accurately measured epidural depth. This subsequently allowed clinicians to select the correct equipment preemptively, decreased the risk for an accidental thecal puncture, and improved success of combined spinal epidural anesthesia on first needle insertion [31, 34]. A Cochrane analysis reviewed 31 clinical trials and one meta-analysis and consistently found increased success, ease of performance, and reduced rate of traumatic procedures when using ultrasound for neuraxial anesthesia compared to landmark palpation alone [35].

Vascular Access

Another popular use of ultrasound in hospitals and ambulatory surgery centers is to aid vascular access and other percutaneous procedures. The practice of starting peripheral intravenous (PIV) catheters to obtain vascular access is the most common invasive procedure performed worldwide, with an estimated 200 million performed in North America each year [36]. In a 2012 systemic review and meta-analysis, ultrasound guidance was superior to the standard technique in achieving successful peripheral cannulation in difficult-to-access patients [37]. Multiple studies have demonstrated that ultrasound-guided venous access, such as PIVs, midline catheters, and peripherally inserted central catheters, had significantly lower failure rates and complications compared to conventional methods [36, 37, 45]. Facilitating adequate, safe, and efficient IV access in the ambulatory setting can help to minimize delays, improve productivity, enhance patient safety, and increase patient satisfaction in the perioperative ambulatory setting.

Sterilization

Lastly, patient safety and patient care can be improved with the increasing use of ultrasound in the ambulatory setting by paying attention to sterilization and prevention of the risk of infection of contaminated probes in the ambulatory setting – several hospitals have come to realize the importance of this fact in ambulatory surgery centers [38, 40, 42, 44].

Summary

This chapter has provided a comprehensive review of the numerous ways how ultrasound is used in ASCs. Ultrasound use in ASCs can help maximize efficiency, increase profits, enhance patient care, and improve patient safety. There continues to be a broad field of research evaluating the use of POCUS-assisted physical exams to help guide clinical management. As this field continues to evolve with emerging scientific evidence, practitioners in the perioperative setting need to have ultrasound use in their clinical armamentarium.

References

1. Hagen K, Iohom G. Pain management for ambulatory surgery: what is new? Curr Anesthesiol Rep. 2014;4(4):326–33.
2. Manchikanti L, Singh V, Hirsch JA. Saga of payment systems of ambulatory surgery centers for interventional techniques: an update. Pain Physician. 2012;15(2):109–30.
3. Hamad MMAA, Connolly VM. Ambulatory emergency care – improvement by design. Clin Med J R Coll Physicians London. 2018;18(1):69–74.
4. Salinas FV, Joseph RS. Peripheral nerve blocks for ambulatory surgery. Anesthesiol Clin. 2014;32(2):341–55.
5. Vadivelu N, Kai AM, Kodumudi V, Berger JM. Challenges of pain control and the role of the ambulatory pain specialist in the outpatient surgery setting. J Pain Res. 2016;9:425–35.
6. Dahlhamer J, Lucas J, Zelaya C. Pain Awareness Month — September 2018 Prevalence of Chronic Pain and High-Impact Chronic Pain Among Adults — United States, 2016. MMWR Morb Mortal Wkly Rep. 2018;67(36):1001.
7. Perrine DC, Votta-Velis G, Borgeat A. Ultrasound indications for chronic pain management: an update on the most recent evidence. Curr Opin Anaesthesiol. 2016;29(5):600–5.
8. Guay J, Suresh S, Kopp S. The use of ultrasound guidance for perioperative neuraxial and peripheral nerve blocks in children. Cochrane Database Syst Rev. 2019;2(2):CD011436.
9. Sehmbi H, Madjdpour C, Shah UJ, Chin KJ. Ultrasound guided distal peripheral nerve block of the upper limb: a technical review. J Anaesthesiol Clin Pharmacol. 2015;31(3):296–307.
10. Zhang XH, Li YJ, He WQ, et al. Combined ultrasound and nerve stimulator-guided deep nerve block may decrease the rate of local anesthetics systemic toxicity: a randomized clinical trial. BMC Anesthesiol. 2019;19
11. Bagaphou TC, Santonastaso D, Gargaglia E, et al. Ultrasound guided continuous sciatic nerve block for acute herpetic neuralgia. Case Rep Anesthesiol. 2019;2019:1.
12. Salinas FV. Ultrasound and review of evidence for lower extremity peripheral nerve blocks. Reg Anesth Pain Med. 2010;35(2 Suppl):S16–25.
13. Bischoff JM, Koscielniak-Nielsen ZJ, Kehlet H, Werner MU. Ultrasound-guided ilioinguinal/iliohypogastric nerve blocks for persistent inguinal postherniorrhaphy pain: a randomized, double-blind, placebo-controlled, crossover trial. Anesth Analg. 2012;114:1323.
14. Riain SC, Donnell BO, Cuffe T, Harmon DC, Fraher JP, Shorten G. Thoracic paravertebral block using real-time ultrasound guidance. Anesth Analg. 2010;110:248.
15. Looney M, Doran P, Buggy DJ. Effect of anesthetic technique on serum vascular endothelial growth factor C and transforming growth factor β in women undergoing anesthesia and surgery for breast cancer. Anesthesiology. 2010;113(5):1118–25.
16. Elvir-Lazo OL, White PF. The role of multimodal analgesia in pain management after ambulatory surgery. Curr Opin Anaesthesiol. 2010;23(6):697–703.
17. Liu SS. Evidence basis for ultrasound-guided block characteristics onset, quality, and duration. Reg Anesth Pain Med. 2016;41:205.
18. Neal JM. Ultrasound-guided regional anesthesia and patient safety: update of an evidence-based analysis. Reg Anesth Pain Med. 2016;41:195.
19. El-Boghdadly K, Pawa A, Chin KJ. Local anesthetic systemic toxicity: current perspectives: Dove Medical Press Ltd; 2018.
20. Jeng CL, Torrillo TM, Rosenblatt MA. Complications of peripheral nerve blocks. Br J Anaesth. 2010;(suppl 1):i97–107.
21. Barrington MJ, Kluger R. Ultrasound guidance reduces the risk of local anesthetic systemic toxicity following peripheral nerve blockade. Reg Anesth Pain Med. 2013;38(4):289–99.
22. Rosenblatt MA, Abel M, Fischer GW, Itzkovich CJ, Eisenkraft JB. Successful use of a 20% lipid emulsion to resuscitate a patient after a presumed bupivacaine-related cardiac arrest. Anesthesiology. 2006;105(1):217–8.
23. Fredrickson MJ, Kilfoyle DH. Neurological complication analysis of 1000 ultrasound guided peripheral nerve blocks for elective orthopaedic surgery: a prospective study. Anaesthesia. 2009;64:836.
24. Hewson DW, Bedforth NM, Hardman JG. Spinal cord injury arising in anaesthesia practice: Blackwell Publishing Ltd; 2018.
25. Marshall SI, Chung F. Discharge criteria and complications after ambulatory surgery. Anesth Analg. 1999;88(3):508–17.
26. Oks M, Cleven KL, Cardenas-Garcia J, et al. The effect of point-of-care ultrasonography on imaging

studies in the medical ICU: a comparative study. Chest. 2014;146(6):1574–7.
27. Hadzic A, Dilberovic F, Shah S, et al. Combination of intraneural injection and high injection pressure leads to fascicular injury and neurologic deficits in dogs. Reg Anesth Pain Med. 2004;29:417.
28. Kristensen MS, Teoh WH, Graumann O, Laursen CB. Ultrasonography for clinical decision-making and intervention in airway management: from the mouth to the lungs and pleurae. Berlin: Springer; 2014.
29. Urmey WF, McDonald M. Hemidiaphragmatic paresis during interscalene brachial plexus block: effects on pulmonary function and chest wall mechanics. Anesth Analg. 1992;74(3):352–7.
30. Pontet J, Yic C, Díaz-Gómez JL, et al. Impact of an ultrasound-driven diagnostic protocol at early intensive-care stay: a randomized-controlled trial. Ultrasound J. 2019;11(1)
31. Jain K, Jaiswal V, Puri A. Lumbar ultrasound scan: a guide to the epidural space: Wolters Kluwer Medknow Publications; 2019.
32. White PF. The role of non-opioid analgesic techniques in the management of pain after ambulatory surgery: Lippincott Williams and Wilkins; 2002.
33. White PF, Song D. New criteria for fast-tracking after outpatient anesthesia: a comparison with the modified Aldrete's scoring system. Anesth Analg. 1999;88(5):1069–72.
34. Jain K, Puri A, Taneja R, Jaiswal V, Jain A. Preprocedural ultrasound as an adjunct to blind conventional technique for epidural neuraxial blockade in patients undergoing hip or knee joint replacement surgery: a randomised controlled trial. Presented at: Indian Journal of Anaesthesia.: Wolters Kluwer Medknow Publications; 2019.
35. Perlas A, Chaparro LE, Chin KJ. Lumbar neuraxial ultrasound for spinal and epidural anesthesia: a systematic review and meta-analysis. Reg Anesth Pain Med. 2016;41(2):251–60.
36. Alexandrou E. The one million global catheters PIVC worldwide prevalence study. Br J Nurs. 2014;23(SUPPL. 8):S16.
37. Egan G, Healy D, O'Neill H, Clarke-Moloney M, Grace PA, Walsh SR. Ultrasound guidance for difficult peripheral venous access: Systematic review and meta-analysis: BMJ Publishing Group Ltd and the British Association for Accident & Emergency Medicine; 2013.
38. Carrico RM, Furmanek S, English C. Ultrasound probe use and reprocessing: results from a national survey among U.S. infection preventionists. Am J Infect Control. 2018;46(8):913–20.
39. Margale S, Marudhachalam K, Natani S. Clinical application of point of care transthoracic echocardiography in perioperative period. Indian J Anaesth. 2017;61(1):7.
40. Bancroft EA, English L, Terashita D, Yasuda L. Outbreak of Escherichia coli infections associated with a contaminated transesophageal echocardiography probe. Infect Control Hosp Epidemiol. 2013;34(10):1121–3.
41. Cowie B. Focused cardiovascular ultrasound performed by anesthesiologists in the perioperative period: feasible and alters patient management. J Cardiothorac Vasc Anesth. 2009;23(4):450–6.
42. Akpochafor MO, Eze CU, Adeneye SO, Ajekigbe AT. Assessment of ultrasound equipment as a possible source of nosocomial infection in Lagos state hospitals and radio-diagnostic centres. Radiography. 2013;21(2):154–9.
43. Kratz T, Steinfeldt T, Exner M, et al. Impact of focused intraoperative transthoracic echocardiography by Anesthesiologists on Management in Hemodynamically Unstable High-Risk Noncardiac Surgery Patients. J Cardiothorac Vasc Anesth. 2017;31(2):602–9.
44. Ai A, Anderson L, Safdar N, Shirley D. Barriers and facilitators to standardization of ultrasound use and probe disinfection in the ambulatory setting. Infect Control Hosp Epidemiol. 2020;41(4):469–71.
45. Dakhil B, Couineau F, Hernigou J, Bardet J, Tella E, Bagan P. Is ultrasound guidance contributive to vascular access in endovascular therapy? J Med Vascular. 2017;42(4):229–33.

14 Use of Regional Anesthesia/ Neuraxial Anesthesia in Ambulatory Surgery Centers

Vanessa Moll, Amit Prabhakar, Dirk Ubmann, Lukas J. Kandler, Petra Piccolruaz, Max Antonio Thomasius, Elyse M. Cornett, and Alan David Kaye

Abstract

Regional anesthesia-based practice in ambulatory surgery is an effective means of providing excellent postoperative analgesia and is associated with a low rate of PONV, regional anesthesia-associated side effects, and unexpected admissions [1]. With the advent of short-acting local anesthetics licensed for neuraxial anesthesia, spinal and epidural anesthesia have gained some traction in outpatient surgery. Fascial blocks such as the erector spinae, serratus anterior, or rectus sheath blocks are valuable tools in the armamentarium of the ambulatory anesthesiologist. Complications of regional anesthesia techniques remain sparse. Practicing blocks to assure fast room turnovers and excellent surgical anesthesia is of utmost importance for a successful ambulatory regional anesthesia practice.

V. Moll
University Hospital Zurich, Zurich, Switzerland

Department of Anesthesiology, Division of Critical Care Medicine, Emory University School of Medicine, Atlanta, GA, USA
e-mail: vanessa.moll@usz.ch

A. Prabhakar
Department of Anesthesiology, Division of Critical Care Medicine, Emory University School of Medicine, Atlanta, GA, USA

D. Ubmann · L. J. Kandler · P. Piccolruaz · M. A. Thomasius
University Hospital Zurich, Zurich, Switzerland
e-mail: dirk.ubmann@usz.ch; lukas.kandler@usz.ch; petra.piccolruaz@usz.ch; maxantonio.thomasius@usz.ch

E. M. Cornett (✉)
Department of Anesthesiology, Louisiana State University Health Shreveport, Shreveport, LA, USA
e-mail: ecorne@lsuhsc.edu

A. D. Kaye
Departments of Anesthesiology and Pharmacology, Toxicology, and Neurosciences, LSU Health Shreveport, Shreveport, LA, USA
e-mail: akaye@lsuhsc.edu

Introduction

The first outpatient operation was performed as early as 1898 by James Henderson Nicoll [2]. Almost a century later, patient-related benefits and economic significance underscore the growing importance of outpatient surgery centers.

In health economics, costs are rising, necessitating a rethinking. The anesthesiologist is increasingly taking a leading role in optimizing process structures and costs without compromising patient safety or satisfaction [3].

Advances in medicine and patient demand are leading to a shift from inpatient interventions to outpatient care [4, 5]. Despite older patient age, advances in minimally invasive surgical tech-

K. Rajput et al. (eds.), *Pain Control in Ambulatory Surgery Centers*,
https://doi.org/10.1007/978-3-030-55262-6_14

niques and improvements in anesthesia procedures led to an overall lower potential for side effects and fewer postoperative complications [6]. Ambulatory surgery promotes patient-centered care: providing care that is respectful of and responsive to individual patient preferences, needs, and values and ensuring that patient values guide all clinical decisions [7]. Psychological stress is reduced with recovery at home instead of sterile clinical settings.

Designed to enhance patient satisfaction and reduce healthcare costs, enhanced recovery after surgery (ERAS) or enhanced recovery programs (ERP) are gaining traction in the ambulatory setting. These programs utilize evidence-based protocols to a standardize care and decrease healthcare expenditures, hospital length of stay (LOS), and morbidity associated with surgical stress [8, 9]. In outpatient surgery, the goals of ERPs relate to optimizing analgesia, minimizing opioid use, reducing postoperative nausea and vomiting (PONV), early ambulation, and improved quality of recovery. Many of these goals the anesthesiologist can directly influence. The multimodal approach to analgesia has rendered many more surgical procedures amenable to outpatient care [10]. Regional anesthesia to optimize perioperative pain control and thereby aid in recovery can be used well in the outpatient sector, partly due to the progress made in the field of sonography (and peripheral nerve stimulation), and the introduction of new short-acting drugs such as 2-chloroprocaine. A distinction is made between neuraxial and peripheral nerve blocks. A well-considered indication for performing nerve block requires good knowledge of the medical contraindications, and the will of the patient to have the desired operation performed under regional anesthesia. Achieving sufficient analgesia is a high priority in outpatient surgery. Patients undergoing regional anesthesia might require less opioid analgesic medications leading to less PONV. Discharging patients from the PACU requires stable vital signs and sufficient analgesia and the lack of PONV [11].

Earlier discharge times have been shown in patients having received regional anesthesia [12]. Utilizing nerve block analgesia in anterior cruciate ligament reconstruction surgery, the PACU could be bypassed, and unplanned hospital admission could be decreased. Costs could be significantly reduced by eliminating personnel-intensive postoperative pain treatment and PONV therapy, and the possible need for inpatient treatment [13].

PACU scoring systems are helpful to achieve standardized patient treatment and discharge criteria, thereby generating a low number of inpatient admissions. The WAKE score and the zero tolerance criteria are PACU discharge scoring systems useful for patients having received regional anesthesia procedures and tailored to the outpatient setting [14, 15]. These scores use modified Aldrete criteria. The original Aldrete score requires, among other things, the mobility of both extremities to be laterally identical with the same qualities and is therefore not suitable for patients after regional anesthesia in the outpatient sector [3]. See Table 14.1.

Complications after peripheral regional anesthesia are rare and temporary. To perform peripheral blockades, ultrasound-guided puncture is current practice aided by peripheral nerve stimulation when necessary. A distinction is made between in-plane and out-of-plane puncture techniques using sonography. This requires a good anatomical understanding, experience with ultrasound, and good hand, eye, and needle coordination. To establish technical proficiency in regional anesthesia techniques, more than eight sessions, and sometimes many more are necessary to establish technical proficiency [16–18]. Possible complications when performing a neuraxial blockade include permanent paraplegia, hematoma, micturition, or post-puncture headache. Peripheral nerve blocks can result in permanent nerve damage, hematoma, or abscess. With both peripheral nerve blocks and neuraxial techniques, there is the possibility that the effect may be incomplete or even completely absent and that it may be necessary to switch to general anesthesia.

Table 14.1 WAKE score and zero tolerance criteria adapted from [3]

WAKE score – criteria	Score
Movement of at least one upper (UE) and one lower (LE) extremity	0 – No targeted movement 1 – Targeted movement of at least one UE and no LE 2 – Targeted movement of at least one UE and one LE
Blood pressure (sitting and lying on the back)	0 – Less than 40% of preoperative baseline and/or orthostatic symptoms 1 – 20–40% of preoperative baseline and no orthostatic symptoms 2 – Within 20% of preoperative baseline and no orthostatic symptoms
Awareness	0 – Somnolent, ± protective reflexes 1 – Awakening to constant stimulus; protective reflexes present; requests are followed 2 – Awake; responds adequately to requests; easily awakened when addressed
Respiration	0 – Tachypnea, dyspnea, or apnea and/or airway support required 1 – Coughs involuntarily; no respiratory support necessary 2 – Coughing and deep breathing possible and/or on request
Oxygen saturation	0 – <95% (or preoperative value minus 2) ± O2 administration 1 – ≥95% (or preoperative value minus 2) with O2 administration 2 – ≥95% (or preoperative value minus 2) without O2 administration
Score >8 and zero tolerance criteria met allow discharge; score >9 and zero tolerance criteria met in patients with obstructive sleep apnea syndrome and no observed apnea for 30–60 minutes allow discharge	
Zero tolerance criteria	
Pain: adequately adapted to the baseline pain scale of the patient	
PONV: Yes or no	
Shivering, itching, and/or orthostatic symptoms (dizziness and/or hypotension while sitting)	

Local Anesthetics

Short-, intermediate-, and long-acting local anesthetics can be used to perform regional anesthesia. Due to the side effects, in particular neuro- and cardiotoxicity, the use of bupivacaine has given way to levobupivacaine and ropivacaine. The dose varies according to the procedure and clinician's experience. Ultrasound guidance has further enabled dose reduction for some peripheral nerve blocks. Clinicians can now optimize perineural placement of the needle tip and the spread of LA. LA can be combined with adjuvants to increase effectiveness. Adjuvants are medications that work synergistically with LA to enhance the duration and quality of analgesia in RA. Examples of adjuvants to LA are [19, 20]:

Epinephrine: Epinephrine is the most widely applied adjunct. It reduces local anesthetic systemic toxicity, prolongs the duration of sensory and motor blockade, detects intravascular injection, and increases block density [21, 22]. Caution must be used as hypertension, tachycardia, and/or arrhythmias may occur.

Alpha-2 agonists (clonidine or dexmedetomidine): Both have an analgesic effect and dexmedetomidine has been used in regional anesthesia as an adjunct to local anesthetics by prolonging the density and duration of peripheral nerve blocks [23–26]. The main adverse effects of dexmedetomidine are alterations in hemodynamic status, which include hypertension bradycardia, and hypotension via pre- and postsynaptic $\alpha 2$-receptor activation. This can lead to vasoconstriction, vasodilatation, and reflex bradycardia [27].

Dexamethasone: The exact mechanism of action is unclear, but it may be decreased nociceptive C-fiber activity from a direct effect on the glucocorticoid receptor [28], vasoconstrictive effects leading to a reduction of local anesthetic vascular uptake [29, 30], and/or delivering systemic anti-inflammatory effects [31]. Combined with bupivacaine and clonidine, dexamethasone can prolong sensory block. Additive and/or synergistic effects are seen with the combination of dexmedetomidine with dexamethasone in combination with local anesthetics resulting in even longer duration of analgesia. See Table 14.2.

Table 14.2 Various local anesthetics for peripheral nerve block, dosage, and duration of action (mod. according to [19, 32, 33])

Drug	Onset	Duration	Max dose (mg/kg BW)	Max dose with epinephrine (mg/kg BW)
2-Chloroprocaine	Rapid	Short (45–90 min)	10	15
Lidocaine	Rapid	Intermediate (90–180 min)	4.5	7
Prilocaine	Rapid	Intermediate (90–180 min)	6	9
Mepivacaine	Medium	Intermediate	5	7
Bupivacaine	Slow	Long	2.5	3
Levobupivacaine	Slow	Long	3	N/A
Ropivacaine	Slow	Long	4	N/A
Tetracaine	Slow	Long	1.5	N/A

Short duration, 45–90 minutes; intermediate duration, 90–180 minutes; long duration, 4–18 hours

Upper Extremity Blocks

Regional anesthesia (RA) is important in the provision of patient-centered care in ambulatory surgery. Pain control in outpatient surgery is crucial. Uncontrolled postoperative pain can delay discharge from the post-anesthesia care unit (PACU), inhibit physical activity, increase the risk of chronic postsurgical pain, and potentially lead to re-admissions. Regional anesthesia enhances perioperative pain control, decreases postoperative nausea and vomiting (PONV), and improves patient satisfaction [34]. RA also increases the value of care by reducing the length of stay, improving operating department throughput (and increasing patient satisfaction) [35]. A recent perioperative observational study of 16,222 patients demonstrated that predictors of patient dissatisfaction were severe pain, drowsiness, sore throat, and PONV, all of which can potentially be eliminated using RA [36]. For the first seven postoperative days there may be potential benefits of regional over general anesthesia; however, rebound pain can be seen at 24 h and when the block wears out if the patient does not take any additional analgesic medication [37]. Patients with comorbidities such as obesity, obstructive sleep apnea syndrome (OSAS), or heart disease can benefit from regional anesthesia. The manipulation of the airway is avoided, pain management can be performed by continuous catheters avoiding opioid analgesics, and nerve blocks provide hemodynamic stability [38, 39]. However, evolving standards for the prevention of perioperative venous thromboembolism (VTE) and the introduction of increasingly potent antithrombotic medications have resulted in concerns regarding the heightened risk of bleeding with regional anesthesia procedures, especially in the neuraxial space. It is critical for clinicians to be aware of the associated risks and proper management of patients taking these medications. Both the American Society of Regional Anesthesia and Pain Medicine (ASRA) and the European Society of Anesthesiology (ESA) have laid out recommendations regarding anticoagulant use and neuraxial/regional techniques [40, 41].

Peripheral nerve stimulation (PNS) to aid optimal perineural injection has been surpassed by ultrasound technology. Today it is used as an adjunct when sonographic visualization is poor. The identification of nerves, visualization of the needle tip throughout the entire passage, application of continuous catheters, and deposit and spread of the injectate can and should all be observed by ultrasound. Various ultrasound probes are suitable for regional anesthesia. Most frequently, linear probes in the high-frequency range of 5–14 MHz are used (for deeper structures such as sciatic blocks, a curved transducer with 2–8 MHz is appropriate).

If PNS is performed, the lower limit of the stimulation current should be set at 0.5 mA with a frequency of 2 Hz. Good PNS results are obtained in healthy nerves with current intensities from 0.5 mA to 1.0 mA. Comorbidities such as diabetes mellitus, polyneuropathy, or renal insufficiency may reduce the excitability of nerves. Similarly, the application of local anesthetics (LA) or sodium chloride solution for hydro-localization increases the stimulation threshold. Intraneural injections should be avoided since even small injected volumes consistently cause long-term electrophysiologic changes indicating nerve injury. While ultrasound can help to avoid this intraneural injection, the increased pressure upon injection might also be a sign of intraneural injection, and the needle tip should be adjusted again before injection [42].

In 1911 the first supraclavicular block was described by D. Kulenkampff. The most popular upper extremity blocks today are the interscalene, supra- and infraclavicular, and axillary blocks [43].

Interscalene Nerve Block

Indication: Shoulder and upper arm operations.

Anatomy and performance: This block is performed at the level of the posterior triangle of the neck, lateral to the clavicular head of the sternocleidomastoid muscle, and next to the sixth or seventh cervical vertebra using an in-plane or out-of-plane ultrasound technique aided by PNS if necessary. The lateral edge of the sternocleidomastoid muscle serves as the outer landmark. The patient's head is turned slightly to the opposite side, and the ultrasound probe is placed in the area of the supraclavicular fossa at an oblique coronal angle. The large cervical vessels and the scalenus anterior and medius muscles, through which the axillary plexus passes, serve as an orientation. There are many anatomical variations, the most frequent being one or more roots running intramuscularly through or in front of the anterior scalene muscle [44]. The needle is inserted from the lateral side of the ultrasound transducer so that the needle tip can be well visualized and the spread of the LA can be easily observed. The distribution of LA should be observed between the anterior scalene, the medial scalene muscles, and the nerve roots C5–C7. It significantly reduces the perioperative use of opiates and improves rehabilitation potential. The continuous technique reduces pain after rotator cuff repair and can also be performed in an outpatient setting [12, 32].

Dosage local anesthetic: LA 4–10 ml; ropivacaine 0.25–0.5% or bupivacaine 0.25–0.5%, continuous catheters 4–6 ml/h with ropivacaine 0.1–0.4%, bupivacaine 0.125–0.15%, and levobupivacaine 0.1–0.125%.

Undesirable side effects: Nearly 100% transient blockade of the ipsilateral phrenic nerve with about 25% reduction of lung function. Frequent occurrence of a Horner symptom with enophthalmos, miosis, and ptosis due to co-blocking of cervical ganglia.

Contraindications: Severe lung disease, contralateral phrenic, and/or recurrent laryngeal nerve paresis.

Supraclavicular Nerve Block

Indication: Operations of the upper extremity from the distal humerus to the hand.

Anatomy and procedure: In the supraclavicular region, the nerve structures near to each other are often described as a "bunch of grapes". They are located lateral to the subclavian artery, just anterior to the first rib and pleura. The ultrasound probe is placed in the supraclavicular fossa parallel to the clavicle. Internal guiding structures include the subclavian artery, first rib, pleura, and the anterior and middle scalene muscles. For in-plane puncture entering the lateral ultrasound side, the head is positioned slightly to the opposite side. The multiple injection technique is not superior to the single-shot technique at the junction between the artery and the first rib [45, 46], and the single-shot technique has the advantage of being easier to perform. When injecting, it is important to ensure that the injected LA pushes the nerve structures anteriorly and that all nerves are surrounded by the LA at the end of the injection.

Dosage local anesthetic: LA 15–30 ml; ropivacaine 0.25–0.5% or bupivacaine 0.25–0.5%, continuous catheters 4–6 ml/h with ropivacaine 0.1–0.4%, bupivacaine 0.125–0.15%, and levobupivacaine 0.1–0.125%.

Undesirable side effects: Phrenic nerve is less affected in comparison to the interscalene approach, pneumothorax.

Contraindications: Although there are fewer blockages of the phrenic nerve than with IPM, special care should be taken in patients with a pulmonary predisposition.

Infraclavicular Nerve Block

Indication: Operations from the elbow to the hand.

Anatomy and procedure: With this approach, the three fascicles of the brachial plexus located around the subclavian artery are targeted. External landmarks include the jugular fossa, the acromion, and the coracoid process. For internal orientation, the subclavian artery and vein, the pectoralis minor and major muscles, and the pleura serve as landmarks. A single injection point located posterior to the axillary artery can diffuse LA to all fascicles [47, 48]. A fascial click is felt just before reaching the posterior aspect of the artery and signals that the needle tip is in the right location [47]. For a successful infraclavicular block, a U-shaped spread posterior to the artery should be observed from the beginning of the injection.

Dosage local anesthetic: LA 20–30 ml; ropivacaine 0.25–0.5% or bupivacaine 0.25–0.5%, continuous catheters 4–6 ml/h with ropivacaine 0.1–0.4%, bupivacaine 0.125–0.15%, and levobupivacaine 0.1–0.125%.

Undesirable side effects: There is a risk of pneumothorax. It should be borne in mind that compression of the subclavian artery in case of vascular injury is not sufficiently feasible. The risk of ipsilateral phrenic nerve block or Horner's syndrome is rare compared to interscalene block or supraclavicular block.

Axillary Plexus Anesthesia

Indication: Surgical procedures of the hand up to the elbow.

Anatomy and procedure: This block targets the end branches of the brachial plexus. In the axillary area, the median, radial, and ulnar nerves are all bundled around the axillary artery. The musculocutaneous nerve is usually found in the coracobrachialis muscle or between that muscle and the brachialis biceps muscle. A puncture can be performed in-plane and out-of-plane on the arm abducted by 90 degrees. Internal landmarks are the axillary artery and vein and the biceps brachii, triceps brachii, and coracobrachialis muscles. Furthermore, the common tendon of the musculus teres major and the musculus latissimus dorsi serve as a lower boundary. The variability of the nerves around the axillary artery is high. Classically, the radial nerve is located between the axillary artery and the fascia of the musculus teres major but should not be confused with a possible dorsal sound amplification below the artery. PNS might be helpful for identification. The median nerve is usually located above the artery and the ulnar nerve between the artery and the vein. The echographic appearance of the various nerves and the number of blood vessels in the axillary fossa also vary. The musculocutaneous nerve is usually hyperechogenic, round-shaped, flat, or triangular. The median, ulnar, and radial nerves can be slightly hypoechogenic or appear hyperechogenic, making their identification more difficult. Two injections with one around the musculocutaneous nerve and another posterior to the axillary artery seem to provide an equivalent success rate to the identification and injection of each of the four major nerves [49, 50]. This technique not only reduces the time needed to perform the block but also simplifies the block: only the musculocutaneous nerve has to be identified. The injection should be done very proximally, where the conjoint tendon of the latissimus dorsi and teres major muscles can be located. This block is particularly suitable for patients with preexisting pulmonary disease or anticoagulated patients, due to its easy ultrasound anatomy and distal approach to the brachial plexus.

Dosage local anesthetic: LA 20–30 ml; ropivacaine 0.25–0.5% or bupivacaine 0.25–0.5%, continuous catheters 4–6 ml/h with ropivacaine 0.1–0.4%, bupivacaine 0.125–0.15%, and levobupivacaine 0.1–0.125%.

Undesirable side effects: Accidental puncture or injury to the axillary artery or vein.

Singular Block of the Radial Nerve, Ulnar Nerve, or Median Nerve

Blocking of individual nerves distal to the division into the individual end branches in the area of the axillary fossa or below can serve as a rescue block. Rarely singular nerve blocks will be performed for surgeries in more distant areas than the block. Surgeons can also perform rescue blocks.

Intravenous Regional Anesthesia

With the advent of ultrasound, intravenous regional anesthesia (IVRA) or the Bier block has fallen out of favor. This block can be used for brief surgical procedures or manipulations of the upper or lower extremity. However, the Bier block is best used for the upper extremities because tourniquet problems and other safety issues seem to arise more frequently on the lower extremities. The Bier block can be used for small operations in the forearm and hand areas, for example, carpal tunnel splitting or ganglion excision. Complications of IVRA are drug or equipment (i.e., tourniquet) related and can potentially be fatal (local anesthetic systemic toxicity (LAST)). The necessity of exsanguinating the extremity using an Esmarch bandage which might cause pain can also preclude certain procedures from being undertaken with this technique. The LA usually used is lidocaine, and sufficient anesthesia can be achieved 20–40 minutes. This form of anesthesia is not as profound in its effect as direct nerve anesthesia. Two tourniquets are generally used to block the blood flow to the affected extremity, with the distal one being inflated when the patient feels tourniquet pain from the distal one, which will then be deflated. The use of longer-acting LAs allows for approximately 20 minutes of postoperative analgesia after opening the tourniquet [39]. For potentially more painful procedures, performing direct peripheral nerve blocks, such as axillary plexus anesthesia, is recommended to insure long-lasting anesthesia for the postoperative period.

Lower Extremity Blocks

Lower extremity blocks offer many advantages in an ambulatory setting compared with general anesthesia with a focus on patient care, satisfaction, and cost containment, which derives even more importance because of the rising treatment numbers of outpatients in hospitals. On the other hand, there are facility limitations, e.g., no dedicated space or a room for regional anesthesia induction or surgery-specific barriers due to habits or poor understanding of the surgeons, e.g., of a fully sedated, paralyzed patient.

The range of useful indications rises with more and more operations turning from inpatient to an outpatient setting, e.g., knee arthroscopy, varicose veins, or foot surgery. Regional anesthesia advantages include better perioperative analgesia, decreased incidence of postoperative nausea and vomiting, and earlier subsequent hospital discharge [51]. A large advantage of regional anesthesia arises when treating patients suffering from chronic pain. Orthopedic surgeries have the highest incidence of postoperative pain [52, 53] and might benefit most from peripheral nerve blocks. Compared with neuraxial procedures, the use of peripheral blockade can provide prolonged postoperative analgesia and can mostly be utilized even in patients under antithrombotic therapy [40]. To attain proper surgical anesthesia, the peripheral blocks require longer injection to procedure starting times.

Lower extremity blocks should be avoided in patients with local infection, edema, burn, soft tissue trauma, or distorted anatomy with scarring in the area of block placement.

Femoral Block

Indication: Surgical procedures involving the anteromedial thigh, anterior knee, and medial calf (i.e., knee surgeries like arthroscopy or fractures of the mid-femoral shaft).

Anatomy and procedure: The femoral nerve is the largest branch of the lumbar plexus. It passes through the psoas muscle, deep to the iliaca fascia, above the iliacus muscle, and below the inguinal ligament to enter the femoral triangle lateral to the femoral artery and vein. The thigh is slightly abducted with external rotation.

The femoral artery will be localized at the level of the femoral crease. When the femoral artery and the deep artery of the thigh are both seen, the transducer should be moved proximally until only the femoral artery is visualized. The femoral nerve lies lateral to the artery. It is enveloped by two layers of the fascia iliaca and is typically hyperechoic and roughly triangular or oval in shape. The femoral nerve typically is visualized at a depth of 2–4 cm. LA is injected adjacent to the femoral nerve.

Literature: Patel and colleagues were the first to describe the benefit of good perioperative anesthesia and faster discharge with femoral nerve block compared to general anesthesia in knee arthroscopy [54]. The high analgesic potential may be enhanced when used for more painful surgical procedures. Mulroy and colleagues compared a femoral nerve block added to epidural anesthesia with epidural analgesia only (and a sham femoral block) in anterior cruciate ligament repair of outpatient surgery. Significantly lower pain scores were found in the femoral block group postoperatively [55]. An alternative to longer-acting LA such as bupivacaine is mepivacaine 0.2% reducing the prolonged motor weakness with fall risks leading to delayed discharges [56]. Using mepivacaine for extended operations of the knee still remains controversial, and a combination with a sciatic nerve block showed much better results in pain control [57, 58]. The femoral block can be combined with a lateral femoral cutaneous nerve block for varicose veins surgery which has shown comparable satisfaction scores to epidural analgesia for the same surgery [59, 60].

Dosage local anesthetic: LA 15–20 ml; ropivacaine 0.25–0.5% or bupivacaine 0.25–0.5%, continuous catheters 4–6 ml/h with ropivacaine 0.1–0.4%, bupivacaine 0.125–0.15%, and levobupivacaine 0.1–0.125%.

Undesirable side effects: Accidental puncture or injury to the femoral artery or vein.

Adductor Canal Block

Indication: Supplementation for medial foot/ankle surgery in combination with a sciatic nerve block and analgesia for knee surgery in combination with multimodal analgesia and saphenous vein stripping or harvesting.

Anatomy and procedure: The sartorius muscle descends in a lateral to the medial direction across the anterior thigh and forms the "roof" of the adductor canal in the lower half of the thigh. The sides of the triangular canal are formed by the vastus medialis laterally and the adductor longus or magnus medially (depending on how proximal or distal the scan is). The sensory only saphenous nerve can be seen as a small, round, hyperechoic structure anterior to the artery. The femoral vein accompanies the artery and saphenous nerve, which can usually be identified at a depth of 2–3 cm. The needle tip should be visualized anterolateral to the artery and slightly deep to the posterior fascia of the sartorius muscle when injecting LA [61].

Literature: Comparable sensory block and analgesia was achieved with the injection of 10 versus 30 mL of 0.1% ropivacaine without causing significant motor weakness [62]. The simple technique and the isolated sensory block have advantages compared to the femoral nerve block for postoperative pain control in knee arthroscopies and facilitate discharge due to the lack of motor weakness [63].

Dosage local anesthetic: LA 5–10 ml; ropivacaine 0.25–0.5% or bupivacaine 0.25–0.5%, continuous catheters 4–6 ml/h with ropivacaine 0.1–0.4%, bupivacaine 0.125–0.15%, and levobupivacaine 0.1–0.125%.

Undesirable side effects: Accidental puncture or injury to the femoral artery or vein.

Proximal Sciatic Nerve Block

Indication: Foot and ankle surgery, below-knee amputation, analgesia following knee surgery involving the posterior compartment.

Anatomy and procedure:

Anterior approach: This approach can be useful in patients who cannot be positioned in the lateral position due to pain, trauma, the presence of external fixation devices that interfere with positioning, or other issues. The sciatic nerve is imaged approximately at the level of the minor trochanter. A curved transducer is placed transverse on the anteromedial aspect of the thigh imaging the adductor longus muscle, adductor magnus muscle, adductor brevis muscle, femoral artery, and femur. Deep and medial to the femoral artery is the deep artery of the thigh. Both can be identified with color Doppler ultrasound for orientation. Medial to the femur is the adductor magnus muscle. The sciatic nerve is visualized as a hyperechoic oval structure beneath the adductor magnus muscle. The nerve is typically visualized at a depth of 6–8 cm.

Transgluteal and subgluteal approach: With the transgluteal approach, the sciatic nerve is approached deep to the gluteus maximus muscle, where it is identified between the ischial tuberosity and the greater trochanter. To obtain view of the sciatic nerve and the osseous structures at this level, the curvilinear probe is typically needed. With the subgluteal approach, the nerve can be imaged just below the level of the gluteal crease where it lies more superficial (can often be imaged with a linear probed). The preference of one approach over the other is based on the patient's anatomical characteristics and the clinician's preference. The subgluteal approach may be a better choice for most patients and indications, including the obese patients.

At the transgluteal level, the sciatic nerve is visualized in the short axis between the two hyperechoic bony prominences of the ischial tuberosity and the greater trochanter of the femur. The ultrasound probe is positioned transverse on the posterior buttock. The most superficial muscular layer is the gluteus maximus muscle bridging the two osseous structures, typically several centimeters thick. The sciatic nerve is located immediately deep to the gluteus maximus muscle and superficial to the quadratus femoris muscle. The nerve is seen as an oval or roughly triangular hyperechoic structure. At the subgluteal level, the sciatic nerve is visualized between the long head of the biceps femoris muscle and the posterior surface of the adductor magnus with the ultrasound probe transverse on the gluteal crease. With either approach, LA spread should be seen within the sciatic nerve sheath.

Dosage local anesthetic: LA 10–20 ml; ropivacaine 0.25–0.5% or bupivacaine 0.25–0.5%, continuous catheters 4–6 ml/h with ropivacaine 0.1–0.4%, bupivacaine 0.125–0.15%, and levobupivacaine 0.1–0.125%.

Undesirable side effects: Accidental puncture or injury to vessels.

Popliteal Sciatic Nerve Block

Indication: Foot, ankle Achilles tendon surgery.

Anatomy and procedure: The anatomy of the sciatic nerve in the popliteal fossa is variable, and the division into the tibial nerve and common peroneal nerve occurs at an inconstant distance from the popliteal crease. The most common approaches to the popliteal sciatic block are the lateral approach (patient in the supine or lateral position) and the posterior approach (patient being in the prone or lateral position). With the ultrasound transducer in the transverse position at the popliteal crease, the popliteal artery is identified. Color Doppler ultrasound can aid visualization. The popliteal vein is positioned just superficial (posterior) to the artery. Lateral to the popliteal artery are the biceps femoris muscles and medially the semimembranosus and semitendinosus muscles. The tibial nerve is positioned superficial and lateral to the vein and is seen as a hyperechoic, oval, or round structure with a honeycomb pattern. The common peroneal nerve is localized slightly more superficial and lateral to the tibial nerve. The nerves should be followed proximally until the tibial and peroneal nerves are visualized coming together to form the sciatic nerve. LA is deposited within the sheath of the popliteal sciatic nerve.

Literature: Due to its easy access in the popliteal region, the distal sciatic nerve block is the preferable point for blockade, because the proximal block targets nerves that are usually deep with a higher risk of prolonged motor weakness of the hamstring muscles with a risk of a delayed discharge. This block when done in the popliteal fossa is safe and easily achieved and has high patient satisfaction. The nerves can be approached from either the classic posterior approach described by Rorie [64] or the lateral approach described by Hadzic, which offers more possible ways of optimal positioning for the patients [65]. Faster onset of popliteal fossa block within 7 min was demonstrated using both 0.5% ropivacaine and 1% mepivacaine [66].

Using a continuous popliteal catheter for up to 48 h after surgery led to significantly decreased postoperative pain and less need for opioid analgesic rescue medication and improved quality of recovery and patient satisfaction after foot and ankle surgery [67]. Zaric et al. confirmed similar benefits with the use of continuous popliteal catheters [68].

Dosage local anesthetic: LA 10–20 ml; ropivacaine 0.25–0.5% or bupivacaine 0.25–0.5%, continuous catheters 4–6 ml/h with ropivacaine 0.1–0.4%, bupivacaine 0.125–0.15%, and levobupivacaine 0.1–0.125%.

Undesirable side effects: Accidental puncture or injury to the popliteal artery or vein.

Ankle Block

Indication: Distal foot and toe surgery.

Anatomy and procedure:
While this ankle block can be performed by landmark technique only, the use of ultrasound increased clinical efficacy with improved surgical anesthesia, a lower need for rescue systemic opioids, and smaller postoperative opioid doses [69].

Ankle block involves anesthetizing five separate nerves: two deep and three superficial nerves. The two deep nerves are the tibial nerve and the deep peroneal nerve, and the three superficial nerves are the superficial peroneal, sural, and saphenous nerves. All nerves, except the saphenous, are terminal branches of the sciatic nerve; the saphenous nerve is a sensory branch of the femoral nerve. If the smaller superficial nerves (sural, saphenous, and superficial peroneal) cannot be imaged by ultrasound, these nerves can be blocked simply by injecting LA into the subcutaneous tissue as a "skin wheal"; for the sural nerve, inject from the Achilles tendon to the lateral malleolus; for the superficial peroneal and the saphenous, inject anteriorly from one malleolus to the other (avoid injuring the great saphenous vein). This block can also be used as a "rescue block" in case of a failure from the more cranial distal sciatic nerve block.

Dosage local anesthetic: LA 3–5 ml per nerve; lidocaine 1–2%, ropivacaine 0.25–0.5%, or bupivacaine 0.25–0.5%.

Undesirable side effects: Accidental puncture or injury to the femoral artery or vein.

Neuraxial Techniques

Spinal anesthesia (SPA) is a cost-effective and convenient anesthesia technique in the ambulant setting. Several aspects must be met to be successful (happy patient) and fast (happy surgeon).

Ambulatory anesthesia often is mistaken as the easier version of inpatient anesthesia as surgeries performed are shorter and less invasive and patients are generally healthier. Several factors make SPA more challenging in the outpatient setting. Time and timing are key. While the anesthesiologist is initially pressured to perform a fast spinal puncture leading to a fast and dense block to get the surgery started without delays, the block also needs to vane swiftly after surgery ends for the patient to be discharged from the post-anesthesia care unit (PACU).

While the clinician's experience is key for a fast and successful start, the selection of the right LA agent is critical for the block density and resolution.

Legal Aspects

Patients who are planned for neuraxial blocks must consent to this procedure. They should know that they might be awake and able to hear and smell during the surgery. Many issues with an unhappy patient can be avoided by a thorough preoperative explanation. The general risks of SPA are very small [70] but must be explained carefully according to local guidelines for receiving informed patient consent (see complications of regional and neuraxial anesthesia below).

Local Anesthetics

In theory, lidocaine seems to be perfect for ambulatory spinal anesthesia. This short-acting amide LA presents a relatively fast recovery time, but the occurrence of transient neurologic symptoms (TNS) [71] prohibits its intrathecal use. Since the risk of TNS is relatively high with lidocaine, it is no longer approved for intrathecal use in many countries [72].

The well-established hyperbaric bupivacaine 0.5%, an amide LA with an acceptable onset time of 6 to 8 minutes but a longer-acting time (dose depending between 90 and 180 minutes), seems to be a good LA alternative. Therefore, low-dose and unilateral approaches are widely spread. While a saddle or unilateral block is possible with 4 to 6 mg hyperbaric bupivacaine 0.5% (positioning the patient with the operative side down for 12 to 16 minutes), a long recovery time until the patient finally can be discharged remains [72].

The ester LA 2-chloroprocaine has advantages in the ambulatory setting. A previously reported, high TNS occurrence was deemed to be due to additives in the formulation, and plain 2-chloroprocaine now has been accepted as a good LA choice for SPA. The dose-dependent very-short-acting time of 75 to 150 minutes makes it a fitting agent for ambulant spinal anesthesia. 2-Chloroprocaine's isobaricity might be one limitation, and a profound saddle block is hard to archive. 40 to 50 mg of 1% 2-chloroprocaine are common dosages and achieve a level of sensory block up to T10, and an off-label dose of 60 mg has been successfully used [72]. 50 mg 2-chloroprocaine led to a better anesthetic result with similar recovery time as compared to 40 mg providing 50–60 minutes of surgical anesthesia [73].

Prilocaine is an amide LA with fast onset, intermediate potency, and intermediate duration of action and a low incidence of TNS [71]. Currently 2% hyperbaric prilocaine is licensed in the UK but at present not approved for intrathecal use in the USA [72]. 40 to 60 mg prilocaine seems adequate for lower abdominal and leg surgery lasting up to 1.5 hours. Doses of 10 to 20 mg might be sufficient for perineal surgery [74]. Irrespective of what LA is available, contraindications such as allergies to LA or the risk of methemoglobinemia in patients with sickle cell anemia (prilocaine) need to be assessed preoperatively.

Fentanyl and sufentanil are widely used off-label in conjunction with intrathecal LA with the goal of improving the quality of intraoperative anesthesia by reducing visceral pain. While there are reports of superior postoperative analgesia, the addition of opioids is associated with higher rates

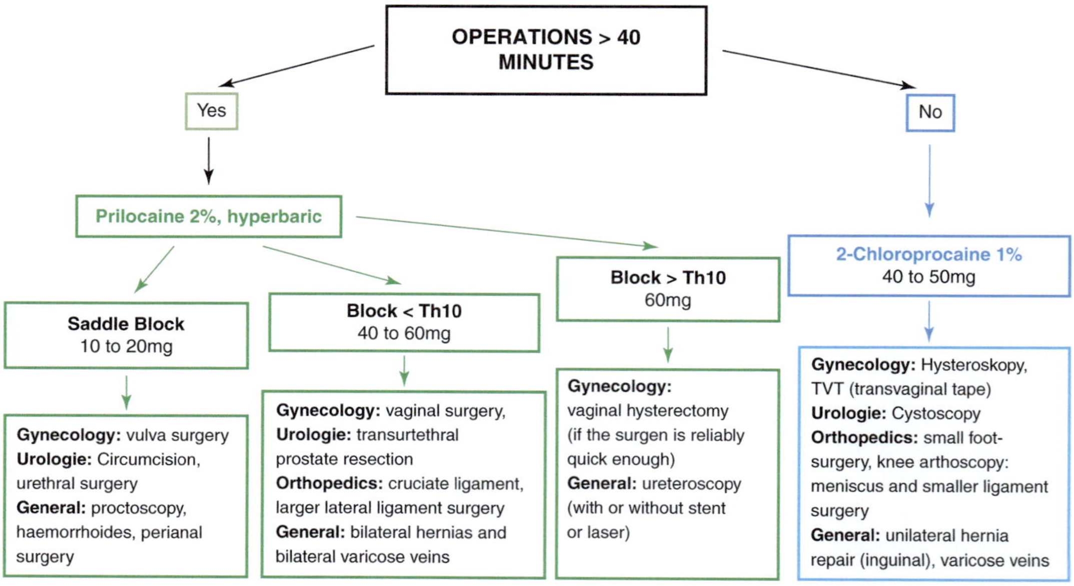

Fig. 14.1 Which surgeries can be considered for ambulant SPAs? (Adapted from [72])

of opioid-induced adverse effects, including pruritus, PONV, and postoperative urinary retention [75]. For ambulatory surgery, SPA can be supplemented by early oral analgesia and locoregional techniques making routine addition of intrathecal opioids unnecessary. Many ambulatory surgeries can be performed with SPA. To aid in the decision-making of what surgeries can be considered for SPA, a flowchart is shown in Fig. 14.1.

Anatomy and procedure:
Patient positioning is the key to a successful, atraumatic, and fast procedure. Taking time to explain the position to the patient will eventually save time during the puncture. The aseptic technique when performing neuraxial anesthesia is mandatory [76]. When preparing for SPA, it is important to accurately identify landmarks on the patient. The midline is identified by palpating the spinous processes, and the iliac crests usually are at the same vertical height as the fourth lumbar spinous process. Depending on the level of anesthesia necessary for the surgery and the ability to feel for the interspace, the L3–L4 or the L4–L5 interspace can be used to introduce the spinal needle. Because the spinal cord commonly ends at the L1-to-L2 level, it is conventional not to attempt spinal anesthesia at or above this level. The process of injecting LA (typically lidocaine 1%) with a smaller subcutaneous needle can be utilized to scout the anatomy. With the median approach, the following layers are penetrated before entering the intrathecal space: skin, subcutaneous fat, supraspinous ligament, interspinous ligament, ligamentum flavum, dura mater, subdural space, arachnoid mater, and finally the subarachnoid space.

Penetration of the dura gives a typical feel of a click, and cerebrospinal fluid (CSF) slowly appears after removing the stylet. CSF usually confirms entry into the correct space, and the LA can be applied. However, an issue especially with pencil-point needles is that the opening, being much longer than the bevel of a Quincke needle, may "straddle" the dura so that some LA reaches the CSF and some the epidural space. This may be exaggerated by the dura acting as a "flap" valve across the needle opening. Initially, CSF pressure pushes the dura outward so that aspiration is successful but subsequent injection pushes the dura forward and the solution is misplaced in the epidural space.

These eventualities are impossible to identify at the actual time of SPA, but a rotation of the needle through 360° after the initial appearance of CSF, and before CSF aspiration is checked, has been advocated as a way of minimizing a failed spinal [77, 78]. We recommend using a simpler version, the 180° rotational test, minimizing the risk of needle displacement when switching hand positions. See Fig. 14.2.

After having rotated the spinal needle back to the starting position, aspirate CSF before injecting the LA. Two or three aspirations (beginning/end or beginning/middle/end) during the injection to ensure ongoing intrathecal placement of the needle tip are debatable. Even more, frequent aspirations can cause displacement on its own. To prevent displacement at any stage, it has been advocated that the dorsum of one hand should be anchored firmly against the patient's back and the fingers used to immobilize the needle, while the other hand is used to manipulate the syringe [79]

Other factors that affect intrathecal spread are solution density and patient position after LA injection. LA with a density within the normal range of that of CSF ("isobaric") will guarantee a block of the lower limbs with little risk of thoracic nerve block and thus hypotension [80]. When hyperbaric LA solutions are used, the level of the SPA can be modulated by tilting the operating room table or positioning the patient. Although testing the SPA level appears to be the easiest part of the entire procedure, it can be performed more or less efficient. Explaining to the patient that you are going to test the level of the block and that a) it is normal that the SPA is not at the final level at the time of the first test and b) that the patient doesn't need to be worried that the operation will start before the SPA has reached a sufficient blockade will make for a satisfied patient.

Epidural Anesthesia in the Ambulant Setting

Lumbar epidural anesthesia can be used in outpatient procedures involving lower abdomen laparoscopy, hernia repair, lower extremity surgery, and vascular procedures below the umbilicus [81–84].

In France ambulatory epidural analgesia has become a common option for women in labor

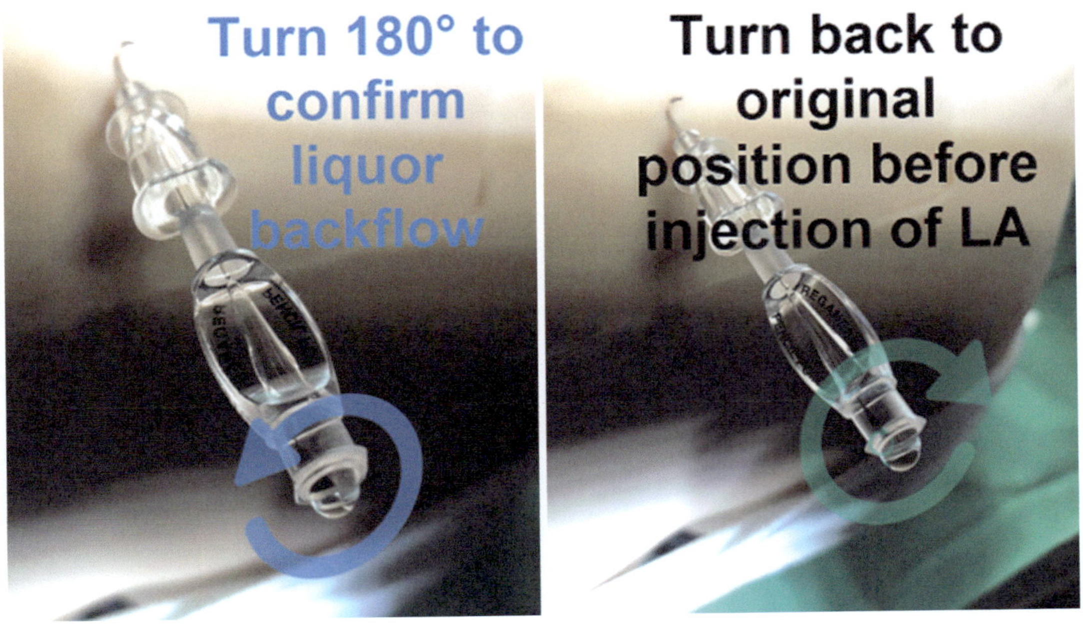

Fig. 14.2 180° test to confirm CSF flow and avoid a failed spinal. (This is an original figure created by the author: Lukas J. Kandler, MD)

[85]. Furthermore, an epidural with a short-acting LA can be very appealing for operations with uncertain duration. A faster discharge from PACU might be achieved with epidural when compared to spinal anesthesia due to a lower risk of urinary retention [81–84].

Complications/Limitations of Regional/Neuraxial Anesthesia in ASCs

Complications of regional anesthesia can be divided into consequences of needle trauma such as accidental vascular puncture (hematoma) or trauma to nerves leading to minor or major sensory deficits and impacts of the LA and use of adjuncts such as epinephrine. Inadvertent injection of LA into the nerve can cause a chemical neuropathy leading to minor or major sensory deficits, and accidental injection of LA directly into vasculature can lead to local anesthetic systemic toxicity (LAST). Nerve injury is usually temporary and with full recovery expected over the following weeks to months. The estimated incidence of serious long-term nerve injury is 2–4/10000 peripheral blocks [86, 87].

Previously used surface anatomy-based techniques, such as PNS, the palpation of landmarks, fascial "clicks," paresthesias, and transarterial approaches, did not allow for monitoring of the needle path or the disposition of the LA injectate. Ultrasound guidance, nowadays the gold standard for performing peripheral nerve blocks, offers safety and other practical advantages. It can shorten block performance, block onset times, reduce the number of needle passes, and reduce the amount of LA injected [88]. A positive impact of ultrasound guidance on the risk of neurological complications following regional anesthesia has yet to be conclusively demonstrated. This is not surprising given the multifactorial etiology and relatively low incidence of perioperative peripheral nerve injury [89].

Peripheral nerve blocks performed by ultrasound guidance alone, or in combination with PNS, display an improved sensory and motor block with reduced need for LA supplementation and fewer minor complications [90].

Some important aspects before discharging patients who received regional anesthesia should be considered to avoid unnecessary complications. Upper extremity peripheral nerve blocks: Patients must be advised to avoid any injury or pressure to the extremity during the period of numbness and should be sent home with a sling until arm numbness has recovered [39]. Lower extremity blocks and neuraxial anesthesia lead to a fall risk when the motor blockade has not yet fully receded. Patients must be able to ambulate safely before discharge. When utilizing continuous catheters for postoperative analgesia, patients must be capable to follow instructions, ambulate independently, and care for the pump and catheter site when at home. Patients need to understand the signs of complications after discharge enabling them to follow up when indicated.

Complications of Regional Anesthesia of the Upper Extremity

A retrospective review of over 600 patients receiving axillary blocks for outpatient hand surgery showed no serious complications including no neurological complications. Six patients out of 600 (6/600) in this group complained of postoperative nausea [2]. Pneumothorax can be a complication of supraclavicular and infraclavicular nerve blocks with an incidence of 0.6–6.1% without the utilization of ultrasound [91]. Ultrasound guidance and constant needle tip visualization likely decrease this risk [39]. The interscalene block can lead to an ipsilateral phrenic nerve block and consequently a hemidiaphragmatic paresis, Horner's syndrome, and recurrent laryngeal nerve block. Injecting a lower volume of LA (5 ml versus 20 ml) decreases the incidence of diaphragmatic paralysis in ultrasound-guided interscalene blocks significantly [92]. See Table 14.3.

Table 14.3 Side effects and complications of peripheral nerve blocks (Adapted from [93])

Side effect or complication	Nerve block	Further information
Phrenic nerve block	Supraclavicular nerve block Interscalene nerve block	Side effect (common)/complication (rare) May rarely cause respiratory compromise
Horner's syndrome	Supraclavicular nerve block Interscalene nerve block Infraclavicular nerve block	Side effect (rare) Causes meiosis, partial ptosis, and anhidrosis on the ipsilateral side
Recurrent laryngeal nerve block	Supraclavicular nerve block Interscalene nerve block	Side effect (rare) Causes hoarse voice
Inadvertent arterial puncture	All	Complication
Hematoma	All	Complication (rare) More common in continuous catheters vs single-shot techniques
Pneumothorax	Supraclavicular nerve block Interscalene nerve block Infraclavicular nerve block Truncal blocks such as PECS, serratus anterior, erector spinae blocks	Complication (rare)
Local anesthetic systemic toxicity (LAST)	All	Complication (rare) From mild systemic symptoms to life-threatening central nervous and cardiovascular collapse
Infections	All	Complication (rare) Appropriate aseptic precautions have to be taken
Nerve injury	All	Complication (rare) Transient, rarely permanent paresthesia, hypoesthesia, paresis

Complications of Regional Anesthesia of the Lower Extremity

The motor weakness caused by lower extremity blocks is the most obvious and potentially dangerous side effect leading to an increased fall risk [3]. The neural blockade persists for a longer time in the lower extremity, and thus motor block may be present for almost twice as long as in the upper extremity leading to a potentially longer time to discharge [39]. The weakness of femoral and obturator nerve function after a lumbar plexus block leads to the loss of both hip and knee flexion and extension, loss of hip adduction, and loss of proprioception making ambulation difficult. The combination of sciatic with femoral nerve blocks can lead to foot drop. All weaknesses of the lower extremity lead to an increased fall risk [3, 39].

The addition of multimodal perineural analgesia (short-acting LA combined with oral/intravenous analgesic such as NSAID, COX2 inhibitors, acetaminophen, metamizole, and if needed opioids) may provide a useful patient-centered solution to the unwanted and prolonged risks of motor block by significantly reducing required LA concentrations. Targeting nerves at their branches and most distal sites allows for increased mobilization and can facilitate same-day discharge. Adductor canal block or infiltration between the popliteal artery and capsule of the knee (IPACK) might be regional anesthesia options more suitable to ambulatory settings as they spare motor nerves [94–97].

Complications of Continuous Peripheral Nerve Blocks (CPNB)

Continuous peripheral nerve blocks might have some advantages such as preservation of motor and at least partial sensory function due to the use of more dilute LA solutions (while ensuring excellent anesthesia for performing the surgery and postoperative analgesia) and potentially lowering the incidence and/or severity of chronic, persistent postsurgical pain [39, 98]. An obvious complication specific to the use of catheters is dislodgement and secondary block failure; others are muscle weakness, hematoma, and infection [3, 87]. Secondary block failure rates have been reported at 19% and 26% for infra- and supraclavicular blocks, respectively [99]. Pump malfunction and disconnection, catheter dislodgement, catheter obstruction, and infusate leak around the insertion site can all result in block failure [100].

Complications of Neuraxial Anesthesia

Spinal anesthesia has become increasingly popular for inpatient surgery, but, until recently, its use has been limited in ambulatory surgery by the lack of a safe, licensed short-acting LA agent. However, as described above, hyperbaric prilocaine and plain 2-chloroprocaine present good short-acting LA options for SPA in the ambulatory setting. Technically epidural anesthesia is the more difficult procedure. It takes longer to perform and longer to develop the block. The challenges in EA are the operating room turnover time, post-anesthesia recovery, and time to discharge, and the need to demonstrate the ability to void before discharge in risk groups [101].

Limiting factors for the use of spinal anesthesia are post-dural puncture headache (PDPH), transient neurologic symptoms (TNS), urinary retention, delayed mobilization, neurotoxicity, and nerve injury [72].

PDPH can occur due to a leak of cerebrospinal fluid (CSF) at the dural puncture site, resulting in a decrease of CSF pressure, causing gravitational traction on the brain structures and a painful neurovascular response of the meninges [102]. However, with the small-gauge, pencil-point (27–29 G) needles used nowadays, the incidence of this complication has decreased to less than 1% [103]. Though a smaller gauge lowers the incidence, there is an increased failure rate with needles smaller than 27 gauge due to increased procedural challenges such as a slower return of cerebrospinal fluid [39, 104]. It is estimated that PDPH follows about 1% of all neuraxial blocks for labor and delivery [105].

1. TNS reflects significant back pain that radiates into the buttocks or legs. It may or may not be associated with dysesthesias. Pain typically lasts 3–4 days and is treated with NSAID and other analgesics [39]. TNS can occur with almost any spinal anesthetic, but lidocaine, which is no longer licensed for intrathecal use in the UK and USA, has the highest, not dose-dependent, incidence >15%. Lidocaine remains a safe and popular choice for epidural anesthesia [72]. Bupivacaine has a low and preservative-free 2-chloroprocaine has no reported incidence of TNS [101]. Potential contributing factors are patient position (such as knee arthroscopy or lithotomy), early ambulation, and use of pencil-point needles.
2. Urinary retention. The long duration of the anesthetic drugs can cause over-distension of the bladder, and thus bladder catheterization is often required following resolution of the block. In general, intravenous volume administration should be restrictive. Risk factors for urinary retention are older age, male sex, pelvic surgery, rectal and inguinal hernia operations, prolonged surgery, and history of previous urologic dysfunction. These patients should be required to void before discharge [39]. Patients with a low risk for bladder dysfunction and over-distension who received a short-acting neuraxial LA can likely be safely discharged prior to spontaneous voiding [81–84]. Urinary retention requiring catheterization following general anesthesia has been reported in 1/229 patients [106], whereas voiding was delayed after short-acting neuraxial blockade in 3 of 201 patients [84]. Interestingly, unilateral low-dose spinal anesthesia does not decrease the incidence of urinary retention in high-risk patients [107].
3. Delayed mobilization and discharge have been an issue with the use of bupivacaine in SPA. Full return of sensory and motor func-

tion is required for mobilization. Prilocaine and 2-chloroprocaine have a faster block resolution than bupivacaine [72, 74, 108]. After the return of normal motor and sensory function, patients should be mobilized with direct supervision.

4. Neuraxial complications are extremely rare, but when they occur, they often result in life-altering injuries. Spinal hematoma is the most common cause of neuraxial injuries that proceed to litigation, and these injuries are often permanent. Infectious complications have a higher likelihood of at least partial recovery. The incidence of neuraxial injury associated with regional anesthetic techniques varies widely, and this makes it extremely difficult to cite an overall risk for injury. The risk of an epidural hematoma is higher with EA than with SPA and increases in the presence of coagulation issues, increased age, or female sex. Preexisting neurologic diseases or spinal stenosis may worsen injury severity. Neuraxial injury risk due to infection rises with immunocompromised patients, with prolonged epidural catheterization or omission of aseptic techniques [86]. Cases of arachnoiditis caused directly by the neuraxial anesthetic are extremely rare and most likely relate to an idiosyncratic reaction following an unknown provocation. Concern has been raised regarding the possibility that antiseptic solutions, particularly chlorhexidine and alcohol mixtures, might cause arachnoiditis. A retrospective cohort study of more than 12,000 patients however reported no increased risk in neuraxial complications utilizing chlorhexidine as the skin disinfectant [86, 109].

Truncal blocks have a high safety profile.
There has been a rise in the popularity of truncal fascial plane blocks as they can be simpler and safer alternatives to thoracic epidural and paravertebral blockade [110, 111]. The anatomy of these blocks makes them relatively safe techniques with minimal risk of serious needle-related complications. Erector spinae, serratus anterior plane, transversus abdominis plane, ilioinguinal, iliohypogastric, and rectus sheath blocks all have a low side effect profile. However, pneumothorax has been described in case reports as a complication of erector spinae and serratus anterior blocks [112–114]. The use of ultrasound while performing these blocks has improved efficacy and safety. Truncal blocks can be a valuable regional anesthesia tool for ambulatory surgery.

Important Clinical Findings

Recently high-value basic ultrasound-guided regional anesthetic techniques were proposed [115] (see Table 14.4). We will be discussing recent developments in the literature looking at "Plan A" blocks.

A recent systematic review evaluated the available literature on the effects of analgesic and surgical interventions on pain after rotator cuff repair. Interscalene brachial plexus blockade was recommended as the first-choice regional analgesic technique. The suprascapular nerve block, with or without axillary nerve block, was sug-

Table 14.4 High-value basic ultrasound-guided regional anesthetic techniques adapted from [115]; IPACK, interspace between the popliteal artery and the capsule of the posterior knee; PECS, pectoral nerves

Anatomical location	Plan A (basic blocks)	Plan B/C/D (advanced blocks)
Upper limb		
Shoulder	Interscalene brachial plexus block	Superior trunk block, combined axillary and suprascapular nerve blocks
Below shoulder	Axillary brachial plexus block	Infraclavicular block, supraclavicular block
Lower limb		
Hip	Femoral nerve block	Fascia iliaca block, lumbar plexus block
Knee	Adductor canal block	Femoral nerve block ± IPACK block
Foot and ankle	Popliteal sciatic block	Ankle blocks, proximal sciatic nerve block
Trunk		
Chest wall	Erector spinae plane block	Paravertebral block, serratus plane block, PECS blocks
Abdominal midline	Rectus sheath block	Quadratus lumborum blocks

gested as an alternative [116]. The anterior suprascapular block provides noninferior analgesia compared to the interscalene approach for major arthroscopic shoulder surgery without the frequent side effect of hemidiaphragmatic paralysis as seen in the interscalene approach [117].

The axillary approach to the brachial plexus nerve block was first described by Dr. Halstead et al. in 1884 [118]. Before the advent of ultrasound, its superficial location and low risk of complications made it a useful block for outpatient hand and arm surgery. Real-time ultrasound guidance, however, improves the success rate and reduces the meantime to the onset of anesthesia and the time of block performance for the axillary brachial plexus [119].

Ambulatory arthroscopic anterior cruciate ligament reconstruction (ACLR) is associated with moderate pain, even when nonopioid oral analgesics such as acetaminophen and nonsteroidal anti-inflammatory drugs are used. Recently, the Society for Ambulatory Anesthesia (SAMBA) evaluated the analgesic efficacy and associated risks of supplemental femoral nerve block, adductor canal block, and local installation analgesia. SAMBA recommends local instillation analgesia as part of a multimodal analgesic regimen for ACLR [120]. This recommendation goes in hand with a recent systematic review that did not support the routine use of femoral nerve blocks for analgesia in patients having ACLR [121].

The adductor canal block (ACB) for minor ambulatory arthroscopic knee surgery provides modest analgesic benefits, including improved relief for rest pain and reduced opioid consumption for up to 8 and 24 hours, respectively, as demonstrated in a recent systematic review and meta-analysis. The analgesic benefits of ACB are not different from placebo or FNB after ambulatory ACLR [120, 121], suggesting a limited role of both blocks in this procedure. In a third systematic review by Yung et al. [122], the use of LIA by the surgeon reduced pain scores and analgesic consumption for patients having ACLR when compared to placebo. Until the results of larger pragmatic studies or population-based data have been published, the general use of peripheral nerve blocks for either knee arthroscopy or ACLR should not be routine use especially when carefully placed periarticular LIA has already been used by the surgeon [123].

Popliteal block: A recent meta-analysis comparing single-shot to continuous catheter popliteal sciatic block confirmed the safety and efficacy in outpatient foot and ankle surgery. The continuous popliteal block was associated with lower visual analog scale (VAS) scores up to 48 hrs [124].

Thoracic fascial blocks represent a novel and rapidly expanding facet of regional anesthesia. These recently described techniques have the potential for excellent analgesia, enhanced technical safety profiles, and reduced physiological side effects. Many of these blocks can be and are already utilized in ambulatory surgery.

1. The erector spinae plane (ESP) block is a recently described ultrasound-guided technique in which LA is injected into a fascial plane between the tips of the thoracic transverse processes and the overlying erector spinae muscle (longissimus thoracis) [125]. Large randomized controlled trials evaluating the ESP block are still lacking. Tsui et al. recently performed a pooled review of 242 cases relating to the ESP block: 90.5% of publications were either case reports or case series, 5.5% were anatomical cadaver studies, and only 2.4% were randomized controlled trials (RCT) [126]. ESP blocks are showing promise as a regional technique for breast surgery. Small randomized controlled trials have shown effective analgesia and reduced postoperative opioid consumption when compared with standard care in patients undergoing surgery for breast cancer (including mastectomy) [127, 128]. However, one prospective randomized trial in radical mastectomy surgery showed lower pain scores and postoperative tramadol consumption if a modified pectoral nerve block was performed rather than an ESP block [129]. A perceived key benefit of the ESP block over other interfascial blocks for abdominal procedures (rectus sheath, transverse abdominis blocks) is the anterior spread

of injectate into the paravertebral and epidural space. This would block not only spinal nerve roots but also rami communicantes transmitting sympathetic fibers, thus leading to relief from visceral pain. This was highlighted in the small case series with significant relief of visceral pain after ESP blocks seen in three bariatric patients undergoing laparoscopic abdominal surgery [130]. In an RCT comparing ESP and subcostal TAP blocks in laparoscopic cholecystectomy, both techniques were found to lower rest and dynamic pain scores and analgesic requirements [131]. In hysterectomy patients, lower fentanyl consumption in the first 24 postoperative hours and significantly lower pain scores in the first 12 hours were reported [132]. Other reports have highlighted using the ESP block in thoracic, hip, and spine surgery [133–137].

2. Rectus sheath block (RSB): Bilateral RSBs are indicated in surgeries requiring midline skin incisions: umbilical hernia repair, open gastrectomy, laparoscopic procedures, and open abdominal surgical cases. The RSB, however, does not provide visceral analgesia. Bilateral RSB for open gastrectomies showed reduced opioid requirements during surgery and postoperatively [138]. RSB analgesia with repeated doses (versus single-shot and continuous infusions) had an opioid-sparing effect in a small RCT in patients undergoing midline laparotomy [139].

Summary

Regional anesthesia techniques offer significant advantages in the ambulatory surgery setting. Side effects of nausea, vomiting, and pain that frequently delay discharge or cause admission can be avoided. These techniques can provide prolonged analgesia and offer, with continuous catheters, the promise of a pain-free perioperative period. The choice of drugs must be carefully adjusted, especially with neuraxial techniques. Despite frequently requiring additional time at the outset, regional anesthesia techniques have consistently been shown to provide competitive discharge times and costs when compared with general anesthesia.

References

1. Malchow RJ, Gupta RK, Shi Y, Shotwell MS, Jaeger LM, Bowens C. Comprehensive analysis of 13,897 consecutive regional anesthetics at an ambulatory surgery center. Pain Med. 2018;19(2):368–84.
2. Fleisher LA. Ambulatory anesthesia: the innovating edge of perioperative medicine? Anesthesiol Clin. 2019;37(2):xiii–xiv.
3. Moore JG, Ross SM, Williams BA. Regional anesthesia and ambulatory surgery. Curr Opin Anaesthesiol. 2013;26(6):652–60.
4. Jani SR, Shapiro FE, Gabriel RA, Kordylewski H, Dutton RP, Urman RD. A comparison between office and other ambulatory practices: analysis from the National Anesthesia Clinical Outcomes registry. J Healthc Risk Manag. 2016;35(4):38–47.
5. Seligson E, Beutler SS, Urman RD. Office-based anesthesia: an update on safety and outcomes (2017–2019). Curr Opin Anaesthesiol. 2019;32(6):756–61.
6. PricewaterhouseCoopers. Ambulant vor stationär – Oder wie sich eine Milliarde Franken jährlich einsparen lassen. [cited 2020 Jun 7]; Available from: https://www.pwc.ch/de/insights/gesundheitswesen/ambulant-vor-stationar-oder-wie-sich-eine-milliarde-franken-jahrlich-einsparen-lassen.html
7. Institute of Medicine, Committee on Quality of Health Care in America. Crossing the quality chasm: a new health system for the 21st century: National Academies Press; 2001. 360 p.
8. Whang EE, Stopfkuchen-Evans MF. Enhanced recovery after surgery: a new standard for perioperative care [Internet]. J Laparoendoscop Adv Surg Tech. 2017;27:859. Available from: https://doi.org/10.1089/lap.2017.29023.eew
9. Fawcett WJ. Anesthetic management and the role of the anesthesiologist in reducing surgical stress and improving recovery [Internet]. Enhanced Recovery Surg. 2020. p. 131–40. Available from: https://doi.org/10.1007/978-3-030-33443-7_14
10. Afonso AM, Tokita HK, McCormick PJ, Twersky RS. Enhanced recovery programs in outpatient surgery. Anesthesiol Clin. 2019;37(2):225–38.
11. International Association for Ambulatory Surgery. Discharge process and criteria [Internet]. [cited 2020 Jun 7]. Available from: https://www.iaas--med.com/index.php/iaas-recommendations/discharge-process-and-criteria
12. Ardon AE, Prasad A, McClain RL, Melton MS, Nielsen KC, Greengrass R. Regional anesthesia for ambulatory anesthesiologists. Anesthesiol Clin. 2019;37(2):265–87.
13. Williams BA, Kentor ML, Vogt MT, Vogt WB, Coley KC, Williams JP, et al. Economics of nerve block pain

management after anterior cruciate ligament reconstruction: potential hospital cost savings via associated postanesthesia care unit bypass and same-day discharge. Anesthesiology. 2004;100(3):697–706.
14. Lee JH. Anesthesia for ambulatory surgery. Korean J Anesthesiol. 2017;70(4):398–406.
15. Williams BA, Kentor ML. The WAKE© score: patient-centered ambulatory anesthesia and fast-tracking outcomes criteria. Int Anesthesiol Clin. 2011;49(3):33–43.
16. Rosenblatt MA, Fishkind D. Proficiency in interscalene anesthesia-how many blocks are necessary? J Clin Anesth. 2003;15(4):285–8.
17. Barrington MJ, Wong DM, Slater B, Ivanusic JJ, Ovens M. Ultrasound-guided regional anesthesia: how much practice do novices require before achieving competency in ultrasound needle visualization using a cadaver model. Reg Anesth Pain Med. 2012;37(3):334–9.
18. Kopacz DJ, Neal JM, Pollock JE. The regional anesthesia “learning curve”: what is the minimum number of epidural and spinal blocks to reach consistency? Reg Anesth. 1996;21(3):182–90.
19. Bruce BG, Green A, Blaine TA, Wesner LV. Brachial plexus blocks for upper extremity orthopaedic surgery. J Am Acad Orthop Surg. 2012;20(1):38–47.
20. Prabhakar A, Lambert T, Kaye RJ, Gaignard SM, Ragusa J, Wheat S, et al. An assessment of the role of non-opioid adjuvants in regional anesthesia practice. Best Pract Res Clin Anaesthesiol [Internet]. 2019.; Available from: http://www.sciencedirect.com/science/article/pii/S1521689619300412
21. Albért J, Löfström B. Bilateral ulnar nerve blocks for the evaluation of local anesthetic agents. 3. Tests with a new agent, prilocaine, and with lidocaine in solutions with and without epinephrine. Acta Anaesthesiol Scand. 1965;9(4):203–11.
22. Dogru K, Duygulu F, Yildiz K, Kotanoglu MS, Madenoglu H, Boyaci A. Hemodynamic and blockade effects of high/low epinephrine doses during axillary brachial plexus blockade with lidocaine 1.5%: a randomized, double-blinded study. Reg Anesth Pain Med. 2003;28(5):401–5.
23. Kirksey MA, Haskins SC, Cheng J, Liu SS. Local anesthetic peripheral nerve block adjuvants for prolongation of analgesia: a systematic qualitative review. PLoS One. 2015;10(9):e0137312.
24. Chad M, Brummett BAW. Additives to local anesthetics for peripheral nerve blockade. Int Anesthesiol Clin. 2011;49(4):104.
25. Emelife PI, Eng MR, Menard BL, Myers AS, Cornett EM, Urman RD, et al. Adjunct medications for peripheral and neuraxial anesthesia. Best Pract Res Clin Anaesthesiol. 2018;32(2):83–99.
26. Vorobeichik L, Brull R, Abdallah FW. Evidence basis for using perineural dexmedetomidine to enhance the quality of brachial plexus nerve blocks: a systematic review and meta-analysis of randomized controlled trials. Br J Anaesthes. 2017;118(2):167–81.
27. Weerink MAS, Michel M R, Hannivoort LN, Barends CRM, Absalom AR, Colin P. Clinical pharmacokinetics and pharmacodynamics of dexmedetomidine [Internet]. Clin Pharmacokinet. 2017;56:893–913. Available from: https://doi.org/10.1007/s40262-017-0507-7
28. Johansson A, Hao J, Sjölund B. Local corticosteroid application blocks transmission in normal nociceptive C-fibres. Acta Anaesthesiol Scand. 1990;34(5):335–8.
29. Marks R, Barlow JW, Funder JW. Steroid-induced vasoconstriction: glucocorticoid antagonist studies. J Clin Endocrinol Metab. 1982;54(5):1075–7.
30. Shishido H, Kikuchi S, Heckman H, Myers RR. Dexamethasone decreases blood flow in normal nerves and dorsal root ganglia. Spine. 2002;27(6):581–6.
31. Barnes PJ. Anti-inflammatory actions of glucocorticoids: molecular mechanisms. Clin Sci. 1998;94(6):557–72.
32. Steinfeldt T, Volk T, Kessler P, Vicent O, Wulf H, Gottschalk A, et al. Peripheral nerve blocks on the upper extremity: technique of landmark-based and ultrasound-guided approaches. Anaesthesist. 2015;64(11):846–54.
33. Hadzic A. Hadzic's peripheral nerve blocks and anatomy for ultrasound-guided regional anesthesia: McGraw Hill Professional; 2011.
34. Chou R, Gordon DB, de Leon-Casasola OA. Management of postoperative pain: a clinical practice guideline from the American pain society, the American Society of Regional Anesthesia and Pain Medicine, and …. The Journal of [Internet]. 2016.; Available from: https://www.sciencedirect.com/science/article/pii/S1526590015009955
35. Hutton M, Brull R, Macfarlane AJR. Regional anaesthesia and outcomes [Internet]. BJA Edu. 2018;18:52–6. Available from: https://doi.org/10.1016/j.bjae.2017.10.002
36. Walker EMK, Bell M, Cook TM, Grocott MPW, Moonesinghe SR, Central SNAP-1 Organisation, et al. Patient reported outcome of adult perioperative anaesthesia in the United Kingdom: a cross-sectional observational study. Br J Anaesth. 2016;117(6):758–66.
37. Héroux J, Belley-Côté E, Echavé P, Loignon M-J, Bessette P-O, Patenaude N, et al. Functional recovery with peripheral nerve block versus general anesthesia for upper limb surgery: a systematic review protocol. Syst Rev. 2019;8(1):273.
38. Grewal G, Joshi GP. Obesity and obstructive sleep apnea in the ambulatory patient. Anesthesiol Clin. 2019;37(2):215–24.
39. Mulroy MF, McDonald SB. Regional anesthesia for outpatient surgery [Internet]. Anesthesiol Clin North Am. 2003;26:289–303. Available from: https://doi.org/10.1016/s0889-8537(02)00071-8
40. Horlocker TT, Vandermeulen E, Kopp SL, Gogarten W, Leffert LR, Benzon HT. Regional anesthesia in the patient receiving antithrombotic or thrombolytic therapy: American Society of Regional Anesthesia and

Pain Medicine Evidence-Based Guidelines (Fourth Edition). Reg Anesth Pain Med. 2018;43(3):263–309.

41. Neal JM, Barrington MJ, Brull R, Hadzic A, Hebl JR, Horlocker TT, et al. The second ASRA practice advisory on neurologic complications associated with regional anesthesia and pain medicine: executive summary 2015. Reg Anesth Pain Med. 2015;40(5):401–30.
42. Vlassakov K, Lirk P, Rathmell JP. Intraneural injection Is the jury still out? Anesthesiology. 2018;129(2):221–4.
43. Nadeau M-J, Lévesque S, Dion N. Ultrasound-guided regional anesthesia for upper limb surgery. Can J Anaesth. 2013;60(3):304–20.
44. Gutton C, Choquet O, Antonini F, Grossi P. Ultrasound-guided interscalene block: influence of anatomic variations in clinical practice. Ann Fr Anesth Reanim. 2010;29(11):770–5.
45. Roy M, Nadeau M-J, Côté D, Levesque S, Dion N, Nicole PC, et al. Comparison of a single- or double-injection technique for ultrasound-guided supraclavicular block: a prospective, randomized, blinded controlled study. Reg Anesth Pain Med. 2012;37(1):55–9.
46. Tran DQH, Muñoz L, Zaouter C, Russo G, Finlayson RJ. A prospective, randomized comparison between single- and double-injection, ultrasound-guided supraclavicular brachial plexus block [Internet]. Reg Anesthesia Pain Med. 2009;34:420–4. Available from: https://doi.org/10.1097/aap.0b013e3181ae733a
47. Desgagnés M-C, Lévesque S, Dion N, Nadeau M-J, Coté D, Brassard J, et al. A comparison of a single or triple injection technique for ultrasound-guided infraclavicular block: a prospective randomized controlled study. Anesth Analg. 2009;109(2):668–72.
48. Tran DQH, Bertini P, Zaouter C, Muñoz L, Finlayson RJ. A prospective, randomized comparison between single- and double-injection ultrasound-guided infraclavicular brachial plexus block. Reg Anesth Pain Med. 2010;35(1):16–21.
49. Imasogie N, Ganapathy S, Singh S, Armstrong K, Armstrong P. A prospective, randomized, double-blind comparison of ultrasound-guided axillary brachial plexus blocks using 2 versus 4 injections [Internet]. Anesthesia Analgesia. 2010:1. Available from: https://doi.org/10.1213/ane.0b013e3181cb6791
50. Bernucci F, Gonzalez AP, Finlayson RJ, Tran DQH. A prospective, randomized comparison between perivascular and perineural ultrasound-guided axillary brachial plexus block. Reg Anesth Pain Med. 2012;37(5):473–7.
51. Liu SS, Strodtbeck WM, Richman JM, Wu CL. A comparison of regional versus general anesthesia for ambulatory anesthesia: a meta-analysis of randomized controlled trials. Anesth Analg. 2005;101(6):1634–42.
52. Chung F, Ritchie E, Su J. Postoperative pain in ambulatory surgery. Anesth Analg. 1997;85(4):808–16.
53. Beauregard L, Pomp A, Choinière M. Severity and impact of pain after day-surgery. Can J Anaesth. 1998;45(4):304–11.
54. Patel NJ, Flashburg MH, Paskin S, Grossman R. A regional anesthetic technique compared to general anesthesia for outpatient knee arthroscopy. Anesth Analg. 1986;65(2):185–7.
55. Mulroy MF, Larkin KL, Batra MS, Hodgson PS, Owens BD. Femoral nerve block with 0.25% or 0.5% bupivacaine improves postoperative analgesia following outpatient arthroscopic anterior cruciate ligament repair. Reg Anesth Pain Med. 2001;26(1):24–9.
56. Ambrosoli AL, Chiaranda M, Fedele LL, Gemma M, Cedrati V, Cappelleri G. A randomised controlled trial of intrathecal blockade versus peripheral nerve blockade for day-case knee arthroscopy. Anaesthesia. 2016;71(3):280–4.
57. Williams BA, Kentor ML, Vogt MT, Williams JP, Chelly JE, Valalik S, et al. Femoral-sciatic nerve blocks for complex outpatient knee surgery are associated with less postoperative pain before same-Day discharge. A review of 1,200 consecutive cases from the period 1996–1999. Anesthesiology. 2003;98(5):1206–13.
58. Harbell MW, Cohen JM, Kolodzie K, Behrends M, Braehler MR, Kinjo S, et al. Combined preoperative femoral and sciatic nerve blockade improves analgesia after anterior cruciate ligament reconstruction: a randomized controlled clinical trial. J Clin Anesth. 2016;33:68–74.
59. Vloka JD, Hadzic A, Mulcare R, Lesser JB, Koorn R, Thys DM. Combined popliteal and posterior cutaneous nerve of the thigh blocks for short saphenous vein stripping in outpatients: an alternative to spinal anesthesia [Internet]. J Clin Anesthesia. 1997:9;618–22. Available from: https://doi.org/10.1016/s0952-8180(97)00150-5
60. Lee J, Roh W, Chung J, Park C, Kim B, Cho C, et al. A comparison of the patient satisfaction of femoral and popliteal sciatic nerve blocks with that of epidural anesthesia for greater saphenous vein stripping surgery [Internet]. Eur J Anaesthesiol. 2006;23:128–9. Available from: https://doi.org/10.1097/00003643-200606001-00459
61. Rasouli MR, Viscusi ER. Adductor canal block for knee surgeries: an emerging analgesic technique. Arch Bone Jt Surg. 2017;5(3):131–2.
62. Jæger P, Koscielniak-Nielsen ZJ, Hilsted KL, Fabritius ML, Dahl JB. Adductor canal block with 10 mL versus 30 mL local anesthetics and quadriceps strength: a paired, blinded, randomized study in healthy volunteers. Reg Anesth Pain Med. 2015;40(5):553–8.
63. Ludwigson JL, Tillmans SD, Galgon RE, Chambers TA, Heiner JP, Schroeder KM. A comparison of single shot adductor canal block versus femoral nerve catheter for total knee arthroplasty [Internet]. J Arthrop. 2015;20:68–71. Available from: https://doi.org/10.1016/j.arth.2015.03.044
64. Rorie DK, Byer DE, Nelson DO, Sittipong R, Johnson KA. Assessment of block of the sciatic nerve in the popliteal fossa. Anesth Analg. 1980;59(5):371–6.

65. Hadzic A, Vloka JD. A comparison of the posterior versus lateral approaches to the block of the sciatic nerve in the popliteal fossa. Anesthesiology. 1998;88(6):1480–6.
66. Fernández-Guisasola J, Andueza A, Burgos E, Plaza A, Porras MC, Reboto P, et al. A comparison of 0.5% ropivacaine and 1% mepivacaine for sciatic nerve block in the popliteal fossa. Acta Anaesthesiol Scand. 2001;45(8):967–70.
67. White PF, Issioui T, Skrivanek GD, Early JS, Wakefield C. The use of a continuous popliteal sciatic nerve block after surgery involving the foot and ankle: does it improve the quality of recovery? Anesth Analg. 2003;97(5):1303–9.
68. Zaric D, Boysen K, Christiansen J, Haastrup U, Kofoed H, Rawal N. Continuous popliteal sciatic nerve block for outpatient foot surgery–a randomized, controlled trial. Acta Anaesthesiol Scand. 2004;48(3):337–41.
69. Chin KJ, Wong NWY, Macfarlane AJR, Chan VWS. Ultrasound-guided versus anatomic landmark-guided ankle blocks: a 6-year retrospective review. Reg Anesth Pain Med. 2011;36(6):611–8.
70. Agarwal A, Kishore K. Complications and controversies of regional anaesthesia: a review. Indian J Anaesth. 2009;53(5):543–53.
71. Zaric D, Pace NL. Transient neurologic symptoms (TNS) following spinal anaesthesia with lidocaine versus other local anaesthetics. Cochrane Database Syst Rev. 2009;2:CD003006.
72. Rattenberry W, Hertling A, Erskine R. Spinal anaesthesia for ambulatory surgery. BJA Edu. 2019;19(10):321–8.
73. Goldblum E, Atchabahian A. The use of 2-chloroprocaine for spinal anaesthesia. Acta Anaesthesiol Scand. 2013;57(5):545–52.
74. Saporito A, Ceppi M, Perren A, La Regina D, Cafarotti S, Borgeat A, et al. Does spinal chloroprocaine pharmacokinetic profile actually translate into a clinical advantage in terms of clinical outcomes when compared to low-dose spinal bupivacaine? A systematic review and meta-analysis. J Clin Anesth. 2019;52:99–104.
75. Nair GS, Abrishami A, Lermitte J, Chung F. Systematic review of spinal anaesthesia using bupivacaine for ambulatory knee arthroscopy. Br J Anaesth. 2009;102(3):307–15.
76. Practice Advisory for the Prevention, Diagnosis, and Management of Infectious Complications Associated with Neuraxial Techniques: An Updated Report by the American Society of Anesthesiologists Task Force on Infectious Complications Associated with Neuraxial Techniques and the American Society of Regional Anesthesia and Pain Medicine. Anesthesiology. 2017;126(4):585–601.
77. Mechanisms and Management of Failed Spinal Anesthesia–NYSORA[Internet].NYSORA.2019[cited 2020 Jun 5]. Available from: https://www.nysora.com/foundations-of-regional-anesthesia/complications/mechanisms-management-failed-spinal-anesthesia/
78. Fettes PDW, Jansson J-R, Wildsmith JAW. Failed spinal anaesthesia: mechanisms, management, and prevention. Br J Anaesth. 2009;102(6):739–48.
79. Tarkkila PJ. Incidence and causes of failed spinal anesthetics in a university hospital: a prospective study. Reg Anesth 1991;16(1):48–51.
80. Wildsmith JAW, Mcclure JH, Brown DT, Scott DB. Effects of posture on the spread of isobaric and hyperbaric amethocaine [Internet]. Br J Anaesthesia. 1981;53:273–8. Available from: https://doi.org/10.1093/bja/53.3.273
81. Schuricht AL, McCarthy CS, Wells WL, Kumor RJ, Cwik J. A comparison of epidural versus general anesthesia for outpatient endoscopic preperitoneal herniorrhaphy. JSLS. 1997;1(2):141–4.
82. Dahl V, Gierløff C, Omland E, Raeder JC. Spinal, epidural or propofol anaesthesia for out–patient knee arthroscopy? Acta Anaesthesiol Scand. 1997;41(10):1341–5.
83. Mulroy MF, Larkin KL, Hodgson PS, Helman JD, Pollock JE, Liu SS. A comparison of spinal, epidural, and general anesthesia for outpatient knee arthroscopy. Anesth Analg. 2000;91(4):860–4.
84. Mulroy MF, Salinas FV, Larkin KL, Polissar NL. Ambulatory surgery patients may be discharged before voiding after short-acting spinal and epidural anesthesia. Anesthesiology. 2002;97(2):315–9.
85. Karraz MA. Ambulatory epidural anesthesia and the duration of labor. Int J Gynaecol Obstet. 2003;80(2):117–22.
86. Neal JM, Barrington MJ, Brull R, Hadzic A, Hebl JR, Horlocker TT, et al. The second ASRA practice advisory on neurologic complications associated with regional anesthesia and pain medicine [Internet]. Reg Anesthes Pain Med. 2015;40:401–30. Available from: https://doi.org/10.1097/aap.0000000000000286
87. Jeng CL, Torrillo TM, Rosenblatt MA. Complications of peripheral nerve blocks. Br J Anaesth. 2010;105(suppl_1):i97–107.
88. Koscielniak-Nielsen ZJ. Ultrasound-guided peripheral nerve blocks: what are the benefits? Acta Anaesthesiol Scand. 2008;52(6):727–37.
89. Barrington MJ, Kluger R. Ultrasound guidance reduces the risk of local anesthetic systemic toxicity following peripheral nerve blockade. Reg Anesth Pain Med. 2013;38(4):289–99.
90. Albrecht E, Chin KJ. Advances in regional anaesthesia and acute pain management: a narrative review. Anaesthesia. 2020;75 Suppl 1:e101–10.
91. Bhatia A, Lai J, Chan VW, Brull R. Pneumothorax as a complication of the ultrasound-guided supraclavicular approach for brachial plexus block. Anesth Analg. 2010;111(3):817.
92. Riazi S, Carmichael N, Awad I, Holtby RM, McCartney CJL. Effect of local anaesthetic volume (20 vs 5 ml) on the efficacy and respiratory consequences of ultrasound-guided interscalene brachial plexus block. Br J Anaesth. 2008;101(4):549–56.

93. Kusre S, Mc Ewen A, Matthew G. Ultrasound-guided supraclavicular brachial plexus block. WFSAHQ [Internet]. 2018;(Tutorial 384). Available from: https://www.wfsahq.org/components/com_virtual_library/media/2ffc0a053d75e1cae94f93f57cddb8ff-atow-384-00-01.pdf
94. Gao F, Ma J, Sun W, Guo W, Li Z, Wang W. Adductor canal block versus femoral nerve block for analgesia after total knee arthroplasty. Clin J Pain. 2017;33(4):356–68.
95. Zhao X-Q, Jiang N, Yuan F-F, Wang L, Yu B. The comparison of adductor canal block with femoral nerve block following total knee arthroplasty: a systematic review with meta-analysis. J Anesth. 2016;30(5):745–54.
96. Kim DH, Beathe JC, Lin Y, YaDeau JT, Maalouf DB, Goytizolo E, et al. Addition of infiltration between the popliteal artery and the capsule of the posterior knee and adductor canal block to periarticular injection enhances postoperative pain control in total knee arthroplasty: a randomized controlled trial. Anesth Analg. 2019;129(2):526–35.
97. Kandarian B, Indelli PF, Sinha S, Hunter OO, Wang RR, Kim TE, et al. Implementation of the IPACK (infiltration between the popliteal artery and capsule of the knee) block into a multimodal analgesic pathway for total knee replacement. Korean J Anesthesiol. 2019;72(3):238–44.
98. Neal JM, Brull R, Horn J-L, Liu SS, McCartney CJL, Perlas A, et al. The Second American Society of Regional Anesthesia and Pain Medicine Evidence-Based Medicine Assessment of Ultrasound-Guided Regional Anesthesia [Internet]. Reg Anesthes Pain Med. 2016;41:81–94. Available from: https://doi.org/10.1097/aap.0000000000000331
99. Ilfeld BM. Continuous peripheral nerve blocks: an update of the published evidence and comparison with novel, alternative analgesic modalities. Anesth Analg. 2017;124(1):308–35.
100. Ahsan ZS, Carvalho B, Yao J. Incidence of failure of continuous peripheral nerve catheters for postoperative analgesia in upper extremity surgery. J Hand Surg Am. 2014;39(2):324–9.
101. Alley EA, Mulory MF. Neuraxial anesthesia for outpatients. Anesthesiol Clin. 2014;32(2):357–69.
102. Liu SS, McDonald SB. Current issues in spinal anesthesia. Anesthesiology. 2001;94(5):888–906.
103. Awad IT, Chung F. Factors affecting recovery and discharge following ambulatory surgery. Can J Anaesth. 2006;53(9):858–72.
104. Flaatten H, Rodt SÅ, Vamnes J, Rosland J, Wisborg T, Koller ME. Postdural puncture headache A comparison between 26- and 29-gauge needles in young patients. Anaesthesia. 1989;44(2):147–9.
105. Loures V, Savoldelli G, Kern K, Haller G. Atypical headache following dural puncture in obstetrics. Int J Obstet Anesth. 2014;23(3):246–52.
106. Pavlin DJ, Janet Pavlin D, Pavlin EG, Gunn HC, Taraday JK, Koerschgen ME. Voiding in patients managed with or without ultrasound monitoring of bladder volume after outpatient surgery [Internet]. Anesthesia Analgesia. 1999;89:90–7. Available from: https://doi.org/10.1213/00000539-199907000-00016
107. Voelckel WG, Kirchmair L, Rehder P, Garoscio I, Krappinger D, Luger TJ. Unilateral anesthesia does not affect the incidence of urinary retention after low-dose spinal anesthesia for knee surgery [Internet]. Anesthesia Analgesia. 2009;109:986–7. Available from: https://doi.org/10.1213/ane.0b013e3181af406e
108. Manassero A, Fanelli A. Prilocaine hydrochloride 2% hyperbaric solution for intrathecal injection: a clinical review [Internet]. Local Reg Anesth. 2017;10:15–24. Available from: https://doi.org/10.2147/lra.s112756
109. Sviggum HP, Jacob AK, Arendt KW, Mauermann ML, Horlocker TT, Hebl JR. Neurologic complications after chlorhexidine antisepsis for spinal anesthesia [Internet]. Reg Anesth Pain Med. 2012;37:139–44. Available from: https://doi.org/10.1097/aap.0b013e318244179a
110. Kandarian BS, Elkassabany NM, Tamboli M, Mariano ER. Updates on multimodal analgesia and regional anesthesia for total knee arthroplasty patients [Internet]. Best Pract Res Clin Anaesthesiol. 2019;33:111–23. Available from: https://doi.org/10.1016/j.bpa.2019.02.004
111. Chin KJ, McDonnell JG, Carvalho B, Sharkey A, Pawa A, Gadsden J. Essentials of our current understanding [Internet]. Reg Anesth Pain Med. 2017;43:133–83. Available from: https://doi.org/10.1097/aap.0000000000000545
112. Desai M, Narayanan MK, Venkataraju A. Pneumothorax following serratus anterior plane block. Anaesth Rep. 2020;8(1):14–6.
113. Ueshima H. Pneumothorax after the erector spinae plane block. J Clin Anesth. 2018;48:12.
114. Hamilton DL. Pneumothorax following erector spinae plane block. J Clin Anesth. 2019;52:17.
115. Turbitt LR, Mariano ER, El-Boghdadly K. Future directions in regional anaesthesia: not just for the cognoscenti [Internet]. Anaesthesia. 2020;75:293–7. Available from: https://doi.org/10.1111/anae.14768
116. Toma O, Persoons B, Pogatzki-Zahn E, Van de Velde M, Joshi GP, PROSPECT Working Group collaborators. PROSPECT guideline for rotator cuff repair surgery: systematic review and procedure-specific postoperative pain management recommendations. Anaesthesia. 2019;74(10):1320–31.
117. Auyong DB, Hanson NA, Joseph RS, Schmidt BE, Slee AE, Yuan SC. Comparison of anterior suprascapular, supraclavicular, and interscalene nerve block approaches for major outpatient arthroscopic shoulder surgery: a randomized, double-blind, noninferiority trial. Anesthesiology. 2018;129(1):47–57.
118. de Jong RH. Axillary block of the brachial plexus. Anesthesiology. 1961;22:215–25.
119. Qin Q, Yang D, Xie H, Zhang L, Wang C. Ultrasound guidance improves the success rate of axillary

plexus block: a meta-analysis. Braz J Anesthesiol. 2016;66(2):115–9.
120. Abdallah FW, Brull R, Joshi GP, Society for Ambulatory Anesthesia (SAMBA). Pain management for ambulatory arthroscopic anterior cruciate ligament reconstruction: evidence-based recommendations from the Society for Ambulatory Anesthesia. Anesth Analg. 2019;128(4):631–40.
121. Vorobeichik L, Brull R, Joshi GP, Abdallah FW. Evidence basis for regional anesthesia in ambulatory anterior cruciate ligament reconstruction: part I—femoral nerve block. Anesth Analg. 2019;128(1):58.
122. Yung EM, Brull R, Albrecht E, Joshi GP, Abdallah FW. Evidence basis for regional anesthesia in ambulatory anterior cruciate ligament reconstruction: part III: local instillation analgesia—a systematic review and meta-analysis. Anesth Analg. 2019;128(3):426.
123. McCartney CJL, McIsaac D. Are peripheral nerve blocks indicated in ambulatory knee surgery? Anesth Analg. 2019;128(1):3–4.
124. Prasad A, Perlas A, Ramlogan R, Brull R, Chan V. Ultrasound-guided popliteal block distal to sciatic nerve bifurcation shortens onset time: a prospective randomized double-blind study. Reg Anesth Pain Med. 2010;35(3):267–71.
125. Forero M, Adhikary SD, Lopez H, Tsui C, Chin KJ. The erector Spinae plane block: a novel analgesic technique in thoracic neuropathic pain. Reg Anesth Pain Med. 2016;41(5):621–7.
126. Tsui BCH, Fonseca A, Munshey F, McFadyen G, Caruso TJ. The erector spinae plane (ESP) block: a pooled review of 242 cases [Internet]. J Clin Anesth. 2019;53:29–34. Available from: https://doi.org/10.1016/j.jclinane.2018.09.036
127. Gürkan Y, Aksu C, Kuş A, Yörükoğlu UH, Kılıç CT. Ultrasound guided erector spinae plane block reduces postoperative opioid consumption following breast surgery: a randomized controlled study. J Clin Anesth. 2018;50:65–8.
128. Altıparmak B, Toker MK, Uysal Aİ, Demirbilek SG. Comparison of the efficacy of erector spinae plane block performed with different concentrations of bupivacaine on postoperative analgesia after mastectomy surgery: randomized, prospective, double blinded trial [Internet]. BMC Anesthesiol. 2019;19. Available from: https://doi.org/10.1186/s12871-019-0700-3
129. Altıparmak B, Korkmaz Toker M, Uysal Aİ, Turan M, Gümüş DS. Comparison of the effects of modified pectoral nerve block and erector spinae plane block on postoperative opioid consumption and pain scores of patients after radical mastectomy surgery: a prospective, randomized, controlled trial. J Clin Anesth. 2019;54:61–5.
130. Chin KJ, Malhas L, Perlas A. The erector Spinae plane block provides visceral abdominal analgesia in bariatric surgery: a report of 3 cases. Reg Anesth Pain Med. 2017;42(3):372–6.
131. Tulgar S, Kapakli M, Kose H, Senturk O, Selvi O, Serifsoy T, et al. Evaluation of ultrasound-guided erector spinae plane block and oblique subcostal transversus abdominis plane block in laparoscopic cholecystectomy: randomized, controlled, prospective study [Internet]. Anesthesia. 2019;13:50. Available from: https://doi.org/10.4103/aer.aer_194_18.
132. Hamed MA, Goda AS, Basiony MM, Fargaly OS, Abdelhady MA. Erector spinae plane block for postoperative analgesia in patients undergoing total abdominal hysterectomy: a randomized controlled study original study. J Pain Res. 2019;12:1393–8.
133. Zhang T-J, Zhang J-J, Qu Z-Y, Zhang H-Y, Qiu Y, Hua Z. Bilateral erector Spinae plane blocks for open posterior lumbar surgery. J Pain Res. 2020;13:709–17.
134. Singh S, Choudhary NK, Lalin D, Verma VK. Bilateral ultrasound-guided erector spinae plane block for postoperative analgesia in lumbar spine surgery: a randomized control trial. J Neurosurg Anesthesiol [Internet]. 2019. Available from: https://doi.org/10.1097/ANA.0000000000000603
135. Yayik AM, Cesur S, Ozturk F, Ahiskalioglu A, Ay AN, Celik EC, et al. Postoperative analgesic efficacy of the ultrasound-guided erector Spinae plane block in patients undergoing lumbar spinal decompression surgery: a randomized controlled study. World Neurosurg. 2019;126:e779–85.
136. Righetti R, Zani G, Piraccini E, Terenzoni M, Fusari M. Lumbar ultrasound-guided erector Spinae plane block to reduce perioperative opioid consumption in particular high-risk patients undergoing peripheral vascular surgery. J Cardiothorac Vasc Anesth. 2020;34(6):1707–8.
137. Zhao H, Xin L, Feng Y. The effect of preoperative erector spinae plane vs. paravertebral blocks on patient-controlled oxycodone consumption after video-assisted thoracic surgery: a prospective randomized, blinded, non-inferiority study. J Clin Anesth. 2020;62:109737.
138. Hong S, Kim H, Park J. Analgesic effectiveness of rectus sheath block during open gastrectomy: a prospective double-blinded randomized controlled clinical trial. Medicine. 2019;98(15):e15159.
139. Purdy M, Kinnunen M, Kokki M, Anttila M, Eskelinen M, Hautajärvi H, et al. A prospective, randomized, open label, controlled study investigating the efficiency and safety of 3 different methods of rectus sheath block analgesia following midline laparotomy. Medicine. 2018;97(7):e9968.

15 Ketamine Infusions: Role and Use in Ambulatory Surgery Centers

Sathya Kikkeri, Luke Mosel, Shilpadevi S. Patil, Harish Siddaiah, and Rinoo Vasant Shah

Abstract

As many patients are refractory to traditional methods of treatment for chronic neuropathic pain and psychiatric illness, physicians and researchers looked to other avenues for alternative treatment possibilities. Ketamine, which has actually been around for over 50 years, is a dissociative anesthetic, used historically mostly for induction of anesthesia and functions via N-methyl-d-aspartate receptor complex inhibition. While the undesired dissociative effects have caused it to have limited, but necessary, utility as an induction agent, ketamine delivered at subanesthetic doses has shown to improve pain and depressive symptoms in patients suffering from chronic pain or depression refractory to standard treatment. Ketamine infusions are quickly becoming more popular among patients and providers as treatment alternatives for pain or depression that is not responding to the traditional method of treatment. Patients across the United States continue to be at risk of opioid abuse as the search for powerful non-opioid analgesia is still ongoing. Ketamine infusions delivered at subanesthetic doses may also be a possibility as treatment for patients suffering from opioid addiction. Currently, ketamine infusions are offered around the United States as an off-label treatment for chronic pain, post-traumatic stress disorder (PTSD), depression, and a variety of other psychiatric and neuropathic pain conditions. In this chapter, we discuss the role of ambulatory surgery centers in ketamine infusions and benefits for patients and providers.

S. Kikkeri
Alabama College of Osteopathic Medicine, Dothan, AL, USA

L. Mosel · S. S. Patil · H. Siddaiah
Department of Anesthesiology, Louisiana State University Health Science Center – Shreveport, Shreveport, LA, USA
e-mail: lmosel@lsuhsc.edu; spati1@lsuhsc.edu; hbanga@lsuhsc.edu

R. V. Shah (✉)
Louisiana State University Health Science Center – Shreveport School of Medicine, Shreveport, LA, USA

Introduction

Ketamine, a phencyclidine derivative, received FDA approval for clinical use in 1970. It has been a uniquely useful anesthetic over the last 50 years, but lately interest has grown exponentially for its uses outside the realm of the operating room. Ketamine is becoming a more popular treatment option for neuropathic pain refractory to traditional treatments and is also fast becoming an alternative route and treatment option for psychi-

K. Rajput et al. (eds.), *Pain Control in Ambulatory Surgery Centers*,
https://doi.org/10.1007/978-3-030-55262-6_15

atric illnesses refractory to traditional methods [1–4]. As the opioid crisis came to a peak, the search for non-opioid analgesic medication led to renewed interest and use of ketamine. Ambulatory surgery centers (ASC) are commonly the setting of choice for the administration of ketamine infusions. Although costs for the patient might be slightly higher than if administered in-office, the safety benefits for the patient and provider heavily outweigh what is offered in an office or clinic setting. In an ASC, patients receive some of the highest levels of care, monitoring, access to personnel, and equipment available in modern medicine. ASCs provide a setting that allows patients to avoid excessive hospital fees and time wasted in a hospital system. ASCs as a setting for ketamine infusions not only lessens the financial burden on the patient, but it also wastes less healthcare dollars as patients are not inpatient in most cases.

Pharmacology

Ketamine is a commonly used intravenous anesthetic producing its effect through inhibition of the N-methyl-D-aspartate receptor complex [5]. Ketamine has two clinically relevant forms that have been shown to induce NMDA-mediated sensory blockade. (S)-Ketamine is about four times more potent than (R)-Ketamine [6, 7]. The (S)-Ketamine isomer has also been shown to be associated with a reduction of adverse effects without reducing or altering its analgesic and anesthetic properties. Ketamine is oxidatively metabolized in the liver into norketamine, which is considered to be the major metabolite in humans, although recent studies have begun to refute that. Eventually it is hydrolyzed and conjugated to a water-soluble inactive glucuronide metabolite excreted by the kidneys [8]. Norketamine can be measured in plasma about 2–3 minutes of intravenous ketamine bolus with a maximum plasma concentration reaching after 30–60 minutes [5]. Ketamine is rapidly distributed throughout the body with a distribution half-life of 11 to 16 minutes. The elimination half-life of ketamine is 2–3 hours, and it is cleared at 12–17 mL/kg/min [9]. A single induction dose of ketamine is generally 1–2 mg/kg intravenous (IV) or 4–8 mg/kg intramuscular (IM). Patients lose consciousness in 30–60 seconds after IV administration and 2–4 minutes after being given IM injection. Patients can regain consciousness after 10–20 minutes, but they might take 60–90 minutes to fully recover from the dissociative effects. Repeated dose and repeated infusions of ketamine will result in the accumulation of the drug as it has a context-sensitive half-life comparable to that of propofol. Ketamine has a large volume of distribution at 3 L/Kg. Infusions can run anywhere from 45 minutes to several hours as a standard infusion protocol has not been established yet [10, 11]. Ketamine can also be administered as a nasal spray called esketamine; however, it is still quite new and currently very expensive and not cost-effective for the management of treatment-resistant depression unless the price is lowered by 40% or more [12].

Use in Surgery Centers

Our primary concern as healthcare providers is patient safety and consideration of all contributing factors *to minimize harm*. Treatments must be individualized to patients and that includes choosing the optimal setting for treatment administration. The use of ketamine is expanding beyond the idea of just being an anesthetic, and physicians must take heed of multiple factors such as contraindications to ketamine and location of administration of infusion when considering treatment protocols involving the use of ketamine.

Ambulatory surgery centers provide a safe environment where ketamine infusions can be administered because of the level of care they are required to provide. The ASA has created practice guidelines for non-anesthesiologists for the delivery of medications for moderate and deep sedation. The recommendations include ensuring NPO status, use of supplemental oxygen during deep sedation, monitoring of patient consciousness level, hemodynamics, ventilation, and oxygenation prior, during, and after the infusion.

Discharge occurs once certain criteria have been met [13]. Ketamine is associated with adverse psychomimetic effects such as dysphoria, hallucinations, nightmares, and vivid dreams. It is also associated with negative GI symptoms [14, 15]. Proper monitoring of the patient during infusion can possibly help limit the severity of these adverse effects and prevent other more serious adverse effects.

Consensus guidelines and recommendations on the use of intravenous ketamine infusions for acute and chronic pain management have been created by the American Society of Regional Anesthesia and Pain Medicine (ASRA), the American Academy of Pain Medicine (AAPM), and the American Society of Anesthesiologists (ASA) [11, 16]. The evidence was evaluated according to the US Preventive Services Task Force grading of evidence defining the levels of evidence based on magnitude and certainty of benefit [17]. The ASRA/AAPM/ASA recommend that the setting of administration must contain resuscitative equipment and immediate access to rescue medications and personnel trained in treating emergencies. The supervising clinician should be experienced with ketamine, such as an anesthesiologist, who is ACLS certified and trained in administering moderate sedation. The administering clinician is a registered nurse or physician assistant who has completed formal training in safe administration of moderate sedation [11]. While these recommendations hold true for ketamine infusions offered in clinic settings, an ambulatory surgery center (ASC) provides access to far superior resources. Infusions administered in office-based settings are not always under the supervision of an anesthesiologist or individuals trained in moderate to deep sedations. These situations are not always the safest of environments for patients under moderate to deep sedation and are not always set up properly in case of unintended adverse sequelae.

Ambulatory surgery centers must have written transfer agreements with a local hospital, or all physicians who perform surgery at that surgery center must have admitting privileges at a designated hospital. In an ASC, in case of emergencies, patients can be transported to the operating room and managed till emergency transportation arrives to transport to a hospital. If patients experience an aspiration or airway event, patients can be taken to the operating room and have a protected airway till emergency services can transport them to a hospital. If patients were to suffer from an unexpected cardiac event, surgery centers generally have more space for medical staff and personnel to work around and maneuver leading to easier access of the patient. The level of care provided by an ambulatory surgery center (ASC) is greater than what is typically available in a standard clinic setting as conversion to the operating room and maintenance on volatile gasses are options while emergency transportation is on their way to the facility. While surgery centers have many safeguards and backups in place, complications resulting in hospital admissions are rare.

Surgery centers are a "goldilocks" option for patients and providers as the location for the administration of ketamine infusion. Many providers performing ketamine infusions prefer to only perform the treatment at an ASC as it guarantees a higher level of monitoring and confidence in the availability of properly trained and equipped personnel. Patient safety is maximized by the increased level of care and monitoring provided by an ASC while costing less out-of-pocket payment from the patient versus if it were performed at a hospital inpatient setting [18].

Typical Workflow of an Infusion

An example of a typical patient workflow of a ketamine infusion in an ASC is as follows. The patient should arrive 30 minutes prior to their scheduled appointment time to check in at the front desk. This time will allow for any necessary paperwork to be filled out by the patient and allows time for the pre-op nurses to admit the patient including obtaining a history and vital signs. The patient must have fasted for a minimum of 6 hours. Patients should have been instructed to take any medication they currently take daily for comorbidities such as blood pressure control and asthma. A thorough review of any medications taken that day and reconfirmation of nothing to eat or drink are performed again. Any remaining paperwork and consent forms must be discussed and signed. Next, the patient is taken to the area where they will be seated for the duration of the procedure. Many facilities have comfortable reclining chairs set up in the post-anesthesia care unit or near the preoperative area. It is recommended that patients be placed in an area with soft, dim lighting away from any loud or sudden noises. As the medication can have adverse psychoactive effects, it is best to create an environment in which the patient can relax. Many providers have calming music playing in the background of the facility, or they provide noise-cancelling headphones for the patients. Some providers allow their patients to bring their own music; however, it is recommended patients choose soothing music as this experience can trigger emotions. Artwork can also evoke a soothing feeling or calmness for some patients, and as such facilities should be aware when adding artwork to rooms.

When the patient is seated comfortably, they will then be attached to monitors and an initial reading of their vital signs including blood pressure, heart rate, respiratory rate, and oxygenation recorded. The supervising anesthesiologist will then perform a focused preoperative evaluation including a history and physical. Once they have cleared the patient and have ruled out any contraindications to the procedure that day, they can next obtain intravenous access. The nurse or qualified individual will obtain peripheral intravenous access with an 18-gauge or 20-gauge needle, and an IV line will be attached to the patient and to an infusion pump from which the ketamine is administered. Pump settings are chosen based on the IV pump and confirmed by the supervising physician before leaving the patient. As the patient is now beginning to settle down for their treatment, they are then given a sleep mask and offered ear plugs or headphones or just listen to the sound of the room if it has soothing music. The infusion is run through a liter of normal saline. The nurse will continue to monitor the patient, and the supervising anesthesiologist will also monitor the patient and will check in on them from time to time as the patient is receiving their infusion. Once the infusion is completed, the nurse will then disconnect and remove the IV from the patient. The IV site is sometimes left if the patient is to return for another infusion in the next few days. If it is the case, the patient is instructed to avoid tampering with it at all costs and to shower and bathe with it protected and covered with plastic. If the IV site is to be removed, the nurse can remove it and clean the site with alcohol and place a band aid or tape with gauze over the puncture site.

Discharge from the ASC after infusion can follow a modified Post Anesthesia Discharge Scoring System as follows in Fig. 15.1. Other post-anesthesia care unit discharge scoring systems can be used; this is mostly dependent on provider experience and/or protocol set by the ASC. The patient should expect to feel relaxed and calm after the infusion and can resume eating and drinking normally. Patients must have a ride home as they are not allowed to drive themselves home or operate heavy machinery for 12 to 24 hours post-infusion. They should also receive instructions to not operate any kitchen equipment or power tools. They should avoid any strenuous activities and any recreational activities such as swimming, hiking, hunting, fishing, etc. for the next 12–24 hours. They should be instructed to avoid alcohol consumption for the next few days and avoid any recreational substances they might take. Any medications that were stopped prior to the procedure can now be resumed. Some providers will prescribe a very weak benzodiazepine for sleep aid, and others might recommend the use of over-the-counter diphenhydramine if they have trouble sleeping. Patients might be slightly nauseous and/or fatigued after the infusion but should be able to communicate more clearly than when they were receiving the infusion. If patients notice any unusual side effects or changes, they should contact their physician or call 911 if it is an emergency.

Fig. 15.1 Modified Post Anesthesia Discharge Scoring System (PADS)

Vital Signs	2= within 20% of preoperative values 1= 20% to 40% of preoperative values 0= 40% or more of preoperative values
Activity and Mental Status	2= and oriented to time, person, place, AND has steady gait 1= oriented to time, person, place, OR has steady gait 0= unable to ambulate
Nausea/Vomiting	2= Minimal to none, treated with oral medication 1= moderate nausea, treated with parenteral/Intravenous medication 0= persistent nausea/vomiting refractory to medication
Surgical Bleeding	2= Minimal requiring no dressing change 1= Moderate 0= Severe requiring 3 or more dressing changes
Intake and Output	2= voiding with input 1= difficulty voiding 0= retention of fluids
Total Pads Score=10	Consider for discharge when score is ≥ **9**

Future and New Directions in Pain Management and Beyond

New avenues in the study of pain management, neurology, psychiatry, and other specialties have shown potential uses for ketamine. Neuropathic pain is highly prevalent and is estimated between 6% and 10% of the population [1]. It has been shown that low-dose intravenous ketamine reduces opioid consumption by 40% while also reducing pain scores in patients receiving a continuous infusion or boluses of low-dose ketamine for postoperative analgesia [15]. It is known that excessive activation of glutamate receptors enhances excitatory transmission of nociceptive pain pathways in chronic pain. Comprehensive review of literature has shown that NMDA receptor antagonists can help treat neuropathic pain [19]. Producing significant analgesia when delivered at anesthetic doses, recently ketamine infusions administered at subanesthetic doses have produced long-term and effective pain relief in patients with complex regional pain syndrome type 1 (CRPS-1) refractory to standard pain treatments [4, 20]. (S)-Ketamine administered as a multiple-day infusion has been shown to reduce pain in chronic CRPS-1 patients [4]. New evidence also shows possible neuroprotective effects of (S) -Ketamine [21]. Ketamine provides a new therapeutic option for patients with depression refractory to standard treatment. Several publications have shown ketamine infusions demonstrating efficacy in the treatment of major depressive disorder and marked improvement of depressive symptoms [2, 22]. Ketamine in its current use should not be viewed as a "one-and-done" cure, but as an alternative treatment management option to traditional methods for treating psychiatric disease. A single infusion of ketamine has shown very rapid efficacy in treatment for major depressive disorder and bipolar disorder for a week [22]. Patients with chronic migraines or new daily persistent headache might also benefit from treatment with subanesthetic ketamine infusions [23] Concern regarding NMDA receptor antagonism impairing neurodevelopment has been a question, and now with an increase in ketamine use, further studies are warranted on the specific mechanism of ketamine-induced structural changes in the central nervous system synapses and brain [24] As the use of ketamine expands, facilities such as ambulatory surgery centers will be used more due to the medical direction of an anesthesiologist, thus allowing for a safe environment in which the medication can be administered.

As the cost of healthcare continues to rise, physicians and other allied professionals working in healthcare must do their share to adopt cost-saving measures in their practice. Physicians and providers should maximize cost-saving tactics without compromising on the safety of patients. In an ASC, costs are significantly reduced as patients are ambulatory and are discharged the same day versus inpatient settings resulting in unnecessary cost and burden on the patient and healthcare system. Even during the COVID-19 pandemic, ASCs were demonstrated to be safe locations for patients to undergo elective surgery if patients received proper preoperative screening [25].

Economics

While the cost of ketamine is relatively low (solution (ketamine HCl injection) 10 mg/mL (per mL), $1.21; 50 mg/mL (per mL), $0.43–$0.98; 100 mg/mL (per mL), $1.97–$2.78), the cost of any infusion treatment can vary from $300 to $800 with some even exceeding $1000. Multiple treatments are often recommended to achieve the best outcomes. While this may seem excessive when compared to the cost of the drug, it tends to be similar to the cost of other intravenous infusion treatments. This is primarily due to the need for monitoring and staff that must be present for an infusion, particularly a sedative. While ketamine infusion treatment claims can be submitted to insurance companies, they are usually not approved as chronic pain and psychiatric treatments and are off-label uses. Esketamine as an intranasal treatment is usually cheaper than an IV ketamine infusion due to elimination of IV supplies. While ketamine is usually readily available, the Food and Drug Administration does list it as currently in a shortage, particularly the 100 mg/mL 5 mL vial. This will continue to change as COVID-19 and other circumstances evolve.

Summary

Ketamine is revealing itself to be much more useful than previously thought. An infusion of ketamine delivered at subanesthetic levels is still considered administration of an anesthetic, and as such, extra care and precautions must be taken while monitoring patients. Ambulatory surgery centers as compared to a standard physician clinic or office are much more equipped for emergencies, since they generally have to adhere to different building and staffing requiring more space, allowing for easier maneuvering, and availability of medical staff experienced in airway management such as a physician anesthesia supervisor. Ambulatory surgery centers offer providers peace of mind knowing their patients are monitored by an anesthesiologist with the facility having all the tools to convert to an operating room environment if need be, albeit unlikely. Ambulatory surgery centers have all the tools a physician would want in a facility where they choose to administer their ketamine infusions. Further, more long-term studies are needed to determine the incidence of adverse events possibly leading to hospitalization in patients receiving ketamine infusions and then comparison of rates of unexpected admission from patients receiving infusions at a clinic versus ambulatory surgery centers.

References

1. van Hecke O, Austin SK, Khan RA, Smith BH, Torrance N. Neuropathic pain in the general population: a systematic review of epidemiological studies [Internet]. Pain. Elsevier B.V.. 2014 [cited 2020 Jul 11];155:654–62. Available from: https://pubmed.ncbi.nlm.nih.gov/24291734/
2. Segmiller F, Rüther T, Linhardt A, Padberg F, Berger M, Pogarell O, et al. Repeated S-ketamine infusions in therapy resistant depression: a case series. J Clin Pharmacol. 2013;53(9):996–8.
3. Murrough JW, Iosifescu DV, Chang L, al Jurdi RK, Green C, Perez A, et al. P.2.f.028 Antidepressant efficacy of ketamine in treatment-resistant major depression: a two-site, randomised controlled trial. Eur Neuropsychopharmacol. 2013;23:S411–2.
4. Sigtermans MJ, van Hilten JJ, Bauer MCR, Arbous MS, Marinus J, Sarton EY, et al. Ketamine produces effective and long-term pain relief in patients with Complex Regional Pain Syndrome Type 1. Pain. 2009;145(3):304–11.
5. Peltoniemi MA, Hagelberg NM, Olkkola KT, Saari TI. Ketamine: a review of clinical pharmacokinetics and pharmacodynamics in anesthesia and pain therapy. Clin Pharmacokinet. Springer International Publishing. 2016;55:1059–77.
6. Oye I, Paulsen O, Maurset A. Effects of ketamine on sensory perception: evidence for a role of N-methyl-D-aspartate receptors. J Pharmacol Exp Ther. 1992;260(3)
7. Sinner B, Graf BM. Ketamine BT – Modern aesthetics. In: Schüttler J, Schwilden H, editors. Handbook of experimental pharmacology [Internet]. Springer Berlin Heidelberg; 2008 [cited 2020 Jul 17]. p. 313–33. Available from: https://doi.org/10.1007/978-3-540-74806-9_15
8. Stoelting R, Hillier S. Pharmacology and physiology in anesthetic practice [Internet]. 2012 [cited 2020 Jul 25]. Available from: https://books.google.com/books?hl=en&lr=&id=lHhGtkvOoM0C&oi=fnd&pg=PT11&ots=MkY1banSg-&sig=VGXPkR5jEgvH-js02EDOA-0BnDU
9. Gorlin AW, Rosenfeld DM, Ramakrishna H. Intravenous sub-anesthetic ketamine for perioperative analgesia [Internet]. J Anaesthesiol Clin Pharmacol. Medknow Publications. 2016 [cited 2020 Jul 25];32:160–7. Available from: /pmc/articles/PMC4874067/?report=abstract.
10. Zanos P, Moaddel R, Morris PJ, Riggs LM, Highland JN, Georgiou P, et al. Ketamine and ketamine metabolite pharmacology: Insights into therapeutic mechanisms. Pharmacol Rev [Internet]. 2018 Jul 1 [cited 2020 Jul 25];70(3):621–60. Available from: /pmc/articles/PMC6020109/?report=abstract.
11. Cohen SP, Bhatia A, Buvanendran A, Schwenk ES, Wasan AD, Hurley RW, et al. Consensus Guidelines on the Use of Intravenous Ketamine Infusions for Chronic Pain From the American Society of Regional Anesthesia and Pain Medicine, the American Academy of Pain Medicine, and the American Society of Anesthesiologists [Internet]. Reg Anesth Pain Med. Lippincott Williams and Wilkins. 2018 [cited 2020 Jul 17];43:521–46. Available from: /pmc/articles/PMC6023575/?report=abstract.
12. Ross EL, Soeteman DI. Cost-effectiveness of esketamine nasal spray for patients with treatment-resistant depression in the United States. Psychiatr Ser [Internet]. 2020 [cited 2020 Jul 25];1–10. Available from: https://pubmed.ncbi.nlm.nih.gov/32631129/
13. Practice Guidelines for Sedation and Analgesia by Non-Anesthesiologists | Anesthesiology | ASA Publications [Internet]. [cited 2020 Jul 18]. Available from: https://anesthesiology.pubs.asahq.org/article.aspx?articleid=1944958
14. Laskowski K, Stirling A, McKay WP, Lim HJ. A systematic review of intravenous ketamine for postoperative analgesia [Internet]. Can J Anaesth. 2011 [cited 2020 Jul 10];58:911–23. Available from: https://pubmed.ncbi.nlm.nih.gov/21773855/
15. Jouguelet-Lacoste J, la Colla L, Schilling D, Chelly JE. The use of intravenous infusion or single dose of low-dose ketamine for postoperative analgesia: a review of the current literature. Pain Med (United States). 2015;16(2):383–403.
16. Schwenk ES, Viscusi ER, Buvanendran A, Hurley RW, Wasan AD, Narouze S, et al. Consensus guidelines on the use of intravenous ketamine infusions for acute pain management from the American Society of Regional Anesthesia and Pain Medicine, the American Academy of Pain Medicine, and the American Society of Anesthesiologists. Reg Anesth Pain Med. 2018;43(5):456–66.
17. Grade Definitions | United States Preventive Services Taskforce [Internet]. [cited 2020 Jul 18]. Available from: https://www.uspreventiveservicestaskforce.org/uspstf/grade-definitions
18. AAOS Now September 2019: Ambulatory Surgery Centers Versus Hospital-based Outpatient Departments: What's the Difference? [Internet]. [cited 2020 Jul 18]. Available from: https://www.aaos.org/aaosnow/2019/sep/managing/managing02/
19. Aiyer R, Mehta N, Gungor S, Gulati A. A systematic review of NMDA receptor antagonists for treatment of neuropathic pain in clinical practice [Internet]. Clin J Pain. Lippincott Williams and Wilkins. 2018 [cited 2020 Jul 11];34:450–67. Available from: https://pubmed.ncbi.nlm.nih.gov/28877137/
20. Schwartzman RJ, Alexander GM, Grothusen JR, Paylor T, Reichenberger E, Perreault M. Outpatient intravenous ketamine for the treatment of complex regional pain syndrome: a double-blind placebo controlled study. Pain. 2009;147(1–3):107–15.
21. Himmelseher S, Pfenninger E. Die klinische anwendung von S-(+)-ketamin - Eine standortbestimmung [Internet]. Anasthesiologie Intensivmedizin Notfallmedizin Schmerztherapie. Anasthesiol Intensivmed Notfallmed Schmerzther. 1998 [cited

2020 Jul 19];33:764–70. Available from: https://pubmed.ncbi.nlm.nih.gov/9893910/
22. Kishimoto T, Chawla JM, Hagi K, Zarate CA, Kane JM, Bauer M, et al. Single-dose infusion ketamine and non-ketamine N-methyl-d-aspartate receptor antagonists for unipolar and bipolar depression: a meta-analysis of efficacy, safety and time trajectories. Psychol Med [Internet]. 2016 [cited 2020 Jul 13];46(7):1459–72. Available from: /pmc/articles/PMC5116384/?report=abstract.
23. Pomeroy JL, Marmura MJ, Nahas SJ, Viscusi ER. Ketamine infusions for treatment refractory headache. Headache. 2017;57(2):276–82.
24. Nader ND, Iacobucci GJ, Visnjevac O, Pourafkari L. Literature review Ketamine: an update on cellular and subcellular mechanisms with implications for clinical practice. Pain Physician [Internet]. 2017;20:285–301. Available from: www.painphysicianjournal.com
25. RA C, TC W, WP A. Evaluating postoperative outcomes of patients undergoing elective procedures in an ambulatory surgery center during the COVID-19 pandemic. Aesthet Surg J [Internet]. 2020 [cited 2020 Jul 25]; Available from: https://pubmed.ncbi.nlm.nih.gov/32598480/

Management of Perioperative Nausea and Intractable Pain in Outpatient Surgery: Mechanisms, Strategies, and Clinical Considerations

16

Chizoba Mosieri, Debbie Chandler, Rhett M. Reynolds, Alex D. Pham, Harish Siddaiah, Shilpa Patil, Taylor Smith, Katherine Cox, Gabriel Stapleton, Laura Edwards, Lindsey Cieslinski, Elyse M. Cornett, and Alan David Kaye

Abstract

Outpatient surgery centers are used instead of hospitals to schedule procedures more conveniently. Patients are able to make appointments more quickly and return to the comfort of their home on the day of surgery. Intractable pain and perioperative nausea are two challenges that outpatient surgery centers face. Patients can feel extreme discomfort which can lead to unnecessary emergency room visits. In this chapter we discuss the benefits of the outpatient surgery center and challenges associated with postoperative nausea and intractable pain. The paper will also address the pivotal role that anesthesia plays in the success of an outpatient surgery and preventing perioperative nausea and intractable pain.

C. Mosieri · D. Chandler · S. Patil · T. Smith
E. M. Cornett (✉)
Department of Anesthesiology, Louisiana State University Health Shreveport, Shreveport, LA, USA
e-mail: cmosie@lsuhsc.edu; dchan3@lsuhsc.edu; spati1@lsuhsc.edu; tsmi29@lsuhsc.edu; ecorne@lsuhsc.edu

R. M. Reynolds
Louisiana State University Shreveport Health Science Center, Shreveport, LA, USA
e-mail: rreyn3@lsuhsc.edu

A. D. Pham
Department of Anesthesiology, Louisiana State University Health New Orleans, New Orleans, LA, USA
e-mail: apham5@lsuhsc.edu

H. Siddaiah
Department of Anesthesiology, LSU Health Shreveport, Shreveport, LA, USA
e-mail: hbanga@lsuhsc.edu

K. Cox · L. Edwards · L. Cieslinski
Department of Anesthesiology, Tulane University School of Medicine, New Orleans, LA, USA
e-mail: kscox@tulane.edu; ledwards1@tulane.edu; lcieslinski@tulane.edu

G. Stapleton
Department of Internal Medicine, Tulane University School of Medicine, New Orleans, LA, USA
e-mail: staplet@tulane.edu

A. D. Kaye
Departments of Anesthesiology and Pharmacology, Toxicology, and Neurosciences, Louisiana State University Health Shreveport, Shreveport, LA, USA
e-mail: akaye@lsuhsc.edu

K. Rajput et al. (eds.), *Pain Control in Ambulatory Surgery Centers*,
https://doi.org/10.1007/978-3-030-55262-6_16

Introduction

An outpatient surgery center, also known as an ambulatory surgery center, is a healthcare facility that offers surgical procedures to be performed outside the hospital setting and does not require an overnight stay. Outpatient surgery centers are used instead of hospitals to schedule procedures more conveniently, improve quality and customer service, and reduce the costs of surgery. Physicians are able to assemble teams of highly skilled staff and ensure that the equipment and supplies are best suited for them. These centers benefit physicians and greatly benefit the patient. Patients are able to make appointments more quickly and return to their home on the day of surgery, all at a much lower cost compared to the hospital surgery setting.

To help treat pain after surgery, outpatient surgery centers may have a focused ambulatory pain specialist on site, who, in addition to providing safe anesthesia, could intervene early once problematic pain issues are recognized, thus preventing emergency room visits, and readmissions for uncontrolled pain [1]. Intractable pain and perioperative nausea are two challenges that outpatient surgery centers face when discussing anesthesia.

Intractable pain is defined as pain that cannot be controlled with standard medical care and is difficult to treat or manage. This type of pain is not curable; therefore, a physician's focus is to reduce discomfort, which can be challenging in an outpatient center setting. Intractable pain and nausea are the two most common reasons for delayed discharge and unexpected admissions to the hospital. Therefore, control of pain in the ambulatory setting is important [1].

Peri-/postoperative nausea and vomiting (PONV) is used to describe nausea and vomiting in the post-anesthesia care unit (PACU) or in the immediate 24 postoperative hours. Patients can feel extreme discomfort which can lead to unnecessary emergency room visits. Therefore, a goal of outpatient surgery centers is to achieve effective analgesia with medications that decrease nausea and/or with the utilization of regional anesthesia techniques in conjunction with non-opioid therapies [1].

In this chapter, we discuss the benefits of outpatient surgery centers and some of the challenges that they cause physicians to face. We will focus specifically on the topics of perioperative nausea and intractable pain and discuss how to best treat these patients. This paper will also discuss the important role that anesthesia plays in the success of an outpatient surgery center, including, how to properly manage postoperative nausea and pain.

Intractable Pain in Outpatient Surgery

The number of ambulatory surgeries has increased, however, appropriate pain control of patients undergoing surgery has remained unmatched [1]. Up to 70% of patients experience moderate -to -severe pain after surgery and postoperative pain is a frequent reason for prolonged post-anesthesia care unit (PACU) stays and hospital admissions [1]. Clinicians will inevitably encounter patients who experience intractable postoperative pain, therefore they should understand the available treatments and when they should be used.

Intractable pain is defined as ongoing, severe, debilitating, and unyielding pain that progressively fails escalation of medical management [2]. Although no set guidelines exist to treat intractable postoperative pain, there are several options recommended by both the American Pain Society (APS), the American Society of Regional Anesthesia and Pain Medicine (ASRA), and the American Society of Anesthesiology (ASA) to treat severe postoperative pain.

Clinicians should educate patients and their families on the available management options and expectations for postoperative pain. This includes how pain is assessed and when it is reported. Treatment plans should be individually tailored to the patient including their medical, psychiatric, chronic pain, substane abuse, and surgical postoperative treatment history. This tailored plan can decrease postoperative opioid consumption, reduce preoperative anxiety, and decrease in stay after surgery [3]. The presence of bleeding disorders or a history of spinal surgery can be contraindications for spinal or epidural pain interventions. Prior opioid dependence can lead to a higher opioid requirement and prolong the postoperative recovery period leading to a change in analgesic choice [3]. Psychiatric factors including depression may be associated with greater postoperative pain and must be recognized and addressed [4].

Clinicians should adjust their pain treatment plan based on the patient's pain response and history. Because pain is subjective there are several available treatment. If patients have cognitive deficits or are sedated, clinicians can use behavioral assessment tools and include the caregiver's input on the patient's level of pain. Objective measures such as vital signs, can be included however, it is not recommended that the diagnosis rely solely on objective measures. Pain assessment modalities are available to accurately assess and quantify the intensity of pain. This includes the visual analog scales, numeric or verbal rating scales, and symbols among others. Because no one particular pain assessment tool is superior, selecting a pain assessment modality must be based on the patient including cognitive ability, developmental status, level of education, and language. If it is indicated that the patient's pain intensity is consistently high despite continued or escalation of therapy, there may be a new medical insult or surgical complication present. Further assessing for delirium, sedation, and nausea will also assist in adjusting for postoperative pain treatment [3].

Based on the recommendations by the APS, ASRA, and ASA, a multimodal analgesic plan including medications and techniques combined with non-pharmacological treatments can be used for postoperative pain. This can lead to additive, synergistic, and more effective pain control compared to one intervention. For example, the clinician may employ regional anesthesia including neural axial and peripheral analgesic modalities while placing the patient on systemic opioids with other analgesic medications. There are a variety of non-opioid analgesics and non-pharmacological modalities that can be utilized which will be discussed later. As a general approach, it is highly recommended that regional anesthesia techniques be implored for surgeries of the thorax, abdomen, and extremities due to prior trials showing positive results with the addition of systemic analgesics [3].

Opioids are commonly used for postoperative pain. Although oral and IV forms are available for severe pain, it is recommended that oral administration be pursued over IV if patient is able to swallow. Prior evidence suggest that IV administration of opioids is not superior to oral. In addition, it is not recommended to give opioids preoperatively as a means to decrease postoperative pain. It is also not recommended to give analgesic through the intramuscular route as it has shown to have unreliable absorption and cause further pain [3].

Because opioids are a significant component of postoperative pain treatment, much research has been conducted in its use to decrease PACU stay. It was found that 5 mg of morphine (1 mg/ml) soaked in geofoam placed in the epidural space reduced PACU stay, decreased analgesia use, and extended pain relief after spinal surgery. In addition, the effects of perineural fentanyl additive to ropivacaine had shown a reduction in VAS score at 30 minutes after being given in the PACU [5].

If the parenteral route is needed, the use of a patient-controlled analgesia (PCA) is highly recommended. This can be considered in patients who can't take oral medications due to ileus and aspiration or from the surgery itself. PCA are recommended for patients who will need pain relief for several hours given that they understand how to use the device. Basal infusion with PCA is not recommended [3].

In addition to opioids, there are several non-opioid options available. It is highly recommended by APS, ASRA, and ASA that acetaminophen and NSAIDs be utilized in the postoperative period if tolerated. When both were used with the addition of opioids, it was associated with decreased postoperative pain and opioid use versus opioids alone. This may be attributed to the fact that acetaminophen and NSAIDs reduce pain via different pathways versus opioids [3]. IV acetaminophen given 15 minutes prior to endotracheal intubation for a cesarean section under general anesthesia reduced administration of pain postoperatively [5]. When compared to fentanyl, IV ketorolac was equivocal to reducing postoperative pain at 30 minutes and 150 minutes; however, fentanyl was superior at 15 minutes [5]. Furthermore, IV ketorolac, when used perioperatively, assisted in early discharge from the PACU after laparoscopic bypass surgery. Although NSAIDs are shown to be beneficial, the clinician must be aware of the side effects including adverse cardiovascular events, gastrointestinal ulceration, and renal insult. Due to this, the use of celecoxib might be a reliable alternative as it is a selective cyclooxygenase-2 inhibitor. It is highly recommended that preoperative celecoxib be given to patients without contraindications as it is associated with decreased opioid use after surgery with lower postoperative pain. Most trials use a dose of 200 to 400 mg 30 minutes to 1 hour prior to surgery. Of note, celecoxib should be avoided in patients undergoing surgery for coronary artery bypass graft [3].

It is highly recommended that the clinician utilize pregabalin and gabapentin as part of the multimodal regimen as both medications are associated with decreased opioid use after surgery with associated decreased pain scores. From prior studies, it would seem that giving these medications preoperatively is more effective. Knowing this, the clinician must be aware that with increasing doses, there will be a high risk for sedation and possible delayed discharge from the PACU [3, 5].

IV ketamine has also been recommended for the management of postoperative pain. Ketamine, an NMDA antagonist, can assist with analgesia and attenuate central sensitization and opioid tolerance [5]. Ketamine infusions were associated with a reduction in the use of pain medication after surgery and reduction in persistent postsurgical pain [3]. Ketamine, when given intraoperatively as an infusion, provided superior postoperative pain control compared to placebo after a laparoscopic cholecystectomy [5]. If ketamine is used, it is recommended to give a 0.15–2 mg/kg bolus prior to surgery and then begin an intraoperative infusion at a rate of 10 μg/kg/minute [3]. Clinicians should use ketamine in major surgeries and may have utility in patients who have a strong tolerance to opioids. Side effects of ketamine include neurotoxicity, hallucinations, and nightmares [3, 5].

Dexmedetomidine can also be a useful adjunct therapy for postoperative pain relief and has been shown to decrease opioid need after surgery. This has been shown when given intraoperatively. In the PACU, IV dexmedetomidine was shown to decrease severe pain and prevent emergence agitation. Dexmedetomidine has been shown beneficial as both an intrathecal adjuvant and epidural adjuvants in providing postoperative pain relief. It has also been shown that when given as an adjunct in an ilioinguinal/iliohypogastric nerve block, it provided decreased pain after pediatric inguinal hernia surgery. It also extended the time to the demand of the first analgesia [5].

The use of dexamethasone and its effect on postoperative pain have been researched. Through prior meta-analysis, it was indicated that one perioperative dose of IV dexamethasone provided a strong benefit to reducing pain after surgery, decreasing opioid use, and prolonging the time to the first dose of analgesic while decreasing stay at the PACU. It was also shown that one dose of IV dexamethasone prior to induction of anesthesia strengthened the postoperative analgesia provided by ketamine. It has also been reported that IV dexamethasone can increase the duration of analgesia of postoperative interscalene blocks after arthroscopic shoulder surgery [5].

The APS, ASRA, and ASA recommend that clinicians consider the use of IV lidocaine infusions for patients undergoing either laparoscopic or open abdominal surgery. Prior studies have shown that if given intraoperatively or perioperatively, they were associated with a decrease in duration of ileus time and improved the quality of analgesia versus placebo. It is recommended that an induction dose be given at 1.5 mg/kg followed with an infusion of 2 mg/kg/h during the operation [3].

The use of infiltrative techniques has been frequently studied. The use of surgical site-specific local anesthetic infiltration of long-acting local anesthetic has shown positive results when given as part of a multimodal approach in specific procedures. It was effective in many surgical procedures including arthroscopic knee surgeries, total knee replacement, cesarean section, hemorrhoid surgeries, and laparotomies. It is recommended that the use of infiltrative techniques should be utilized only if shown benefit in specific procedures but not to be used routinely [3].

Peripheral regional anesthesia is highly recommended with high-quality evidence supporting its use for treating postoperative pain. It has shown positive results as part of the multimodal approach especially with several surgeries including thoracotomies, lower extremity joint surgeries, cesarean section, hemorrhoid surgery, circumcision, and shoulder surgery. Clinicians should consider this especially for surgeries on the extremities [3]. Lumbar plexus blocks given preoperatively lead to a decrease in pain scores in the PACU after patient underwent total hip arthroplasty [5]. It has also been shown that a single femoral nerve block for total hip arthroplasty leads to reduced PACU stay postoperatively [5]. The use of ropivacaine 0.5% was found to be superior to bupivacaine 0.25% and ropivacaine 0.2% for femoral nerve blocks and reducing postoperative pain [5]. If the need for analgesia is predicted to exceed a single injection of peripheral regional analgesia, then the clinician should pursue a continuous local anesthetic-based peripheral regional analgesic technique [3].

Neuroaxial techniques are commonly used including epidural or spinal analgesia with local anesthetics. This can be given with or without opioids. It is highly recommended that the clinician employ neuroaxial techniques as it is associated with decreased pain after surgery and analgesic use versus a placebo injection or systemic opioid use. Older studies suggested that using epidural or spinal analgesia was associated with a reduction in risk of venous thromboembolism, myocardial infarction, postoperative mortality, reduction in duration of ileus compared to systemic analgesia, and reduction in mortality after surgery. This can be particularly helpful in patients who had undergone abdominal and thoracic surgeries, cesarean section, and lower extremity procedures who have a high risk of cardiopulmonary adverse events. The advantage of epidural analgesia is that it can be given as a PCA or as an infusion. Spinal analgesia only allows opioids as a single dose [3].

Finally, the use of physical modalities have been suggested. One systemic review demonstrated that a transcutaneous electrical nerve stimulation (TENS) is associated with nearly 25% less postoperative analgesic use compared to the no TENS group. Therefore, the TENS unit should be included as a postoperative pain treatment adjuvant therapy.

The number of ambulatory surgeries has been increasing; however, appropriate pain control of patients undergoing surgery has remained unmatched [1]. In fact, it is reported that up to 70% of patients experience moderate to severe pain after surgery [1]. Considering this, it is inevitable that clinicians will encounter patients suffering from severe and intractable pain after surgery. It can be challenging to achieve optimum pain control in these patients as appropriate treatment plans can be complex. It is our hope that current guidelines and recommendations on treating severe postoperative pain can be applied to patient experiencing both severe and intractable postoperative pain.

Perioperative Nausea in Outpatient Surgery

PONV is one of the most difficult complications that surgeons and anesthesiologists face in a surgical setting. Studies have demonstrated that up to 30% of patients suffer from PONV, with that number getting to as high as 80% in high-risk patients [6]. Outside of patient discomfort and delayed discharge, PONV can lead to complications such as electrolyte abnormalities, wound dehiscence, esophageal rupture, and increased intracranial pressure. For these reasons, it is vital to identify high-risk patients early on to implement prophylactic treatment. Ultimately, treating and preventing the onset of PONV leads to higher patient satisfaction, fewer unexpected hospital admissions, and lower healthcare costs across the perioperative period.

The possible five afferent pathways causing nausea and vomiting studied are the chemoreceptor trigger zone (CTZ), the vagal mucosal pathway of the gastrointestinal (GI) system, vestibular neuronal pathways, reflex afferent pathways of the cerebral cortex, and afferents from the midbrain. If any of these pathways are stimulated, the sensation of nausea and vomiting is triggered. There are various receptors involved in these pathways including serotonergic, histaminergic, dopaminergic, neurokinin-1 (NK-1), and cholinergic muscarinic receptors. Generally, the caudal hindbrain or the brainstem reticular formation is well known anatomically as a primary emesis center for the human body. It is termed as "vomiting center" and is an important emesis-generating locations in the brain. This center receives input from all the afferent pathways mentioned above. These pathways may trigger emesis by interaction with the nucleus tractus solitarius (NTS). Along with these pathways, various neurotransmitters such as serotonin, dopamine, substance P, histamine, and acetylcholine are associated with these pathways to trigger emesis from the NTS [7]. But how do they work? The gastrointestinal system is a good example. As discussed in L. Veiga-Gil et al., when neuroendocrine cells release serotonin in response to toxins or caustic substances in the GI tract, vagal afferent fibers are stimulated and feed back to the NTS [8]. As the NTS is stimulated, a cascade of other pathways become involved leading to nausea, cold sweats, salivation, and diaphragmatic contraction leading to retching and vomiting. The other pathway to discuss with regard to emesis centers is the area postrema (AP). The AP is also located in the caudal hindbrain and is connected to the NTS. The lack of the blood-brain barrier is what differentiates the AP from the NTS, making it more sensitive to toxic stimulation and substances in the blood such as drugs. The efferent signals are transmitted through glossopharyngeal, trigeminal, accessory, hypoglossal, and spinal segmental nerves. The coordinated contraction of the muscles supplied by these nerves leads to vomiting. The pathophysiology behind PONV is complex and will need to be continuously researched.

The physiology and factors that influence PONV are complex. These factors can be broken up into different categories: patient, preoperative, intraoperative, and postop. The intraoperative factors include either anesthetic or surgical factors. The challenge is being able to identify those factors that have been statistically proven to be predictors of PONV. Patient-specific factors include sex, smoking history, age, obesity, history of motion sickness, history of PONV, and patient-specific comorbidities. Of these listed, the strongest patient-specific factor is female sex [9]. Patient-dependent comorbidities or conditions with delayed gastric emptying are other strong predictors which increase their chances for PONV [9]. For example, patients with diabetes, hypothyroidism, abdominal pathology, full stomach or presence of blood in the stomach, and pregnancy are likely to be at high risk for PONV. Nonsmokers are more prone to PONV than smokers, most likely related to gradual desensitization of the CTZ among smokers. Preoperative factors include fear or anxiety of surgery and perioperative fasting. Intraoperative anesthetic factors such as procedures under general anesthesia, use of nitrous oxide, inhalation agents, etomidate, ketamine, and opioids increase the incidence of PONV. Next, postop factors that lead to PONV are pain, ambulation, and opioids. Pain has always been a common cause of PONV, and adequate analgesia is an important approach to avoid this complication. Opioids are commonly used for pain control; however, their use is associated with an increased risk for PONV [9]. Patients receiving opioids for postop pain control are also at increased susceptibility to motion sickness during ambulation in the early postop period [9]. These factors have led physicians to explore other medications and modalities of analgesia in the postoperative settings such as use of nonsteroidal anti-inflammatory drugs and regional analgesia. The surgical factors include the duration and type of surgery that heavily contribute to PONV. As per Gan et al., reported that cholecystectomy, gynecological surgery, and laprascopic surgeries increase patient risk of PONV [10]. Increasing surgery length by even 30 minutes can also increase incidence of PONV by 60% [9]. In addition, certain pharmacogenetic factors are thought to be associated with PONV. Homozygous patients with A118 variant of OPRM1 are at higher risk of having PONV.

The anesthesia provider should establish whether the patient is a candidate for regional anesthesia or general anesthesia, what organ systems will be stimulated during the operation, which anesthetic needs to be used, and which to avoid. When these factors are identified, a physician can risk score each patient before a surgical procedure. A widely used scoring system is the Apfel scoring system for PONV [11]. This system uses four factors to determine a patient's 24-hour risk of PONV. Table 16.1 shows the factors involved and the scoring system used to risk stratify a patient in the postoperative period.

Treatment: Many strategies with many different medications have been attempted, with some "gold standards" being identified. One main class of drugs used are the serotonin receptor antagonists (5HT-3). This is the most widely used class of drugs in the perioperative setting with some examples including ondansetron, granisetron, dolasetron, ramosetron, tropisetron, and palonosetron. Of these drugs, ondansetron is currently considered the "gold standard" as compared to other antiemetic medications [8]. It is started at 4 mg and has been shown to decrease PONV by 25% when given prophylactically [7]. The side effect profile is quite safe with headache and constipation being its most common side effects, but at higher doses, ondansetron (16 mg or more) and other 5HT-3 antagonists have been associated with QT prolongation. This warrants one to be cautious when treating high-risk cardiac patients with the drug. Another promising drug in this class is palonosetron. With a much higher half-life of 40 hours as compared to other in this class, this drug may be more effective than ondansetron in high-risk patients [7]. More extensive studies will be needed to further compare palonosetron to other antiemetic classes.

Table 16.1 Apfel scoring for postoperative nausea and vomiting

Risk factors	Apfel points
Female gender	1 point
Non-smoker	1 point
Positive history of motion sickness	1 point
Use of postoperative opioids	1 point
Interpretation	
Apfel score	**24-hour risk**
0	10%
1	21%
2	39%
3	61%
4	79%

Histamine (H1) reeptor antagonsts: This class is not as effective as 5HT-3 antagonists but has also not been widely studied. In the proper setting or in combination therapy with other drugs, they can be quite useful. Two drugs in this class are promethazine and dimenhydrinate. These drugs are dosed at 12.5–25 mg IV and 1–2 mg/kg IV, respectively, and they both have a similar side effect profile of dry mouth, constipation, drowsiness, urinary retention, and blurred vision [9]. Meclizine, chlorpromazine, diphenhydramine, and perphenazine are other such drugs in this class.

Corticosteriods: Dexamethasone is quite effective across many clinical trials. One trial in particular called the DREAMS trial explored the benefit of preoperative administration of dexamethasone for PONV [12]. This trial showed that not only does a single 4–8 mg dose IV of preoperative dexamethasone significantly reduce the incidence of PONV but it decreases administration of additional antiemetics in the postoperative period [13].

A 2018 study investigating adverse side effects of dexamethasone in surgical patients found that a single dose of dexamethasone "probably does not increase the risk for postoperative infection" [14]. However, it is uncertain whether dexamethasone has an effect on delayed wound healing in surgical patients.

Dopamine (D2) receptor antagonists: Droperidol is considered to be as effective as other "gold standard" drugs such as ondansetron and dexamethasone. However, its side effect profile is what prevents it from being used on a larger scale. At one point, the FDA issued a black box warning against all doses due to its QT prolongation [7]. Further studies have shown droperidol to be safer at lower doses and pose little risk for cardiac arrhythmias. Droperidol is also associated with increased restlessness postoperatively which could pose an issue for its use in an outpatient setting [7]. Another dopamine antagonist to be mentioned is amisulpride. It is a potent D2/D3 antagonist with potential for monotherapy indications in PONV patients. It has a very favorable side effect profile, and compared to droperidol, it has shown to cause minimal QT prolongation making it a more desirable option [15]. One randomized controlled study by Candiotti et al. displayed significant results with the use of amisulpride. Compared to placebo, a 5 mg or 10 mg dose of the medication showed to be efficacious in the treatment of established PONV making it a promising medication going forward [15]. One last dopamine receptor antagonist to include is metoclopramide. It promotes gastric emptying, increases duodenal peristalsis, increases gastroesophageal sphincter tone, and decreases pyloric sphincter tone leading to faster movement of digestive contents of the bowel. It has a weak antiemetic effects and, when given at a dose of 10 mg, it has shown promise in its ability to reduce the incidence of PONV [7]. Domperidone, chlorpromazine, and haloperidol are other examples of dopamine (D2) receptor antagonists. Side effects include extrapyramidal symptoms or dyskinesia, sedation, headache, and dizziness.

Neurokinin receptor 1 (NK-1) antagonists: The most commonly used drug from the NK-1 class is aprepitant. This class works by inhibiting the actions of substance P, which prevents vagal afferent projections stimulating the NTS and ultimately prevents the onset of nausea and vomiting [8]. Studies have shown that a typical 80 mg oral dose given in the preoperative setting can significantly reduce PONV and be on a therapeutic level close to that of ondansetron making it a challenger for another "gold standard" in PONV therapy [7]. However, the prohibitive cost of aprepitant may be a hindrance for more widespread use.

Current data shows that the proper therapy to treat and prevent PONV is available for the majority of patients. Yet, the problem still exists on a large scale. Identifying those at risk in the outpatient setting is the first step. One review on prophylaxis administration showed that at an ambulatory surgery center, 8% of high-risk patients were not given any antiemetic prophylaxis [16]. This same study suggests that computer algorithms be implemented to identify these patients early on in the preoperative setting [16]. With today's healthcare moving to full electronic records, this change could help downscale PONV in the outpatient setting. Regardless of new changes and revolutionary therapies, it seems that the threshold upon which physicians administer prophylaxis is not set in stone, and stronger guidelines may be required going forward.

Role of Anesthesia in Outpatient Surgery

Patient Selection

A successful ambulatory surgery requires that the patient and the procedure are both suitable for ambulatory anesthesia. Therefore, several factors must be considered when planning anesthesia in an outpatient care facility, such as the type of surgery, patient selection, and elective versus emergent surgery. Considering that ambulatory surgeries involve early discharge and fast recovery, perhaps the most important factor is determining the method of anesthesia followed by patient selection, with both playing a key component in the success of an ambulatory surgery.

Preoperative assessment and optimization are fundamental to assure a good outcome in patient selection. In general, most patients are eligible for ambulatory surgery unless the type of surgery itself is deemed an overnight stay. Several factors intervene for patient selection such as medical, surgical, and anesthetic factors [17].

Medical Considerations

Patients with unstable medical conditions should not have surgery in an ambulatory care setting, but rather in a hospital care facility. Patients with chronic and stable illnesses might be good candidates for ambulatory care surgery for faster discharge home and back to their daily routine and lifestyle management. Patient selection should be based on their actual functional status at the time of assessment, but not necessarily based on age, ASA status, or BMI. However, one should be cautious about managing morbidly obese patients in an outpatient facility due to obesity- related comorbidities which might limit the goals of ambulatory care surgery of faster recovery and discharge. In such cases, hospital setting surgery might be the safest choice to handle anesthesia and surgical complications associated with obesity [1].

Social Considerations

Before committing a patient for ambulatory care surgery, the anesthesia provider must have a clear understanding from the patient about certain social considerations including, the patient should agree and understand that they cannot drive for 24 hours following anesthesia; therefore, a responsible adult must be available for transportation and communication with the surgery facility. The patient understanding the procedure, anesthetic techniques, postoperative care, and pain management is essential to the success of surgery in the setting of ambulatory care surgery [18].

Surgical Considerations

When considering ambulatory surgery, a key component is to avoid all types of interventions that might carry a risk of major complications (bleeding, stroke, cardiovascular instability). Postoperative pain control should be carefully planned, and the patient should be mobile to some extent prior to discharge. Early discharge is optimal with return to baseline functions. If abdominal or thoracic surgery is performed, a minimally invasive approach should be considered [18].

How to Plan Anesthesia in an Ambulatory Care Setting and How to Control Intractable Pain and Prevent Nausea and Vomiting

Providing safe and optimum anesthesia/analgesia for ambulatory surgery patients preoperatively, intraoperatively, and postoperatively is essential to prevent withdrawal syndromes and pain flare-ups and to safely discharge patients in a timely manner. Therefore, to achieve these goals, an anesthesia provider should preferably use medications causing less nausea and/or use techniques in conjunction with non-opioid medications. Such techniques include regional anesthesia, neuraxial anesthesia, and local infiltrations combined with non-opioid medications.

Regional Anesthesia

Regional anesthesia can be used as a single injection nerve block or a continuous peripheral nerve block. It provides excellent pain relief without opioid requirements. This can be achieved by peripheral nerve blocks or local infiltration. There is a broader use of regional anesthesia which can now be used in most types of upper or lower extremities surgeries and breast surgeries. Regional anesthesia provides a fast recovery, effective pain control with excellent analgesia, a highly reduced risk of nausea and vomiting, and reduced risks of cognitive impairment in the elderly patient. Serious but rare complications include, local anesthetic toxicity, nerve damage, and prolonged sensory or motor deficit [19].

Neuraxial Anesthesia

Epidural, caudal, and spinal anestheisa are increasingly used in an ambulatory care setting. Spinal anesthesia is mostly used in the adult population and keeps the patient free of pain and protects the patient from nausea and vomiting that can occur with general anesthesia. Also, there is a lower incidence of postoperative pain with spinal analgesia and the incidence of complications is rare [20].

Choice of Analgesia

Acetaminophen

Combined with nonsteroidal anti-inflammatory drugs, acetaminophen provides better analgesia than used alone. Its forms of administration are oral, parenteral, or rectal. Intravenous acetaminophen reduces morphine consumption by 22–46% in patients undergoing major orthopedic surgeries [17, 21].

Nonsteroidal Anti-inflammatory Drugs (NSAIDs)

Parenteral NSAIDs provide analgesic effect comparable to traditional opioid analgesia without opioid-associated side effects. These include piroxicam, diclofenac, and ketorolac. In addition to their analgesic property, they have antipyretic and anti-inflammatory properties. NSAIDs are mostly used as part of multimodal analgesia to control postoperative mild to moderate pain. They act by blocking prostaglandins synthesis through COX-1 and COX-2 inhibition, thereby decreasing the production of acute inflammatory mediators and reducing peripheral nociception and central response. Studies have found that ketorolac provides improved postoperative analgesia and patient comfort compared to fentanyl [22]. While tramadol and ketorolac have comparable analgesic effects, ketorolac also decreased the risk of post-anesthesia nausea and vomiting. It was shown that in pediatric populations, ketorolac provides comparable pain control than caudal block with bupivacaine; recovery was faster with a shorter time to void, leading to early ambulation and early discharge. However, despite their great analgesic property, NSAIDs might cause gastrointestinal bleeding, platelet dysfunction, and kidney damage in high doses or after repetitive exposure.

COX-2 Inhibitors

COX-2 inhibitors can be used in combination with non-opioid analgesics for multimodal analgesia. Compared with NSAIDS, they have a less prominent effect on platelet function and a lower risk of bleeding. The use of COX-2 inhibitors results in a significant opioid-sparing effect and increases overall patient satisfaction. However, because of rofecoxib's adverse cardiovascular effects, it was withdrawn from the market. Celecoxib is still in use, and a newer drug, etoricoxib, has also been in use and has proven to provide pain relief associated with certain type of surgeries.

Gabapentin

Gabapentin is a well-known anticonvulsant (gamma amino-butyric acid analog (GABA)) with some analgesic property. Though it has a GABA-like structure, its mechanism of action involves binding to α2-d subunits of voltage-dependent pre-synaptic calcium channels, therefore reducing excitatory neurotransmitter release and subsequent postsynaptic calcium influx [23]. When administered preoperatively, a dose of 600 mg of gabapentin reduced postoperative pain and opioid consumption. Gabapentin is also associated with a decreased incidence of nausea and vomiting in patients undergoing mini-laparoscopic cholecystectomy [24].

Ketamine

A single dose of intravenous use of ketamine has been shown to provide a significant opioid-sparing analgesic effect in orthopedic and intra-abdominal surgery.

Ketamine is a non-competitive NMDA (N-methyl-D-aspartate) receptor antagonist; it acts by modulating central sensitization induced by incision and tissue damage. Intramuscular use of ketamine even in small dose also provides opioid-sparing analgesic effects, less occurrence of nausea and vomiting, and a better patient and physician relationship. Studies show that the rate of nausea and vomiting was lower in patients who were given 0.4 mg/kg of ketamine and 8 mg of dexamethasone than those on placebo [25].

Alpha-2 Adrenergic Agonists

Dexmedetomidine is an alpha-2 adrenergic agonist. Administration of 1 μg/kg IV dexmedetomidine followed by a continuous infusion of 0.4 μg/kg/h is associated with a significant decrease of PCA morphine need in patients undergoing major surgeries. However, its use in an ambulatory setting has not been widely studied. Dexmedetomidine has significant anesthetic and analgesic-sparing effects. It also reduces anxiety and intraoperative opioid requirement. The most common side effect is sedation and bradycardia.

Opioids

The use of opioids has to be done very wisely in the setting of ambulatory care surgery. Although opioids provide optimal pain relief, they are, however, associated with a broad spectrum of side effects such as PONV, urinary retention, prolonged sedation, and respiratory depression which might defeat the goal of outpatient surgeries as far as early discharge and recovery and reducing nausea and vomiting are concerned. Shorter-acting opioids such as fentanyl might be more indicated for day surgery with a lower incidence of nausea and vomiting compared to morphine. Also, the use of opioids for perioperative pain management might cause an acute opioid-induced hyperalgesia in some patients; therefore, it is more suitable to use a multimodal analgesia approach in the setting of outpatient care facility.

Choice of Antiemetic Agent

PONV might occur in up to 80% of patients without antiemetic prophylaxis. Nausea and vomiting after ambulatory surgery remain the major cause of delayed discharge after outpatient surgery. PONV is also associated with a decrease in patient satisfaction, and increased morbidity and healthcare costs. For these reasons, routine use of antiemetic prophylaxis is highly recommended during outpatient surgery to minimize the risk of developing PONV and improve patient outcomes.

Because of the multifactorial etiology of PONV, and at least four different neurotransmitter systems involved in the physiology of PONV, there is no single antiemetic drug that can prevent PONV in all patient populations. Therefore, a combination of antiemetic therapy that acts at different neuroreceptor sites is preferred in patients with high risk of PONV. Antiemetic prophylaxis with a combination of ondansetron, metoclopramide, and droperidol is highly effective in minimizing PONV after office-based surgery [26]. Studies demonstrate that a combination of dexamethasone with a 5-HT3 receptor antagonist provides a greater antiemetic efficacy and this combination therapy provides an optimal choice for prophylaxis against PONV [27]. Other studies reporte that dexamethasone enhanced the antiemetic efficacy of other antiemetics (e.g., dopamine antagonists) when administered as part of a combination therapy.

To summarize, eight antiemetics, ondansetron, dolasetron, granisetron, tropisetron, dexamethasone, droperidol, cyclizine, and metoclopramide, are commonly used in the prevention of PONV, and each antiemetic reliably prevents nausea and vomiting after surgery. However, although no drug is found to be especially better than another, when combined, their antiemetic effects are additive [28]. Many experts have promoted the idea of administering three different classes of antiemetics for additive and/or synergistic effects for high-risk patients, and this strategy is commonly employed as a treatment strategy.

Challenges for Pain Management in Outpatient Surgery

Poorly controlled pain negatively affects quality of life, functional recovery, sleep, causes persistent postsurgical pain, and leads to delayed discharge of patients and unanticipated hospital admissions following surgery ultimately increasing consumption of healthcare resources [29]. Patients with chronic pain present a specific type of challenge. In one study, patients with preexisting chronic pain using opioids reported considerably greater levels of postoperative pain than the control group undergoing general and orthopedic surgery [1]. Patients taking even modest amounts of opioids preoperatively will need their baseline opioid dose in addition to two- to threefold the dose of opioids regularly given for well-controlled pain in opioid-naïve patients [30, 31]. Some recommend inpatient admission for 24 hours following surgery to determine the amount of oral opioid to be administered. When employing regional anesthesia as a multimodal means of anesthesia, it should be noted that epidural opioids do not cover the systemic need created by chronic oral opioid administration [32]. However, overall regional anesthesia techniques serve a critical role in multimodal analgesia while reducing opioid use. Underreporting the usage of drugs is more predominant in female patients and in patients taking opioid analgesics in comparison to other drugs [33]. As a result, inadequate management perioperatively may go overlooked and may cause withdrawal [32]. Additionally, caregivers can overemphasize addiction, tolerance, and sedation due to analgesics, but underestimate the effects of non-opioid adjuncts and underestimate dependence. These factors make the management of chronic pain patients even more difficult. Studies report the importance of perioperative evaluation, including a risk stratification questionnaire, to formulate an individualized patient pain treatment program.

Additionally, intractable pain can be especially harmful in patients financially and physiologically. Patients with ischemic heart disease or those with chronic respiratory conditions are the most susceptible to the increased cardiovascular requirements caused by pain [34]. There are economic and healthcare costs associated with inadequately treated acute pain that develops into chronic pain. Cost should also be considered when using new or different interventions to treat intractable pain to make these innovation strategies viable in the long term.

PONV/PDNV is a multifactorial complication of surgery and anesthetics that has an incidence of 20–40%, with some high-risk patients experiencing rates up to 80% [35]. Furthermore, the development of post-discharge nausea and vomiting is more frequent. Up to 35% of surgical outpatients experience PDNV, many of whom did not develop such symptoms in the recovery unit [36]. It can lead to a poor surgical experience and recovery and other physiologic abnormalities such as dehydration, electrolyte disturbances, wound dehiscence, pulmonary aspiration, delayed hospital discharge, and/or hospital readmission. The pathophysiology of PONV is comprised of multiple neurophysiologic pathways and can be stimulated by cholinergic, dopaminergic, histaminergic, and/or serotonergic receptors. As previously mentioned, there are multiple classes of agents that target specific pathways. There are many studies that recommend a multimodal approach, which includes several medications from different classes, rather than monotherapy. The goal is to understand each patients individual risk by using validated risk scores and tailoring an antiemetic plan [11]. As same-day surgery is becoming more popular, the use of other modalities outside of antiemetic medications is of interest. Most of these modalities aim to reduce the risk of developing PONV or PDNV. The risk for PONV was nine times less among patients receiving regional anesthesia than those receiving general anesthesia [9]. Non-pharmacologic devices have also been studied such as acupressure devices and aromatherapy in the pediatric surgery suites. One study by White et al. illustrated that using Pressure Right, a disposable, non-invasive acupressure device, enhanced the efficacy of the commonly used anti-emetic prophylactic regimen (droperidol, ondansetron, and dexamethasone) for preventing PONV symptoms for the first 24 hours after major laparoscopic surgery [37].

It also important to consider the effects that PONV can have on the daily operations of the ambulatory surgery center. Parra-Sanchez et al. conducted a time-motion economic analysis of PONV that evaluated the overall cost in terms of additional time spent with patients, additional supplies used, recovery time, use of rescue treatments, and quality of life through the third post-operative day. In 100 ambulatory patients they found that patients with PONV spent 1 hour longer in the post-anesthesia care unit (PACU). After itemizing the expenses of caring for patients with PONV, they found an incremental cost of $75 per patient (US dollars in 1999). The cost difference was not driven by physician expense or by the cost of additional antiemetic medications, but by the additional PACU minutes [38]. Other studies mirrored these results and suggested decreasing the maximum numbers of patients in the PACU by rearranging the operating room schedule as a way to optimize the PACU admission rate. These studies shine a light on the additional strains as a result of PONV to not only the patients and those who care for them but also on the healthcare system overall.

Clinical Considerations

Identifying patient groups at the highest risk for intractable pain can allow for targeted interventions to reduce the likelihood of prolonged pain after surgery. A 2019 single-institution retrospective study of outpatients with intractable chronic pain found that patients with chronic intractable pain who were identified as having higher self-efficacy had lower pain disability and depression [39]. The authors of this study contextualized these results using the fear-avoidance model, proposing that patients who have higher self-efficacy can confront their pain and begin the process of recovery. Likewise, those who were identified as having high anxiety and depression scores measured by the Hospital Anxiety and Depression Scale (HADS) in this model move from a fear of pain toward pain anxiety and hypervigilance. The authors suggest that this leads to disuse, disability, and depression which only further exacerbates their chronic pain.

The findings in this study reinforce a Japanese 2017 retrospective study in an outpatient pain liaison clinic investigating the factors that lead to prolonged, intractable pain among patients receiving outpatient pain treatment. This study found that severe depression on initial visit was correlated with prolonged pain after treatment [40]. A multidisciplinary team including anesthesiologists, orthopedic surgeons, and psychiatrists worked with patients experiencing chronic pain to come up with a treatment plan that addressed both the physical and psychological components of pain. In their analysis of the results, the study authors found that patients who had low HADS scores at the beginning of treatment had much better relief than those with higher HADS after this multidisciplinary intervention. These findings reinforce that depressed patients tend to have a harder time recovering from pain. However, even in the patients with high HADS scores, there were improvements in depression and pain scores seen after 6 months of treatment.

These two studies suggest that there are a high-risk group of patients identified by depression scores who are more likely to have prolonged and intractable pain. These patients may be able to be screened in the preoperative clinic visit to allow for early referral to a multidisciplinary pain liaison treatment team for close follow-up that addresses the psychological barriers to recovering from postoperative pain. Furthermore, cognitive behavioral therapy (CBT) was a recommended treatment strategy by both groups, which can lead to an improvement in negative symptoms, mood, and anxiety, and may ultimately prevent intractable pain postoperatively.

Another clinical consideration is the treatment of patients with either current or prior opiate use disorders. Several new advances in perioperative pain management focus on non-opiate adjuncts to either reduce or take the place of opiates in pain management. A 2017 single-center, prospective, randomized, blinded trial found that intraoperative ketamine infusion reduced immediate postoperative opioid consumption after spinal fusion surgery in chronic pain patients with opioid dependency [41]. Ketamine was used as an adjunct to routine opioid intraoperative management, and notably in this study at 6 months follow-up, the ketamine group reported significantly less pain and increased activity. This study was done in an inpatient setting; however, multimodal pain control techniques have also been shown to be successful in the outpatient setting in reducing opioid requirements postoperatively. A 2018 cohort study at a head and neck surgery service performing outpatient thyroid and parathyroid surgery found that multimodal anesthesia including acetaminophen, NSAIDs, and gabapentin preoperatively followed by acetaminophen and ibuprofen postoperatively was associated with a significant decline in the prescription of postoperative opioid analgesics [42]. Another 2018 retrospective review of outpatient breast surgery procedures found that multimodal analgesia given preoperatively decreased both narcotic use and pain scores postoperatively [43]. By reducing opioids in this way, high-quality pain control can be achieved in a way that limits potential opioid misuse a well as the potential emetic effects of opioid medication. Perioperative management of opiate-tolerant patients is covered in-depth elsewhere in this text.

Alongside pain, nausea and vomiting are the top reasons that patients are unable to be discharged following outpatient surgery [44]. Therefore, a systematic PONV protocol must be in place to mitigate the need for prolonged stay in the ambulatory surgery center following a procedure. For PONV as well, reducing opioids can be an important tool to decrease nausea and vomiting. Current consensus guidelines from the Society for Ambulatory Anesthesiology recommend risk stratifying patients and applying a sliding scale of treatment that range from waiting and seeing to a multimodal approach including multiple interventions [10]. Given that nausea and vomiting are more easily prevented and treated, special consideration should be given to those patients who are at the highest risk of PONV [45].

Delayed discharges due to perioperative nausea and vomiting are not the only considerations in the ambulatory setting. Managing post-discharge nausea and vomiting is also paramount in increasing patient satisfaction and decreasing emergency room visits after surgery. There have been several recent studies investigating the role of the anesthesiologist in decreasing post-discharge nausea and vomiting (PDNV) via a multimodal intraoperative and postoperative medication regimen. A 2003 systematic review on the routine prophylactic use of antiemetics on the incidence of post-discharge nausea and vomiting following ambulatory surgery found that combination management of PONV with more than one drug leads to a reduction of the relative risk of post-discharge nausea and vomiting [46]. This study suggests that perioperative prophylactic management in high-risk patients helps not only with PONV but after discharge as well, making the anesthesiologists' role doubly important.

Overall, in perioperative pain, nausea, and vomiting control, there are several patients who can be identified in the preoperative period who have a high risk of intractable pain and PONV/PDNV. These patients should be tar-

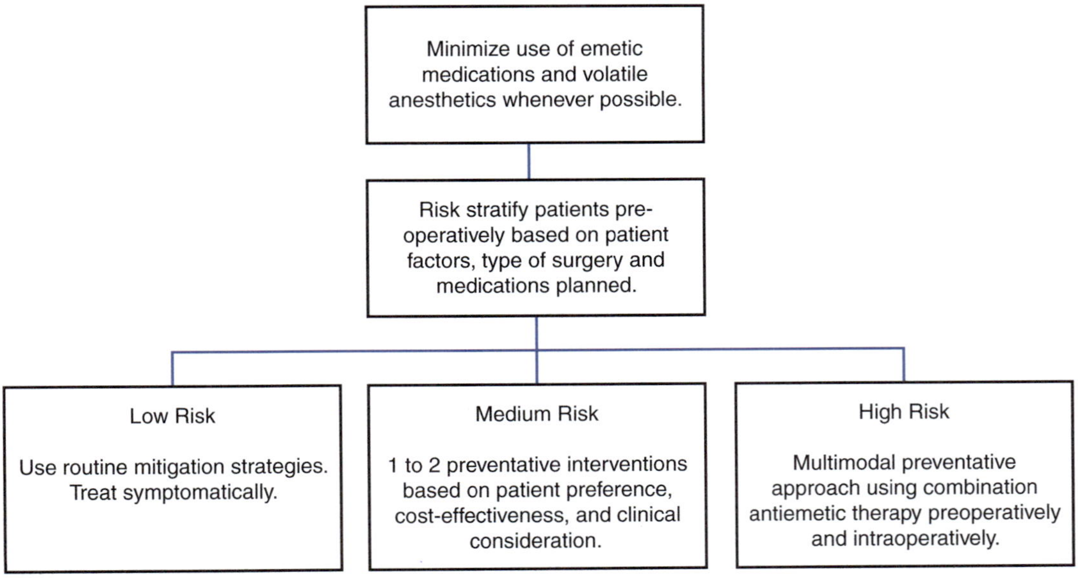

Fig. 16.1 Algorithm for the management of PONV. (Adapted from guidelines provided by Gan et al. [10])

geted with combination treatments that seek to prevent common barriers to discharge and patient satisfaction in the ambulatory surgery center. By focusing on prevention in high-risk groups, the side effects of these treatments can be minimized while improving outcomes. See Fig. 16.1.

Summary

Ambulatory surgery aims to facilitate early recovery, safe discharge, and early resumption of normal daily activies after elective surgery. To achieve these aims, it is necessary to optimally manage various issues that can derail the positive outcome of a safe and effective outpatient surgery. These include perioperative management of nausea, vomiting, and intractable pain. Postoperative nausea and vomiting (PONV) are common and very distressing to patients. If unresolved, it can lead to prolonged post-anesthesia care (PACU) stay and unplanned hospital admission, resulting in significant healthcare costs.

Pain also has negative implications on postoperative recovery including prolongation of the time to recovery milestones, delayed discharge, and unplanned admissions in an outpatient setting. Inadequate pain control has negative effects on quality of life, function, and functional recovery. Therefore, the optimal management of postoperative pain is key. Multimodal analgesia is the use of more than one analgesic modality to achieve effective pain control while reducing opioid-related side effects. Multimodal analgesia has become the bedrock of enhanced recovery after surgery (ERAS). Assuring safe and optimum anesthesia/analgesia perioperatively is necessary to avoid withdrawal syndromes and pain flare-ups and to safely discharge patients in a timely manner. Therefore, the anesthesia provider should use medications that induce less nausea and try to use a combination of non-opioid drugs. These methods include regional anesthesia, neuraxial anesthesia, and local penetration of non-opioid medicines.

Finally, pain management is multidisciplinary and should include the patient, members of the patient family, and the healthcare team. Pain management should tailored to the individual and facilitated by the healthcare team and the patients family. These overall suggestions will help facilitate postoperative recovery and prevent postoperative nausea and intractable pain.

Bibliography

1. Vadivelu N, Kai AM, Kodumudi V, Berger JM. Challenges of pain control and the role of the ambulatory pain specialist in the outpatient surgery setting. J Pain Res. 2016;9:425–35.
2. Tennant F, Hermann L. Intractable or chronic pain: there is a difference. West J Med. 2000;173(5):306.
3. Chou R, Gordon DB, De Leon-Casasola OA, Rosenberg JM, Bickler S, Brennan T, et al. Management of postoperative pain: a clinical practice guideline from the American pain society, the American society of regional anesthesia and pain medicine, and the American society of anesthesiologists' committee on regional anesthesia, executive commi. J Pain [Internet]. 2016;17(2):131–57. Available from: https://doi.org/10.1016/j.jpain.2015.12.008
4. Ghoneim MM, O'Hara MW. Depression and postoperative complications: an overview visceral and general surgery. BMC Surg [Internet]. 2016;16(1):1–10. Available from: https://doi.org/10.1186/s12893-016-0120-y
5. Luo J, Min S. Postoperative pain management in the postanesthesia care unit: an update. J Pain Res. 2017;10:2687–98.
6. Tateosian VS, Champagne K, Gan TJ. What is new in the battle against postoperative nausea and vomiting? Vol. 32, Best Pract Res. Bailliere Tindall Ltd; 2018. p. 137–48.
7. Horn CC, Wallisch WJ, Homanics GE, Williams JP. Pathophysiological and neurochemical mechanisms of postoperative nausea and vomiting. Vol. 722, Eur J Pharmacol. Elsevier; 2014. p. 55–66.
8. Veiga-Gil L, Pueyo J, López-Olaondo L. Postoperative nausea and vomiting: Physiopathology, risk factors, prophylaxis and treatment. Rev Española Anestesiol y Reanim (English Ed). 2017;64(4):223–32.
9. Shaikh S, Nagarekha D, Hegade G, Marutheesh M. Postoperative nausea and vomiting: a simple yet complex problem. Anesth Essays Res. 2016;10(3):388.
10. Gan TJ, Diemunsch P, Habib AS, Kovac A, Kranke P, Meyer TA, et al. Consensus guidelines for the management of postoperative nausea and vomiting. Anesth Analg. 2014;118(1):85–113.
11. Apfel CC, Läärä E, Koivuranta M, Greim C-A, Roewer N. A simplified risk score for predicting postoperative nausea and vomiting. Anesthesiology. 1999;91(3):693.
12. Dexamethasone versus standard treatment for postoperative nausea and vomiting in gastrointestinal surgery: randomised controlled trial (DREAMS Trial). BMJ. 2017;357:j1455.
13. Chen Q, An R, Zhou J, Yang B. Clinical analgesic efficacy of dexamethasone as a local anesthetic adjuvant for transversus abdominis plane (TAP) block: a meta-analysis. Choi S, editor. PLoS One. 2018;13(6):e0198923.
14. Polderman JAW, Farhang-Razi V, Van Dieren S, Kranke P, Devries JH, Hollmann MW, et al. Adverse side effects of dexamethasone in surgical patients. Vol. 2018, Cochrane Database of Systematic Reviews. John Wiley and Sons Ltd; 2018.
15. Candiotti KA, Kranke P, Bergese SD, Melson TI, Motsch J, Siddiqui N, et al. Randomized, double-blind, placebo-controlled study of intravenous amisulpride as treatment of established postoperative nausea and vomiting in patients who have had no prior prophylaxis. Anesth Analg. 2019;128(6):1098–105.
16. McCaul C, Buckley M, Hegarty A. Ambulatory anesthesia and postoperative nausea and vomiting: predicting the probability. Ambul Anesth. 2016;3:27–35.
17. Tasmuth T, Kataja M, Blomqvist C, Von Smitten K, Kalso E. Treatment-related factors predisposing to chronic pain in patients with breast cancer: a multivariate approach. Acta Oncol (Madr). 1997;36(6):625–30.
18. Prabhakar A, Cefalu JN, Rowe JS, Kaye AD, Urman RD. Techniques to optimize multimodal analgesia in ambulatory surgery. Vol. 21, Current Pain and Headache Reports. Current Medicine Group LLC 1; 2017. p. 1–6.
19. Mukherju RA. Postoperative pain relief for ambulatory surgery. Indian J Anaesth. 2006;50(5):355.
20. Lee JH. Anesthesia for ambulatory surgery. Vol. 70, Korean Journal of Anesthesiology. Korean Society of Anesthesiologists; 2017. p. 398–406.
21. Shea RA, Brooks JA, Dayhoff NE, Keck J. Pain intensity and postoperative pulmonary complications among the elderly after abdominal surgery. Hear Lung J Acute Crit Care. 2002;31(6):440–9.
22. Iskandar H, Rakotondriamihary S, Dixmérias F, Binje B, Maurette P. Analgesie par bloc axillaire continu apres chirurgie des traumatismes graves de la main: Auto-administration versus injection continue. Ann Fr Anesth Reanim. 1998 Oct;17(9):1099–103.
23. Pyati S, Gan TJ. Perioperative pain management. CNS Drugs. 2007;21(3):185–211.
24. Bang Y-S, Park C, Lee S-Y, Kim M, Lee J, Lee T. Comparison between monitored anesthesia care with remifentanil under ilioinguinal hypogastric nerve block and spinal anesthesia for herniorrhaphy. Korean J Anesthesiol. 2013;64(5):414.
25. Hassanein A, Mahmoud E. Effect of low dose ketamine versus dexamethasone on intraoperative nausea and vomiting during cesarean section under spinal anesthesia. Egypt J Anaesth. 2015;31(1):59–63.
26. Tang J, Chen X, White PF, Wender RH, Ma H, Sloninsky A, et al. Antiemetic prophylaxis for office-based surgery: are the 5-HT3 receptor antagonists beneficial? Anesthesiology. 2003;98(2):293–8.
27. Henzi I, Walder B, Tramèr MR. Dexamethasone for the prevention of postoperative nausea and vomiting: a quantitative systematic review. Anesth Analg. 2000;90(1):186–94.
28. Carlisle J, Stevenson CA. Drugs for preventing postoperative nausea and vomiting. Vol. 2006, Cochrane

Database of Systematic Reviews. John Wiley and Sons Ltd; 2006.
29. Jafra A, Mitra S. Pain relief after ambulatory surgery: Progress over the last decade. Vol. 12, Saudi Journal of Anaesthesia. Wolters Kluwer Medknow Publications; 2018. p. 618–25.
30. De Leon-Casasola OA, Lema MJ. Epidural sufentanil for acute pain control in a patient with extreme opioid dependency. Anesthesiology. 1992;76(5):853–6.
31. Tennant F. The physiologic effects of pain on the endocrine system. Pain Ther. 2013;2(2):75–86.
32. Savage R. Cyclo-oxygenase-2 inhibitors: when should they be used in the elderly? Vol. 22, Drugs and Aging. Drugs Aging; 2005. p. 185–200.
33. Schwarzer A, Kipping K, Maier C, Bussemas HH. Cross-sectional study medication compliance in patients with chronic pain. Pain Physician. 2014;17:81–94.
34. Kehlet H, Jensen TS, Woolf CJ. Persistent postsurgical pain: risk factors and prevention. Lancet. 2006;367(9522):1618–25.
35. Cao X, White PF, Ma H. An update on the management of postoperative nausea and vomiting. J Anesth. 2017;31:617–26.
36. Carroll NV, Miederhoff P, Cox FM, Hirsch JD. Postoperative nausea and vomiting after discharge from outpatient surgery centers. Anesth Analg. 1995;80(5):903–9.
37. White PF, Zhao M, Tang J, Wender RH, Yumul R, Sloninsky AV, et al. Use of a disposable acupressure device as part of a multimodal antiemetic strategy for reducing postoperative nausea and vomiting. Anesth Analg. 2012;115(1):31–7.
38. Parra-Sanchez I, Abdallah R, You J, Fu AZ, Grady M, Kenneth, et al. Reports of original investigations. Can J Anesth/J Can Anesth. 2012;59:366–75.
39. Tsuji H, Tetsunaga T, Tetsunaga T, Nishida K, Misawa H, Ozaki T. The factors driving self-efficacy in intractable chronic pain patients: a retrospective study. J Orthop Surg Res. 2019;14(1)
40. Tetsunaga T, Tetsunaga T, Nishida K, Tanaka M, Sugimoto Y, Takigawa T, et al. Short-term outcomes of patients being treated for chronic intractable pain at a liaison clinic and exacerbating factors of prolonged pain after treatment. J Orthop Sci. 2017;22(3):554–9.
41. Nielsen RV, Fomsgaard JS, Siegel H, Martusevicius R, Nikolajsen L, Dahl JB, et al. Intraoperative ketamine reduces immediate postoperative opioid consumption after spinal fusion surgery in chronic pain patients with opioid dependency. Pain. 2017;158(3):463–70.
42. Militsakh O, Lydiatt W, Lydiatt D, Interval E, Lindau R, Coughlin A, et al. Development of multimodal analgesia pathways in outpatient thyroid and parathyroid surgery and association with postoperative opioid prescription patterns. In: JAMA Otolaryngology – Head and Neck Surgery. American Medical Association; 2018. p. 1023–1029.
43. Barker JC, Di Bartola K, Wee C, Andonian N, Abdel-Rasoul M, Lowery D, et al. Preoperative multimodal analgesia decreases postanesthesia care unit narcotic use and pain scores in outpatient breast surgery. Plast Reconstr Surg. 2018;142(4):443E–50E.
44. Aubrun F, Ecoffey C, Benhamou D, Jouffroy L, Diemunsch P, Skaare K, et al. Perioperative pain and post-operative nausea and vomiting (PONV) management after day-case surgery: the SFAR-OPERA national study. Anaesth Crit Care Pain Med. 2019;38(3):223–9.
45. Sizemore DC, Grose BW. Postoperative nausea. 2020;
46. Gupta A, Wu CL, Elkassabany N, Krug CE, Parker SD, Fleisher LA. Does the routine prophylactic use of antiemetics affect the incidence of postdischarge nausea and vomiting following ambulatory surgery? A systematic review of randomized controlled trials. Anesthesiology. 2003;99(2):488–95.

Part III

NORA Locations

17 Sedation for Interventional Pain Procedures

Warren Southerland, Meredith L. Gioe, Alexandra Fonseca, Anna C. Rogers, Mason E. Triay, Mark R. Jones, Elyse M. Cornett, and Alan David Kaye

Abstract

Many patients undergoing interventional techniques may require mild to moderate sedation, related to the nature of chronic pain and anxiety. Since the patient cannot communicate acute changes in symptoms, deep sedation and/or general anesthesia for most interventional procedures is considered as unsafe, thus resulting in increased morbidity and mortality, and creating compliance issues. For patients undergoing interventional pain procedures, sedation is a critical aspect and requires competence and defined standards of experience and expertise. Along with the monitoring standards established by the American Society of Anesthesiologists (ASA), including temperature, blood pressure, EKG, pulse oximetry, and quantitative end tidal CO2, other considerations are warranted by the anesthesiologist for a safe and successful procedure, including perioperative medications and fasting.

W. Southerland · A. Fonseca
Department of Anesthesia, Critical Care, and Pain Medicine, Beth Israel Deaconess Medical Center, Harvard Medical School, Boston, MA, USA
e-mail: wsouther@bidmc.harvard.edu; Acfonsec@bidmc.harvard.edu

M. L. Gioe
Louisiana State University Health New Orleans, School of Medicine, New Orleans, LA, USA
e-mail: mgioe@lsuhsc.edu

A. C. Rogers · M. E. Triay
Louisiana State University Health Shreveport, School of Medicine, Shreveport, LA, USA
e-mail: arog11@lsuhsc.edu; mtriay@lsuhsc.edu

M. R. Jones
Department of Anesthesia, Critical Care, and Pain Medicine, Beth Israel Deaconess Medical Center, Harvard Medical School, Boston, MA, USA

Weill Cornell Medical College, Department of Anesthesia, New York, NY, USA

E. M. Cornett
Department of Anesthesiology, Louisiana State University Health Shreveport, Shreveport, LA, USA
e-mail: ecorne@lsuhsc.edu

A. D. Kaye (✉)
Departments of Anesthesiology and Pharmacology, Toxicology, and Neurosciences, Louisiana State University Health Shreveport, Shreveport, LA, USA
e-mail: akaye@lsuhsc.edu

Introduction

Thousands of patients undergo interventional pain procedures each year in the USA [1–4], many of which have comorbid states and take daily medications that have significant effects during the perioperative period. Procedural sedation is a tool used by anesthesia providers to decrease patient anxiety and increase patient cooperativity during interventional pain procedures. Not all interventional pain procedures require the use of additional sedation techniques for the patient to remain still and calm during the

K. Rajput et al. (eds.), *Pain Control in Ambulatory Surgery Centers*,
https://doi.org/10.1007/978-3-030-55262-6_17

procedure. However, the use of sedation is helpful during more complicated procedures such as sympathetic blocks, chemical ablations, percutaneous discectomies, permanent spinal cord stimulator and lead implantation, and intrathecal pump implantations [5].

Procedural sedation allows the patient to remain motionless but also communicate acute changes in symptoms to the anesthesia provider, resulting in fewer complications from the procedure. This is important because patients can suffer from permanent neurologic injury, hypoxic brain injury, and even death as a result of oversedation, hypoventilation, and spinal cord injury [6–13]. It is important that providers deliver sedation in alliance with the established standards of care laid out by the American Society of Anesthesiologists (ASA) and the American Society of Interventional Pain Physicians (ASIPP) [14–17]. In this chapter, we will outline relevant guidelines for performing procedural sedation during interventional pain procedures.

Locations

Related to the varying degree of complexity and difficulty of interventional pain procedures, there is a wide range of locations where procedures are performed. Examples of locations where interventional procedures can be performed include but are not limited to operating rooms, outpatient management centers, diagnostic centers, and physician offices. Physicians should understand the specific characteristics of the procedure locations to ensure patient safety and realize that standards of care are unchanged regardless of practice setting.

A survey of the site prior to the commencement of a procedure is necessary to ensure that adequate care is delivered in a controlled and routine manner.

The ASA supports the notion of providing anesthetic care in ambulatory settings but has also established guidelines for physicians to follow to provide high-quality patient care and maintain patient safety. The *ASA Guidelines for Ambulatory Anesthesia and Surgery* state that "the facility must be established, constructed, and equipped and operated in accordance with applicable local, state, and federal laws and regulations" [18]. The ASA also delineates more specific standards that a facility must adhere to in their *Statement on Nonoperating Room Anesthetizing Locations*. There are not only requirements that demand adequate size, lighting, and ventilation of the room used for procedures, but there are also medical and anesthesia equipment requirements for oxygen, suction, and resuscitation measures [19]. These guidelines set out by the ASA ensure a standardized level of safety for all pain procedures despite the varying degree of medical locations in which the procedures are performed. Additionally, the Joint Commission on Accreditation of Healthcare Organizations (JCAHO) and the Occupational Safety and Health Administration (OSHA) provide guidelines on the utilization of intravenous procedural sedation in any location [20].

Established Standards of Care

The established standard of care when undergoing anesthesia for an interventional pain procedure is outlined by the ASA in their statements on the *Basic Standards for Preanesthesia Care* [21], *Standards for Basic Anesthetic Monitoring* [22], *Standards for Postanesthesia Care* [23], and *Guidelines for Ambulatory Anesthesia and Surgery* [18]. The concept of anesthesia delivery in the office, as is used for many interventional pain procedures, is referred to as office-based anesthesia (OBA) and is considered a subset of ambulatory anesthesia. Unlike hospital or licensed ambulatory surgical facilities, physician offices that provide OBA have little regulatory control by government agencies. Because of this, pain practitioners must be confident that they have addressed the requirements for delivering sedation for pain procedures to reduce risk and liability.

The ASA's *Guideline for Office-Based Anesthesia* summarizes the perioperative care requirements. It states that there should be an anesthesiologist present in the intraoperative period and being available (at least by telephone) when discharged from anesthetic care.

Resuscitation equipment and emergency transfer should be immediately available to the facility. An appropriate written consent, patient education regarding follow-up, and discharge instructions are necessary and apply to all patients undergoing these procedures. It also expresses that the discharge of the patient is a physician's responsibility and that personnel with advanced resuscitative techniques should be available until all patients are discharged home [24].

As stated by the ASA, patients should need only local anesthesia for interventional pain procedures unless unique circumstances are present. If a procedure is particularly painful or prolonged, physicians should follow the guidelines for sedation or monitored anesthesia care (MAC), which are discussed later in this chapter. It is important to recognize that patients undergoing sedation, MAC, or local anesthesia for pain procedures, especially elective cervical spine procedures, must be aware enough to be able to communicate with the practitioner should they experience pain when a needle is misplaced intraneurally, within the spine itself, or in another aberrant location.

JCAHO and OSHA also have healthcare and patient safety goals that must be met to receive accreditation to perform outpatient anesthesia and pain procedures. Some of JCAHO's goals aim to improve the accuracy of patient identification, improve safety of using medications by reconciling medication information, and reduce risks of healthcare-associated infections [25]. JCAHO's *Accreditation Handbook for Office-Based Surgery* underscores that a practitioner who administers sedation must be able to rescue the patient from any depth of anesthesia (e.g., "when the patient slips from moderate into deep sedation or from deep sedation into full anesthesia") [20]. It further specifies that a cardiorespiratory rescue team is not an acceptable replacement of a practitioner who is qualified to administer sedation and thus also qualified to rescue a patient from any depth of anesthesia. These guidelines further increase patient safety during OBA and pain procedures. OSHA's compliance standards focus on protecting employees from hazards and pathogens through the use of personal protective equipment hazard communication [26]. OSHA guidelines cover safety items such as radiation exposure, high sound levels, and heavy mechanical equipment, which can all be applicable to the practice of pain management. It is crucial to be in compliance with organizations such as JCAHO and OSHA to provide the adequate standard of care for interventional pain procedures.

Facilities and Equipment

When performing procedures that require ambulatory anesthesia, clinicians must consider the basic monitoring of the patient. The "Standards of Basic Anesthetic Monitoring" outlines the fundamental monitoring equipment needed for any procedure requiring anesthesia. Basic monitoring equipment should include automatic non-invasive blood pressure device, electrocardiogram, pulse oximeter, capnography for both quantitative and end tidal $CO2$, and respiratory monitoring devices [27]. Monitoring the perioperative state of the patient allows for quick recognition of many impending complications. Detecting acute changes in the stability of the patient before a procedure, in particular, can prevent the development of possible life-threatening conditions.

In the *Statement on Nonoperating Room Anesthetizing Locations*, the ASA lists the minimally necessary equipment for procedure completion outside of the standard operating room [19]. As listed, the location should have an oxygen supply to last the length of the procedure. There should also be a back-up supply of oxygen, which is encouraged to be at least a full E cylinder. Additionally, there should be a reliable source of suction in each of the procedure locations. If inhaled anesthetic is used, there should be a reliable system for scavenging waste anesthetic gases. Other important equipment includes a self-inflating hand resuscitator bag that is capable of administering at least 90 percent oxygen to deliver positive pressure ventilation. Also remember to prepare adequate anesthesia drugs, supplies, and equipment for the intended procedure [19]. Including IV fluid in your supplies is prudent, as many patients may benefit from fluid resuscitation throughout the duration of their procedure. It is the responsibility of the provider administering anesthesia and monitoring the patient to ensure that all equipment and supplies are present and functional; this may include making an equipment checklist, if warranted [27].

In the case of an emergency, there should be a cart prepared with a defibrillator, emergency drugs, and other necessary equipment to provide adequate cardiopulmonary resuscitation [19]. Once the procedure is completed, there also should be adequate equipment and supplies to support the patient in the post-anesthesia state – monitoring must continue until the patient reaches a stable state or is back to baseline. In addition to the basic equipment listed, it also important to consider every patient's individual needs and risks. One should therefore tailor preparations for the patient and the procedure being performed [27].

Any facility providing patient care outside of the operating room must follow the federal and state safety regulations. No facility can be adequately prepared if the structural integrity or fire safety standards are not met [18]. Assuring these basic requirements will provide a safe environment for all personnel and patients. In the outpatient clinic, away from the hospital resources, more delicate care should be taken in the preparation process [27].

With regard to individual procedure rooms, the location should provide ample space for personnel and equipment. The anesthetic and monitoring machines and the patient must be readily accessible [24]. Next, there should be an adequate number of electrical outlets capable of supporting the needed anesthetic and monitoring equipment. In addition to these basic outlets, there should be clearly labeled outlets with direct connection to the emergency power supply [24]. Lighting is one of the most important considerations in preparation for the procedure. Adequate lighting should be provided for the anesthetic and monitoring machines and the patient and procedural field; a form of back-up battery-powered lighting should be immediately available [19]. Finally, two-way communication from within the procedure room to request assistance must be immediately available [19]. In the case of electrically powered equipment, these devices should have a back-up power source immediately available or should be battery-powered. Interventional pain procedures often require fluoroscopy; thus, radiation safety is of the utmost importance. Advanced preparation should be made for proper storage and handling of machines, lead aprons or glass shields, and thyroid shields. Dosimetry data should comply with state and federal regulations.

Personnel and Staffing

The ASA has provided the *Guidelines for Ambulatory Anesthesia and Surgery*, which outlines the staff needed for all procedures performed in this setting. The primary staff member is the physician or other practitioner that holds a valid license and is qualified for the specific procedure [18]. Licensed nurses are also an essential component throughout the entire process, from preprocedural phase until the patient has safely recovered. The ASA states that it is also important to consider the housekeeping and maintenance staff. These staff members provide a sterile and consistently safe environment as multiple patients utilize the same facilities [18]. Importantly, all staff present should be prepared to efficiently handle emergent situations. The ASA states that the most common causes of morbidity associated with sedation/analgesia are drug-induced respiratory depression and airway obstruction. In the event a patient's condition deteriorates, the patient will need to be rapidly transferred to an acute care facility. Any delay of this transfer could be detrimental to the patient's functional status [18]. Therefore, personnel should be qualified and adequately prepared to rescue a patient from any level of sedation [27].

The ASA has issued detailed recommendations as to the personnel responsible for delivering anesthesia, which requires an understanding that sedation and general anesthesia exist on a continuum. In the ambulatory setting, taking additional precautionary steps when delivering any type of sedation is imperative. Both the ASA and the Joint Commission have defined each level of sedation and the type of practitioner that is able to safely administer the various levels of sedation. The ASA believes that in all deep sedation cases, it is safest for the sedative to only be administered by the physician anesthesiologist [28]. Deep sedation achieves a state of awareness just below the level of general anesthesia, a state in which the patient is no longer aroused to repeated or painful stimulation [28]. Deep sedation incurs significant risk of the patient deepening to a general anesthetic state. If the practitioner is not equipped to quickly recognize and recover the patient from this state, the patient could experience adverse events such as cardiopulmonary decline or aberrant procedural complications.

Although the physician anesthesiologist is preferred in most cases of deep sedation, non-anesthesiologist physicians play an important role in the delineation of sedation services. The Centers for Medicare & Medicaid Services (CMS) has defined non-anesthesiologist physicians as providers such as licensed physicians, dentists, oral surgeons, or podiatrists who are qualified to administer anesthesia under state law but who have not completed postgraduate training in anesthesiology. These providers must be able to recognize when a patient has advanced from deep sedation to general anesthesia and maintain appropriate hemodynamic and respiratory function of the patient until they return to the intended level of sedation [28].

Non-anesthesiologist physicians may safely provide mild and moderate sedation but must still be qualified for the intended procedure. They must be able to recognize states of deeper/unintended levels of sedation and rescue the patient from these states. It is also advised to have a dedicated staff member who is responsible for monitoring the patient's vitals for the duration of the procedure [27]. It is prudent to ensure that staff members can assist in patient resuscitation, if needed, and all staff should ideally obtain training in Basic Life Support (BLS) or Advanced Cardiac Life Support (ACLS).

All staff and personnel must continually update their qualifications and certifications to provide anesthesia. All staff should be prepared for every possible outcome, as patients may exhibit significant variability in response to sedation. Always anticipate emergency situations by constantly monitoring the patient and be able to contact emergency services rapidly. Following these major guidelines for all personnel involved in the patient's care will provide a safe environment for any type of sedation-requiring procedure.

Patient Evaluation

All patients receiving anesthesia care should undergo a preprocedural evaluation. Assessing the patient's history and physical status prior to delivering sedation allows the provider to develop an anesthetic plan specific to the patient's physical status and comorbidities. In accordance with ASA guidelines for ambulatory anesthesia and surgery, evaluation and administration of anesthesia or sedation may be performed by anesthesiologists and by "other qualified physicians or nonphysician anesthesia personnel medically directed by an anesthesiologist" [18]. Non-anesthesiologist physicians serving this role must be deemed qualified after completing appropriate training and licensure and credentialing by the facility [18]. The provider administering sedation should, at a minimum, review the patient's available medical record and inquire as to the patient's medical history and prior anesthetic experiences [21]. Such investigations are geared toward revealing any comorbidities, prior adverse experiences with anesthesia or sedation, or history of difficult airway that may affect the anesthetic plan [29]. It is also important to obtain an updated list of current medications at the time of interview to assess for potential drug interactions [29]. Allergies to medications should be ascertained to prevent the administration of any drugs that may elicit an adverse reaction [29]. The patient's social history, including tobacco, alcohol, and illicit substance use, should also be discussed at this time [29].

A focused physical examination, including vital signs, heart and lung auscultation, and airway evaluation, should be performed [29]. Further components of the physical exam should be dictated by the patient's comorbid conditions [29]. Any available laboratory tests should be reviewed; should the provider have specific concerns based on the patient's physical condition or comorbidities, testing should be ordered in advance and reviewed prior to the delivery of sedation [21]. Similarly, any consultations that may be deemed necessary may be requested and completed, presuming the patient is being evaluated well in advance of the procedure date [21]. Preoperative medications may be ordered by the provider and administered at this time [21]. The patient interview and evaluation conclude with the provider developing a plan for sedation, discussing this plan with the patient, and then gaining the patient's approval and consent to deliver care; this discussion should be documented in the medical record [18]. Patients should also be evaluated for aspiration risk and NPO status prior to the administration of sedation. A minimum fasting period of 2 hours prior to a procedure for clear liquids, 4 hours for light meals, and 8 hours for all other meals is the current consensus [14].

Consent should be obtained prior to administration of sedation for the pain procedure. During the consent process, patients should be made aware that they may feel portions of the procedures, such as local anesthesia injection. This level of awareness is required by local, regional, and national standards to prevent injections into the wrong areas. In addition, patients should be informed that more invasive techniques may be required to proceed with a procedure if sedation fails. Rare occurrences, such as acute reactions to medications like anaphylactic reactions, may lead to loss of the airway, cardiovascular collapse, and possibly death. The risks and benefits of all types of anesthetic care should be explained and questions answered to ensure that the patient clearly understands the plan of action. It is recommended that procedures will not be performed if a responsible adult is not available to accompany the patient home after the procedure.

Monitoring

Depth of anesthesia is often referred to as existing on a continuum from minimal sedation to general anesthesia; it is imperative for the practitioner to understand not only the differences between the varying depths of anesthesia but also the anticipated physiologic changes inherent to each. Under minimal or moderate sedation, a patient's cardiovascular function and ability to maintain adequate spontaneous ventilation with a patent airway are often maintained [30]. However, deep sedation is characterized by a patient that is difficult to arouse and potentially unable to maintain ventilatory function independently; as such, intervention may be required to prevent hypoventilation [30]. General anesthesia describes the deepest level of sedation, in which patients are often unable to maintain ventilatory function, lack a patent airway, and experience depressed spontaneous ventilation, in addition to potentially impaired cardiovascular function [30]. Those delivering sedation must be qualified and prepared to manage one level of sedation deeper than that which is intended for the patient [31].

While the ASA's policy documents the need for an anesthesiologist to administer all anesthetics, it also explains that it does not oppose licensed nonphysician anesthesia providers as long as they are medically supervised by a licensed physician [32]. In regard to Anesthetic Care During Interventional Pain Procedures for Adults, the ASA recognizes the provision of sedation or anesthesia as a separate service form the pain procedure and requires specific credentialing [5]. It is important to note that there is a distinction between anesthesia services and moderate (conscious) sedation which each require specific training. According to the Continuum of Depth and Sedation: Definition of General Anesthesia and Levels of Sedation/Analgesia, "Moderate Sedation/Analgesia ("Conscious Sedation") is a drug-induced depression of consciousness during which patients respond purposefully to verbal commands, either accompanied by light tactile stimulation or alone. No interventions are required to maintain a patent airway, and spontaneous ventilation is adequate. Cardiovascular function is usually maintained" [30]. This is in contrast to monitored anesthesia care, which is defined by the ASA to include all aspects of anesthesia care – a preprocedural assessment and optimization, intraprocedural care, and postprocedural management that is inherently provided by a qualified anesthesia provider as part of the bundled specific service [33]. Both moderate sedation and MAC require credentialing to perform and to supervise their administration by nonphysician anesthesia providers.

A leading cause of morbidity with sedation is drug-induced respiratory depression. With appropriate monitoring of the patient and an understanding of the anticipated consequences of each level of sedation, providers can deliver sedation in an effective and safe manner. ASA standards for any patient receiving sedation require monitoring of blood pressure, cardiac rate and rhythm with ECG, pulse oximetry, quantitative end tidal CO2 monitoring, and possibly temperature [14]. As sedation is accompanied by the risk of significant respiratory depression, which carries with it significant morbidity, it is important to detect inadequate ventilation early [34]; *this makes end tidal CO2 monitoring of particular importance*, as it allows for prompt delivery of additional airway support in the setting of hypoventilation [14]. In addition to the abovementioned physiologic monitoring, clinicians may choose to monitor a patient's level of sedation. Assessing depth of sedation allows the provider to balance prevention of awareness and excessive depth of anesthetic [35]. Various methods exist for such monitoring, including but not limited to the bispectral index (BIS), entropy of the electroencephalographic (EEG) signal, Narcotrend, and patient state index (PSI) [36]. Additional tools to grade sedation are the Ramsay Sedation Scale (RSS) and Richmond Agitation-Sedation Scale (RASS) [27]. RSS is scaled 1 (anxious and agitated) to 6 (nonresponsive), while RASS is from +4 (combative) to −5 (unarousable). A patient's comfort level can also be assessed by the visual analog scale (VAS).

Any patient receiving sedation, including monitored anesthesia care, regional anesthesia, or general anesthesia, should also receive postanesthesia care management [23]. As patients recover from sedation, they should be observed with monitoring of oxygenation, circulation, ventilation, temperature, and level of consciousness [23].

Drugs

Clinicians can use a variety of sedatives, opioids, and dissociative agents while performing interventional pain procedures. Listed below are the main categories and most commonly used sedatives for pain procedures. Appropriate dose titration is dependent upon the sedation needs for a procedure and the patients' age, comorbidities, and active medications. Immediate access to airway equipment is necessary when using these medications. In addition, intravenous access is required for administration of these medications. Intravenous access should be maintained throughout the periprocedural period until the patient is awake, alert, and hemodynamically stable.

Benzodiazepines (Table 21.1) selectively act upon gamma-aminobutyric acid (GABA) recep-

Table 21.1 Benzodiazepines [37, 38]

Drug name (brand name)	Mode of administration	Doses	Pharmacokinetics
Midazolam (Versed)	Intravenous, oral	0.5–1 mg repeated	Onset: 1–2.5 min Peak: 3–5 min Duration: 1–5 h Elimination: 1.7–3.5 h
Diazepam (Valium)	Intravenous, oral	2 mg repeated (up to max dose of 20 mg IV)	Onset: 1–2 min Peak: 8 min Elimination: 20–50 h
Lorazepam (Ativan)	Intravenous, oral	0.25 mg repeated	Onset: 15–20 min Peak: 60–90 min Elimination: 11–22 h

tors (specifically $GABA_A$ receptors), augmenting fast inhibitory synaptic transmission in the central nervous system. This action produces a hypnotic, sedative, anxiolytic, amnesic, and centrally produced muscle-relaxing effect [37]. These drugs have a dose-dependent continuum of effect from mild to deep sedation [38]. Benzodiazepines can cause cardiac and respiratory depression, along with a blunted response to hypercarbia [37]. Midazolam is the most commonly used benzodiazepines, mainly due to its fast onset, short duration, and high amnesic properties. Other commonly used benzodiazepines include diazepam and lorazepam.

Opioids (Table 21.2) act upon μ-opioid receptors to produce an analgesic effect and sedation. Commonly used opioids for pain control during interventional pain procedures include fentanyl and alfentanil. These drugs have high lipid solubility, as seen in their rapid onset of action and short duration of action [27]. Compared to fentanyl, alfentanil is one-fifth as potent with one-third the duration of action, making it valuable for office-based procedures [27]. Longer-acting opioids, such as morphine and hydromorphone, can also be utilized. These drugs produce respiratory depression in a dose-dependent manner and decrease the hypoxic and hypercarbic respiratory drive. These effects are synergistic with benzodiazepines.

Other side effects include constipation, bradycardia, nausea, and vomiting. Rapid administration of these drugs has been noted to cause chest wall rigidity, which can lead to difficulty ventilating.

Other commonly used intravenous anesthetics include propofol, ketamine, and dexmedetomidine. Propofol, an induction agent for general anesthesia, can provide sedation at lower doses. It typically has a short duration of action, has fast recovery times, and exhibits antiemetic properties as well; however, propofol oftentimes exhibits significant variability in patient response due to its potency and side effect profile and has no known antidote. As most interventional pain procedures are performed in the prone position, episodes of respiratory depression and resultant hypoxia are rendered all the more difficult to remedy. Secondary to its potency and side effect profile, propofol is recommended for use only for the most stimulating interventional pain procedures wherein providers do not require patient feedback or participation. Related to its potential to decrease arterial blood pressure and cause apnea, the current recommendations of the ASA mandate that it can only be provided by clinicians trained in the administration of general anesthesia, emergency resuscitation, and airway management [24].

Ketamine, a phencyclidine, antagonizes the NMDA receptor and provides dissociative anesthesia, rendering the patient unable to process sensory information [37]. It also acts as an analgesic and can be used for hyperalgesia and opiate tolerance [37]. Differing from other anesthetic agents, ketamine causes an increase in blood pressure and heart rate. The respiratory system is minimally affected, aside from the drug acting as a bronchodilator, which can be useful in asthmatics. Psychotropic effects are common with the use of ketamine, including illusions and delirium, and patients should be educated about these potential side effects.

Dexmedetomidine, a selective alpha-2 agonist, has sedative and analgesic properties. This

Table 21.2 Opioids [38, 39]

Drug name (brand name)	Mode of administration	Doses	Pharmacokinetics
Fentanyl (Sublimaze)	Intravenous	25–100 μg as initial dose with repeated boluses of 25–50 μg per patient response	Onset: 3–5 min Duration: 3 h
Alfentanil (Alfenta)	Intravenous	25–50 μg/kg initial bolus with 5–10 μg/kg intermittent boluses or 0.5–2.0 μg/kg/min infusion	Onset: 1–2 min Duration: 10 min
Morphine (Duramorph)	Intravenous	1–2 mg boluses as needed	Onset:20 min Duration: 4–5 h
Hydromorphone (Dilaudid)	Intravenous	0.25–0.5 mg boluses as needed	Onset: 10–20 min Duration: 4–5 h

drug does not produce significant respiratory depression but can cause bradycardia, hypotension, and nausea [40]. Therefore, the practitioner should exercise caution when using this drug on patients with cardiac comorbidities requiring beta-blockade or vasodilation.

The use of these medications can lead to cardiorespiratory complications and oversedation. Knowledge of reversal agents and their indications are required to safely perform procedures and provide sedation. Flumazenil is a competitive benzodiazepine receptor antagonist. It is given in 0.2 mg intravenous doses (maximum dose 1 mg) until adequate response is achieved [38]. It is important to note that, due to its antagonism, patients who are dependent upon benzodiazepines may experience seizures if given the drug [38]. Flumazenil's duration of action is shorter than most benzodiazepines (plasma half-life of 1 hour), and as a result of this rapid clearance, patients may become resedated. This is less likely to occur with midazolam, due to its short half-life [37]. Its side effects include anxiety, nausea, and vomiting.

Naloxone is an opioid antagonist that competes for mainly μ-receptors without causing an opioid effect. It can restore spontaneous ventilation after opioid overdose and reverse other opioid-induced symptoms, such as urinary retention, nausea, vomiting, and pruritus [39]. It is given in 0.08 mg–0.2 mg intravenous doses every 2–3 minutes until adequate patient response and ventilation [38]. With this reversal, the analgesia provided by the opioids is lost, leading to perception of pain and increased sympathetic stimulation. Also, as with flumazenil, naloxone is more rapidly cleared than some opioids (duration of action: 45 minutes), resulting in the reappearance of narcosis. Acute opioid withdrawal symptoms have been noted in patients with opioid dependency.

Along with reversal agents, medications for abrupt loss of consciousness, seizure, allergic reaction, and adverse procedural outcomes should be readily available for emergent use. These emergency rescue drugs include epinephrine, diphenhydramine, and dexamethasone.

Procedures

A variety of procedures are available for chronic pain patients, given their pathophysiology (Table 21.3) [27]. Pain procedures usually consist of a local anesthetic that can provide quick pain relief and a corticosteroid to reduce inflammation. The type and volume of injected medication will vary based on the type of pain procedure being performed. The analgesic effect of a local anesthetic is usually immediate, with the majority of patients experiencing partial or complete pain relief within minutes. The expected duration from the local anesthetic alone will vary based on the type of medication administered, but typi-

Table 21.3 List of common pain procedures [27]

Procedure
Short duration (15–30 minutes)
Diagnostic blocks and infusions
Trigger-point/myofascial injections
Cryoablation injection
Facet joint injections
Epidural steroid injections, including cervical, thoracic, and lumbar
Transforaminal nerve root injections
Caudal injections
SIJ injections
Hip injections
RF thermocoagulation (RFTC)
Pulsed electromagnet field injections (PEMF)
Knee injections
Sympathetic/ganglion blocks, including sphenopalatine ganglion, stellate ganglion, dorsal root ganglion, splanchnic nerve, celiac plexus block, thoracic and lumbar sympathetic, hypogastric plexus, and ganglion impar
Intercostal nerve blocks
Suprascapular nerve blocks
Long duration (30–60 minutes)
Discograms: cervical, thoracic, lumbar
Epidurolysis/epiduroscopy
Augmentation techniques, including SCS (dorsal column stimulation testing and permanent implantation) of the occipital nerve and cervical, thoracic, lumbar, or sacral spinal cord
Intrathecal implantation
Neurolytic and neurolysis blocks, including ethyl alcohol, phenol, hypotonic, hypertonic, and glycerol injections
Decompressive neuroplasty (Racz procedure)
Vertebroplasty

Table 21.4 Intravenous anesthetics [37]

Drug name (brand name)	Mode of administration	Doses	Pharmacokinetics
Propofol (Diprivan)	Intravenous	0.5–1 mg/kg initial bolus with repeated boluses of 0.25–0.5 mg/kg until appropriate level of sedation reached, maintenance sedation with 25–75 μg/kg/min	Onset: 40 sec Duration: 6 min
Ketamine (Ketalar)	Intravenous, intramuscular	IV: 1–2 mg/kg initial bolus with repeated boluses of 0.25–1 mg/kg until appropriate level of sedation reached IM: 4–5 mg/kg single dose	Onset: 30 sec (IV), 3–4 min (IM) Duration: 5–10 min (IV), 12–25 min (IV)
Dexmedetomidine (Precedex)	Intravenous	0.2–1 μg/kg/hr	Onset: 5–10 min Duration: 60–120 min

cally does not persist beyond 1–2 days. As the effects from the local anesthetic diminish, the anti-inflammatory action of an added corticosteroid will take effect (10–14 days may be needed for full effect) and provide patients with 3–6 months of sustained relief [41].

Clinicians should have a good understanding of these procedures to safely and confidently administer sedation. A time-out is necessary prior to the start of any interventional pain procedure, ensuring that the correct procedure on the correct side is being performed. Many of the interventions listed in Table 21.4 can be performed effectively under moderate sedation. To ensure a successful procedure, appropriate monitoring, careful titration of drugs, and effective communication between the providers are essential. Personnel should document vital signs throughout the periprocedural period and develop skills for early recognition in oversedation. Important anesthetic considerations include availability of supplemental oxygen, tools for intravenous access and airway equipment, and emergency personnel.

Patient Recovery

After the pain procedure is completed, the patient is then placed in supine position in a recovery area for roughly 15 minutes and monitored for any side effects of motor or sensory deficits. Supplemental oxygen and monitors may be needed for transport if traveling a long distance to the recovery area. Patients should be assessed in the recovery area, noting their vital signs, level of sedation, and pain score. Patients may continue to be at risk for developing complications in recovery and should be continuously observed in an appropriately staffed and equipped area until they are near their baseline level of consciousness and no longer at risk for hypoxemia and cardiorespiratory depression. Prior to discharge, the patient should have returned to baseline mental status and stable vital signs. A responsible adult must be with the patient when he or she is discharged, and the patient should have discharge instructions provided, specifying appropriate diet, medications, acceptable activities, and contact information in case of emergency.

Reported complications from these procedures are typically minor and relatively infrequent, consisting mostly of facial flushing, increased transient pain or numbness, and vasovagal reactions that occur immediately after treatment but tend to rapidly resolve with minimal supportive care [42]. Patient discharge from the facility should be delayed until symptoms have resolved and the patient is able to ambulate without any difficulty.

Patients may return to a regular diet as tolerated. However, diabetic patients must pay close attention to their blood sugar levels checking it frequently. Epidural steroid injections were noted to cause a significant increase in the blood glucose levels in diabetics but should not last longer than 2 days [43].

More grave but rare complications can occur. Dural puncture and unintentional misadministration of medication into the thecal space may result in spinal anesthesia, which can lead to hypotension, motor blockade, and bowel and bladder incontinence [41]. Fortunately, these symptoms also tend to be temporary and usually only require observation with minimal supportive care. However, persistent or worsening symptoms, development of chest pain, shortness of breath, fever, difficulty walking, changes in mental status, or severe headache may indicate need for emergent evaluation.

Special Considerations

When providing sedation, it is important to recognize certain types of patients who are at an increased risk for developing complications. Patients with underlying medical conditions, such as severe cardiac, pulmonary, hepatic, or renal disease, should be seen by an appropriate medical specialist (cardiologist, pulmonologist, etc.) to mitigate the risks associated with moderate and deep sedation. Anesthesiologists should be consulted for patients with significant sedation-related risk factors, such as morbid obesity, potentially difficult airway, and sleep apnea, and may be asked to be immediately available should problems arise.

Regarding interventional pain procedures, three major potential complications should be acknowledged by the interventional pain practitioner. First, if the patient is under deep or general anesthesia, a patient cannot express sudden paresthesias, dysesthetic pain, or any other aberrant sensations to the interventional pain practitioner if a needle is inserted into an incorrect location (e.g., the spinal cord). The practitioner needs this feedback information from the patient to safely perform the procedure and reduce potential for severe and permanent complications. For example, if a needle is inserted into the spinal cord inappropriately, intramedullary deposition of as little as 0.5–1 mL of injectate will most likely result in neurologic deficit due to syrinx formation and disruption of neuronal pathways [11, 44].

Second, the prone position, which is utilized for most interventional pain procedures, can increase risk and complicate life-saving measures when adverse events do occur. The prone position during surgery is typically reserved for posterior spinal procedures, craniotomies, rectal and buttock procedures, and procedures on the posterior extremities [45]. Most patients are anesthetized on a stretcher while supine and then rolled into the prone position onto the operating table after intubation. Prone positioning can have some variable effects on cardiovascular physiology. Most commonly, during prone positioning, there can be a reduction in the cardiac index, due to a decrease in venous return back to the heart. Abdominal compression from the prone position increases intrathoracic pressure and reduces left ventricular compliance [45]. This can also lead to vena caval compression and reduction in venous return with resultant hypotension, venous stasis, and increased pressure in the epidural venous plexus. It was found that prone position did not significantly affect the respiratory system compliance or the lung and chest wall compliance. Respiratory resistance slightly increased in the prone position, mainly due to the chest wall resistance, but both functional residual capacity (FRC) and PaO2 increased from the supine to the prone position, whereas PaCO2 was unchanged [46]. Due to the prone positioning, if cardiovascular and/or respiratory failure occurs, resuscitation measures are more difficult, even with proper personnel, equipment, and monitors.

Third, sedation is a continuum, from mild sedation to general anesthesia, and can result in hypoventilation, pulmonary compromise, anoxic brain states, and/or death if not carefully monitored. In the setting of sedation and anesthesia, hypoxia from hypoventilation is the most likely cause of hypoxemia which is indicated by a low PaO_2 and an elevated $PaCO_2$. Hypoventilation can result from not only respiratory depression but also airway obstruction. Benzodiazepines and opioids used in moderate sedation typically produce mild degrees of respiratory depression. Far more significant in the development of hypoventilation is when a relaxed patient develops an anatomical airway obstruction from soft tissues like tongue, tonsils, or adenoids [47].

Prompt detection of hypoventilation using pulse oximetry is generally less reliable when patients are provided supplemental oxygen, as the higher inspired oxygen concentration will allow arterial oxygenation to remain adequate for considerably longer despite progressive hypoventilation. Patients breathing room air instead of supplemental oxygen will desaturate faster as they begin to hypoventilate [34]. For this reason, it is recommended to utilize a continuous capnographic waveform to assess the patient's respiratory status during the procedure. Deep sedation should be avoided to allow feedback of new occurrences of pain or paresthesia and to allow patient cooperation with positioning during the procedure [48]. Of note, oversedation in the immediate pre- or post-anesthesia period can result in severe hypoventilation, atelectasis, or worsening hypoxemia and hypercapnia in spontaneously breathing COPD patients [49].

Summary

Sedation for interventional pain procedures requires careful planning and decision-making and can be challenging yet rewarding. Proper location of procedure, facility equipment, and staff are also required to meet minimum standards of care outlined by the ASA [32]. Sedation must be provided by either qualified anesthesia or non-anesthesia providers, with appropriate understanding of the medications, drug interactions, and resuscitative protocols [50]. Along with the monitoring standards established by the ASA, including temperature, blood pressure, EKG, pulse oximetry, and quantitative end tidal CO2, other factors the anesthesiologist must consider to ensure patient safety include perioperative medications and fasting. For safe and successful sedation, defined standards of experience and proficiency of the providers are essential. Failure to meet these guidelines needlessly incurs heightened risk of significant morbidity and mortality for chronic pain patients undergoing sedation.

References

1. Manchikanti L, Soin A, Mann DP, Bakshi S, Pampati V, Hirsch JA. Reversal of growth of utilization of interventional techniques in managing chronic pain in medicare population post affordable care act. rn [Internet]. 2017;20(7):551–67. Available from: http://www.ncbi.nlm.nih.gov/pubmed/29149139.
2. Manchikanti L, Soin A, Mann DP, Bakshi S, Pampati V, Hirsch JA. Comparative analysis of utilization of epidural procedures in managing chronic pain in the medicare population: pre and post affordable care Act. Spine (Phila Pa 1976) [Internet]. 2019;44(3):220–32. Available from: http://www.ncbi.nlm.nih.gov/pubmed/30005043.
3. Hirsch JA, Chandra RV, Pampati V, Barr JD, Brook AL, Manchikanti L. Analysis of vertebral augmentation practice patterns: a 2016 update. J Neurointerv Surg [Internet]. 2016;8(12):1299–304. Available from: http://www.ncbi.nlm.nih.gov/pubmed/27799375.
4. Lad SP, Babu R, Bagley JH, Choi J, Bagley CA, Huh BK, et al. Utilization of spinal cord stimulation in patients with failed back surgery syndrome. Spine (Phila Pa 1976) [Internet]. 2014;39(12):E719–27. Available from: http://www.ncbi.nlm.nih.gov/pubmed/24718057.
5. Statement on Anesthetic Care During Interventional Pain Procedures for Adults | American Society of Anesthesiologists (ASA).
6. Rathmell JP, Michna E, Fitzgibbon DR, Stephens LS, Posner KL, Domino KB. Injury and liability associated with cervical procedures for chronic pain. Anesthesiology [Internet]. 2011 Apr;114(4):918–26. Available from: http://www.ncbi.nlm.nih.gov/pubmed/21386702.
7. Bhananker SM, Posner KL, Cheney FW, Caplan RA, Lee LA, Domino KB. Injury and liability associated with monitored anesthesia care: a closed claims analysis. Anesthesiology [Internet]. 2006;104(2):228–34. Available from: http://www.ncbi.nlm.nih.gov/pubmed/16436839.
8. Heran MKS, Smith AD, Legiehn GM. Spinal injection procedures: a review of concepts, controversies, and complications. Radiol Clin North Am [Internet]. 2008;46(3):487–514, v–vi. Available from: http://www.ncbi.nlm.nih.gov/pubmed/18707959.
9. Bartynski WS, Grahovac SZ, Rothfus WE. Incorrect needle position during lumbar epidural steroid administration: inaccuracy of loss of air pressure resistance and requirement of fluoroscopy and epidurography during needle insertion. AJNR Am J Neuroradiol [Internet]. 2005;26(3):502–5. Available from: http://www.ncbi.nlm.nih.gov/pubmed/15760856.
10. Cucuzzella TR, Delport EG, Kim N, Marley J, Pruitt C, Delport AG. A survey: conscious sedation with epidural and zygapophyseal injections: is it necessary? Spine J [Internet]. 6(4):364–9. Available from: http://www.ncbi.nlm.nih.gov/pubmed/16825040.
11. Epstein NE. Neurological complications of lumbar and cervical dural punctures with a focus on epidural injections. Surg Neurol Int [Internet]. 2017;8:60. Available from: http://www.ncbi.nlm.nih.gov/pubmed/28540126.
12. Elder BD, Goodwin CR, Abu-Bonsrah N, Sciubba DM. Intramedullary steroid injection of the cervical spine with incidental vertebral artery dissection. Spine J [Internet]. 2016;16(11):e725–6. Available from: http://www.ncbi.nlm.nih.gov/pubmed/27012650.

13. Lee J-H, Lee J-K, Seo B-R, Moon S-J, Kim J-H, Kim S-H. Spinal cord injury produced by direct damage during cervical transforaminal epidural injection. Reg Anesth Pain Med [Internet]. 33(4):377–9. Available from: http://www.ncbi.nlm.nih.gov/pubmed/18675752.
14. Kaye AD, Jones MR, Viswanath O, Candido KD, Boswell M V, Soin A, et al. ASIPP guidelines for sedation and fasting status of patients undergoing interventional pain management procedures. Pain Physician [Internet]. 2019;22(3):201–7. Available from: http://www.ncbi.nlm.nih.gov/pubmed/31151329.
15. The National Uniform Claims Committee. Specialty Designation for Interventional Pain Management- 09.
16. Medicare Payment Advisory Commission. 2001. Report to the Congress: Paying for interventional pain services in ambulatory settings 2001.
17. Manchikanti L, Abdi S, Atluri S, Benyamin RM, Boswell M V, Buenaventura RM, et al. An update of comprehensive evidence-based guidelines for interventional techniques in chronic spinal pain. Part II: guidance and recommendations. Pain Physician [Internet]. 2013;16(2 Suppl):S49–283. Available from: http://www.ncbi.nlm.nih.gov/pubmed/23615883.
18. Guidelines for Ambulatory Anesthesia and Surgery | American Society of Anesthesiologists (ASA).
19. American Society of Anesthesiologists (ASA). Statement on Nonoperating Room Anesthetizing Locations. Park Ridge, IL;
20. The Joint Commission. Accreditation Handbook for Office-Based Surgery: What You Need to Know About Obtaining Accreditation. [Internet]. [cited 2020 Mar 31]. Available from: www.jointcommission.org/assets/1/18/2011_OBS_Hdbk.pdf
21. Basic Standards for PreAnesthesia Care | American Society of Anesthesiologists (ASA).
22. Standards for Basic Anesthetic Monitoring | American Society of Anesthesiologists (ASA).
23. Standards for Postanesthesia Care | American Society of Anesthesiologists (ASA).
24. Guidelines for Office-Based Anesthesia | American Society of Anesthesiologists (ASA).
25. Ambulatory Health Care: 2020 National Patient Safety Goals | The Joint Commission.
26. Safety and Health Topics | Healthcare - Standards and Enforcement | Occupational Safety and Health Administration.
27. Kaye ADML. Interventional pain management procedures. In: Urman RDKA, editor. Moderate and deep sedation in clinical practice. 2nd ed. Cambridge: Cambridge University Press; 2017. p. 321–9.
28. (ASA). 1. American Society of Anesthesiologists. Advisory on Granting Privileges for Deep Sedation to Non-Anesthesiologist Physicians. Park Ridge, IL; 2010.
29. Practice Guidelines for Moderate Procedural Sedation and Analgesia 2018: A Report by the American Society of Anesthesiologists Task Force on Moderate Procedural Sedation and Analgesia, the American Association of Oral and Maxillofacial Surgeons, American. Anesthesiology [Internet]. 2018;128(3):437–79. Available from: http://www.ncbi.nlm.nih.gov/pubmed/29334501
30. Continuum of Depth of Sedation: Definition of General Anesthesia and Levels of Sedation/Analgesia | American Society of Anesthesiologists (ASA).
31. Waugh JB, Epps CA, Khodneva YA. Capnography enhances surveillance of respiratory events during procedural sedation: a meta-analysis. J Clin Anesth [Internet]. 2011;23(3):189–96. Available from: http://www.ncbi.nlm.nih.gov/pubmed/21497076.
32. Statement on Qualifications of Anesthesia Providers in the Office-Based Setting | American Society of Anesthesiologists (ASA).
33. Position on Monitored Anesthesia Care | American Society of Anesthesiologists (ASA).
34. Fu ES, Downs JB, Schweiger JW, Miguel RV, Smith RA. Supplement oxygen impairs detection of hypoventilation by pulse oximetry. Chest. 2004;
35. Das S, Ghosh S. Monitored anesthesia care: an overview. J Anaesthesiol Clin Pharmacol [Internet]. 31(1):27–9. Available from: http://www.ncbi.nlm.nih.gov/pubmed/25788769.
36. American Society of Anesthesiologists Task Force on Intraoperative Awareness. Practice advisory for intraoperative awareness and brain function monitoring: a report by the american society of anesthesiologists task force on intraoperative awareness. Anesthesiology [Internet]. 2006;104(4):847–64. Available from: http://www.ncbi.nlm.nih.gov/pubmed/16571982.
37. Vuyk J, Sitsen E, MR. Intravenous anesthetics. In: Gropper MA, Cohen NH, Eriksson LI, Fleisher LA, JPW-K KL, editors. Miller's anesthesia. 9th ed. Philadelphia, PA: Elsevier; 2020. p. 638–79.
38. Arjun Reddy KM. Sedation in the endoscopy suite. In: Urman RDKA, editor. Moderate and deep sedation in clinical practice. 2nd ed. Cambridge: Cambridge University Press; 2017. p. 206–20.
39. Mark Shumacher KF. In: Gropper MA, Cohen NH, Eriksson LI, Fleisher LA, JPW-K KL, editors. Opioids, Miller's anesthesia. 9th ed: Cambridge; 2020. p. 680–741.
40. Belleville JP, Ward DS, Bloor BC, Maze M. Effects of intravenous dexmedetomidine in humans. I. Sedation, ventilation, and metabolic rate. Anesthesiology [Internet]. 1992;77(6):1125–33. Available from: http://www.ncbi.nlm.nih.gov/pubmed/1361310.
41. Iannuccilli JD, Prince EA, Soares GM. Interventional spine procedures for management of chronic low back pain-A primer. Semin Intervent Radiol. 2013;
42. Post-Procedure Instructions | Pain Management | Dr. Dhanani.
43. Even JL, Crosby CG, Song Y, McGirt MJ, Devin CJ. Effects of epidural steroid injections on blood glucose levels in patients with diabetes mellitus. Spine (Phila Pa 1976). 2012;
44. Singh R, Panagos A. Quadriparesis following cervical epidural steroid injections. Spine J [Internet]. 6(3):349. Available from: http://www.ncbi.nlm.nih.gov/pubmed/16651233.

45. Courington FW, Little DM. The role of posture in anesthesia. Clin Anesth 1968.
46. Pelosi P, Croci M, Calappi E, Cerisara M, Mulazzi D, Vicardi P, et al. The prone positioning during general anesthesia minimally affects respiratory mechanics while improving functional residual capacity and increasing oxygen tension. Anesth Analg. 1995;
47. Edrich T, Sadovnikoff N. Anesthesia for patients with severe chronic obstructive pulmonary disease. Curr Opin Anaesthesiol 2010.
48. Visser WA, Lee RA, Gielen MJM. Factors affecting the distribution of neural blockade by local anesthetics in epidural anesthesia and a comparison of lumbar versus thoracic epidural anesthesia. Anesthesia and Analgesia. 2008.
49. Lumb AB, Nunn JF. Respiratory function and ribcage contribution to ventilation in body positions commonly used during anesthesia. Anesth Analg. 1991;
50. Practice Guidelines for Sedation and Analgesia by Non-Anesthesiologists | Anesthesiology | ASA Publications.

18 Sedation and Analgesic Considerations for Gastrointestinal Procedures

Mitchell C. Fuller, Kyleigh Harrison, Erin Tullis, Mark R. Jones, Elyse M. Cornett, and Alan David Kaye

Abstract

Gastrointestinal (GI) procedures are performed in various settings and are important for prevention and treatment of various disease states. For many years, these procedures were commonly performed with a combination of opioids and benzodiazepines. However, in recent years, there has been a significant shift to propofol, allowing for both moderate and deep sedation. Propofol has been popular with patients and has sedative effects with no known antidote. Baseline vital signs, physical examination, and past medical history are always required for any patient who is to receive anesthesia. Further, sedation involving propofol requires airway expertise, since its delivery can result in hypoxia and respiratory depression. Of note, standard monitoring nationwide requires temperature, blood pressure, electrocardiogram, pulse oximetry, and quantitative continuous end tidal CO_2 monitoring. Given that many GI procedures are performed in the lateral and prone positions, it is essential for safety to utilize all five standards monitors to provide safe anesthesia for these patients. While midazolam and fentanyl remain popular for many patients needing moderate sedation, a deeper level of sedation is most typically achieved with propofol related to increased patient satisfaction and ideal pharmacokinetics. New anesthetic agents such as the alpha-2 agonist dexmedetomidine are being evaluated to aid GI sedation. To reduce potential adverse events during GI procedural anesthesia, anesthesiology services are recommended for most patients and particularly in high-risk populations requiring deep sedation. In summary, the strongest emphasis should be placed on utilization of ASA standard monitors for all patients undergoing GI procedures. Continuous quantitative end tidal CO_2 monitoring must be employed for safe delivery of sedation for any GI procedure.

M. C. Fuller · K. Harrison · E. Tullis
Medical College of Wisconsin, Wauwatosa, WI, USA
e-mail: mfuller@mcw.edu; khar12@lsuhsc.edu; etulli@lsuhsc.edu

M. R. Jones
Beth Israel Deaconess Medical Center, Harvard Medical School, Department of Anesthesia, Critical Care, and Pain Medicine, Boston, MA, USA

Weill Cornell Medical College, Department of Anesthesia, New York, NY, USA

E. M. Cornett
Department of Anesthesiology, Louisiana State University Health Shreveport, Shreveport, LA, USA
e-mail: ecorne@lsuhsc.edu

A. D. Kaye (✉)
Departments of Anesthesiology and Pharmacology, Toxicology, and Neurosciences, Louisiana State University Health Shreveport, Shreveport, LA, USA
e-mail: akaye@lsuhsc.edu

K. Rajput et al. (eds.), *Pain Control in Ambulatory Surgery Centers*,
https://doi.org/10.1007/978-3-030-55262-6_18

Introduction

Among all medical procedures performed across the globe, gastrointestinal endoscopies comprise the single largest group with over 51 million being performed in the United States in 2017 [1]. The goal of procedural sedation and anesthesia (PSA) is to reduce the patients' consciousness and pain recognition while retaining their continuous independent ventilation and protective reflexes [2]. The role of PSA in GI procedures is growing as sedation outside the operating room, in GI suites, without anesthesiologist assistance is becoming commonplace. A comparison of GI procedures in the United States between 2003 and 2009 found sedation outside the operating theatre without anesthesiologist assistance rose from 13.5% to 30.2% [2]. As the administration and management of GI PSA expands in scope and setting, a standardized multi-disciplinary guideline is lacking; nearly all current published guidelines are written by gastroenterologists without anesthesia provider input. The UK has a stronger set of guidelines, where more than 2.5 million cases are performed under either benzodiazepines or opioids for less invasive procedures and propofol most commonly for deeper sedation needs [3]. To bridge this gap and recapitulate the UK model, a coordinated effort by both anesthesia and GI endoscopy societies is required to devise safe practice sedation guidelines. In all cases, the anesthetist or endoscopist should conduct a comprehensive pre-procedural evaluation, appropriate explanation of procedural risks, and obtain consent before initiating sedative measures. Unfortunately, in many centers workload pressures constrain time available for evaluations and as a result evaluations are often limited to a focused history and examination [4].

Additionally, a plan and all necessary equipment should be in place to manage complications such as aspiration and hypoxemia; all staff should be briefed and cognizant of processes in such an event. The evidence used to generate these guidelines attempts to meet the need of an ever-enlarging gastrointestinal procedural arsenal including complex cases including endobariatrics and submucosal resection, among others. The ensuing chapter provides a review of existing recommendations regarding patients undergoing GI procedures under sedation.

Pre-sedation Patient Assessment

Sedation is defined as a depressed level of consciousness achieved through drug administration. Pre-sedation patient assessment includes four core components: (1) Pre-procedural medical history and American Society of Anesthesiologists physical status classification, (2) Vital signs, (3) Informed consent and guardianship, and (4) Sedation-related education. First, a previous medical history must probe for cardiopulmonary disease, neurological disease, sleep apnea, medications, alcohol and illicit drug abuse, and compliance with fasting timeline. Of note, American Society of Anesthesiologists and other guidelines similarly recommend a minimum fasting period of 2 hours for clear fluids, 4 hours for light solid food, and 8 hours for lipid-rich solid food [5]. Additionally, the American Society of Anesthesiologists classification is critical for intraoperative risk stratification and quality control measures outside clinical responsibility [6]. Of particular importance, the patient must be accurately assessed for level of consciousness before endoscopic sedation is given. Since sedative agents lower the level of consciousness, a score of 5/5 from the modified observer's assessment of alertness and sedation scale (MOAA/S) should be recorded to ensure patient safety.

The second step is to review vital signs such as the blood pressure, heart rate, respiratory rate, and oxygen saturation. Sedative and analgesic agents administered during endoscopic sedation commonly cause drops in blood pressure, respiratory depression, and occasionally arrhythmias; establishing a baseline is essential for intraoperative safety.

Third, informed consent and guardianship must be obtained. The current recommended format for consent is as follows: purpose and necessity for sedation, explanation of sedative endoscopic procedure, processes and methodology of sedation, risks and possible complications of endoscopic sedation, alternative options aside from endoscopic sedation, and prognosis if left untreated. Guardianship is required such that in the setting of prolonged sedative drift after the procedure, the patient will be under the care of a guardian.

Fourth, sedation-related education must be provided to cover life-threatening adverse events (e.g., cardiopulmonary dysfunction). All endoscopists, nurses, and other assistants are trained to complete sedation-related evaluation of symptoms prior to each procedure, during the procedure, and after the procedure to ensure patient safety [7].

A thorough physical airway exam should be conducted prior to the procedure, which consists of Mallampati score, thyro- and hyomental distances, dentition assessment, mouth opening, and neck range of motion. Mallampati score is graded I–IV, with grade I suggesting the easiest endotracheal intubation and IV the most difficult. Before beginning endoscopic sedation, an airway exam and Mallampati score should be verified and if the patient is deemed a potentially difficult airway, anesthesia assistance is recommended [8]. Further, physical examination not only accentuating the head and neck, including the airway, but as well, the heart and the lungs is required for all patients undergoing anesthesia. Moreover, as GI procedures are more commonly performed outside the operating theatre and in less comprehensively supported settings such as GI suites, it is recommended that the ratio of examination room beds-to-recovery room beds is at least 2:1 [9, 10]. When emergencies occur in the GI suite, the appropriate personnel, areas, and equipment to facilitate rapid response must be easily accessible and ready to respond.

Personnel and Equipment

There is much thought and careful planning that goes into designing a gastroenterological endoscopy facility. Much of this planning is guided by the type of facility; there are hospital endoscopy suites, single-specialty or multispecialty ambulatory surgery centers, or an office endoscopy suite.

Some basic equipment that should be in the facility includes endoscopes, electrocautery units, hemostasis units, devices for monitoring pulse oximetry, blood pressure, and cardiac function, catheters, forceps, snares, brushes, endoscopic report writer with photo generator and image manager, esophageal dilators, height-adjustable rolling procedural stretcher carts, suction equipment, sedation and analgesic agents, benzodiazepine antagonist, glucagon, atropine, intravenous equipment, solutions, needles, syringes, disinfecting solutions, an emergency cart, resuscitation equipment, high-level disinfection equipment, instrument storage cabinets, blanket warmer, eyewash station, and an audio/music system. A typical endoscopy suite will have the following rooms and spaces: waiting room, reception/business area, pre-/post-procedure area, procedure area, reprocessing area for soiled instruments, storage room, utility room, IT room, biohazard/soiled linen/trash room, medical gas room, staff area with locker rooms, a shower and staff restrooms, parking, and a canopy extending to the curb.

The patient procedure preparation area and post-procedure area should be in the same area, allowing for an efficient use of the space. This area should also contain a nurses' station with an unobstructed view of the patients, a nutrition area, medication area, storage for patient belongings, handwashing sinks, restrooms and areas for patient changing, and an exam/consult room. Facility Guidelines Institute guidelines state that the procedure rooms must be a minimum of 200 clear square feet; however, more complex endoscopy procedures may require 300 square feet. The floors of the procedure rooms must be clear of all wires, cords, and cables. The room must contain all endoscopic accessories, oxygen, supplies, resuscitation equipment, and an emergency call button.

Near the procedure rooms, there should be an emergency crash cart. To improve efficiency, the reprocessing for soiled instruments should be located near the procedure rooms. Overall, it is important to consider the flow of the patients, staff, physicians, and equipment throughout the facility to design a space that will maximize efficiency and provide satisfaction to patients, staff, and physicians [11].

The administration of sedatives in the United States is largely predominated by an anesthesia provider. In patients undergoing routine endoscopic procedures without an ASA class 3 or above, severe sleep apnea, morbid obesity, gastric outlet obstruction, gastroparesis, or achalasia, nurse-administered propofol sedation has shown to be safe and achievable [12, 13]. Similarly, gastroenterologist-directed propofol sedation has also been shown to be a safe and efficient means of sedation for endoscopic procedures in this patient population. These methods of sedation can offer a more cost-effective means of sedation in low-risk patients with American Society of Anesthesiologists monitoring standards [13]. Monitored anesthesia care (MAC) remains the sedation method for the majority and, in particular, for higher-risk patients. Emergency equipment must be available regardless of who is administering the sedation. Propofol has no reversal agents; thus, it is imperative to have a way to manage patients airways until its effects wear off. Emergency equipment includes oxygen, oral suction, laryngoscope, an air-mask-bag unit, and a defibrillator [14].

Patient Monitoring for GI Endoscopy

Continuous monitoring during and after the administration of sedatives detects early signs of distress and allows for timely intervention and rescue. Standard American Society of Anesthesiologists non-invasive monitoring includes monitoring a patient's oxygenation, ventilation, circulation, and temperature, if wide ranges in periprocedural temperature are anticipated. This can be achieved with electrocardiogram, a non-invasive blood pressure monitor, pulse oximetry, a temperature monitor, and continuous quantitative capnography [15]. In this regard, quantitative continuous capnography monitoring is a *standard monitoring requirement* related to its ability to detect inadequate respiratory efforts and/or apnea [16, 17]. The MOAA/S is used to quantify a patient's level of unconsciousness. This scale accounts for the patient's level of responsiveness, speech, facial expression, and eyes to arrive at a score ranging from 1 to 5. A score of 1–2 represents unconsciousness and 3–4 represents a moderate level of sedation [18].

In moderate sedation of patients undergoing GI procedures outside of the OR, monitoring ventilation according to current standards is identical to that of a hospital. The American Society of Anesthesiologists issued an amendment in 2011 stating that ventilation should be evaluated by continually observing qualitative signs and by quantitatively monitoring exhaled CO_2. CO_2 exhalation monitoring requires a nasal cannula, and to achieve accurate measurements, the prongs must be carefully placed. In GI procedures, the patient's movement and the placement of the scopes can interfere with this precise prong placement. One quality improvement project proposed the use of a non-invasive, thoracic, impedance-based respiratory volume monitor as a means of monitoring ventilation. This method of monitoring uses an adhesive electrode PadSet and provides a real-time respiratory curve and measurements of minute ventilation, tidal volume, and respiratory rate. In this study, patient's end-tidal CO2 (ETCO2) and minute ventilation were recorded before, during and after GI procedures using the nasal cannula and impedance device respectively. After initial placement, the nasal cannula and electrodes were not repositioned or adjusted. These researchers found that the impedance device was a more dependable method of revealing decreased ventilation and did so more rapidly than the nasal cannula [19]. Given the rapid and reliable information it provides, impedance-based ventilation monitors in GI procedures outside of the OR should be further considered.

MAC for GI endoscopic sedation has significantly increased in fee-for-service environments and in the Veteran's Health Administration (VHA), which operates as a capitated system. A retrospective cohort study published in 2017 discussed the use of monitored anesthesia care in over 2,000,000 veterans that underwent outpatient GI endoscopy. This study found that despite the absence of financial incentives there was still unsuitable utilization of MAC in VHA facilities. They found only a slight increase in the odds of MAC use in patients with obesity (class III), obstructive sleep apnea (OSA), and those with the highest comorbidity scores. Similarly, the probability of MAC use in patients with an opioid or benzodiazepine prescription within 6 months of their GI procedure was only slightly increased compared to those without. Additionally, the influence of provider-level predictors and geographic location also showed a small influence on MAC utilization in VHA facilities. These factors such as facility-specific organizational factors, unrelated to patients directly, seem to have a large effect on MAC utilization and require further investigation to ensure that MAC is allocated to patients that will benefit from it. [20] Thus, both facility- and provider-level factors heavily influence whether patients receive moderate versus deep sedation as well as procedure sedation nurses, CRNAs, and/or anesthesiologists. This further reflects the importance of dosing of sedative medications, proper monitoring, identification of high-risk patients, and level of expertise of person providing sedation.

Common Procedures in GI Endoscopy

Common procedures in GI endoscopy include esophagogastroduodenoscopy (EGD), sigmoidoscopy, proctoscopy, colonoscopy, and endoscopic retrograde cholangiopancreatography and pancreatic cytology (ECRP). Sedation and anesthesia play various roles in these procedures. In an EGD, an endoscope is inserted in the mouth and passes through the esophagus, stomach, pylorus, and upper duodenum to evaluate these areas for any tissue abnormalities [21]. Colonoscopies are performed as a routine screening for the presence of polyps or tumors. During this procedure, an endoscope is placed in the rectum and then passed through the colon. EGDs and colonoscopies also allow for a tissue biopsy to be taken during the procedure if necessary. Patient's requiring moderate sedation for upper GI endoscopies (EGDs) or colonoscopies may receive a combination of a benzodiazepine and an opioid analgesic. Previously, the most commonly used combination was midazolam and fentanyl. This form of sedation may be administered by non-anesthesia clinicians. MAC is another option for the sedation of these patients and provides for moderate or deep sedation with an anesthesiologist. This generally involves the administration of propofol and has shown increased procedural success rates, patient cooperation, and post-sedation recovery scores. It has also shown decreased complications, reduced recovery times and reduced discharge times. More specifically, in colonoscopies, propofol decreases the odds of cardiopulmonary complications with proper monitoring and personnel [12]. Flexible sigmoidoscopy is performed to evaluate the sigmoid colon, the anus, and the rectum, while proctoscopy allows for viewing of only the anus and rectum. During both procedures, physicians investigate for any tissue abnormalities. Flexible sigmoidoscopy also allows for the monitoring of inflammatory bowel disease, polyp detection, and the evaluation and treatment of lower GI bleeds [21]. Generally speaking, most patients require sedation for either of these procedures related to a patient's level of anxiety.

Endoscopic retrograde cholangiopancreatography and pancreatic cytology is typically used to evaluate and treat conditions involving the bile ducts and the pancreas. During this procedure, the patient is in the prone or semi-prone position and a moderate to deep level of sedation is required. The mode of sedation is dependent on whether or not the patient is at a high risk of sedation-related adverse events (SRAEs). These include OSA, abdominal ascites, BMI >35 kg/m^2, chronic obstructive pulmonary disease, American Society of Anesthesiologists class ≥3, and moderate to heavy alcohol use. In those without this risk, the use of deep sedation-analgesia with a nasal trumpet connected to a Mapleson C circuit is recommended.

However, in patients with a high risk for sedation-related adverse events the recommended method is general endotracheal anesthesia

(GEA). One study found that patients at high risk of SRAEs that underwent propofol-based monitored anesthesia care had an increased incidence of hypoxemia and required more airway maneuvers; for this reason GEA is a preferred method in this patient population [22].

Choice of Sedation Agents

Endoscopic sedation is routinely employed to facilitate optimal gastrointestinal procedure performance. Sedation practices in GI procedures have changed significantly over the past decade as the number of procedures has risen and anesthesiologists have responded to new literature showing improved patient satisfaction with deeper sedation. The general principle of endoscopic sedation is to limit untimely patient movement and decrease pain response, thereby increasing safety and quality of the procedures [23].

Sedation agents, sedation levels, and the need for an anesthesiologist are commonly determined by the length and complexity of procedure and the patients' comorbidities. Patient response to sedation and to tolerance of the endoscopic procedure ranges considerably as well [24]. The most commonly used level of sedation in endoscopic procedures is moderate sedation, defined as purposeful response to visual or tactile stimuli by the patient. Many procedures require deep sedation or general anesthesia. Benzodiazepine agents used alone or combined with opiate agents were the classic sedative combination given to these patients for successful moderate sedation delivery. Recently, a sedative technique rapidly gaining popularity in practice is a deeper level of sedation achieved with propofol.

Various sedatives, opioids, and dissociative agents have been used in the management of patients undergoing endoscopic procedures. An ideal sedative agent in this setting should meet all of the following characteristics: rapid onset of action, practical means of delivery, short half-life with rapid recovery, safe sedative response, minimal respiratory and cardiovascular effects, and pain-free cooperative patient. Previously, the most utilized class of drugs in the endoscopy suite were benzodiazepines. Midazolam (Versed) and diazepam (Valium) have a comparable efficacy although midazolam is the agent of choice owing to a more rapid onset, short half-life, and amnestic properties [25]. Benzodiazepines, in general, have discrete interactions in the cerebral cortex; they have no analgesic properties, but they do have amnesic, sedative, and anxiolytic properties. Of particular clinical relevance, the high potency of midazolam necessitates careful titration to avoid overdose and apnea, particularly in the elderly population.

Because of their powerful analgesic properties, opioids are frequently administered to endoscopic patients along with midazolam. The two most popular drug choices are fentanyl and meperidine, albeit meperidine has fallen out of favor in recent years due to its side effect profile, including tachycardia, and potential drug interactions [26]. These drugs work by inhibiting noxious stimuli in peripheral nociceptors. One unique property of opioids is their lipid solubility which correlates with a rapid onset of action and short duration of action. The duration of action for fentanyl is 30–45 minutes whereas the duration of action for meperidine is 2–4 hours. If the patient requires a prolonged analgesia, multidosing of opioids can result in suppression of ventilation either from direct opioid actions or through drug-drug additive or synergistic effects.

Concurrent use of opioids and benzodiazepine agents, even in small incremental doses of fentanyl, can therefore result in significant sedative-related effects, which renders careful ventilatory monitoring a critical aspect in GI sedation delivery [26]. Other common side effects of opioids include cross reactivity with the mu-opioid receptors of the gastrointestinal tract, which causes decreased gut peristalsis and ileus. Opioids are not known to depress cardiac functionality, but they can lead to vagus nerve-mediated bradycardia and chest wall rigidity in some patients.

In any circumstance when a standard moderate sedation technique is not sufficient, deep sedation can be achieved with propofol. Propofol has widely gained popularity in the last decade related to its favorable pharmacokinetic qualities (i.e., rapid onset of action and short half-life) and superior patient satisfaction rating [27]. Propofol is a combined hypnotic and antiemetic agent with a prompt recovery period allowing patients to safely go home the day of a GI procedure in most instances. Propofol has historically been administered via manual bolus or continuous infusion, although new target-controlled infusion techniques have also proven useful [28–30]. Unfortunately, the predominate risk of propofol sedation in GI procedures is the narrow therapeutic range and inadvertent entry into a deeper level of general anesthesia, defined as an unarousable state with painful stimulus. In this inadvertent state, profound respiratory depression and apnea can devolve into harrowing complications; prevention of such events requires standard American Society of Anesthesiologists monitors, including quantitative continuous end tidal CO_2. Failing to employ quantitative continuous $EtCO_2$ is below any local, regional, or national standard of care and can result in hypoxia, brain damage, cardiopulmonary collapse, and/or death. Because of this very real risk, it is recommended that an anesthesia provider administer propofol sedation to ensure careful titration and comprehensive patient monitoring.

In general, guidelines suggest gastroenterologists can in most instances maintain a low to moderate level of sedation without anesthesia assistance, while delivering combinations of benzodiazepine and/or opioid. In this regard, gastroenterologists should not attempt to deliver propofol, in general, because they do not possess airway management skills which can guarantee patient safety. Sedation nurses, as well, do not typically possess airway management skills and should not deliver propofol in most instances. Though studies documented in this chapter have shown efficacy and safety with non-anesthesia personnel and the delivery of propofol, very real facts include that most non-anesthesia providers lack airway skillsets that can be essential in the management of over-sedated patients with propofol.

Three newer agents have recently bolstered the sedative arsenal for endoscopic procedures: remimazolam, fospropofol, and dexmedetomidine. Remimazolam, the newest pharmaceutical innovation in anesthesia, is an ester based benzodiazepine designed for ultra-short duration of action and organ independent metabolism via tissue esterases [31]. Remimazolam safety profile has already been recognized as superior to that of midazolam, with no serious adverse effects found on clinical trial and a moderate level of sedation that is readily managed by the gastroenterologist [32]. Moreover, fospropofol was an innovation that intended to create a water soluble propofol prodrug with desirable prolonged duration of action (half-life of 30 min). Fospropofol has not gained popularity due to controversial early published literature, yet phase II and III clinical trial data suggests that is generally well tolerated [33]. Finally, dexmedetomidine is an alpha 2-agonist with anxiolytic, sedative, and analgesic effects. It can be administered intranasally or intravenously and is not known to cause respiratory depression, making it an attractive sedative agent. Dexmedetomidine causes bradycardia and a biphasic change in blood pressure, although dexmedetomidine alone or with meperidine and midazolam has demonstrated less respiratory depression and a higher patient satisfaction for routine/advanced endoscopic procedures than midazolam and meperidine alone [23].

Pediatric endoscopic sedation often employs ketamine related to its preferable route of administration, rapid onset of action, short duration of action, and safe pediatric profile [34]. Ketamine works predominately by inhibiting NMDA receptors in the central nervous system [35]. In turn, ketamine produces a dissociative state of anesthesia characterized by hypnosis, intense analgesia, increased sympathetic activity, and maintenance of airway tone and respiration. More recent anesthesia advances have combined ketamine with dexmedetomidine as a potent sedative cocktail for pediatric GI procedures.

It is the responsibility of the practitioner to have reversal agents (competitive antagonists) at the ready such as naloxone and flumazenil. Naloxone acts as an opioid reversal agent that can save patients from opioid overdose and respiratory depression. Flumazenil is a benzodiazepine reversal agent that antagonizes the hypnotic effects more potently than the amnestic effects. Side effects of these reversal agents includes withdrawal of all analgesic effect and sudden agonizing pain response for naloxone, and anxiety reactions such as nausea and vomiting with flumazenil [36]. In this regard, there is no known reversal agent for propofol.

Endoscopic Sedation in Special Patient Populations

The choice of sedation for patients with comorbidities is often paramount and requires close attention by the anesthesiologist or gastroenterologist. Patients with cirrhosis are one of the most prevalent indications for emergent endoscopy. As liver dysfunction reduces plasma protein binding and hepatic drug metabolism by the cytochrome P450 enzymes, in patients with liver failure it is imperative to correlate anesthesia planning with sedative agents that can be cleared by the kidneys [37]. Several studies investigating endoscopy procedure efficacy in cirrhotic patients found propofol to exhibit faster sedation recovery when compared to midazolam [38]. On the other hand, endoscopy procedures in pregnant patients are deemed high risk and should only be performed for the most convincing indications such as significant GI bleeding, biliary pancreatitis or cholangitis, severe nausea and vomiting, severe diarrhea, and dysphagia. These procedures should be deferred to the second trimester when possible to limit fetal exposure to the sedative agents. Maternal hypoxemia and hypotension result in harm to the mother and fetal hypoxia and fetal demise [39]. Anesthesia services are strongly recommended to be involved in endoscopic procedures involving pregnant patients due to the teratogenic and hypoxic risk in addition to an increased risk of aspiration. To mitigate risk of fetal demise as best possible, fetal monitoring should be made a priority before and, if possible, after the operation. A final important patient population are obese patients.

Obese patients are at risk for obstructive apnea and adverse cardiovascular events during the procedure. The STOP-BANG tool is a widely accepted stratification for high- and low-risk OSA patients (snoring, tiredness, observed apnea, blood pressure, body mass index, age, neck circumference, and gender) [40]. Amplification of these risks is apparent when delivering moderate or deep sedation in the prone position, further demonstrating the critical importance of quantitative continuous EtCO2 monitoring as a nonstop measure of respiration.

Recovery

All patients who receive sedation, regional anesthesia, or general anesthesia should be transferred to a Post Anesthesia Care Unit (PACU), or some equivalent, for appropriate post-procedural monitoring and care. Post-procedural care begins with patient transport from OR to PACU. The patient should be accompanied by a member of the anesthesia care team while being transported from OR to PACU. Prior to transport, the patient's need for oxygenation, ventilation, medications, and any additional equipment such as a cardiac monitor should be addressed. During transport, the patient should be continuously monitored, and the patient should receive supplemental oxygen and other necessary treatment as needed [41, 42].

Upon arrival to PACU, the patient should be immediately re-evaluated by the accompanying anesthesia care team member, and the patient's status at that time should be relayed to the PACU team assuming responsibility of the patient. The PACU nurse should document the status of the patient at that time. A handoff report should be conducted between the anesthesia care team member and the PACU team member. This is the time to report any essential information regarding the patient history, the procedure performed, complications that occurred, medications given, fluids administered, and status of the patient. Once the PACU team is briefed on the patient, care is then turned over to the PACU team. Upon arrival to the PACU, the patient should be reassessed continually. Specifically, the patient's oxygenation, ventilation, circulation, level of consciousness, temperature, and analgesia should be monitored closely. Pulse oxygenation and heart rate should be continuously monitored. Blood pressure should be monitored regularly. The patient should also be monitored for post-operative nausea and vomiting. A detailed written record of patient's course in PACU should be kept [41, 42].

While in the PACU, the patient should be monitored for emergence delirium (ED), a potential adverse effect of anesthesia. In high-risk populations, ED can be seen in significant numbers of patients, especially those under general endotracheal anesthesia, less so with propofol only, though the literature varies in terms of incidence. ED is generally defined as a change in behavior, such as disorientation, agitation, hypoactivity, or hyperactivity, during the emergence or recovery from anesthesia [43]. Patients that experience ED may end up injuring themselves or others and tend to require more nursing resources, longer hospital stay durations, and more frequent hospital readmissions [43, 44]. The hypoactive form of ED has been associated with long-term cognitive and physical deterioration. General and inhaled anesthetics have been more commonly associated with ED when compared with other types. A few risk factors have been identified and include anesthesia duration greater than 1.5 hours, anxiety, depression, PTSD, history of combat or deployment, long-term benzodiazepine or antidepressant use, smoking, social alcohol use, and surgeries involving the abdomen, breast, ear, nose, and throat [43]. Delirium in the first few hours postoperatively may be associated with recurrence of delirium in the following days postoperatively, and increased morbidity and mortality [44]. Prevention is considered most effective in improving outcomes and includes preoperative education, emotional support, and avoidance of inhaled anesthetics when possible. Once ED is identified in a patient, the first step should be to address any triggers such as hypoxia, catheters, or pain. The next steps should be to provide the patient reassurance and allow a family member to be present at bedside. If these attempts fail, the practitioner should be prepared to administer an anxiolytic, antipsychotic, or sedative such as haloperidol or dexmedetomidine [43].

The anesthesiologist and PACU team should work together to determine whether the patient is ready for discharge. A commonly used discharge criteria assessment is the Aldrete score. This system scores each patient based on activity level, respiration, circulation, level of consciousness, and oxygen saturation. The score is calculated and then used to determine if the patient is ready for discharge. Another commonly used discharge criteria system is the Post Anesthesia Discharge Scoring System. This system assesses vital signs, surgical bleeding, activity and mental status, intake and output, and pain/nausea/vomiting. The decision to discharge must be approved by the department of anesthesiology. Once the patient is deemed ready for discharge, the PACU staff should provide the patient and caregiver with discharge instructions and specific patient education for the postoperative period [41, 42].

Special Considerations

Anesthesia providers may face many challenges when using sedation in gastrointestinal procedures. Some potential complications of sedation include hypoxemia, respiratory depression, and arrhythmias [45]. Of these, respiratory depression is most common. Many anesthetics cause a resultant decrease in the body's central respiratory drive. Although it is a minimal risk with moderate sedation, it is more likely with deep sedation and general anesthesia [46]. Moderate to deep sedation is associated with increased risk of airway obstruction and hypoventilation [47]. Other potential complications include apnea, laryngospasm, anatomical obstruction, and aspiration. Laryngospasms occur more commonly with deep sedation or general anesthesia, and in children and adult smokers. Apnea with upper airway obstruction is also more common with deep sedation or general anesthesia and may represent a life-threatening emergency [46].

The potential adverse effects associated with sedation are further increased in high-risk patients, such as those with OSA. OSA is a commonly diagnosed disorder where patients experience nocturnal episodes of airway collapse and subsequent hypoxemia. Patients with OSA are at increased risk for difficult airway challenges, such as difficult intubation or difficult mask ventilation. Perioperative risk is potentially increased in patients with OSA because anesthesia alters the ventilatory drive, upper airway anatomy, airway reflexes, and consciousness. Following the use of neuromuscular blocking agents, OSA patients are at increased risk for residual neuromuscular blockade, postoperative respiratory failure, or hypoxemia. Following the use of propofol for sedation, OSA patients may be at increased risk for respiratory compromise and hypoxemic events. Sedation with benzodiazepines is associated with upper airway collapse and therefore must be used with caution in patients with OSA. Frequent and close monitoring of these patients is imperative [48].

Many GI procedures require that the patient be placed in the prone position. This position has been associated with increased risk of adverse events, which may be attributable to the physiological changes the position initiates. Placing the patient in the prone position results in an increase in intra-thoracic pressures and a decrease in stroke volume, left ventricular compliance, and cardiac index. It may also result in obstruction of the inferior vena cava. Additionally, there is an associated increased risk of airway loss when the patient is prone. To minimize accidental extubation, special attention must be given to perfect positioning and frequent rechecks [49].

To minimize the potential for adverse events, the anesthesiologist should employ the standard American Society of Anesthesiologists monitors throughout the procedure. The standard American Society of Anesthesiologists monitors include pulse oximeter, electrocardiography, noninvasive blood pressure device, body temperature monitor, and continuous quantitative end tidal carbon dioxide monitor [50, 51]. Capnography is a method of measuring end tidal carbon dioxide that utilizes the absorptive properties of carbon dioxide in the electromagnetic spectrum. Continuous quantitative end tidal capnography allows for real-time assessment of ventilation, and it can detect alveolar hypoventilation before progression to hypoxemia occurs. It is highly useful in all patients, including in particular high-risk patients, such as those with OSA, BMI >30, significant cardiopulmonary history, and the elderly, and patients undergoing deep sedation with longer procedural times. By closely following the ASA monitors, the anesthesia provider may potentially avoid any adverse outcomes [45].

Summary

In summary, gastrointestinal procedures are rapidly expanding in location, variety, and volume, in turn demanding an updated set of guidelines that adapt to ensure continued patient safety and satisfaction. Albeit controversial, a growing number of endoscopic procedures are conducted each year by non-anesthesia services such as endoscopists. A standardized approach to pre-procedural patient assessment is crucial to avoiding intraoperative complications and an individualized patient approach to sedative drug selection ensures adequate pain control and undesirable movement prohibition. While the classic combination of midazolam and fentanyl remains popular for many patients needing moderate sedation, a deeper level of sedation achieved with propofol is rapidly growing in utilization related to increased patient satisfaction and ideal pharmacokinetics. Moreover, new anesthetic agents such as the alpha-2 agonist dexmedetomidine offer an appealing side effect profile and patient recovery period. As obesity and other cardiovascular comorbidities become more prevalent in the United States, it is imperative that special considerations for intraoperative management are performed.

To minimize potential adverse events during GI procedural anesthesia, anesthesiology services are recommended for most patients and particularly those with high-risk morbidities or who require deep sedation. Finally, a strong emphasis must be placed on the strict utilization of ASA standard monitors for all patients undergoing GI procedures. In particular, the critical role and the current local, regional, and national standard for continuous quantitative end tidal CO_2 monitoring must be employed for safe delivery of sedation for any GI procedure.

References

1. An Astounding 19 Million Colonoscopies are Performed Annually in The United States – iData Research. https://idataresearch.com/an-astounding-19-million-colonoscopies-are-performed-annually-in-the-united-states/. Accessed March 21, 2020.
2. Saunders R, Erslon M, Vargo J. Modeling the costs and benefits of capnography monitoring during procedural sedation for gastrointestinal endoscopy. Endosc Int Open. 2016;04(03):E340–51. https://doi.org/10.1055/s-0042-100719.
3. Sidhu R, Turnbull D, Newton M, et al. Deep sedation and anaesthesia in complex gastrointestinal endoscopy: a joint position statement endorsed by the British Society of Gastroenterology (BSG), Joint Advisory Group (JAG) and Royal College of Anaesthetists (RCoA). Frontline Gastroenterol. 2019;10(2):141–7. https://doi.org/10.1136/flgastro-2018-101145.
4. Goudra B, Singh P. Critical analysis of guidelines for providing sedation to patients undergoing gastrointestinal endoscopy procedures. Anesth Essays Res. 2019;13(4):601. https://doi.org/10.4103/aer.aer_135_19.
5. Kaye AD, Jones MR, Viswanath O, et al. Guidelines ASIPP Guidelines for Sedation and Fasting Status of Patients Undergoing Interventional Pain Management Procedures. 2019. www.painphysicianjournal.com. Accessed March 21, 2020.
6. Daabiss M. American society of anaesthesiologists physical status classification. Indian J Anaesth. 2011;55(2):111–5. https://doi.org/10.4103/0019-5049.79879.
7. Lee JK, Lee YJ, Cho JH, et al. Updates on the sedation for gastrointestinal endoscopy. Clin Endosc. 2019;52(5):451–7. https://doi.org/10.5946/ce.2019.172.
8. Mallampati Score – an overview | ScienceDirect Topics. https://www.sciencedirect.com/topics/medicine-and-dentistry/mallampati-score. Accessed March 21, 2020.
9. Mulder CJJ, Jacobs MAJM, Leicester RJ, et al. Guidelines for designing a digestive disease endoscopy unit: Report of the World Endoscopy Organization. Dig Endosc. 2013;25(4):365–75. https://doi.org/10.1111/den.12126.
10. Pall H, Lerner D, Khlevner J, et al. Developing the Pediatric gastrointestinal endoscopy unit. J Pediatr Gastroenterol Nutr. 2016;63(2):295–306. https://doi.org/10.1097/MPG.0000000000001189.
11. Mergener K, Tanner B. Setting up an endoscopy facility. 2019. doi:https://doi.org/10.1016/B978-0-323-41509-5.00002-5.
12. Lin OS, Weigel W. Nonoperating room anesthesia for gastrointestinal endoscopic procedures. Curr Opin Anaesthesiol. 2018;31:486. https://doi.org/10.1097/ACO.0000000000000610.
13. Wehrmann T, Triantafyllou K. Propofol sedation in gastrointestinal endoscopy: a gastroenterologist's perspective. Digestion. 2010;82:106. https://doi.org/10.1159/000285554.
14. Repici A, Hassan C. The endoscopist, the anesthesiologists, and safety in GI endoscopy. Gastrointest Endosc. 2017;85:109. https://doi.org/10.1016/j.gie.2016.06.025.
15. Tobias JD. Sedation of infants and children outside of the operating room. Curr Opin Anaesthesiol. 2015;28:478. https://doi.org/10.1097/ACO.0000000000000203.
16. Gerstenberger PD. Capnography and patient safety for endoscopy. Clin Gastroenterol Hepatol. 2010;8:423. https://doi.org/10.1016/j.cgh.2010.02.024.
17. Lightdale JR, Goldmann DA, Feldman HA, Newburg AR, DiNardo JA, Fox VL. Microstream capnography improves patient monitoring during moderate sedation: a randomized, controlled trial. Pediatrics. 2006;117:e1170. https://doi.org/10.1542/peds.2005-1709.
18. American Society of Anesthesiologists Martinench A. American Society of Anesthesiologists: ASA physical status classification system. In: Am Soc Anesthesiol Web site Internet; 2014.
19. Ebert TJ, Middleton AH, Makhija N. Ventilation monitoring during moderate sedation in GI patients. J Clin Monit Comput. 2017;31:53. https://doi.org/10.1007/s10877-015-9809-1.
20. Adams MA, Prenovost KM, Dominitz JA, et al. Predictors of use of monitored anesthesia care for outpatient gastrointestinal endoscopy in a capitated payment system. Gastroenterology. 2017;153:1496. https://doi.org/10.1053/j.gastro.2017.08.030.
21. Paz JC. Acute care handbook for physical therapists; 2014. https://doi.org/10.1016/B978-1-4557-2896-1.00008-1.
22. Smith ZL, Mullady DK, Lang GD, et al. A randomized controlled trial evaluating general endotracheal anesthesia versus monitored anesthesia care and the incidence of sedation-related adverse events during ERCP in high-risk patients. Gastrointest Endosc. 2019;89:855. https://doi.org/10.1016/j.gie.2018.09.001.
23. Wadhwa V, Vargo JJ. Sedation and monitoring in endoscopy- clinical gastrointestinal edoscopy. 3rd ed. (Chandrasekhara V, Khashab M, Elmunzer J, Muthusamy R, eds.).; 2019. https://www-clinicalkey-com.proxy.lib.mcw.edu/#!/content/book/3-s2.0-B9780323415095000074. Accessed 21 Mar 2020.
24. Levitzky BE, Lopez R, Dumot JA, Vargo JJ. Moderate sedation for elective upper endoscopy with balanced propofol versus fentanyl and midazolam alone: a randomized clinical trial. Endoscopy. 2012;44(1):13–20. https://doi.org/10.1055/s-0031-1291421.
25. Brouillette DE, Leventhal R, Kumar S, et al. Midazolam versus diazepam for combined esophogastroduodenoscopy and colonoscopy. Dig Dis Sci. 1989;34(8):1265–71. https://doi.org/10.1007/BF01537276.
26. Sedative and Analgesic Drugs for Gastrointestinal Endoscopic Procedure | Amornyotin | Journal

of Gastroenterology and Hepatology Research. http://www.ghrnet.org/index.php/joghr/article/view/779/893. Accessed March 21, 2020.

27. Early DS, Lightdale JR, Vargo JJ, et al. Guidelines for sedation and anesthesia in GI endoscopy ASGE STANDARDS OF PRACTICE COMMITTEE. Gastrointest Endosc. 2018;87:327–37. https://doi.org/10.1016/j.gie.2017.07.018.
28. Effect of target controlled propofol infusion versus intermittent boluses during oesophagogastroduodenoscopy: a randomized controlled trial | African Health Sciences. https://www.ajol.info/index.php/ahs/article/view/192297. Accessed March 21, 2020.
29. Ogawa T, Tomoda T, Kato H, Akimoto Y, Tanaka S, Okada H. Propofol sedation with a target-controlled infusion pump in elderly patients undergoing ERCP. Gastrointest Endosc. 2020;92:301. https://doi.org/10.1016/j.gie.2020.03.002.
30. Mu J, Jiang T, Xu XB, Yuen VM, Irwin MG. Comparison of target-controlled infusion and manual infusion for propofol anaesthesia in children. Br J Anaesth. 2018;120:1049–55. https://doi.org/10.1016/j.bja.2017.11.102.
31. Pambianco DJ, Cash BD. New horizons for sedation: the ultrashort acting benzodiazepine remimazolam. Tech Gastrointest Endosc. 2016;18(1):22–8. https://doi.org/10.1016/j.tgie.2016.02.004.
32. Pastis NJ, Yarmus LB, Schippers F, et al. Safety and efficacy of remimazolam compared with placebo and midazolam for moderate Sedation during bronchoscopy. Chest. 2019;155(1):137–46. https://doi.org/10.1016/j.chest.2018.09.015.
33. Dinis-Oliveira RJ. Metabolic profiles of propofol and fospropofol: clinical and forensic interpretative aspects. 2018. https://doi.org/10.1155/2018/6852857.
34. Eskander AE, El Baroudy NR, El Refay AS. Ketamine sedation in gastrointestinal endoscopy in children. Maced J Med Sci. 2016;4(3):392–6. https://doi.org/10.3889/oamjms.2016.085.
35. Sleigh J, Harvey M, Voss L, Denny B. Ketamine - more mechanisms of action than just NMDA blockade. Trends Anaesth Crit Care. 2014;4(2–3):76–81. https://doi.org/10.1016/j.tacc.2014.03.002.
36. Sivilotti MLA. Flumazenil, naloxone and the 'coma cocktail'. Br J Clin Pharmacol. 2016;81(3):428–36. https://doi.org/10.1111/bcp.12731.
37. Conscious sedation using propofol versus midazolam in cirrhotic patients during upper GI endoscopy: a comparative study – Wahab – 2019 – JGH Open – Wiley Online Library. https://onlinelibrary.wiley.com/doi/pdf/10.1002/jgh3.12098. Accessed March 21, 2020.
38. Mohamed F, Kandil Y. Propofol versus midazolam in sedation for upper gastrointestinal endoscopy. Int J Med Arts. 2019;0(0):0–0. https://doi.org/10.21608/ijma.2019.18082.1037.
39. Rabiee A, Moshiree B. Upper and lower endoscopy for gastrointestinal (GI) bleeding in pregnancy. In: Non-obstetric surgery during pregnancy: Springer; 2019. p. 155–64. https://doi.org/10.1007/978-3-319-90752-9_12.
40. Chung F, Abdullah HR, Liao P. STOP-bang questionnaire a practical approach to screen for obstructive sleep apnea. Chest. 2016;149(3):631–8. https://doi.org/10.1378/chest.15-0903.
41. Standards for Postanesthesia Care | American Society of Anesthesiologists (ASA). Am Soc Anesthesiol. 2019.
42. Postanesthesia Care - Practice Considerations. American Association of Nurse Anesthetists.
43. Stein K. Clarifying the confusion of adult emergence delirium. AANA J. 2017;85(3):223.
44. Cui V, Tedeschi CM, Kronzer VL, McKinnon SL, Avidan MS. Protocol for an observational study of delirium in the post-anaesthesia care unit (PACU) as a potential predictor of subsequent postoperative delirium. BMJ Open. 2017;7(7):e016402. https://doi.org/10.1136/bmjopen-2017-016402.
45. Wadhwa V, Gupta K, Vargo JJ. Monitoring standards in sedation and analgesia: the odyssey of capnography in sedation for gastroenterology procedures. Curr Opin Anaesthesiol. 2019;32(4):453–6. https://doi.org/10.1097/ACO.0000000000000756.
46. Becker DE, Haas DA. Recognition and management of complications during moderate and deep sedation part 1: respiratory considerations. Anesth Prog. 2011;58(2):82–92. https://doi.org/10.2344/0003-3006-58.2.82.
47. Steven E. Abram, MD; Michael C. Francis M. Hazards of sedation for interventional pain procedures – anesthesia patient safety foundation. Anesth Patient Saf Found. 2012;27(2).
48. Memtsoudis SG, Cozowicz C, Nagappa M, et al. Society of anesthesia and sleep medicine guideline on intraoperative management of adult patients with obstructive sleep apnea. Anesth Analg. 2018;127(4):967–87. https://doi.org/10.1213/ANE.0000000000003434.
49. Edgcombe H, Carter K, Yarrow S. Anaesthesia in the prone position. Br J Anaesth. 2008;100(2):165–83. https://doi.org/10.1093/bja/aem380.
50. Standards for Basic Anesthetic Monitoring | American Society of Anesthesiologists (ASA). Am Soc Anesthesiol. 2015.
51. Weaver J. The latest ASA mandate: CO(2) monitoring for moderate and deep sedation. Anesth Prog. 2011;58(3):111–2. https://doi.org/10.2344/0003-3006-58.3.111.

19 Management of Perioperative Pain and Sedation for Interventional Radiology Procedures

Jonathan S. McDougal, Praveen N. Sankrithi, Jonathan B. Kozinn, and Brandt C. Wible

Abstract

Interventional radiology is especially well positioned to succeed in an ambulatory surgery center. While minimally invasive procedures can often be performed with local analgesia and conscious sedation administered by the performing interventionalist, as procedures become increasingly complex or life-threatening, the use of regional nerve blocks, deep sedation, monitored anesthesia care (MAC), or general anesthesia (GA) can improve procedural success rates and patient-perceived experiences. Post-procedural discomfort is a common indication for admission. Effective pain management/anesthesia can be cost-effective by increasing same-day discharge rates. A thorough history and physical exam is necessary before any interventional procedure. High-risk populations include those patients with obesity, chronic obstructive pulmonary disease (COPD), obstructive sleep apnea (OSA), coronary artery disease, chronic renal failure, patients with drug addiction, and elderly/pediatric. Special pre-procedure considerations include risk of bleeding, contrast-induced nephropathy, adverse reactions to contrast, patient-positioning, breath-holding, vascular access site, and recovery planning. Additional considerations are based on the specific procedure planned and the imaging modality utilized.

J. S. McDougal (✉) · B. C. Wible
University of Missouri-Kansas City School of Medicine, Kansas City, MO, USA

Saint Luke's Health System, Department of Radiology, Saint Luke's Hospital, Kansas City, MO, USA
e-mail: mcdougalj@umkc.edu; bwible@saint-lukes.org

P. N. Sankrithi
Kansas City University of Medicine and Biosciences, Kansas City, MO, USA
e-mail: psankrithi@kcumb.edu

J. B. Kozinn
University of Missouri-Kansas City School of Medicine, Kansas City, MO, USA

Saint Luke's Health System, Department of Anesthesiology, Saint Luke's Hospital, Kansas City, MO, USA
e-mail: jkozinn@saint-lukes.org

Abbreviations

GA	General anesthesia
IR	Interventional radiology
MAC	Monitored anesthesia care
PCA	Patient-controlled analgesia
RA	Regional anesthesia/nerve blocks
SA	Spinal anesthesia/paravertebral/epidurals
SIR	Society of Interventional Radiology

K. Rajput et al. (eds.), *Pain Control in Ambulatory Surgery Centers*,
https://doi.org/10.1007/978-3-030-55262-6_19

Introduction

Interventional radiology (IR) specializes in minimally invasive image-guided procedures, and as such, most of the work of IR can be readily performed in an ambulatory/outpatient setting. While most interventional work can be performed with local anesthesia and conscious sedation/analgesia, certain patient factors may warrant further workup by an Anesthesiologist. The typical interventionalist is trained and credentialed to provide up to moderate sedation; however, as procedures become increasingly complex-technically or life-threatening the proceduralist is at risk of becoming distracted from careful titration of sedatives and analgesics and dedicated monitoring by a trained Anesthesiologist may make all of the difference. Additionally, peri-procedural discomfort has been a common indication for admission. However, thanks to the assistance of our anesthesia/pain management colleagues several of the procedures that have historically required an overnight stay can safely, and more cost-effectively, be performed in a controlled manner allowing discharge of the patient to the comfort of their own home the same day.

Pre-Procedure Considerations

Pre-Procedure Imaging

Interventional radiology often has the benefit of cross-sectional and radiographic imaging readily available during pre-procedure planning. Immediate pre-procedural review of the patient's prior imaging is vital, not only for IR-procedure planning purposes, but also for anesthesia planning. It is important to assess for any anatomic variants or abnormalities that may place patient risk at higher risk for sedation or intubation if needed (e.g., a patient with a large thoracic mass compressing the trachea (Fig. 19.1)). Examples of airway challenges in IR include tumors of the head and neck, trismus, SVC syndrome, and Mallampati class IV. Review of imaging can also help to predict the level of intraprocedural patient discomfort which is likely to occur (Fig. 19.2) and plan for appropriate analgesia.

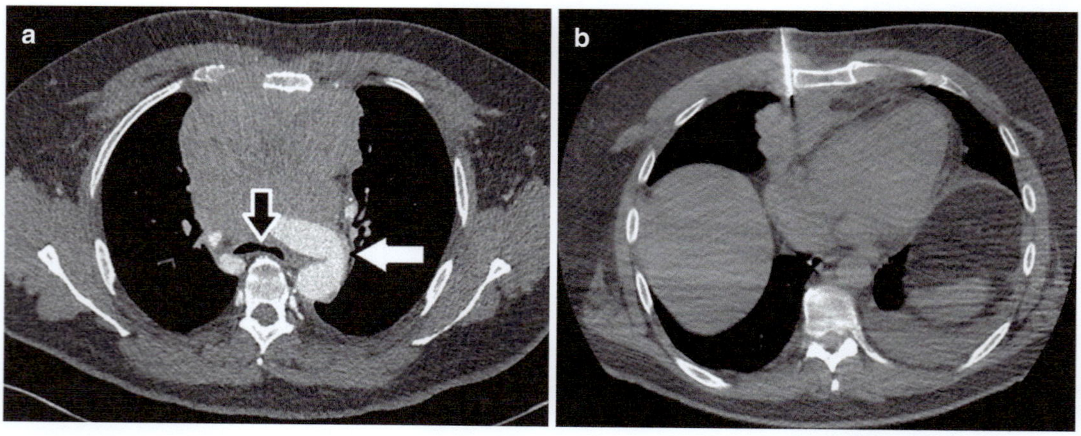

Fig. 19.1 Mediastinal mass biopsy. Contrast-enhanced CT in a patient with a large anterior mediastinal mass (**a**). Notice the significant mass effect with shift of the middle mediastinal structures posteriorly resulting in kinking of the aortic arch [White Arrow] as well as high-grade narrowing of the trachea [Black Arrow]. Discussion and coordinated pre-procedure planning between the interventionalist and anesthetist determined that a lower approach would be preferable (**b**). Even though this approach was closer to the heart, it was felt any increased mass effect from potential post-biopsy bleeding would not further compress the trachea. The procedure was performed as a coordinated effort with Anesthesia at bedside during the procedure and for the recovery. The patient did well and did not require emergent intubation

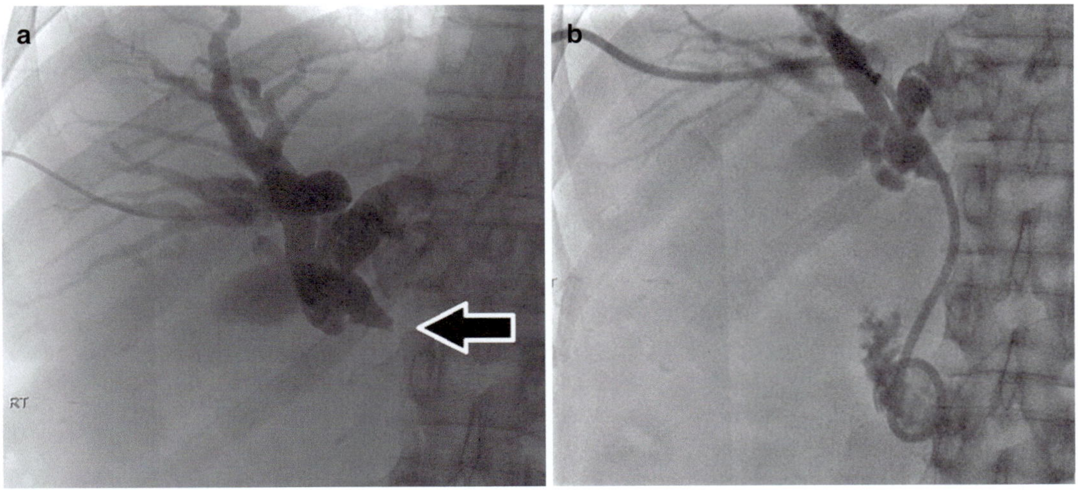

Fig. 19.2 Diagnostic cholangiography and intervention. Cholangiogram (**a**) via right-sided percutaneous access demonstrates a diffusely dilated biliary system with abrupt cutoff at the level of the proximal/mid common bile duct [Arrow] secondary to a known duodenal small bowel carcinoma. Placement of the percutaneous biliary drain (**b**) required initial wire passage and balloon cholangioplasty of the occluded common bile duct, a procedure which many patients find exquisitely painful. In this case, general anesthesia facilitated breath-holding during initial access, plus provided the analgesia necessary to properly position the biliary drain

History and Physical Exam

A thorough history and physical exam is necessary before any interventional procedure. High-risk populations include those patients with obesity, chronic obstructive pulmonary disease (COPD), obstructive sleep apnea (OSA), coronary artery disease, chronic renal failure, patients with drug addiction, and elderly and pediatric populations. Special care must be taken to appropriately manage their anesthetic status during and after interventional procedures.

Obese patients are at increased risk of gastroesophageal reflux and oversedation. Additionally, upper airway obstruction can occur in obese patients at relatively lighter levels of sedation. Obese patients are also more susceptible to the respiratory depressant effects of sedative agents; therefore, drug doses should be estimated based on estimated lean body mass instead of total body mass [1–4].

COPD results in increased risk of adverse respiratory events from sedation and analgesia. Placing these patients in the supine position impairs chest muscle wall function, thus impeding appropriate oxygenation. All prescribed bronchodilators should be given before the procedure is started. Similarly, special care should be taken in patients with a history of dependent sleep apnea or who are prescribed a continuous positive airway pressure (CPAP) machine [2, 4].

Coronary artery disease is commonly present in patients undergoing interventional radiology procedures, particularly when treating peripheral artery and renovascular disease. Inadequate sedation can increase the risk of an acute cardiac event in these patients due to increased cardiac demand. Excessive sedation can precipitate cardiac sequelae by inducing hypotension or hypoxemia. Appropriate anesthesia in coronary artery disease patients will reduce or maintain myocardial oxygen demand and preserve myocardial oxygen supply. Patients should take all routine cardiac medication, such as beta blockers, the day of the procedure [2, 4].

Patients with chronic renal failure are at increased risk for overdose because many anesthetic medications are excreted renally. Special care should be taken in the selection of neuromuscular blockers, as there is increased risk of recurarization in patients receiving renally cleared neuromuscular blocking agents. In these patients longer-acting opioids should be avoided; however, shorter-acting agents such as fentanyl are thought to be safe. Elderly patients can experience longer-lasting and more pronounced effects from sedatives and analgesics because of changes in bioavailability and reduction in drug metabolism. Finally, pediatric patients tend to require higher doses by weight and have more narrow safety margins than adults [2, 4].

Careful attention should also be paid to the patient's medication list and habits, in particular regarding opiates and/or anxiolytics. Patients with drug addiction are at risk for withdrawal and should take all replacement medications (e.g., methadone) the day of their procedure. Chronic use (and abuse) can lead to tolerance of these drugs, requiring greater than typical dosing and narrowing the window between effective moderate and deep sedation. This issue is exacerbated when the proceduralist is also the provider of moderate sedation. When encountering a patient with a potential tolerance to these medications, anesthesia monitoring or alternate forms of pain management should be considered, especially as the degree of complexity and/or the pain associated with the procedure increases.

Physical examination in the pre-procedure setting includes careful assessment of the patient's airway before any level of sedation is administered. Beyond assessing for obesity, COPD, or apnea as previously discussed, the physical examination also includes determination of the Mallampati airway classification, assessment of any facial dysmorphism (e.g., micrognathia), jaw protrusion, and degree of and difficulties with neck flexion and extension. Any potential problems that may inhibit airway management or ventilation must be considered. Additionally the patient should be asked about any previous history of difficult intubations or other events involving anesthesia [2, 4].

ASA Risk Stratification

The American Society of Anesthesiologist (ASA) classification, originally designed for surgical patients, is a relatively simple way to categorize and communicate a patient's pre-anesthesia medical comorbidities and is routinely used in IR [5].

Table 19.1 American Society of Anesthesiologist (ASA) physical classification system

Score	Description
ASA I	Normal, healthy patient
ASA II	Mild systemic disease (e.g., obesity with BMI 30–40, current smoker, well-controlled DM or HTN)
ASA III	Severe systemic disease (e.g., obesity with BMI >40, ESRD on hemodialysis, alcohol dependence, poorly controlled DM or HTN)
ASA IV	Severe illness that is a constant threat to life (e.g., recent stroke or MI, sepsis, severe heart failure)
ASA V	Moribund patient, not expected to survive without operation (e.g., ruptured AAA, massive trauma)
ASA VI	Brain-dead patient; organs being harvested

There should be a low threshold for anesthesiologist consultation when dealing with ASA class III and IV patients based on any number of potentially complicating factors, including procedure type/length, type of patient comorbidities, etc. In general ASA class V patients should not be encountered in the outpatient setting, and if so should be transferred to the nearest emergency department without delay

In most cases, ASA class I or II patients may be managed by the performing interventionalist; any higher may require special considerations. Refer to (Table 19.1) for further details [5–7].

Certain patient populations and procedures may merit risk stratification using additional metrics as well. The Cardiac Risk Index determines the adverse event rate and may prompt a cardiology consultation before the procedure is performed. Metrics of patient performance status used in risk-benefit determination of procedures include the Eastern Cooperative Oncology Group (ECOG) scale commonly used in oncology patients, plus the Model for End-Stage Liver Disease (MELD) and Child-Pugh scores employed with chronic liver disease and HCC patients respectively [8].

Bleeding Risk

A routinely encountered issue is that of pre-procedure coagulation parameters (i.e., PT/INR and CBC with hemoglobin/platelet count) and the determination of if or when anticoagulants and antiplatelet medications should be discontinued, and restarted. Pre-procedure labs can often add significant expense and are generally indicated only in certain patient scenarios. In general, the determination centers around whether a procedure is classified as "low bleeding risk" or "high bleeding risk." Examples of low bleeding risk procedures include: tunneled catheter placements, venous catheter exchanges, superficial biopsies, thoracentesis, paracentesis, diagnostic arteriography, and venography, to name a few. Examples of high-risk procedures include: solid organ percutaneous tumor ablations, arterial interventions, biliary interventions, deep abscess drainage, nephrostomy placement, and vertebral augmentations. The 2019 "Society of Interventional Radiology Consensus Guidelines for the Periprocedural Management of Thrombotic and Bleeding Risk in Patients Undergoing Percutaneous Image-Guided Interventions—Part II: Recommendations" by Patel et al. provides the most comprehensive recommendations generally accepted at this time [9].

In general, for *high-risk* cases pre-procedural routine labs are recommended, and consensus threshold recommendations include: (1) INR, correct to within range of $\leq$1.5–1.8, and, (2) platelets, transfuse if <50 × 10^9/L. In general, for *low-risk* cases pre-procedural routine labs are not recommended. However, if they are obtained consensus thresholds include: (1) INR, correct to within range of $\leq$2.0–3.0, and, (2) platelets, transfuse if <20 × 10^9/L. The guidelines go on to state that low-risk pre-procedural laboratory testing may be indicated for "patients who have an inherently higher bleeding risk, such as those with hematologic disorders, patients receiving certain chemotherapies, or those who are receiving anticoagulant therapy." It is also important to note that these parameters, even if elevated, may not be applicable in patients with chronic liver disease as they may not correlate with true bleeding risk given altered hemostasis in these patients [9].

Guidelines for temporarily stopping preprocedural anticoagulation are based in the same framework. In general, consensus guidelines do not recommend withholding anticoagulants if the procedure is low-risk for bleeding, the exception being the glycoprotein IIb/IIa inhibitors where the long-acting abciximab (ReoPro) should be held for 24 h and the short-acting eptifibatide (Integrilin) and tirofiban (Aggrastat) should be held 4–8 h before the procedure. For high-risk procedures withholding is generally recommended. An exhaustive list of all of the various types of anticoagulants and antiplatelets and how long they should be discontinued before the procedure is beyond the scope of this chapter and the interested reader can refer to the aforementioned 2019 SIR guidelines for further details. Traditional non-steroidal anti-inflammatory drugs (NSAIDs) inhibit platelets transiently and have no recommendation to be held in high-risk procedures. Aspirin irreversibly binds to platelet cyclooxygenase-1 (COX-1) and recommendations are that it be held for 3–5 days prior to the procedure. Reinitiation post-procedure can typically occur the following day assuming the procedure was uncomplicated, although some agents may be started sooner [9].

Contrast-Induced Nephropathy

Assessment of creatinine and calculation of GFR is important in patients undergoing angiographic procedures with intravascular iodinated contrast as baseline renal function and preexisting renal insufficiency is the most predictive risk factor for the development of post-contrast acute kidney injury (PC-AKI) (a correlative diagnosis), and potential contrast-induced nephropathy (CIN) (a causative diagnosis). Definitions vary, but one commonly used criteria has been absolute increase of serum creatinine 0.5 mg/dL over baseline. This is typically transient, peaking at 4–7 days, and <1% of patient's will progress to (often temporary) dialysis or ESRD [10]. Whether CIN is a real entity and contrast is truly an independent risk factor for AKI is currently debated in the literature; however, assuming it is there is little evidence that it poses a significant risk in patients with a stable estimated glomerular filtration rate (eGFR) >30 mL/min/1.73 m^2. On the other hand, the presence of an AKI due to any of the various potential causes before contrast administration may place patients at greater than normal risk of CIN even if their GFR is within "acceptable ranges." Additionally most studies also evaluate volumes of contrast typically utilized for CT, and interventionalists may find themselves using more or less than this. Thus each practice and interventionist must determine their own acceptable criteria, which may need to be evaluated on a case-by-case basis [11, 12].

Regardless of the system, if the patient is determined to be at risk then use of another agent (e.g., CO_2) can be considered. However this is often not possible and if iodinated contrast is required then the general recommendation for prophylaxis is pre- and post-procedure volume expansion (assuming the patient has no contraindications such as CHF) for renal protection. Proposed regimens for outpatients consist of higher than usual oral hydration for 12–24 h before and after the procedure. For elective inpatients (or outpatients admitted overnight pre- or post-procedure) hydration with 1 mL/kg/h for 12 h before and after and/or boluses (e.g., 500 mL) 1 h before and after the procedure can be considered [10]. Nephrotoxic medications have not been proven as independent risk factors for CIN; however, if clinically feasible discontinuing them for 1–2 days pre-procedure may be prudent. Metformin is not a separate risk factor; however, if CIN does develop there is an increased risk of lactic acidosis, therefore recommendations are to withhold metformin for at least 48 h after contrast administration until renal function has been re-evaluated and found to be normal in a select group of patients, namely those with a known AKI, eGFR < 30, or undergoing interventional studies that may result in emboli to the renal arteries [11].

Adverse Reactions to Contrast

A thorough H&P should include any history of adverse reactions to iodinated contrast. Adverse reactions to contrast are uncommon with modern low osmolality iodinated contrast material (LOCM). Combined (physiologic and allergic-like) reaction rates to LOCM are reported at 3.1%. Allergic-like reactions are rare, reported in 0.6% of patient's overall and severe in only 0.04%. A prior allergic-like reaction is the greatest risk factor for future allergic-like reactions, conferring a fivefold increased risk. Other factors, such as asthma, may also increase the risk of an adverse reaction; however, the effect is relatively small and current guidelines do not recommend restricting contrast or pretreating for any factor other than a prior reaction, nor do they recommend pretesting [11, 13].

Various studies have shown that corticosteroid premedication reduces the overall risk of contrast reactions; however, data showing a decreased risk of severe reactions is lacking. Breakthrough reactions are also known to occur, and even when pre-medicated a patient with a history of prior allergic-type reaction has a 3–4 times higher risk than the ordinary reaction rate of the general population. When breakthrough reactions do occur they are usually of similar severity to the index reaction [11]. Therefore, in most practices a previous severe reaction to IV contrast (e.g., laryngeal edema, severe bronchospasm, or hypotension/shock) typically precludes future use of iodinated contrast, and in this scenario an alternate procedure or alternate contrast agent (e.g., CO_2) should be considered. For those with a history of more mild reactions (such as itching or hives) pre-procedure prophylaxis may be considered as listed in (Table 19.2). Select contrast reactions, and recommended treatments, can be found in (Table 19.3).

Patient Positioning and Breath-Holding

Patients must be able to lie still in the necessary position for the duration of the procedure, including peri-procedural preparation and on-table recovery. This should be discussed with patient during the pre-procedure workup, and if the patient is unable to lie flat for a minimum of 20 min or longer depending on the procedure (whether due to pain and discomfort, respiratory issues, or altered mental status), then consider-

Table 19.2 Proposed contrast reaction pretreatment regimens

Outpatient/nonemergent	13-h prep utilizing prednisone 50 mg PO at 13, 7, and 1 h plus diphenhydramine 50 mg PO/IV/IM at 1 h OR methylprednisolone PO at 12 and 2 h (with optional diphenhydramine 50 mg at 1 h).
Urgent	Methylprednisolone sodium succinate (e.g., Solu-Medrol) 40 mg IV or hydrocortisone sodium succinate (e.g., Solu-Cortef) 200 mg IV immediately, and then every 4 h until contrast medium administration. Or if the patient is allergic to both of these dexamethasone sodium sulfate (e.g., Decadron) 7.5 mg IV can be substituted at the same intervals (but is considered less desirable) plus diphenhydramine 50 mg IV 1 h before contrast medium administration.
Emergent situations	Solu-Medrol 40 mg IV or Solu-Cortef 200 mg IV plus diphenhydramine 50 mg IV 1 h before contrast administration may be attempted; however, evidence for efficacy is lacking in the literature.

Adapted from the ACR Manual on Contrast

Note that while studies have shown that pretreatment with corticosteroids decreases the overall incidence of contrast reactions data for efficacy in the setting of severe reactions is limited. Thus extreme care should be taken, or preferably an alternate study performed, in those with a history of severe reactions such as laryngeal edema or anaphylaxis with hypotension/shock

Table 19.3 Common contrast reactions and treatments

Hives	PO/IV diphenhydramine 25–50 mg +/− IM epinephrine (1:1000) 0.1–0.3 mg
Facial/laryngeal edema	O_2 6–10 L/min IM epinephrine (1:1000) 0.1–0.3 mg
Bronchospasm	O_2 6–10 L/min IM epinephrine (1:1000) 0.1–0.3 mg Albuterol nebulizer.
Hypotension with tachycardia (anaphylaxis)	O_2 6–10 L/min, elevate legs Bolus 500–1000 mL normal saline Consider IM epinephrine (1:1000) 0.1–0.3 mg or IV Epi (1:10,000) 0.1 mg
Hypotension with bradycardia (vasovagal)	O_2 6–10 L/min, elevate legs Bolus 500–1000 mL normal saline IV atropine 0.6–1 mg.
Pulmonary edema	O_2 6–10 L/min + elevate head of bed if possible + IV furosemide (Lasix) 20–40 mg
Seizure	O_2 6–10 L/min Protect patient tongue/airway and suction as needed + lay patient on side if possible IV lorazepam (Ativan) 2–4 mg if not spontaneously resolving

Adapted from the ACR Manual on Contrast and Wible

Several of the most commonly encountered contrast reactions with potential treatment responses are listed. In any situation there should be a low threshold for considering calling a rapid response, code blue, or 911 depending on the context, especially if patient shows any sign of potential decompensation.

ation should be given to anesthesia management for patient comfort and safety.

Fluoroscopic and computed tomographic (CT) imaging may require breath-holding to ensure adequate procedural conditions or optimal diagnostic results. Certain invasive procedures are possible through patient-controlled breath-holding (e.g., percutaneous lung biopsy), but more significant procedures often require involuntary breath-holding and deep sedation (e.g., percutaneous biliary drain placement, or transjugular portosystemic shunt (TIPS) placement) not achievable while the patient is responsive.

Diagnostic magnetic resonance imaging (MRI) studies are especially sensitive to patient motion, given the number of required sequences and the length of time of most scans. Patient inability to lie still, whether due to pain, anxiety, or other factors, may require the presence of an anesthetist, who must face certain unique challenges related to the MRI facility and MRI-compatible equipment.

Peri-procedural Considerations: Sedation and Monitoring

The majority of interventional procedures are performed using a combination of local analgesia and moderate sedation administered and monitored by the performing interventionalist. Lighter levels of sedation include local only, regional/nerve blocks and minimal sedation/anxiolysis. Heavier sedation, including deep sedation, monitored anesthesia care (MAC), and general anesthesia (GA) require attendance of a qualified anesthesia provider. The intended level of sedation should be determined as part of the pre-procedure workup to allow time for proper workup and preparation by the anesthesia team if necessary [2].

Moderate sedation is defined as a level of sedation allowing the patient to retain the ability to respond purposefully to verbal/tactile stimuli while also maintaining their cardiovascular and respiratory function and maintaining their own airway. Typical agents include a benzodiazepine plus an opioid given "to effect" which act synergistically to provide adequate pain control and relaxation without loss of vital functions such as airway control [2].

Benzodiazepines result in anxiolysis, anterograde amnesia, sedation, and muscle relaxation, as well as enhancing the effect of gamma-aminobutyric acid (GABA), resulting in decreased neuronal excitability. Midazolam (Versed) is often the preferred agent. Adult doses typically start at 0.5–2 mg as an initial bolus, with 0.5–1 additional boluses as needed based on patient response and procedure length. Onset of effects are seen 2–5 min after injection (therefore one should wait at least 5 min before redosing), and the elimination half-life is 1.5–2.5 h, although this may be prolonged in patients with comorbidities. Care should be taken in debilitated patients, the elderly, or those with respiratory, hepatic, or renal insufficiency. Midazolam is metabolized in the liver and excreted in the urine; thus hepatic or renal dysfunction may cause decreased metabolization or accumulation of byproducts with prolonged effects. In certain patient populations, including children, elderly, and demented patients, a paradoxical reaction may be seen, with agitation, involuntary movements, hyperactivity, hostility, and/or excitement. If needed midazolam can be reversed with flumazenil (a competitive inhibitor at the benzodiazepine binding site on the $GABA_A$ receptor), dosed at 0.2 mg which can be repeated every 45 s for up to three total doses. Flumazenil half-life is 15–30 min and redosing may be needed to avoid resedation. Side effects include lowered seizure threshold and potential agitation [8].

Opioids result in analgesia by acting as an agonist on the opioid receptors (typically targeting the μ receptor). Potential side effects include confusion, somnolence, constipation, nausea, hypoventilation/apnea, bradycardia, pruritus, and chest wall rigidity (especially in pediatric patients). Fentanyl (Sublimaze) is often the preferred agent. Adult doses typically start at 25–50 μg as an initial bolus, with 25–50 μg additional boluses as needed. Onset may be seen immediately to up to 5 min after injection. The termination of the effect of fentanyl is primarily due to redistribution; thus, additional doses tend to have a longer duration due to tissue saturation and care should be taken with longer procedures. If necessary, naloxone (an opioid antagonist) can be given to reverse the effects, in doses of 0.4 mg up to every 4 min as needed [8]. It is important to note that obese patients tend to be more sensitive to the respiratory-depressant actions of narcotics and are also more prone to airway obstruction.

All patients receiving moderate sedation will generally receive supplemental oxygen and should have adequate intravenous access throughout the procedure and until the patient is no longer at risk of cardiopulmonary depression. Patients must be continuously monitored to assess the depth of sedation and to recognize complications of oversedation, including respiratory depression, airway compromise, and cardiovascular instability. A unique consideration with interventional radiology procedures is that the need may arise for patient cooperation during the procedure. For example, during angiography, it may be necessary for a patient to hold his or her breath. It is critical that the degree of sedation be tailored to the needs of the procedure, and that oversedation is avoided when a cooperative patient is required [14].

Vigilant vital sign monitoring is required, both during and after the procedure. Careful monitoring is important to detect sedation related instability early, allowing prevention or swift intervention. Variations in patient vitals may also be indicative of certain procedural complications, which may not be immediately apparent to the performing interventionalist; in such cases where an anesthetist is present they should not hesitate to inform the proceduralist (especially if they are intensely focused on a difficult procedure) so that a pause and careful assessment can occur. For example, an evolving retroperitoneal hemorrhage often will first become apparent by tachycardia, decreasing blood pressure, and increased patient restlessness.

Standard monitoring includes continuous pulse oximetry, capnography, electrocardiogram (ECG), and temperature and blood pressure monitoring. Depending on the procedure, blood pressure can be monitored by either a non-invasive blood pressure cuff or an arterial line. Both respiratory rate and end-tidal CO_2 are monitored by capnography. When using capnography in conjunction with a nasal cannula, an acute increase or decrease in end-tidal CO_2 may indicate hypoventilation or airway obstruction. A pulse oximeter is not a substitute for continuous capnography. Hypoxemia is often a late finding of hypoventilation, especially when supplemental oxygen is used [15].

While there are many types and causes of arrhythmias that an ECG might record, special attention should be paid to any acute onset arrhythmias, especially when working near the heart, as they may indicate a malpositioned wire or catheter. Blood pressure should be considered in relation to the procedure type as well as the other vital signs, e.g., hypotension and desaturation may signify either a contrast reaction, oversedation, or a developing pneumothorax during a procedure near or involving the chest, while hypotension and tachycardia could indicate an allergic reaction, active bleeding, or developing septic shock (in cases dealing with infection) [14].

Post-Procedural Recovery

Recovery length and appropriate discharge criteria may vary depending on the patient, procedure, procedure length, any complications that may have or end up occurring, amount of sedation, and often have institution specific components. Certain procedures may even entail a planned overnight admit, such as if the perceived procedural risk is higher than usual or if a significant amount of pain control is expected (e.g., ablations and embolizations often require PCA pumps at least overnight). The plan for post-procedure monitoring should be determined and documented ahead of time, with the understanding that complications do happen which may need an escalation of care. Each IR facility in which sedation is administered should develop recovery and discharge criteria that are suitable for their patients based on procedure type and level of sedation. Regardless of other factors in the post-procedural period it is important to closely monitor all patients for sedation complications, signs of significant or ongoing blood loss, and signs of developing sepsis in select scenarios [2, 4].

After transfer to the post anesthesia care unit (PACU), patients should be monitored for their level of sedation/responsiveness, heart rate, blood pressure, oxygen saturation, respiratory rate, etc. A proposed schedule would be frequent monitoring every 15 min twice in a row and then every 30 min until the patient has returned to a pre-procedural baseline for at least 30 min (often at least 2–4 h depending on provider or institution).

One should recognize that decreased procedural stimulation and delayed drug absorption/elimination may contribute to residual sedation and cardiorespiratory depression during the recovery period. This is especially important if a reversal agent such as Narcan (naloxone) or

Romazicon (flumazenil) was given and the monitoring time should be extended to at least 1.5–2 h after the last administration so that patients do not become resedated after reversal effects have worn off. Additionally, patients who have undergone general anesthesia should be monitored by an anesthesiologist or trained unit staff member until their airway reflexes are recovered [2, 4].

Special care and certain precautions should be taken when monitoring vascular access sites into arteries and large veins in the post-procedure period, specifically for the development of hematomas or other complications which may delay discharge or require further intervention. This is especially important when larger diameter sheaths are used. Venous access is relatively safe and any bleeding is typically stopped with the application of manual pressure for 2–5 min post-procedure. Significant post-procedure bleeding/hematoma incidence is reported at a rate of only around 0.2%. With upper venous access (e.g., internal jugular) head of bed elevation is recommended in order to decrease venous pressure. For lower access (specifically translumbar, transhepatic, or femoral) at least 2 h of bed rest should be considered [8].

When dealing with arterial access, and higher arterial pressures, extra precautions are necessary. The common femoral artery is the most frequent access site overall. After sheath removal manual compression is needed for a minimum of 15 min, and sometimes much longer than that. Use of sandbags or other weighted devices is not recommended as they may hide a developing hematoma. Even after manual compression is stopped frequent groin checks and close monitoring for any vital sign abnormalities or increasing pain is needed to exclude rebleeding. Bedrest with immobility of the accessed leg is recommended for at least 6 h after the procedure, and then the patient may get out of bed with assistance. Newer closure devices have been released that decrease complication rates and may reduce the required bedrest time to as little as 1–2 h; however, close monitoring should still occur. Patients should avoid heavy lifting or other strenuous activity for a week after the procedure. If the patient has a history of constipation or chronic opioid use, or will be discharged with a prescription for such, consider prescribing a stool softener as well to prevent straining. Hematoma formation will be encountered most frequently following femoral access; however, these are typically minor (2–10% incidence) and only rarely require further treatment in <0.5% of cases. Other complications are much less frequent, with thrombosis and distal embolization occurring <1% of the time and pseudoaneurysms, arteriovenous fistulas, and dissections (which are often self-limiting with retrograde access) occurring in less than 0.2% of cases. The other common site of access is the radial artery, which has the advantage of being more easily compressed and being superficial; thus, developing complications are more noticeable. Inflatable wristbands are available that allow for automatic and adjustable compression to achieve nonocclusive hemostasis for 30–120 min. After the determined time the band can be deflated slowly over 15 min, and easily reinflated if bleeding re-occurs. Patients can be discharged as soon as 30 min after the band is successfully removed. The most commonly encountered complication is radial artery occlusion, occurring in 6–10% of patients; however, this is usually asymptomatic in patients with a patent ulnar-palmar arch (ulnar artery patency should always be confirmed before radial access is obtained). Other access sites either harbor relatively higher complication rates (e.g., brachial artery) or are used only in certain circumstances (direct aortic access or lower leg arteries) and will be encountered much less frequently [8, 16].

The use of scoring systems may increase confidence in appropriateness for discharge. The Aldrete post anesthesia score is an accepted guideline. Refer to (Table 19.4) for further details [17]. Additional considerations may include well-controlled nausea and pain.

Outpatients should be discharged in the care of a responsible adult who will be able to report any complications and safely transfer the patient back home. Patients should be instructed to not drive, operate heavy machinery, or make important decisions for 24 h following the procedure. It is important to note that even if the patient is alert and oriented amnesia can persist for hours after

Table 19.4 Aldrete score

Aldrete post anesthesia recovery score					
Score	Consciousness	Activity	Respiration	Circulation	Color
2	Fully awake, alert	Moves all extremities voluntarily/on command	Breaths deeply/normally and coughs freely	BP within 20% of pre-procedure value	Normal
1	Arousable to voice	Moves two extremities voluntarily/on command	Dyspnea or shallow breathing	BP within 20–50% of pre-procedure value	Pale
0	Not responsive	Does not move	Apnea	BP >50% different from pre-procedure value	Cyanotic

Adapted from Aldrete and Wible
The Aldrete Post Anesthesia Recovery Score is an example of a post-procedural metric which may be used to assess appropriateness for discharge. Each of these parameters is scored from 0 to 2 and a total score of 9 or 10 is generally recommended for appropriate discharge

sedation, and written as well as verbal instructions (including diet, medications, activities, and a phone number to be called in case of emergency) should be provided to the patient/caregiver [2, 4, 14].

Special Considerations by Location

Fluoroscopy Suite

Standard equipment present and regularly maintained includes a nearby crash cart, oxygen supply, and basic airway devices. Ideally, the IR suite would be built and equipped with general anesthesia in mind similar to standard operating theatres; however, this is not always the case. The combination of multiple monitors used by IR, the X-ray tube/image intensifier, anesthesia machines, and/or other specialized equipment may mean space is tight, and the physical layout may limit anesthesiologist access to the patient. Additionally, resources often taken for granted, such as gas supply lines or electrical outlets, may not be as readily available in a procedure room when compared to the OR. Managing a difficult airway may be made even more challenging in the IR suite if specialized airway instruments are unavailable. It is important to note that if needed fluoroscopy is readily available to confirm and sometimes even to facilitate (i.e., with cross-table lateral views) placement of endotracheal tubes or central lines, and the anesthesiologist should not hesitate to ask the interventionalist for a quick visualization if there is any concern [18].

In emergent cases requiring resuscitation, specifically chest compressions, special care should be taken with table positioning. When extended from the neutral position, much of the patient's weight may be centered over free air and not the table base. This unstable positioning may result in a springboard type effect during compressions which has been shown to decrease the overall quality of CPR [19]. Returning the table to the neutral position should also be considered if feasible, to reduce the magnitude of the lever effect.

Ionizing radiation is a unique hazard to not only the patient but the providers in the room as well. In some scenarios, e.g., neurointerventional procedures where the interventionalist is working via groin access, anesthesiologists may even find themselves closer to the detector with higher overall dose than the interventionalist performing the case [20]. At least basic radiation safety training, including fundamental knowledge of the dangers of direct and scattered radiation, should be considered for anyone who may find themselves regularly in the IR suite. Additionally, at a minimum well-maintained appropriate thickness (0.5 mm) lead aprons and thyroid shields should be worn, and standalone glass lead screens should be made available.

CT Suite

CT and CT-fluoroscopy carry many of the same considerations as the regular fluoroscopy suite, with a few exceptions. Available devices may be even more limited, especially when the CT room is used primarily for diagnostic and not procedural purposes. Dealing with multiple lines and tubes, and/or large or difficulty positioned patients, may be even more troublesome than in the regular fluoroscopy suite. Procedures often require patients to move in and out of the scanner repeatedly. Conversation between the anesthetist and interventionalist before the procedure begins will help to ensure a safe and optimal setup.

The radiation dose to staff in the room is often lower in CT versus fluoroscopy, especially in CT only cases where staff may completely leave the room during image acquisition. Regardless, if anesthesia plans to stay in the room, particularly in cases where CT fluoroscopy is to be utilized, proper lead shielding should be worn.

MRI Suite

MRI scanners produce magnetic fields which are powerful enough to draw in oxygen tanks, anesthesia machines, or any other ferromagnetic object at projectile speeds, potentially injuring the patient or healthcare providers. MRI zone safety training should be provided for anyone who may find themselves near the MRI scanner at any point. If acute intervention is required, it is vital to ask the MRI technologist to remove the patient from the MRI room Zone 4 into the Zone 3 area. Zone 3 acts as a buffer area where emergency situations, such as codes or anaphylaxis, can be managed.

MRI scanners are quite loud, and the bore is longer than that of a CT scanner. Patients with claustrophobia, phonophobia, or inability to lay still (e.g., pediatric or demented patients) may not tolerate the typical oral or IV anxiolytics prescribed by the ordering physician. In certain cases, general anesthesia may be needed. If necessary, induction and securing the airway should occur outside of the MRI room, and there should always be a contingency plan for patients receiving lighter levels of sedation in case of acute decompensation. There is a variety of MRI safe hardware, including ventilators, infusion pumps, etc., which may or may not be available in an outpatient/ambulatory setting. Alternatively providers may choose to run plastic tubing from a safe area and manage devices from there. Whatever the setup anesthetists should familiarize themselves with what is available prior to beginning any case.

Special Considerations by Procedure

There are numerous potential procedures interventional radiology may perform in an outpatient/ambulatory setting, and it is not the purpose of this chapter to go into even a brief description of the majority of them. For the routine IR procedure indications and considerations for anesthesia are patient centric, differ very little, and are discussed in more detail above. The goal of the following pages then is to discuss more atypical cases, either because pain management/anesthesia is more frequently asked to be involved, anesthesia can help in a unique way beyond MAC or GA, or there are special considerations during the peri- or post-procedural periods. When MAC is chosen for these more complicated procedures, a plan should be in place as to how to safely convert to GA if a complication arises. This plan should be agreed upon by all team members as it may necessitate movement of the table or the image intensifier.

Complications are of course site-, procedure-, and pathology-specific. However, what qualifies as a complication and how the degree/severity is assigned often differ between individual publications. Where possible, rates reported below are taken from studies or publications utilizing aggregate data. Unless otherwise specified, the qualification of a complication as "Minor" or "Major" will follow the SIR Quality improvement guidelines metrics. Namely, "Minor" complications require nominal or no therapy, and may or may not result in a simple overnight admission for observation. "Major" complications, on the other hand, result in either an unplanned admission or a prolonged hospital stay and may require more significant therapy, additional interventions, and/or other management as needed [21]. The interested reader may refer to the SIR quality improvement guidelines for more complete pooled success and complication rate data for a variety of the most commonly seen procedures (available at JVIR.org). Additionally, the subsequent sections will focus on intraprocedural or immediate post-procedural considerations; more delayed complications will rarely need to be managed by an anesthesiologist.

Non-Vascular Procedures

Chest Interventions—Biopsy and Thoracostomy

Transthoracic interventions carry a risk of pleural injury resulting in pneumothorax or effusion/hemothorax, and of hemoptysis whenever the lung parenchyma is crossed. Pneumothoraces are actually quite common, reported following 12–45% of cases of percutaneous biopsy. The majority are small and can be managed in an expectant manner, with patient reassurance, supplemental oxygen, and placing the patient recumbent in a "puncture side down" position [22]. Follow-up expiratory chest radiographs should be considered at 1 h intervals for 3 h total, or sooner if the patient is symptomatic. Persistently asymptomatic patients without evidence of an enlarging pneumothorax can generally be safely discharged at this time. Thoracostomy tubes are needed in 2–15% of cases after biopsy (typically due to patient symptoms, large size (>30% of the chest cavity), or increasing size on follow-up radiographs). Chest tubes can usually be managed in an outpatient/ambulatory setting (in many cases removed the same day after several hours of observation). Major pneumothoraces requiring further intervention only occur in 1–2% of cases [23, 24]. Minor hemoptysis is also not uncommon, reported to occur in 5–10% of biopsies, but usually self-limited and managed similarly to a small pneumothorax. Major hemorrhage, reported to occur only 0.5% of the time, is the leading cause of mortality following needle biopsy [25].

Drainage of pleural collections results in pneumo-/hemothorax requiring further intervention with an unplanned chest tube/catheter in 0–12% of cases. Attached to a closed system gravity drainage bag these may be safely managed in an outpatient setting as well, although follow-up will depend on output and need for subsequent intervention.

Biopsies of small pulmonary nodules can be challenging, especially when a nodule is in a difficult location such as behind a rib or near the diaphragm. The location of pulmonary lesions changes with patient respiratory motion, and this effect increases in magnitude the closer a lesion lies to the lung bases. These factors as well as the inherent temporal limitations when using CT, even CT fluoroscopy, can affect the biopsy success rate. In routine cases with cooperative patients, practicing breath holds beforehand can be beneficial. Use of a homolateral phrenic nerve block to cause unilateral diaphragm paralysis has also been described, which may help in some cases with nodules especially close to the diaphragm [26].

For patients under GA, mechanical ventilation with the ability to control and pause respiration can provide significant benefit. Lung biopsy using apneic oxygenation techniques (with aid of a paralytic such as rocuronium) has been described, with changes in continuous positive airway pressure in the range of 5–10 cm H_2O allowing for differing levels of lung expansion, thus facilitating access to difficult to reach nodules [27]. It is important to note, however, that some publications recommend against positive pressure ventilation due to a potential increased risk of pneumothorax. Endotracheal anesthesia does appear to increase the risk of air embolism (theorized to occur when either the tip of the needle is placed into a pulmonary vessel, or causes a bronchial-venous or alveolar-venous fistula). However, symptomatic air embolism is rare, described in less than 0.5% of cases [28].

Hepatobiliary Interventions

Cholangiography indications include its use for diagnostic purposes, dilation of strictures, planned decompression of obstructed biliary ducts via biliary stent placement, access for stone removal, access for tissue sampling, or when biliary access is required in a patient with altered post-surgical anatomy. Pain encountered during percutaneous biliary interventions can be severe and is the most commonly encountered adverse event [29]. Biliary procedures have been associated with the highest rates of sedation complications in IR [30]. Patient discomfort can be difficult to manage with moderate sedation and some proceduralists may prefer general anesthesia, particularly in cases where multiple interventions/dilations or placement of larger caliber catheters is anticipated. Other alternatives for pain control that have been described include epidural anesthesia, intercostal nerve block, celiac plexus block, and paravertebral blocks [30].

Obstructed patients commonly experience jaundice, itching, nausea/vomiting, and diarrhea, and are at risk for developing cholangitis and sepsis with hemodynamic instability. Sepsis and hemorrhage are both reported in approximately 2.5% of cases. Bacterial colonization of the obstructed biliary tree is quite common, even before intervention, and prophylactic antibiotics are generally recommended. One study reported positive bile cultures in 43% of patients with malignancy and 68% of patients with benign disease even during initial percutaneous drain placement [31]. Placement of either a percutaneous drain or stent provides an iatrogenic route for enteric bacteria, and colonization of the biliary tree is presumed when repeat procedures and exchanges are performed. Several studies have documented minor infectious complications in half or more of cases, most commonly cholangitis followed by bacteremia [32]. Patients and providers should be warned that, though often transient, fevers, rigors, or other infectious symptoms are not unexpected. Other infectious/inflammatory conditions, including abscess, peritonitis, cholecystitis, or potentially pancreatitis are encountered as a major complication in 1.2% of cases.

SIR practice guidelines recommend that >95% of primary cholecystostomy drainage procedures be performed to manage acute cholecystitis or remove gallstones, and <5% as a route for biliary tract access (transhepatic is the preferred route in this setting). While cholecystostomy is typically a bridge to surgery, in some cases it may be a more permanent measure and recurrent drain exchanges may be needed. Primary cholecystostomy will not often be encountered in an outpatient/ambulatory setting, but the major complication rates for percutaneous cholecystostomy tubes are similar to percutaneous biliary interventions, as follows: sepsis 2.5%, hemorrhage 2.2%, and other infectious inflammatory processes 1.6%. The rate of post-procedural mortality is higher, 2.5% as opposed to 1.7% for biliary drainage, but this may be partially attributable to increased comorbidities in this population [33].

Percutaneous Nephrostomy

Drainage of urinary obstruction (secondary to renal stones, malignancy, and iatrogenic causes) is by far the most common indication for percutaneous nephrostomy placement [34]. Non-infected urinary tract obstruction will constitute the majority of cases in an average practice, with pyonephrosis or infected hydronephrosis (due to lithiasis in >50% of these cases) encountered as the indication only 19% or less of the time. Other less common reasons for nephrostomy placement include urinary diversion, such as in the setting of a urinary leak or fistula, and access for a variety of percutaneous interventions, including diagnostic nephrostogram, stricture dilation, endoscopic procedures, and medication delivery directly to the collecting system, among others [35]. Depending on the clinical scenario IR may place an external (percutaneous) nephrostomy, an internal-external nephroureteral stent or an internalized (double-J) ureteral stent. If a nephrostomy or nephroureteral drain is to be left for any significant length of time routine exchanges are recommended as crystalline components from the urine can deposit on the catheter leading to malfunction. General recommendations for exchange of percutaneous nephrostomy drains and percutaneous nephroureteral stents are 1–2 months after initial placement and then at approximately 3-month intervals thereafter, or sooner if the patient develops signs of collecting system infection or obstruction. Internal ureteral stents are typically removed or exchanged by Urology [34, 36].

Patients undergoing these procedures may have varying degrees of discomfort; some may tolerate exchanges with local anesthetic, while others require significant sedation. Patient pain-tolerance should be assessed and documented during initial placement to aid planning for future drain/stent exchanges. Nephrostomy drains can be placed utilizing ultrasound and fluoroscopy, but at times CT may be required. Patients generally must be able to lie prone or lateral decubitus. A significantly encrusted nephrostomy drain/nephroureteral stent can become adherent to adjacent tissues and therefore quite painful to exchange over a wire. Consideration of MAC or even GA in select cases may be prudent. Use of intercostal and paravertebral nerve blocks as well as epidurals has also been described, and these may be especially useful in patients where percutaneous nephrostomy access is utilized for further procedures such as nephrolithotomy [37].

Major procedural complications include bleeding and infection. A study of non-emergent, outpatient nephrostomy placement noted fevers and chills without hypotension to occur in 21% of patients [38]. Transient peri-procedural bacteremia should be expected in the setting of a known obstruction, even without frank pyonephrosis; another study in a cohort of 160 patients reported at least low-grade fevers in 100% of cases after emergent placement [39]. When encountered, patients with signs of potential infection should be monitored closely for the development of septic shock with hemodynamic instability. Sepsis is reported in approximately 1–3% of cases, but this number increases to 7–9% in the setting of pyonephrosis [34]. Prophylactic antibiotic treatment should be considered before percutaneous nephrostomy procedures.

Patients should be counseled to expect minor transient hematuria following nephrostomy procedures, occurring in up to 95% of cases [34]. Major post-procedural hemorrhage requiring transfusion is rare, reported to occur in 1–4% of patients, while the need for further intervention to halt bleeding (arterial embolization or nephrectomy) is reported to occur in 0.1–1% of cases. This may be due to hematuria or an enlarging retroperitoneal hematoma. Persistent gross hematuria, hypotension, anemia, or increasing flank pain more than 3–5 days after nephrostomy placement should prompt further workup.

Adrenal Mass Biopsy and Interventions

Improvements in CT and MR techniques and protocols resulting in improved accuracy in diagnosing benign adrenal lesions have obviated the need for biopsy in many cases. However, when biopsy of an otherwise indeterminate renal nodule/mass is requested and truly necessary these cases must be approached with care, especially when pheochromocytoma is suspected (e.g., in the setting of uncontrolled secondary hypertension and/or positive urinary catecholamines). Overall, complications for adrenal biopsy are similar to biopsies elsewhere (i.e., hemorrhage is seen most commonly); however, while rare, inadvertent biopsy or intervention on a primary or metastatic pheochromocytoma with resultant catecholamine release may precipitate a severe hypertensive crisis with hemodynamic instability, severe hyperthermia, and/or multiorgan system failure including cardiac (e.g., cardiomyopathy or myocardial infarction) and pulmonary (edema or acute respiratory distress syndrome) manifestations. Careful pre-procedure workup should be performed, and anesthesia involvement is strongly recommended in potential cases. Appropriate pre-procedure prophylaxis is needed with first an α-adrenergic blockade, typically with the non-selective phenoxybenzamine, and then a direct-acting vasodilator, such as nitroprusside, should also be available during the procedure. Later, β1-adrenergic blockade can be considered for persistent tachycardia (non-selective β blockers should not be used as β2 blockade may also precipitate hypertension). Use of alpha-methyl-p-tyrosine, an inhibitor of catecholamine synthesis, has also been described [40–42].

Vascular

Dialysis Fistulas

A basic or complete metabolic panel (BMP or CMP) to assess potassium and HCO_{3-} levels is generally indicated prior to hemodialysis access intervention, especially if the patient has missed one or more dialysis sessions. Serum potassium >6 mmol/L, acidosis, or any evidence of EKG changes is a relative contraindication to access intervention. Additionally, severe fluid overload and pulmonary edema may result in the patient's inability to lay flat without respiratory distress. Each center should work in concert with their local nephrologists to determine local cutoff values and protocols, as a temporary catheter may need to be placed to allow for dialysis and return to acceptable levels before an intervention is performed [8, 43].

The use of regional anesthesia during outpatient treatment of dysfunctional hemodialysis fistulae may be useful as an addition or alternative to intravenous sedation and analgesia. Ultrasound-guided supraclavicular brachial plexus blocks, typically with lidocaine, for arteriovenous hemodialysis access procedures can be performed in the outpatient setting with high technical success with minimal complications and excellent pain control. Use of US-guided techniques improve the procedure time and effectiveness of brachial plexus blocks with fewer inadvertent vascular punctures. The use of US guidance has been shown to lower the known complications of supraclavicular nerve block, including intravascular injection, hematoma, seizure, arrhythmia, pneumothorax, Horner syndrome, inadvertent phrenic nerve involvement, and local anesthetic systemic toxicity [44].

Approximately 1.5 per 10,000 nerve blocks result in seizures and arrhythmias secondary to intravascular injection of local anesthetic. Treatment consists of airway management, benzodiazepines for seizure control, and lipid emulsion therapy for arrhythmia and cardiac toxicity. Phrenic nerve involvement is a known complication of supraclavicular blocks. This can lead to respiratory failure in patients with COPD or who are otherwise frail. The infraclavicular block can be used for most hemodialysis fistula placements without the risk of diaphragmatic paralysis. An axillary block can also be used, which has even a lower risk of pneumothorax, but requires supplementation of the musculocutaneous nerve [44].

Aortoiliac and Peripheral Arterial Disease Interventions

Endovascular interventions to revascularize lower extremity occlusive lesions of peripheral arterial disease (PAD) include angioplasty, placement of a stent or covered stent-graft, mechanical atherectomy, or thrombolysis, often achieved via percutaneous groin access. Endovascular aneurysm repair (EVAR) is a minimally invasive procedure to treat abdominal aortoiliac aneurysms. Patients undergoing aortoiliac EVAR, or lower extremity arterial revascularization, typically have a greater than average incidence of comorbidities including coronary artery disease, diabetes mellitus, COPD, and renal insufficiency. Local, regional, neuraxial, and general anesthesia have all been described for anesthetic management of endovascular and open lower extremity PAD revascularization. Rates of conversion from EVAR to open repair is low (<2%); however, the anesthesiologist must be prepared for the possibility of massive bleeding and emergent open repair. Immediate access to rapid infusion devices and an arterial line should be strongly considered.

The main advantages of regional anesthetic techniques are a blunted stress/inflammatory response, avoidance of mechanical ventilation in a patient with severe cardiopulmonary diseases, and targeted postoperative analgesia. During EVAR, general anesthesia may be more practical than regional anesthesia due to ease of blood pressure control and the ability to aid imaging via involuntary breath-holding. If aneurysm rupture occurs, the patient's airway is already secure. There is so far no overwhelming evidence to demonstrate any mortality or morbidity benefits of one technique over another. Additionally, it is important to note that the procedural success of EVAR does not appear to be related to the mode of anesthesia.

Complications anesthesiologists must be aware of during EVAR include spinal cord ischemia (incidence of 0.21%), post implantation syndrome, and arterial rupture or dissection. Respiratory failure occurs in 2.9% of patients undergoing EVAR. An arterial blood gas can be helpful in guiding intraoperative ventilator management and predicting the likelihood of postoperative mechanical ventilation. Also, it is advisable to convert those on short-acting beta agonists to longer-acting agents in the perioperative period to minimize the potential issues with withdrawal [45].

Transjugular Intrahepatic Portosystemic Shunt (TIPS)

TIPS is a vital noninvasive technique for interventional radiologists to assist in the management of portal hypertension and its sequela, including: recurrent and/or uncontrollable variceal hemorrhage, gastropathy, refractory ascites, hepatic hydrothorax, hepatorenal and Budd-Chiari syndromes, as well as recurrent portal hypertension after liver transplantation. Initial creation of a TIPS can be a relatively long and complex procedure compared to usual cases in IR, and patient cooperation, including with breath holds, can be vital. Due to the nature of the disease, the cirrhotic patient is more likely to have higher than usual perioperative risk (i.e., ASA III or IV) and will often have coagulation impairment in addition to potential cardiac, respiratory, and renal dysfunction. Reduced hepatic and renal function may also affect metabolization and secretion of several preferred agents for sedation and analgesia. Thus, while TIPS may be successfully performed under moderate sedation, many authors recommend a pre-procedural anesthesia consult, with a low threshold for intraprocedural MAC or GA as indicated.

Major procedural complications of TIPS are reported to occur at a rate of approximately 3%. Hemorrhage is the most common. Significant hemobilia is reported in up to 2% of cases, hepatic arterial injury in up to 1%, and hemoperitoneum in up to 0.5% of cases. Significant biliary peritonitis may also occur in up to 1% of cases. Minor complications include contrast related renal injury, access hematoma, and transient fever which is reported in up to 2% of cases. Transient findings related to acute increases in cardiac output as well as central venous and pulmonary pressures such as acute pulmonary edema or congestive heart failure may also be seen and patients should be closely monitored after the procedure until their hemodynamic status stabilizes [8, 46].

Endovascular Embolization and Percutaneous Ablation

Non-emergent endovascular embolization is used throughout the body to treat a variety of pathology including hepatic malignancy, uterine fibroids, hypersplenism, soft tissue vascular malformations, and to decrease the risk of intraoperative bleed, during nephrectomy for instance. Pain control is the foremost peri-procedural concern related to non-emergent endovascular embolization of organs and soft tissues. As the endovascular arterial embolization targets more distal vessels, the amount of organ parenchyma embolized increases, and patient pain may occur sooner and to a greater degree due to organ ischemia. For example, pre-nephrectomy total renal artery embolization is known to be quite painful with onset occurring before completion of the embolization procedure. Even partial organ embolization (e.g., hepatic segmental chemoembolization) or select target embolization (e.g., embolization of a single soft tissue metastasis) may require an overnight admission for pain control. This is in contrast to emergent endovascular embolization of active bleed in which case the primary peri-procedural concern is often related to fluid resuscitation and stabilization rather than pain control, and in which acute treatment of arterial bleed does not typically result in pain since distal organ ischemia does not occur.

Postembolization syndrome is commonly encountered after distal transarterial embolization or chemoembolization and is reported in up to 90% of cases. It consists of a constellation of flu-like symptoms including fever, nausea/vomiting, pain, and sometimes malaise occurring within the first 72 h. It is usually self-limiting and is thought to relate to cell death from hypoxia leading to the release of breakdown products, inflammatory mediators, and vasoactive substances from the tumor and/or adjacent normal tissues [8]. Symptom control is the key to management, with use of antiemetics and oral or IV pain control as needed. Some patients may benefit from a PCA pump. Combination therapy with NSAIDs may be useful to decrease inflammation-associated pain and reduce overall opioid use. Additionally, use of regional and neuraxial anesthesia (such as paravertebral or intercostal nerve blocks for hepatic/renal embolization or epidurals or superior hypogastric nerve block for uterine artery embolization) has been described to decrease opioid use in the post-procedural period [47, 48].

Absolute alcohol may be used to permanently embolize organs or treat certain varieties of arteriovenous malformations. It may also be injected percutaneously, for example to ablate hepatocellular carcinoma within a cirrhotic liver or produce permanent neurolysis of the celiac plexus. If the use of absolute alcohol (especially volumes >10 mL) is planned either intravascularly or percutaneously, anesthesia involvement should be strongly considered. Large volumes of absolute alcohol can result in significant procedural pain, plus potential cardiopulmonary collapse when delivered into the systemic circulation. Careful consideration of whether to utilize MAC or GA should occur as part of a thorough pre-operative assessment in these patients.

Concerning percutaneous ablations, thermal techniques will be encountered most commonly and may be performed using cold (cryoablation) or heat (radiofrequency (RF) or microwave ablation (MWA)) to induce irreversible cellular injury. Postablation syndrome has been described and is analogous to postembolization syndrome; however, postablation syndrome is reported to occur less frequently, in ~50% or less of cases [49].

Cryoablation overall is reported to be less painful than RF or MWA, likely due to freezing of adjacent nerves, and the procedure is often performed under moderate sedation. Cryoablation works by forming an ice ball often several centimeters in diameter. The ice ball is actively or passively thawed before refreezing occurs in a process which can span up to 30 min. Active bleeding can begin from treated tissues as thawing occurs, either at completion of the procedure or during one of the intermediate thawing cycles. Any attempt to forcibly remove the probes before the ice ball has completely thawed (e.g., to reposition a prone patient supine in a code situation) may result in tissue avulsion and hemorrhage (Fig. 19.3). Coordination is essential, and before every freezing event the IR team should alert the anesthesia team, who should assess the patient for any potential signs of a sudden decompensation within the next few minutes.

Anesthesiologists will likely find themselves involved more often with RF and MWA ablations than with cryoablation. In contrast to cryoablation, heat-based RF and MWA techniques typically are more painful, but with less risk of peri-procedural hemorrhage since the mechanism of action results in electrocautery of vessels during tissue ablation. Specific to RF, generators create a closed electrical circuit when an alternating current is applied through

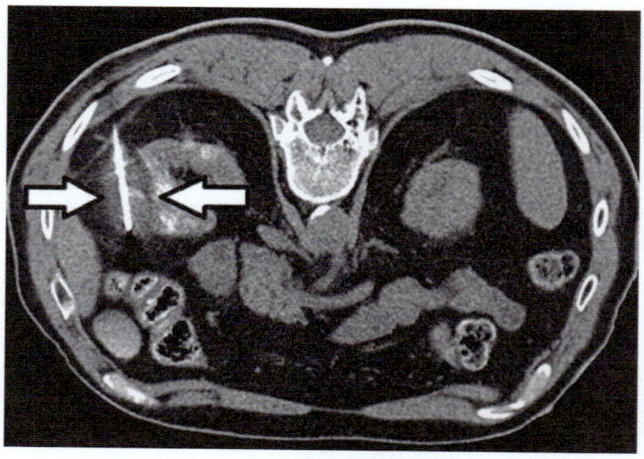

Fig. 19.3 Cryoablation. A non-contrast CT image is shown during renal cryoablation of an interpolar right renal lesion via an intercostal approach. A probe is seen within a peripheral right renal lesion. A 3–4 cm ovoid ice ball (hypodense/darker grey) has formed around the probe [Arrows]. Contrast staining of the right kidney is present, related to a prior angiogram. Inadvertent removal of the probe before thawing is complete can fracture the ice ball, lacerating the kidney or intercostal structures, resulting in severe hemorrhage

the probe, into surrounding soft tissues, and back to the generator through a grounding pad typically applied to the patient's thigh [50]. This electrical circuit can result in complications in regard to cardiac implantable electronic devices, i.e., pacemakers and defibrillators. When used near the heart, potential electromagnetic interference from RF ablation may incorrectly activate tachyarrhythmia modes potentially resulting in asynchronous pacing, inhibition of pacing, inappropriate shocks, or may even reset the device. Certain defibrillators may have an "Electrocautery Protection Mode" or similar setting which disables tachycardia detection and therapy, or they may have an option to directly turn Tachy Mode off or be programmed to asynchronous mode. External pacing support may be beneficial in pacemaker-dependent patients. No matter the type of device, careful review of specific manufacturer recommendations is necessary before any procedure is begun. Additionally, circuits may be formed with other nearby implanted metal devices, e.g., surgical clips or metal orthopedic implants, which when small may result in tissue heating in unintended locations; extra special care should be taken in these cases, especially in patients under GA who are otherwise unable to report burning sensations in a non-target structure.

Microwave ablation is an alternative heating technique which uses a high-hertz alternating electric field to cause oscillation of water molecules around the probe which is positioned within the target tissue. The oscillation of water molecules produces local heat via friction. No grounding pad is necessary, and no electrical circuit is formed. Theoretically, MWA has less chance of interference with other implanted metal (including pacemaker and defibrillators) than does RF, and this has been borne out in some smaller studies. However, device manufacturer recommendations are either limited or advise caution and it may be prudent to take similar precautions as one would with RF ablation in these patients. Each institution/practitioner should develop their own policies [51].

Uterine Artery Embolization

Uterine artery embolization (UAE) for the management of symptomatic uterine fibroids is a minimally invasive alternative to surgical management. Presenting symptoms vary, and include heavy or prolonged bleeding, cramping, pressure, pain, or urinary symptoms. The procedure is commonly associated with significant pelvic pain, historically requiring at least overnight admission for pain control, typically with a combination of NSAIDS and PCA [52]. Regional anesthesia can also play a role as well. Some practitioners may routinely utilize epidural anesthesia. Superior hypogastric nerve block (SHNB), used extensively to control chronic pelvic pain associated with endometriosis and pelvic cancer, can also improve pain control during the first 24 h after UAE [48]. Beyond the general considerations of pain, postembolization syndrome, and complications of arterial access other immediate intra- and post-procedural complications are rarely encountered [53].

Neurointerventional

General Considerations

Both neuroangiography and neurointerventional procedures can be safely performed on an outpatient basis. One study demonstrated the most common indications for both diagnostic and interventional cases in an outpatient setting are cerebral aneurysms (around 50%), followed by vascular malformations [54]. Beyond routine workup, special attention should be paid to the neurological exam, specifically any pre-existing deficits, to be sure of the patient's baseline. Additionally, a careful review of medications as well as a pre-procedure coagulation profile is necessary as many procedures will require specific pre-/intra- and further postoperative anticoagulation (e.g., clopidogrel (Plavix) with intravascular stents) [55].

Non-acute, ambulatory center diagnostic cerebral angiography without planned intervention can be managed using minimal or moderate sedation. Even basic cerebral angiography carries a risk of neurological complications however, occurring in approximately 0.9–4.0% of cases. TIAs are the most common at approximately 2.1%, while complications resulting in permanent disability or death are less common, occurring in approximately 0.2% of patients [56]. Frequent neurological assessments by nursing while in recovery, as well as a dedicated neurological exam by a physician before discharge, should be considered.

Anesthetic considerations specific to neurointerventional procedures include maintaining neuromuscular relaxation during potentially lengthy procedures to improve image quality and reduce the rates of catheter associated complications, the ability for rapid induction and recovery from sedation to enable immediate neurologic examinations, the ability to induce controlled hyper- or hypotension, administration of anticoagulation and/or rapid reversal thereof as needed, and management of emergencies such as bleeding complications and elevated intracranial pressures [57]. Placement of an arterial line should be considered to allow for rapid and accurate adjustment of blood pressure levels. Additionally, in ventilated patients close monitoring of capnography is vital. A rise in $PaCO_2$ while in the range of 20–60 mmHg results in vasodilation and increased cerebral blood flow (CBF), while a lowering of $PaC0_2$ lowers CBF via vasoconstriction. Thus, hyperventilation may be induced when a reduction in CBF is needed [58].

A shared risk of neurointerventional procedures is that of non-targeted vascular occlusion. Potential etiologies include thromboembolism, vessel dissection and injury from catheters or wires, coil migration/misplacement, or vasospasm. Regardless of the etiology when discovered, either on imaging or during intra- or post-procedural neurological exam, the primary goal should be to initiate controlled hypertension, in order to increase the mean arterial pressure (MAP) and promote collateral flow to the ischemic areas. Depending on the etiology further intervention or further medical therapy such as with anticoagulants or even thrombolytic therapy may be necessary [59].

Intracranial Aneurysms

The prevalence of intracranial aneurysms is around 2.3% in adults without specific risk factors, with multiple aneurysms occurring in 20–30% of this population [60, 61]. Most aneurysms are small and incidental. Unruptured aneurysms are typically found during workup for other conditions, with only 10–15% of cases being symptomatic, often due to mass effect of a larger aneurysm with symptoms depending on location (e.g., headache, cranial nerve palsies, strokes and TIAs, seizures, or other poorly defined neurological symptoms) or possibly due to trace bleeding that irritates the meninges but not enough to classify as truly ruptured. Compared to neurosurgical clipping, endovascular coiling of unruptured aneurysms carries a lower morbidity and mortality rate at 1% and 4% respectively and is the preferred treatment in most centers for patients with enough expected remaining life years to see benefit. New medical devices, such as arterial flow diverting devices like the Pipeline Embolic Device, may even further improve these outcomes [62].

General anesthesia is preferred for endovascular coiling of unruptured aneurysms in most centers; however, depending on the preferences of the operator and patient factors successful treatment under MAC as well as conscious sedation has been reported. The primary anesthetic goal during endovascular treatment is prevention of aneurysm rupture. Acute elevations in blood pressure, especially during intubation, emergence, or due to inadequate sedation may increase the risk of rupture and careful monitoring is needed. General recommendations include maintaining systolic blood pressure below 120 mmHg. Clinical signs of a sudden rise in blood pressure should alert the anesthetist to the possibility of a rupture, and the radiologist should be notified to look for a contrast extravasation. If found, immediate goals are to reverse heparin or other coagulation, lower blood pressure and ICP, initiation of osmotic agents, and seizure control. Once bleeding is halted the coiling often continues and blood pressure may be raised to check for extravasation as needed. Rarely further intervention such as ventriculostomy or surgery may be necessary [59]. Further management of complications of subarachnoid hemorrhage, namely re-bleeding and vasospasm, typically warrants admission and management in the intensive care unit or dedicated neurological floor.

AVMs

Arteriovenous malformations (AVMs) are an abnormal, complex, tangle of vessels consisting of feeding arteries, a central nidus and draining veins. Central nervous system locations of AVMs include intracerebral, dural, and spinal. The overall annual rupture rate of brain AVMs is described between 1% and 4%. The most common presenting symptom of AVMs is rupture with hemorrhage (approximately 50%) [63]. Unruptured AVMs may also be found incidentally, or present most commonly with seizures, or with other more vague neurological symptoms including headache, dizziness, or other deficits depending on location [64].

Embolization of larger brain AVMs is commonly performed preoperatively before surgical resection or radiotherapy. However, in many small- to medium-sized AVMs, embolization may be used as definitive treatment with a reported 71–100% obliteration rate of the nidus [65]. Embolizations are commonly performed under GA. Besides the general benefits of a motionless patient when using superselective catheters, GA can provide more precise control of factors which contribute to ICP and cerebral blood blow. Hypocapnia reduces ICP and CBF in normal intracranial vessels; however, flow through the abnormal feeding vessels of an AVM are affected to a lesser degree. Deliberate hypotension can slow flow through all vessels, including the AVM. Both of these conditions may be helpful at the moment of treatment, to increase the shunting of embolic materials toward the AVM and decreasing the overall flow rate so that it arrests there [66].

There are some cases in which MAC is preferred. Specifically, if due to location, vessel tortuosity, or other factors, a superselective catheter is not able to completely reach the lesion and more proximal embolization is being considered or if there is other concern for non-target embolization a superselective anesthesia functional examination (SAFE) may be required. SAFE is reminiscent of the Wada test, with injection of either lidocaine (typically extra-axial arteries) or sodium amytal (intra-axial arteries) (more recent reports using propofol have also been described [67]) through the catheter while positioned at the sight of potential embolization to exclude placement proximal to the origin of normal vessels supplying eloquent cortex or important regions of the brainstem or spine. After injection a repeat neurological examination is performed, which necessitates an awake patient, preferably with minimal or no sedation [68].

Reported treatment complication rates vary, in part related to size and location of the AVM, with complications resulting in permanent morbidity occurring in 3–11% of cases and mortality rates reported as 1–2% [69]. Complications may arise from TIAs or infarction due to non-target embolization, pulmonary embolism due to systemic shunting, hemorrhage, accidental gluing of the catheter to the vessel, and other potential neurological complications such as seizures. Treatment of an AVM shunt can also lead to hyperperfusion, either due to sudden occlusion of a large or high flow AVM shunt or due to venous occlusion of normal brain parenchyma (in cases where there is mutual drainage).

Carotid Angioplasty and Stenting

Ischemic strokes account for the vast majority of cerebral infarcts. Extracranial atherosclerotic disease is implicated in approximately 15–20% of cases. While carotid endarterectomy (CEA) is the gold standard for patients with significant enough stenosis (>60% in asymptomatic and >50% in symptomatic patients based on age/surgical risk), various trials have demonstrated carotid angioplasty and stenting (CAS) to have similar to only mildly inferior outcomes, and this approach may be considered in otherwise poor surgical candidates and based on local provider expertise. In some studies, the subgroup of asymptomatic high surgical risk patients may also show a short-term benefit from CAS over CEA [70, 71].

The preferred route of anesthesia is MAC over GA, allowing for intraprocedural monitoring of neurological function. Hemodynamic instability (HDI), related to stretching of adventitial baroreceptors in the carotid body during treatment, can result in hypotension, bradycardia, hypertension, or asystole potentially necessitating cardiac pacing or other medical treatment. The frequency of HDI has been reported in up to 42% of cases [72]. Prolonged HDI (symptoms lasting >30 min refractory to medical treatment) may necessitate admission to the ICU; described risk factors include plaque calcification, eccentric stenosis, and extensive plaque distribution [73]. Another rare but important to recognize complication is cerebral hyperperfusion syndrome (CHS), characterized by ipsilateral headache, hypertension, seizure, focal neurologic deficits, and/or reperfusion related intracranial hemorrhage. The incidence of CHS and ICH after CAS has been reported from 0.44–11.7% to 0.36–4.5% respectively [74]. Blood pressure control is the key to management, with agents that are not direct vasodilators, such as a calcium channel blocker or nitroprusside, as these also induce cerebral vasodilation and increase cerebral perfusion [55].

References

1. Chau EHL, Lam D, Wong J, Mokhlesi B, Chung F. Obesity hypoventilation syndrome: a review of epidemiology, pathophysiology, and perioperative considerations. Anesthesiology. 2012;117(1):188–205.
2. Martin ML, Lennox PH. Sedation and analgesia in the interventional radiology department. J Vasc Interv Radiol. 2003;14(9):1119–28.
3. Aberle D, Charles H, Hodak S, O'Neill D, Oklu R, Deipolyi AR. Optimizing care for the obese patient in interventional radiology. Diagn Interv Radiol. 2017;23(2):156–62.
4. Moran TC, Kaye AD, Mai AH, Bok LR. Sedation, analgesia, and local anesthesia: a review for general and interventional radiologists. Radiographics. 2013;33(2):E47–60.
5. American Society of Anesthesiologists. American Society of Anesthesiologists: ASA physical status classification system. Am Soc Anesthesiol Website. 2019. https://www.asahq.org/standards-and-guidelines/asa-physical-status-classification-system. Accessed June 2020.
6. Practice Guidelines for Moderate Procedural Sedation and Analgesia 2018: A Report by the American Society of Anesthesiologists Task Force on Moderate Procedural Sedation and Analgesia, the American Association of Oral and Maxillofacial Surgeons, American College of Radiology, American Dental Association, American Society of Dentist Anesthesiologists, and Society of Interventional Radiology. Anesthesiology. 2018;128(3):437–79.
7. American College of Radiology. ACR–SIR practice parameter for sedation/analgesia. ACR Website. 2015. https://www.acr.org/-/media/ACR/Files/Practice-Parameters/Sed-Analgesia.pdf. Accessed June 2020.
8. Wible BC. Diagnostic imaging: interventional procedures. Philadelphia: Elsevier; 2017.
9. Patel IJ, Rahim S, Davidson JC, Hanks SE, Tam AL, Walker TG, et al. Society of Interventional Radiology Consensus Guidelines for the Periprocedural Management of Thrombotic and Bleeding Risk in Patients Undergoing Percutaneous Image-Guided Interventions—Part II: Recommendations: Endorsed by the Canadian Association for Interventional Radiology and the Cardiovascular and Interventional Radiological Society of Europe. J Vasc Interv Radiol. 2019;30(8):1168–1184.e1.
10. Gupta RK, Bang TJ. Prevention of contrast-induced nephropathy (CIN) in interventional radiology practice. Semin Intervent Radiol. 2010;27(4):348–59.
11. American College of Radiology. ACR manual on contrast media. ACR Website. 2020. https://www.acr.org/Clinical-Resources/Contrast-Manual. Accessed June 2020.
12. Davenport MS, Perazella MA, Yee J, Dillman JR, Fine D, McDonald RJ, et al. Use of intravenous iodinated contrast media in patients with kidney disease: consensus statements from the American College of Radiology and the National Kidney Foundation. Radiology. 2020;294(3):660–8.
13. Mervak BM, Davenport MS, Ellis JH, Cohan RH. Rates of breakthrough reactions in inpatients at high risk receiving premedication before contrast-enhanced CT. Am J Roentgenol. 2015;205(1):77–84.
14. American Society of Anesthesiologists Task Force on Sedation and Analgesia by Non-Anesthesiologists. Practice guidelines for sedation and analgesia by non-anesthesiologists. Anesthesiology. 2002;96(4):1004–1.
15. American Society of Anesthesiologists. Standards for basic anesthetic monitoring. Am Soc Anesthesiol Website. 2015. https://www.asahq.org/standards-and-guidelines/standards-for-basic-anesthetic-monitoring. Accessed June 2020.
16. Gradinscak DJ, Young N, Jones Y, O'Neil D, Sindhusake D. Risks of outpatient angiography and interventional procedures: a prospective study. Am J Roentgenol. 2004;183(2):377–81.

17. Aldrete JA. The post-anesthesia recovery score revisited. J Clin Anesth. 1995;7(1):89–91.
18. Arulvelan A, Soumya M, Santhosh K. Fluoroscopy assisted tracheal intubation in a case of anticipated difficult airway: fail safe devices can also fail. Saudi J Anaesth. 2015;9(3):321–3.
19. Yamada T, Ito M, Urai H, Ueda Y, Maki H, Baba R. Effect of using a cardiac catheterization table-stabilizing stick on the quality of cardiopulmonary resuscitation in the cardiac catheterization laboratory: a simulation-based study. J Interv Cardiol. Hindawi. 2019;2019:e6303978. https://www.hindawi.com/journals/jitc/2019/6303978/. Accessed June 2020.
20. Anastasian ZH, Strozyk D, Meyers PM, Wang S, Berman MF. Radiation exposure of the anesthesiologist in the neurointerventional suite. Anesthesiology. 2011;114(3):512–20.
21. Sacks D, McClenney TE, Cardella JF, Lewis CA. Society of Interventional Radiology clinical practice guidelines. J Vasc Interv Radiol. 2003;14:S199–202.
22. Kandarpa K, Machan L, Durham J. Handbook of interventional radiologic procedures. 5th ed. Philadelphia: Wolters Kluwer; 2016. p. 441–4.
23. Gupta S, Hicks ME, Wallace MJ, Ahrar K, Madoff DC, Murthy R. Outpatient management of postbiopsy pneumothorax with small-caliber chest tubes: factors affecting the need for prolonged drainage and additional interventions. Cardiovasc Intervent Radiol. 2008;31(2):342–8.
24. Brown KT, Brody LA, Getrajdman GI, Napp TE. Outpatient treatment of iatrogenic pneumothorax after needle biopsy. Radiology. 1997;205(1):249–52.
25. Protopapas Z, White CS, Miller BH, Miller DL, Westcott JL. Transthoracic needle biopsy practices: results of a nationwide survey. Radiology. 1996;201:770–2.
26. Carrero E, Arguis P, Sánchez M, Sala-Blanch X. Ultrasound-guided phrenic nerve block for CT-guided percutaneous pulmonary fine-needle aspiration biopsy. J Vasc Interv Radiol. 2015;26(4):597–9.
27. Kjaergaard B, Zepernick PR, Bergmann A, Jensen HK, Mladenovic M, Rasmussen BS. CT-guided needle lung biopsy is possible during apneic oxygenation: a case series. Multidiscip Respir Med. 2013;8(1):73.
28. Freund MC, Petersen J, Goder KC, Bunse T, Wiedermann F, Glodny B. Systemic air embolism during percutaneous core needle biopsy of the lung: frequency and risk factors. BMC Pulm Med. 2012;12:2.
29. Venkatanarasimha N, Damodharan K, Gogna A, Leong S, Too CW, Patel A, et al. Diagnosis and management of complications from percutaneous biliary tract interventions. Radiographics. 2017;37(2):665–80.
30. Culp WC, McCowan TC, DeValdenebro M, Wright LB, Workman JL, Culp WC. Paravertebral block: an improved method of pain control in percutaneous transhepatic biliary drainage. Cardiovasc Intervent Radiol. 2006;29(6):1015–21.
31. Yee A, Ho C. Complications of percutaneous biliary drainage: benign vs malignant diseases. Am J Roentgenol. 1987;148(6):1207–9.
32. Khardori N, Wong E, Carrasco CH, Wallace S, Patt Y, Bodey GP. Infections associated with biliary drainage procedures in patients with cancer. Rev Infect Dis. 1991;13(4):587–91.
33. Saad WEA, Wallace MJ, Wojak JC, Kundu S, Cardella JF. Quality improvement guidelines for percutaneous transhepatic cholangiography, biliary drainage, and percutaneous cholecystostomy. J Vasc Interv Radiol. 2010;21(6):789–95.
34. Dagli M, Ramchandani P. Percutaneous nephrostomy: technical aspects and indications. Semin Intervent Radiol. 2011;28(4):424–37.
35. Pabon-Ramos WM, Dariushnia SR, Walker TG, d'Othée BJ, Ganguli S, Midia M, et al. Quality improvement guidelines for percutaneous nephrostomy. J Vasc Interv Radiol. 2016;27(3):410–4.
36. Makramalla A, Zuckerman DA. Nephroureteral stents: principles and techniques. Semin Intervent Radiol. 2011;28(4):367–79.
37. Liu Y, Yu X, Sun X, Ling Q, Wang S, Liu J, et al. Paravertebral block for surgical anesthesia of percutaneous nephrolithotomy: care-compliant 3 case reports. Medicine (Baltimore). 2016;95(28):e4156.
38. Cochran ST, Barbaric ZL, Lee JJ, Kashfian P. Percutaneous nephrostomy tube placement: an outpatient procedure? Radiology. 1991;179(3):843–7.
39. Lee WJ, Patel U, Patel S, Pillari GP. Emergency percutaneous nephrostomy: results and complications. J Vasc Interv Radiol. 1994;5(1):135–9.
40. Sharma KV, Venkatesan AM, Swerdlow D, DaSilva D, Beck A, Jain N, et al. Image-guided adrenal and renal biopsy. Tech Vasc Interv Radiol. 2010;13(2):100–9.
41. Ramachandran R, Rewari V. Current perioperative management of pheochromocytomas. Indian J Urol. 2017;33(1):19–25.
42. Venkatesan AM, Locklin J, Lai EW, Adams KT, Fojo AT, Pacak K, et al. Radiofrequency ablation of metastatic pheochromocytoma. J Vasc Interv Radiol. 2009;20(11):1483–90.
43. Dariushnia SR, Walker TG, Silberzweig JE, Annamalai G, Krishnamurthy V, Mitchell JW, et al. Quality improvement guidelines for percutaneous image-guided management of the thrombosed or dysfunctional dialysis circuit. J Vasc Interv Radiol. 2016;27(10):1518–30.
44. Hull J, Heath J, Bishop W. Supraclavicular brachial plexus block for arteriovenous hemodialysis access procedures. J Vasc Interv Radiol. 2016;27(5):749–52.
45. Kothandan H, Haw Chieh GL, Khan SA, Karthekeyan RB, Sharad SS. Anesthetic considerations for endovascular abdominal aortic aneurysm repair. Ann Card Anaesth. 2016;19(1):132–41.
46. Dariushnia SR, Haskal ZJ, Midia M, Martin LG, Walker TG, Kalva SP, et al. Quality improvement guidelines for transjugular intrahepatic portosystemic shunts. J Vasc Interv Radiol. 2016;27(1):1–7.

47. Midia M, Dao D. The utility of peripheral nerve blocks in interventional radiology. Am J Roentgenol. 2016;207(4):718–30.
48. Rasuli P, Jolly EE, Hammond I, French GJ, Preston R, Goulet S, et al. Superior hypogastric nerve block for pain control in outpatient uterine artery embolization. J Vasc Interv Radiol. 2004;15(12):1423–9.
49. Ahmed M, Brace CL, Lee FT, Goldberg SN. Principles of and advances in percutaneous ablation. Radiology. 2011;258(2):351–69.
50. Piccioni F, Poli A, Templeton LC, Templeton TW, Rispoli M, Vetrugno L, et al. Anesthesia for percutaneous radiofrequency tumor ablation (PRFA): a review of current practice and techniques. Local Reg Anesth. 2019;12:127–37.
51. Swietlik JF, Longo KC, Knott EA, Hinshaw JL, Brace CL, Alexander M, et al. Percutaneous microwave tumor ablation is safe in patients with cardiovascular implantable electronic devices: a single-institutional retrospective review. J Vasc Interv Radiol. 2019;30(3):396–400.
52. Kim M-D. Uterine artery embolization for leiomyomas and adenomyosis: a pictorial essay based on our experience from 1300 cases. Korean J Radiol. 2019;20(10):1462–73.
53. Dariushnia SR, Nikolic B, Stokes LS, Spies JB. Quality improvement guidelines for uterine artery embolization for symptomatic leiomyomata. J Vasc Interv Radiol. 2014;25(11):1737–47.
54. Jeong Y-G, Kim EH, Hwang SM, Lee GY, Kim JW, Choi YJ, et al. Outpatient (same-day care) neuroangiography and neurointervention. Neurointervention. 2012;7(1):17–22.
55. Joung KW, Yang KH, Shin WJ, Song MH, Ham K, Jung SC, et al. Anesthetic consideration for neurointerventional procedures. Neurointervention. 2014;9(2):72–7.
56. Kaufmann TJ, Huston J, Mandrekar JN, Schleck CD, Thielen KR, Kallmes DF. Complications of diagnostic cerebral angiography: evaluation of 19 826 consecutive patients. Radiology. 2007;243(3):812–9.
57. Dash HH, Bhalotra AR. Neurointerventional procedures: anaesthesia or sedation. Eur J Anaesthesiol. 1998;15:32–4.
58. Guercio JR, Nimjee SM, James ML, McDonagh DL. Anesthesia for interventional neuroradiology. Int Anesthesiol Clin. 2015;53(1):87–106.
59. Dorairaj IL, Hancock SM. Anaesthesia for interventional neuroradiology. Contin Educ Anaesth Crit Care Pain. 2008;8(3):86–9.
60. Keedy A. An overview of intracranial aneurysms. Mcgill J Med. 2006;9(2):141–6.
61. Liu H, Park D, Hwang SM, Lee GY, Lim OK, Kim M, et al. Outpatient day-care neuroangiography of unruptured intracranial aneurysms. Neurointervention. 2016;11(1):37–41.
62. Zanaty M, Daou B, Chalouhi N, Starke RM, Samaniego E, Derdeyn C, et al. Same-day discharge after treatment with the pipeline embolization device using monitored anesthesia care. World Neurosurg. 2016;96:31–5.
63. Kim H, Al-Shahi Salman R, McCulloch CE, Stapf C, Young WL. Untreated brain arteriovenous malformation. Neurology. 2014;83(7):590–7.
64. Al-Shahi R, Bhattacharya JJ, Currie DG, Papanastassiou V, Ritchie V, Roberts RC, et al. Prospective, population-based detection of intracranial vascular malformations in adults. Stroke. 2003;34(5):1163–9.
65. Sackey FNA, Pinsker NR, Baako BN. Highlights on cerebral arteriovenous malformation treatment using combined embolization and stereotactic radiosurgery: why outcomes are controversial? Cureus. 2017;9(5):e1266. Published online 2017 May. https://doi.org/10.7759/cureus.1266. Accessed June 2020.
66. Sinha PK, Neema PK, Rathod RC. Anesthesia and intracranial arteriovenous malformation. Neurol India. 2004;52(2):163–70.
67. Jordán González JA, Llibre Guerra JC, Prince López JA, Vázquez Luna F, Rodríguez Ramos RM, Ugarte Suárez JC. Feasibility of the superselective test with propofol for determining eloquent brain regions in the endovascular treatment of arteriovenous malformations. Interv Neuroradiol. 2013;19(3):320–8.
68. Rauch RA, Vinuela F, Dion J, Duckwiler G, Amos EC, Jordan SE, et al. Preembolization functional evaluation in brain arteriovenous malformations: the ability of superselective Amytal test to predict neurologic dysfunction before embolization. AJNR Am J Neuroradiol. 1992;13(1):309–14.
69. Jayaraman MV, Marcellus ML, Hamilton S, Do HM, Campbell D, Chang SD, et al. Neurologic complications of arteriovenous malformation embolization using liquid embolic agents. Am J Neuroradiol. 2008;29(2):242–6.
70. Brott TG, Hobson RW, Howard G, Roubin GS, Clark WM, Brooks W, et al. Stenting versus endarterectomy for treatment of carotid-artery stenosis. N Engl J Med. 2010;363(1):11–23.
71. Ooi YC, Gonzalez NR. Management of extracranial carotid artery disease. Cardiol Clin. 2015;33(1):1–35.
72. Qureshi AI, Luft AR, Sharma M, Janardhan V, Lopes DK, Khan J, et al. Frequency and determinants of postprocedural hemodynamic instability after carotid angioplasty and stenting. Stroke. 1999;30(10):2086–93.
73. Rhim JK, Jeon JP, Park JJ, Choi HJ, Cho YD, Sheen SH, et al. Prediction of prolonged hemodynamic instability during carotid angioplasty and stenting. Neurointervention. 2016;11(2):120–6.
74. Moulakakis KG, Mylonas SN, Sfyroeras GS, Andrikopoulos V. Hyperperfusion syndrome after carotid revascularization. J Vasc Surg. 2009;49(4):1060–8.

Management of Perioperative Pain for Outpatient Bronchoscopy

20

Alec Hendon, Yi Deng,
and Melissa Annette Nikolaidis

Abstract

The growth of hospital-based and freestanding ambulatory surgery centers has enabled a dramatic increase in the variety of procedures being performed on an outpatient basis. Bronchoscopy is a procedure that is fitting for such centers, though the patient population presenting for bronchoscopy can be challenging to manage due to multiple chronic comorbidities. This procedure is generally short and requires minimal medication for pain per se, and thus does not typically require extensive post-procedure monitoring except for standard post-anesthetic care if general anesthesia is used. The aim of this chapter is to present options for periprocedural pain control for outpatient bronchoscopy. Medication regimens to achieve maximal comfort while minimizing potential adverse events and promoting efficient recovery times will be discussed. Common adverse effects of these medications, and some of the remedies available, will also be reviewed.

A. Hendon · Y. Deng · M. A. Nikolaidis (✉)
Department of Anesthesiology, Baylor College of Medicine, Houston, TX, USA
e-mail: Alec.Hendon@bcm.edu; Yi.Deng@bcm.edu; Melissa.Nikolaidis@bcm.edu

Overview of Perioperative Pain Management for Bronchoscopy

Outpatient bronchoscopy can be indicated for both diagnostic and therapeutic purposes. A common indication is definitive diagnosis of incidentally found, yet concerning, nodules identified on computed tomography scans [1]. The improved ability to diagnose lung cancer via bronchial brushings or needle-biopsies has allowed for earlier diagnosis of malignancies while also avoiding the need for surgery [2]. Bronchoscopy can also aid in the diagnosis of stridor, chronic cough, tracheomalacia, and tracheal fistulas. As lung cancer is the most common cause of cancer-associated deaths, bronchoscopy is also frequently employed to manage cancerous lesions along the bronchopulmonary tree. In fact, the field of interventional bronchoscopy includes applications such as tumor debulking via rigid bronchoscope, direct ablation, and/or photocoagulation of tumors utilizing either laser, thermocoagulation (electrocautery), or ionized argon, cryotherapy (which also results in tumor destruction via apoptosis, dehydration, and interrupting blood flow), endobronchial brachytherapy, photodynamic therapy, and even the direct delivery of chemotherapeutic agents into the tumor and/or accessible lymph nodes [1]. These modalities have enhanced treatment for patients that are poor surgical candidates as well as for patients with non-operable (widespread) pulmonary dis-

K. Rajput et al. (eds.), *Pain Control in Ambulatory Surgery Centers*,
https://doi.org/10.1007/978-3-030-55262-6_20

ease [2]. Aside from diagnosis and management of lung cancer, bronchoscopy is useful in the treatment of hemoptysis, balloon-dilation of tracheal stenosis, stenting of the trachea or bronchi, and whole-lung lavage.

Bronchoscopy involves the operator using either a flexible or a rigid scope to enter the airway, via either the oral or the nasal route, to directly visualize the upper and lower airways. As mentioned before, it is performed for both diagnostic and/or therapeutic purposes. In general, flexible fiberoptic bronchoscopy is executed with no sedation to mild sedation. In contrast, rigid bronchoscopy requires general anesthesia with full control of ventilation. With the increasing acuity of patients presenting to outpatient ambulatory surgery centers, although not ideal, it is not uncommon for patients with severe preexisting pulmonary issues with poor pulmonary reserve to present for outpatient bronchoscopy. These cases may also need a general anesthetic with controlled ventilation and may need longer than usual post-procedure monitoring to ensure a return of their pulmonary status to baseline, before discharge. While both flexible and rigid bronchoscopy have become commonplace, the former is more likely to be encountered at an ambulatory surgery center, so this procedure will be the focus of the following discussion.

When considering the treatment of pain associated with bronchoscopy, it is important to appreciate that the procedure itself is not severely painful and therefore does not require large amounts of long-acting analgesic medication. In fact, it is well established that flexible bronchoscopy can be performed with the use of only local anesthetic [3, 4]. However, to achieve optimal pain control, the patient experience must be taken into account. Many physicians view bronchoscopies as a routine procedure and discount the reality that for patients, it can be quite uncomfortable in the short term. Patients' preconceived fear of pain should be sufficient to warrant prophylactic treatment. With this pretreatment, it is also possible to assuage patient anxiety related to other aspects of the procedure such as potential complications. Another important consideration is that this patient population is frequently sicker and frailer than patients presenting for other outpatient procedures, and chronic hypoxemia is not an uncommon finding. There is also the increased risk of experiencing acute hypoxemia during bronchoscopy which can itself cause or exacerbate post-procedure pain. Unfortunately there is a paucity of evidence in the literature describing the relationship between chronic, pre-existing pain related to the indication for bronchoscopy and the acute pain that results from the bronchoscopic procedure.

The most common types of pain and discomfort reported by patients include throat pain, nose pain, dysphagia, coughing, and dyspnea [3, 5, 6]. Though many operators maintain that flexible bronchoscopy is perfectly safe without sedation or analgesia, making sedation and analgesia unnecessary, it is clear that the patient experience can be improved through use of such medication regimens. Patients who have reported appropriate pain control and expressed willingness to return for repeat procedures cite amnesia as the most significant factor influencing their responses [5]. Control of cough also improves patient pain scores [5, 7]. Many medications which control these symptoms with great efficacy, namely benzodiazepines and opioid analgesics, are readily available. Additionally, the portion of the respiratory tract in which stimulation occurs also contributes to post-procedure pain [5]. Manipulation of the upper airway and proximal lower airway is associated with significantly more pain and discomfort after bronchoscopy than the distal lower airways [5]. Bronchoalveolar lavage, for example, generally has better reported control of pain as compared with proximal airway brushings [5]. Knowing the extent and location of planned areas of intervention can help guide the amount and type of medication required to achieve excellent analgesia and optimal patient comfort.

The medication regimen of choice for majority of physicians includes a benzodiazepine such as midazolam, an opioid such as fentanyl, and a local anesthetic, generally lidocaine [3, 5]. This combination in appropriate doses will maximize comfort for the patient and minimize the risks involved in their administration.

Local Anesthetics

Local anesthetics are the cornerstone of anesthesia and analgesia for bronchoscopy [3]. Their use improves patient tolerance for the procedure which in turn improves conditions for the operator, which theoretically decreases the risk of inadvertent injury and procedural complications. From a safety perspective, there is no difference in using local anesthetics alone and using them in combination with sedation. For this reason, many bronchoscopists argue against the use of sedation, especially considering the undesirable respiratory side effects of many sedatives and analgesics [4]. From the patient perspective, however, better satisfaction is consistently reported when sedation is used in conjunction with local anesthetics [3, 5, 7]. When used with sedatives in the pre- and intraprocedural period, local anesthetic reliably reduces the amount of sedation and analgesia required for ideal patient comfort [3].

Lidocaine is the most commonly used local anesthetic used for bronchoscopy. Its side effect profile is the most forgiving when compared to other medications that have been used such as 4% cocaine, 20% benzocaine, and 1% tetracaine (Table 20.1). Further, lidocaine has been found to be equally effective for topical anesthesia when compared to those previously listed in concentrations ranging from 1% to 10%, making 1% lidocaine an excellent choice [3, 9]. Cocaine, for example, is habit forming and has been known to cause coronary artery vasoconstriction possibly leading to myocardial infarction. Benzocaine and tetracaine have narrow therapeutic windows and can lead to the development of methemoglobinemia in the event of an inadvertent overdose. These are severe complications that are challenging to manage appropriately in an ambulatory setting.

Table 20.1 Local anesthetics used for bronchoscopy [3, 8]

	Maximum dose (mg/kg)	Special considerations
Lidocaine	Injectable: 4.5 (plain); 7 (with epinephrine) Topical: 7	Decreased clearance with hepatic dysfunction
Benzocaine	Not currently defined	Methemoglobinemia with large doses
Tetracaine	3	Methemoglobinemia with large doses
Cocaine	3	Habit forming, coronary artery vasospasms, systemic vasoconstriction, hypertension

There are many different techniques that can be used to deliver local anesthetic in bronchoscopy. Soaked pledgets are routinely used in the preoperative setting, as is nebulization. Dropper instillation can be performed as well. Also common is the use of aerosol spray in the "spray-as-you-go" technique. This method involves the operator using the working channel of the bronchoscope to spray local anesthetic into the airway as the bronchoscope is advanced. This is very effective in anesthetizing the areas of the airway that will be manipulated. Transtracheal injection of local anesthetic and nerve blocks (specifically glossopharyngeal and superior laryngeal nerve blocks) produce very dense anesthesia and are generally well tolerated by patients. However, performance of these blocks requires specialized training and are far more invasive than the other choices presented here, so they are not commonly employed. The most effective utilization of local anesthetic is some combination of these techniques. For example, using a soaked pledget or aerosolized spray in the preoperative period with spray-as-you-go supplementation during the procedure [3]. All of these combinations are equally effective, so patient preference should be taken into account as well. For example, when a transnasal approach is to be utilized, most patients reported preference of a nasal gel over aerosolized spray [3, 5]. It is also easy to appreciate that while transtracheal injection might be generally well tolerated, most patients would rather try a less invasive form of local anesthetic administration.

Lidocaine has significant side effects, so it is important to know the maximum safe dose for topical anesthesia as well as be able to recognize signs of toxicity. While the maximum dose for lidocaine for intravenous injection or peripheral nerve block is generally accepted to be somewhere between 3 and 5 mg/kg, for topical dosing, a maximum dose of 7 mg/kg is recommended [3, 10]. This means that a large amount of lidocaine can be utilized for the average patient, particularly if a low concentration is selected. Extra care must be exercised for patients with altered metabolism such as patients with hepatic dysfunction, and those with predisposition to the adverse side effects of lidocaine such as chronic heart failure patients and those of advanced age [3, 10, 11]. Potentially life-threatening effects of particular concern include cardiovascular collapse, arrhythmia, and seizure [10, 11]. Arrhythmias can include, but are not limited to, ventricular tachycardia, torsades de pointes, and ventricular fibrillation. Bradycardia and conduction heart block as well as asystole might be encountered. Lidocaine lowers the seizure threshold in patients and generally leads to tonic-clonic seizures at toxic levels. Seizures are usually encountered prior to any cardiovascular complications with lidocaine toxicity [10]. These are all recognized as part of the LAST syndrome (Local Anesthetic Systemic Toxicity) (Table 20.2). Furthermore, the trachea is an area of high systemic absorption of local anesthetic, making LAST syndrome a possibility when large amounts of local anesthetic are required for patient comfort and good operator conditions [3, 10]. This reality highlights the benefits of using sedation in conjunction with local anesthetic. For more information on LAST and its treatment (Fig. 20.1), refer to the comprehensive guidelines published by the American Society of Regional Anesthesia and Pain Medicine and continuing education from the New York School of Regional Anesthesia [12].

Table 20.2 Signs and symptoms of local anesthetic systemic toxicity (LAST) [10–12]

Central nervous system	Lethargy Agitation Nervousness Tinnitus Slurring of speech Circumoral numbness Muscle twitching Tonic-clonic seizure Loss of consciousness Coma Respiratory arrest
Cardiovascular system	Hypotension Ventricular tachycardia Ventricular fibrillation Torsades de pointes Heart block Negative inotropy Cardiovascular collapse Asystole

Sedatives

Though bronchoscopy is generally well tolerated with equivocal safety outcomes when performed with local anesthetics alone, there is no doubt that both patient satisfaction and post-procedural pain/discomfort are improved with the use of sedative and analgesic medications [3–5, 7]. Several options are available to the anesthesiologist including benzodiazepines, opioid and non-opioid analgesics, and other sedative-hypnotic agents (Fig. 20.1). There is a preference for short-acting medications in ambulatory bronchoscopy as the procedure is not often associated with lasting pain and discomfort. Patients commonly report discomfort or pain solely during the procedure and for a very short period afterward [7]. Additionally, patients without recall of the procedure are more likely to report adequate pain control and willingness to undergo subsequent bronchoscopy [5]. Although the benefits are clear, perioperative sedation is not risk-free.

A large proportion of reported severe complications occurring with fiberoptic bronchoscopy can ostensibly be traced back to the sedation employed [4, 13]. For example, the use of opioids will cause respiratory depression, which could lead to hypoxia and hypercarbia if the patient becomes over-sedated. Benzodiazepines such as midazolam act synergistically to compound this effect. Other medications such as propofol have a cardiovascular depressive effect that, if not judiciously administered, can lead to clinically significant hypotension [3, 13]. Patients receiving propofol may develop difficulty maintaining a patent airway, again increasing risks of hypoxia and hypercarbia. The use of intravenous sedation ultimately prolongs post-procedure recovery

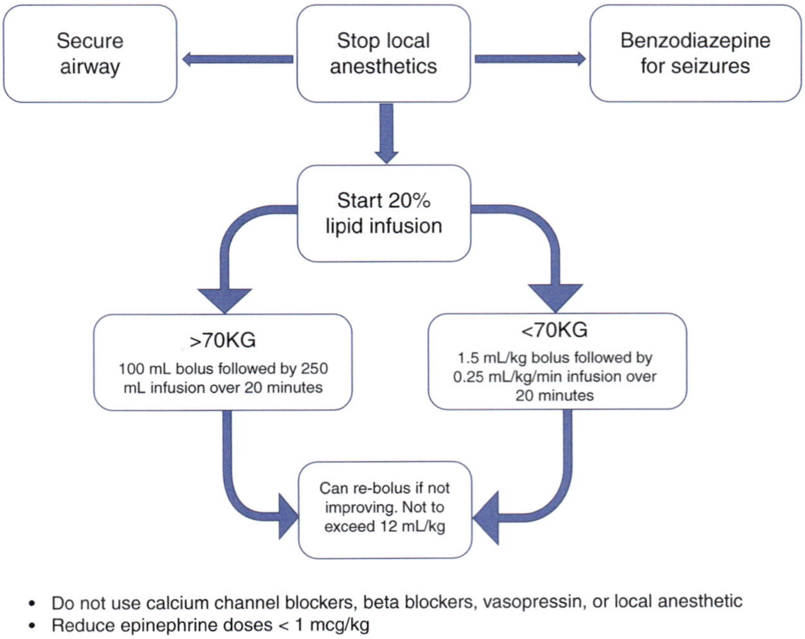

Fig. 20.1 Initial therapy for LAST. Adopted from ASRA LAST checklist [10–12]

time and delays return to baseline functional status when compared with use of lidocaine alone [3]. When utilizing sedation for bronchoscopy, the concern for polypharmacy must be taken into account as no single medication can provide all the desired facets of sedation, namely anxiolysis, analgesia, and amnesia.

The preferred class of medication for providing anxiolysis and amnesia is benzodiazepines [3]. Within this class, midazolam is the most commonly administered. Its relatively short half-life and titratability make it an excellent choice. Patients that receive midazolam report less memory of the procedure, improved comfort, and improved tolerance of bronchoscopy [3, 5, 7]. There is no established ideal dose of midazolam for sedation during bronchoscopy. It should be titrated to the desired effect. Doses ranging from 1 mg to 0.05 mg/kg are common [3, 14] (Table 20.3). Caution should be exercised during the use of benzodiazepines due to possible complications such as increased delirium in elderly patients, respiratory depression, excessive central nervous system depression, and hypotension. Of particular concern to the patient population in question is the ensuing respiratory depression. This effect is synergistic with opioid analgesics, a common component of procedural sedation, and patients presenting for bronchoscopy are more likely to have preexisting chronic pulmonary comorbidities, producing a combination that may to lead to excessive respiratory depression and apnea [3].

Analgesics

Opioid analgesics have many effects compatible with bronchoscopy, particularly when combined with benzodiazepine sedatives. As they are synergistic with benzodiazepines, the concomitant use of the two drug classes allows for achievement of excellent sedation and analgesia with comparatively smaller doses than if each medication was used as a sole agent [3]. Furthermore, opioids have significant antitussive activity, which facilitates improved procedural conditions. Control over cough also results in improved pain control as reported by patients [5, 7]. With many opioid analgesics available for use, again the consideration must be made with respect to the drug's duration of action. As bronchoscopy is not profoundly painful, a short-acting opioid is preferred [3]. This allows precise titration of sedation and analgesia while avoiding over-sedation and profound respiratory depression. For these reasons, fentanyl is the opioid of choice for bronchoscopy. Its rapid peak effect and short half-life make it more attractive than other long-acting agents such as morphine and hydromorphone. It is also very affordable in comparison to other short-acting opioids like remifentanil and sufentanil, though these medications are reasonable alternatives. Fentanyl can be titrated with individual 12.5–50 mcg boluses in combination with midazolam to achieve a chosen level of sedation and analgesia while mitigating respiratory and cardiovascular side effects (Table 20.3).

Other common sedative-hypnotics that can be used for bronchoscopy include propofol and dexmedetomidine. These agents can be used in combination with the previously mentioned medications mentioned above, or as the primary anesthetic agent. Propofol is associated with comparable levels of sedation, amnesia, and procedure tolerance as observed with a benzodiazepine and opioid regimen. If used as the only sedative agent, patients would experience a shorter post-anesthesia recovery as well, freeing up resources in the recovery area. Patients receiving propofol as the sole parenteral sedative in combination with local anesthetic report less anxiety-producing sensations such as feeling asphyxiated, cough, and overall less pain when compared to local anesthetic only, as well as a significant level of amnesia surrounding the procedure [13]. There is no analgesia provided by propofol, however, so care should be taken to fully anesthetize the portions of the airway that will be manipulated during the procedure with local anesthetic and anticipate the possible need for rescue analgesics in the recovery period. In contrast, dexmedetomidine has some inherent analgesic properties in addition to its sedative effects. Both of these medications can lead to soft tissue collapse around the airway, predisposing the patient to develop airway obstruction, so care must be taken to avoid over-sedation. Propofol can be administered via either intermittent bolus or continuous infusion, while dexmedetomidine for procedural sedation is generally given as a 0.5–1 mg/kg bolus over 10–20 minutes followed by a continuous infusion of 0.2 mg/kg/hr to 1 mg/kg/hr, titrated to effect (Table 20.3).

The use of non-opioid analgesics in the postoperative period is desirable as this would help the patient return to pre-procedural functionality more efficiently and provide a multimodal approach to minimize or avoid opioid use and prevent excessive sedation. As the airway is generally well anesthetized, non-opioid analgesics can be reserved for post-operative rescue purposes. NSAIDs and acetaminophen are excellent choices as these can both be administered intravenously to the patient whose oropharynx and posterior pharynx might remain insensate from the topical anesthetic used for the procedure and thus have an impaired swallowing reflex for oral medications.

Table 20.3 Common sedative adjuncts for bronchoscopy [3, 8, 14]

	Dosing (IV)	Time to peak effect	Duration of action	Considerations
Midazolam	0.01–0.1 mg/kg titrated to effect	5–10 minutes	2 hours	Respiratory depression, hypotension
Morphine	0.03–0.15 mg/kg	15–30 minutes	1–6 hours	Respiratory depression, flushing, itchiness, hypotension, no amnestic properties
Fentanyl	0.25–1.5 mcg/kg titrated to effect	5 minutes	1–2 hours	Respiratory depression, hypotension, no amnestic properties
Propofol	0.1–0.5 mg/kg intermittently titrated to effect; 25–100 mcg/kg/min	2 minutes	3–5 minutes	Hypotension, obstructive apnea, bradycardia, pain at injection site
Dexmedetomidine	0.5–1.0 mcg/kg loading dose followed by 0.2–1.5 mcg/kg/hr	15–30 minutes	60–120 minutes	Obstructive apnea, hypertension, hypotension, bradycardia

Adjuncts

Both pharmacological and nonpharmacological adjuncts are commonly used for bronchoscopy. Anticholinergic medications such as atropine and glycopyrrolate have theoretical benefits for bronchoscopy. Their anti-sialagogue properties should help minimize secretions in the airways and provide improved conditions for the bronchoscopist. This, in turn, should lead to improved tolerance of the procedure and reported pain control. However, significant improvement of bronchial secretions when given prior to bronchoscopy has not been definitively shown, and these medications cause significant cardiovascular and central nervous system effects [3]. Pre-bronchoscopy improvements in pulmonary function with these medications are often experienced; however, these have not been shown to persist beyond the procedure to the post-bronchoscopy setting [3]. No significant improvement in the control of patient pain and discomfort has been found with either agent [3]. Because of this, their use is not universally promoted for bronchoscopy.

Nonpharmacological adjuncts that are employed include visual effects and sound effects such sights and sounds of nature, and techniques including structured attention, hypnosis, and distraction therapy [15, 16]. Patients report superior pain control when used in combination with analgesics, while limiting the amount of medication required. This is beneficial given the propensity of our sedative and analgesic medications to cause respiratory depression and cardiovascular instability at higher doses. An intervention as simple as a nature landscape on the curtain surrounding the procedure area can be remarkably effective [15]. These techniques can easily be utilized in an ambulatory surgery setting.

Summary

Bronchoscopy is a routine procedure that can easily be carried out in a freestanding or hospital-based ambulatory surgical center, with no difference in reported patient anxiety or satisfaction [17]. Aspects that improve the patient experience include control of their anxiety and control of the pain associated with the procedure [5, 7]. Given that bronchoscopy is not a profoundly stimulating procedure and that the airways are easily anesthetized with topical local anesthetic, the procedure is uniquely set up for excellent control of these variables. With the use of anxiolytics for amnesia and analgesics for pain and antitussive effects, patients can safely have their procedures performed with excellent pain control. Management of patients presenting for outpatient bronchoscopy can be challenging as they may be sicker than those presenting for other outpatient procedures and are at risk of experiencing hypoxia during the procedure—both of which may exacerbate their experience of post-procedure pain. A multimodal approach to the procedure can lead to success for the operator, anesthetist, and patient.

References

1. Mohan A, Harris K, Bowling MR, Brown C, Hohenforst-Schmidt W. Therapeutic bronchoscopy in the era of genotype directed lung cancer management. J Thorac Dis. 2018;10(11):6298–309.
2. Biswas A, Mehta HJ, Sriram PS. Diagnostic yield of the virtual bronchoscopic navigation system guided sampling of peripheral lung lesions using ultrathin bronchoscope and protected bronchial brush. Turk Thorac J. 2019;20(1):6–11.
3. Wahidi MM, Jain P, Jantz M, Lee P, Mackensen GB, Barbour SY, et al. American College of Chest Physicians Consensus Statement on the use of topical anesthesia, analgesia, and sedation during flexible bronchoscopy in adult patients. Chest. 2011;140(5):1342–50.
4. Colt HG, Morris JF. Fiberoptic bronchoscopy without premedication: a retrospective study. Chest. 1990;96(6):1327–30.
5. Lechtzin N, Rubin HR, Jenckes M, White P, Zhou L, Thompson DA, et al. Predictors of pain control in patients undergoing flexible bronchoscopy. Am J Respir Crit Care Med. 2000;162:440–5.
6. Poi PJ, Chuah SY, Srinivas P, Liam CK. Common fears of patients undergoing bronchoscopy. Eur Respir J. 1998;11(5):1147–9.
7. Diette GB, White P, Terry P, Jenckes M, Wise RA, Rubin HR. Quality assessment through patient self-report of symptoms prefiberoptic and postfiberoptic bronchoscopy. Chest. 1998;114(5):1446–53.
8. Butterworth JF, Mackey DC, Wasnick JD, Morgan GE, Mikhail MS, editors. Morgan & Mikhail's clini-

cal anesthesiology. 6th ed. New York: McGraw-Hill; 2018.
9. Mainland PA, Kong AS, Chung DC, Chan CH, Lai CK. Absorption of lidocaine during aspiration anesthesia of the airway. J Clin Anesth. 2001;13(6):440–6.
10. El-Boghdadly K, Pawa A, Chin KJ. Local anesthetic systemic toxicity: current perspectives. Local Reg Anesth. 2018;11:35–44.
11. Rubin DS, Matsumoto MM, Weinberg G, Roth S. Local anesthetic systemic toxicity in total joint arthroplasty: incidence and risk factors in the United States From the National Inpatient Sample 1998–2013. Reg Anesth Pain Med. 2018;43:131–7.
12. Joseph NM, Barrington MJ, Fettiplace MR, Gitman M, Memtsoudis SG, Morwald EE, et al. The third American society of regional anesthesia and pain medicine practice advisory on local anesthetic systemic toxicity: executive summary 2017. Reg Anesth Pain Med. 2018;43:113–23.
13. Gonzalez R, De-La-Rosa-Ramirez I, Maldonado-Hernandez A, Dominguez-Cherit G. Should patients undergoing a bronchoscopy be sedated? Acta Anaesthesiol Scand. 2003;47:411–5.
14. Sarkiss M. Anesthesia for bronchoscopy. In: Goudra B, Singh P, editors. Out of operating room anesthesia. Cham: Springer; 2017. p. 131–43.
15. Diette GB, Lechtzin N, Haponik E, Devrotes A, Rubin HR. Distraction therapy with nature sights and sounds reduces pain during flexible bronchoscopy: a complementary approach to routine analgesia. Chest. 2003;123(3):941–8.
16. Lang EV, Benotsch EG, Fick LJ, Lutgendorf S, Berbaum ML, Berbaum KS, et al. Adjunctive non-pharmacological analgesia for invasive medical procedures: a randomized trial. Lancet. 2000;355:1486–90.
17. Lunn WW. Office-based bronchoscopy: ready for your practice? Chest. 2006;130(6):1900–5.

Part IV

Special Patient Populations

21 Perioperative Management of Sleep Apnea Patients in an Ambulatory Surgical Setting

Matthew Torre

Abstract

Sleep apnea is a disorder affecting 25–30 million Americans, with significantly more remaining undiagnosed. In fact, it is estimated that 80% of moderate to severe OSA cases are undiagnosed. These patients are of particular interest to anesthesiologists, given that they are at significantly increased risk of perioperative pulmonary and cardiovascular complications. Proper knowledge of the disease, associated risks, comorbid conditions, and an appropriate perioperative management, are vitally important for safe care.

Of the three main types of sleep apnea (Obstructive, Central, and Mixed), Obstructive-type represents the vast majority, and is thus the focus of this section. Given the vastly under-diagnosed nature of OSA, it is commonplace for the anesthesiologist to care for patients with untreated moderate to severe OSA. Therefore, it is imperative to identify these patients at increased risk of perioperative complications prior to the day of surgery in order to risk stratify appropriateness for outpatient surgery, optimize comorbidities, and ensure appropriate equipment and discharge planning are available.

M. Torre (✉)
Virginia Commonwealth University, Richmond, VA, USA
e-mail: Matthew.Torre@vcuhealth.org

Introduction

Patients with obstructive sleep apnea are at a significantly increased risk of developing perioperative complications than those without obstructive sleep apnea. A large meta-analysis including 10 cohort studies with nearly 24,000 patients, demonstrated a complication rate (cardiopulmonary complications are by far the most common) nearly four times that of non-OSA patients. In addition, the length of hospital stay was a full 2-days longer. Others concerns which occur at higher frequency include difficulty with airway management, cardiovascular complications, and postoperative delirium. All of which lead to higher morbidity, longer hospital stays, and increased costs.

In addition to airway difficulties, patients with OSA have a significantly increased prevalence of comorbid conditions such as hypertension, coronary artery disease, myocardial ischemia, congestive heart failure, arrhythmias, stroke, COPD, diabetes mellitus, hyperlipidemia, and GERD. Recent studies have shown as high as 80% of OSA patients have multiple additional comorbidities. It is likely that the number and severity of comorbidities increase with the severity of sleep apnea.

Therefore, it is extremely important to identify which OSA patients are appropriate for ambulatory surgery. There are several important factors known to influence perioperative risk:

K. Rajput et al. (eds.), *Pain Control in Ambulatory Surgery Centers*,
https://doi.org/10.1007/978-3-030-55262-6_21

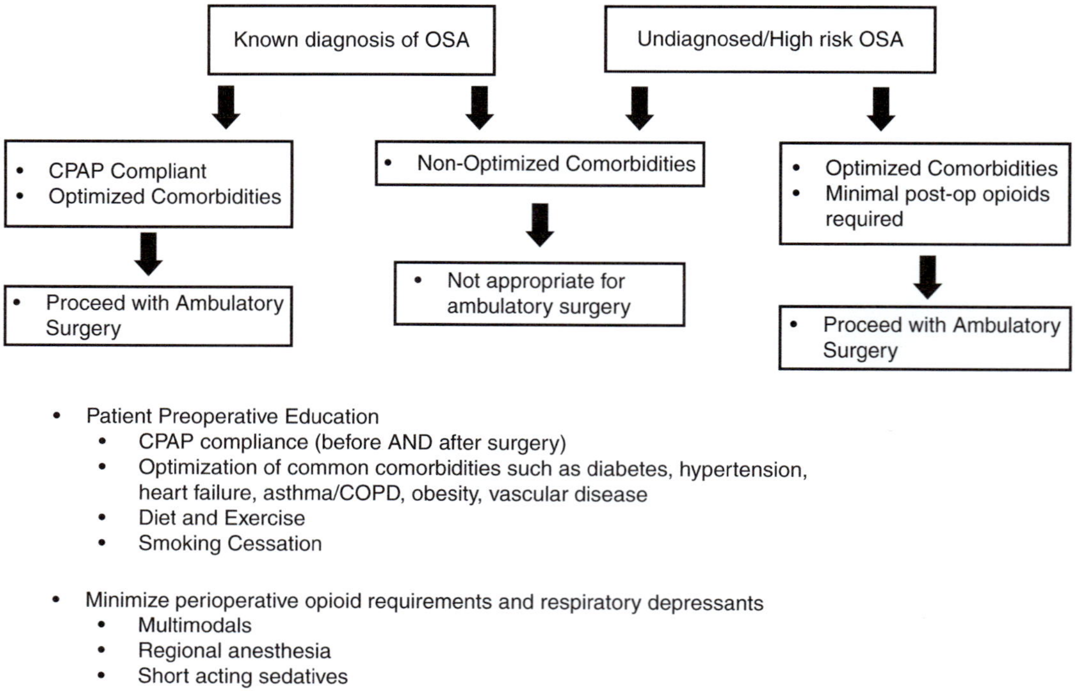

Fig. 21.1 Ambulatory surgery eligibility for obstructive sleep apnea patients

severity of sleep apnea, compliance with CPAP, coexisting diseases, type and location of surgery, type of anesthesia, and need for postoperative opioids. It is also equally important to identify the capabilities of the outpatient facility, such as availability of difficult airway equipment, respiratory care, postoperative monitoring, and inpatient facility relationships for possible transfers.

Several algorithms have been proposed to help simplify the process; however, there are no formal recommendations from the ASA. Therefore, it is recommended that each institution creates their own policy for appropriate risk stratification prior to the day of surgery. An example is shown below (Fig.21.1).

Preoperative Evaluation

The fast-paced environment of ambulatory surgery centers often inhibits the clinician's ability to gather all necessary patient information on the morning of surgery. Safe and effective management of these patients requires proactive planning, and the ability to make any necessary arrangements prior to the day of surgery. Therefore, advanced notice and screening is an essential part of perioperative care.

This is frequently accomplished via preanesthetic clinical evaluations ("PACE" clinics), or advanced notice preoperative phone screens.

An adequate preoperative evaluation of known or suspected OSA patient should include a thorough review of previous medical records, patient interview (in person or remotely), as well as a physical exam. Though the latter of these is less common prior to the day of surgery for many ambulatory centers, it should not be underestimated or overlooked. While this seems intuitive, this consistent approach helps to mitigate any missed or omitted pertinent information.

Prior anesthesia records should also be reviewed to identify any history of difficult intubation or adverse perioperative events. Patients may be unaware of prior intraoperative complications or airway difficulties, making the record review extremely important. Likewise, a discussion with both the patient and family members may be beneficial to help assess the severity of sleep apnea in those who are undiagnosed.

Of note, patients who had previous OSA corrective surgery but have not had a follow-up sleep study are still considered high-risk until proven otherwise.

Patient Screening and Risk Stratification

Multiple screening tools are available, and have evolved over the years. The STOP-BANG and Berlin questionnaires are highly sensitive surveys designed to help categorize the presence or absence of obstructive sleep apnea, as well as provide some insight on severity.

STOP-BANG is the most validated screening tool, and is recommended by the Society for Ambulatory Anesthesia (SAMBA) due to its simplicity, succinctness, and sensitivity. A score of ≥3 indicates a high-likelihood of moderate-severe OSA with ~95–100% sensitivity, and a score of ≤2 essentially rules it out.

STOP – BANG Questionnaire

Item	Yes	No
Snore (Snore Loudly)	○	○
Tired (Daytime fatigue)	○	○
Observed Apnea	○	○
High Blood ***P***ressure	○	○
BMI (>35 kg/m^2)	○	○
Age (>50 years)	○	○
Neck Size (>40 cm/15.75in)	○	○
Gender (Male)	○	○
Total Score 1-Point for each "Yes" Low-Risk OSA *0–2* Moderate-Risk OSA *3–4* High-Risk OSA *5–8*		

In addition to screening for disease severity, the ASA has created a sleep apnea risk-assessment calculator to stratify an individual patients risk for perioperative complications. This algorithm takes into account the severity of sleep apnea, type of surgery being performed, type of anesthesia required, and postoperative opioid consumption (Table21.1). The perioperative implications of the patient's relative risk should always be discussed with both the surgeon and the patient, prior to the procedure.

Table 21.1 Scoring System for Perioperative Risk from OSA

Category	Points
A. Severity Of OSA (0–3 pts)	
None	0
Mild	1
Moderate	2
Severe	3
B. Invasiveness of surgery (0–4 pts)	
Superficial surgery under MAC (mild sedation)	0
Superficial surgery under MAC (moderate sedation) or GA	1
Peripheral surgery under neuraxial anesthesia	1
Peripheral surgery under GA	2
Airway surgery under MAC (moderate sedation)	2
Airway surgery under GA	3
Major surgery under GA	4
C. Requirement for postoperative opioids (0–3 pts)	
None	0
Low dose	1
High dose	3
Other	
CPAP/NIPPV use prior to surgery (and anticipated postoperative use)	-1
Resting PaCo2 > 50mmHg	+1
Estimation of perioperative risk	
Score from category A, plus B or C (whichever is higher, max 6pts)	
Low risk	0–2
Moderate risk	3–5
High risk	4–6

Preoperative Optimization

Healthcare is an ever evolving profession, with more and more focus being placed on "*preventative-medicine*". In regards to surgical preparation, this applies to optimizing modifiable risk factors and comorbidities. Once a patient has been seen, evaluated, and approved for ambulatory surgery, they should be educated on the importance of optimizing comorbid conditions, and how to facilitate a successful and event-free surgery.

Typically, we think of preoperative optimization in terms of blood pressures, blood glucose, thyroid levels, cholesterol, smoking cessation, etc. According to the ASA, several additional modifiable factors have been shown to reduce perioperative morbidity, specifically in sleep apnea patients. These include preoperative initiation of continuous positive airway pressure (CPAP) and/or noninvasive positive pressure ventilation (NIPPV), preoperative use of mandibular advancement devices, and preoperative weight loss.

Patients who began using CPAP prior to surgery have a lower frequency of serious postoperative complications when compared to those without preoperative CPAP. While studies are sparse, these interventions are advocated under the ASA practice guidelines.

Intraoperative Management

One of the biggest concerns in patients with OSA is airway management; before, during, and after surgery. This fear is justifiable, as difficult intubation occurs 4–8 times more frequently than in non-OSA patients. Difficult mask ventilation also occurs at a rate of nearly 4-times that of non-OSA. Fortunately, there is no increase in the failure rate of LMA placement as a rescue device (in case the need arises to progress down the difficult airway algorithm).

Because of this, the ASA recommends all patients with known or suspected OSA to be treated as a potential difficult airway. Proper sniffing positioning with a ramp, shoulder roll, and the head of the bed slightly elevated (20–30 degrees), is essential to improve first chance intubation success.

Medication Selection

OSA patients are significantly more susceptible to the respiratory-depressant effects of opioids, volatile anesthetics, and other sedatives. The anesthetic technique, and medications given, should focus on minimizing risk of respiratory depression and airway compromise. Therefore, pain management should focus on multimodal analgesics, opioid sparing techniques, regional or neuraxial anesthetics, and avoidance of long-acting sedatives.

Nonopioid analgesics such as ibuprofen, celecoxib, ketorolac, and acetaminophen, are the most commonly used, and their efficacy is well documented.

Additional medications such as IV-magnesium, lidocaine, and ketamine, can also be very effective when used properly. Preoperative gabapentin use has been widely debated over recent years, yielding very mixed results. Most recent evidence suggests it has only nominal benefits, but is associated with statistically significant higher incidence of postoperative respiratory depression, naloxone use, and NIPPV requirements.

Ketamine, administered at subhypnotic doses (<0.5 mg/kg), is not known to produce hallucinogenic effects. It provides excellent pain control intraoperatively as well as postoperatively. Studies have demonstrated a significant decrease in postoperative opioid requirements even several days after surgery. In addition, it does not suppress respiratory drive or ventilation (it can actually increase minute ventilation). This makes it a very appealing medication for sleep apnea patients.

Magnesium, while less commonly known for its analgesic benefits, has become more prominent in the days of ERAS (enhanced recovery after surgery) and opioid sparing management. Multiple trials have shown significant benefit from both intraoperative bolus dose alone (30–50 mg/kg), or with infusions (8–15 mg/kg/hr). In addition to improved pain control, magnesium has anxiolytic properties, neuroprotective effects, and decreases overall anesthetic requirements. Caution is advised however in certain patient populations due to its effect on cardiac conduction (pre-existing heart block or arrhythmias), skeletal muscle contraction (neuromuscular diseases such as myasthenia gravis or multiple sclerosis), and accumulation in those with renal failure.

Dexmedetomidine has been shown to be a safe and effective alternative to propofol for procedural sedation. As an alpha-2 adrenergic agonist, it has sympatholytic properties, producing anxiolysis, analgesia, and sedation, with minimal respiratory depression. It also has a very stable hemodynamic profile when given as an infusion, but hypotension and bradycardia may occur with large bolus doses.

The downside of dexmedetomidine, especially in a fast-paced ambulatory center, is its long half-life (90–120 minutes), which may delay PACU discharge due to hypersomnolence. The duration of PACU recovery tends to increase with the length of procedure due to larger total dosage. Adequate titration to minimize this potential delay is largely provider dependent, but may be minimized by a good working relationship and understanding between surgeon and anesthesiologist in regards to surgical and closure time.

Regional Anesthesia

For extremity procedures, sleep apnea patients are excellent candidates for regional anesthetics, including neuraxial anesthesia. However, in regards to neuraxial, the risks/benefits of intrathecal opioids must be weighed.

Mild to moderate sedation is advised, as airway collapse and apnea are an increasing risk with increasing amounts of sedation. There are a multitude of noninvasive adjuncts to help alleviate this risk, such as nasal/oral CPAPs, jaw-thrust devices, or simple head/neck position adjustments. If these are not available, more invasive devices such as oral airways or nasal trumpets are effective. However, these are generally poorly tolerated unless the patient is deeply sedated.

Ideally, avoiding respiratory depression and obstruction are avoided from the start. Medication selection should focus on achieving adequate patient comfort, while maintaining spontaneous respiration.

Regional anesthesia has greatly improved the ability of ambulatory surgery centers to care for such patients who would otherwise require hospital admission, while simultaneously increasing facility efficiency, and decreasing PACU recovery/complications.

Studies have shown dramatic improvements in all these areas, with the majority of patients being fast-tracked home (time from PACU arrival until discharge <30 min), minimal adverse effects (PONV, pain, hypersomnolence, over-sedation, obstruction, desaturation, etc.), and significantly reduced postoperative pain scores and opioid requirements. All of which are vitally important to the efficiency and productivity of the surgery center.

One area of possible concern regarding patients with sleep apnea is the potential phrenic nerve blockade after brachial plexus blocks. This carries the risk of further inhibiting ventilation in a patient population already at risk, predisposing them to additional respiratory complications. While this has been well studied and validated in patients with severe pre-existing pulmonary disease such as COPD, there is currently no evidence to support this in patients with sleep apnea. However, there is a scarcity of literature on this topic, and several clinical trials are currently under way to investigate this.

General Anesthesia

If general anesthesia is necessary, a secured airway with endotracheal tube should be strongly considered over a laryngeal mask airway. Due to body habitus, anatomy, and comorbid conditions, patients with OSA are at higher risk for gastric reflux, aspiration, and potential loss of the airway.

Given that these patients are up to 8-times more likely to be difficult to ventilate and/or intubate, performing a rescue intubation in the middle of surgery, under nonideal circumstances or patient positioning, is a recipe for disaster. Therefore, electing to secure the airway from the start, under ideal conditions, is highly recommended.

Adequate preoxygenation and proper positioning are essential. Preoxygenate with 100% oxygen, with the goal of achieving ETO2>80%. Proper sniffing position along with a ramp or shoulder roll, and placement in a semirecumbent position (30 degree head elevation) provides several very important benefits. Functional residual capacity ("FRC") is increased (as compared to supine), which can significantly increase the time-to-desaturation by maximizing the oxygen reservoir. In healthy patients with normal FRC (2500-3000 cc), this time can approach 9–10 minutes! Secondly, the risk of passive aspiration is decreased (due to gravity), and thirdly, better alignment of the oral and tracheal axis improves vocal cord view and first chance intubation success.

Likewise, extubation should be performed when the patient is awake, fully reversed, and in a head-up position. This ensures the presence of swallow/gag/cough reflex to minimize risk of aspiration and/or laryngospasm, allows time for improved muscular tone of oropharynx/hypopharynx to decrease risk of obstruction, and allows the ability to follow commands during immediate postextubation period where the risks are highest.

Postoperative Management

Sleep apnea patients are very sensitive to the sedating and apneic effects of anesthetic gases, opioids, benzodiazepines, and other sedatives. Because of this, close monitoring in the PACU is required, immediate assistance should be needed.

It is essential to transport all OSA patients with supplemental oxygen, and continue once in the recovery room, with continuous monitoring of ventilation/oxygenation. Unless contraindicated by the surgical procedure, patients who routinely use a CPAP/NIPPV at home should be encouraged to do so in PACU (and continue at home).

Supplemental oxygen should be continued until patient is able to maintain baseline oxygenation while breathing room air, while not being stimulated.

In addition, placement in an inclined/head-up position (rather than supine) helps reduce anatomical risk of airway obstruction, as well as risk of passive aspiration.

Discharge Criteria

In addition to typical PACU discharge criteria, the ASA also recommends that patients at increased risk from OSA not be discharged to an unmonitored setting until they are no longer at risk for perioperative respiratory depression.

This may require longer periods of postoperative observation, ideally in a quiet location, to ensure adequate ventilation with minimal stimulation.

Patient education regarding the importance of continuing their CPAP/BiPAP device at home is essential. Studies have shown that OSA patients experience significant postoperative sleep disturbances, with the greatest increase in apnea/hypopnea episodes on the third postoperative night. This is due to a REM (rapid eye movement) rebound effect, which occurs due to limited or poor REM sleep the first postoperative night, as a result of surgical stress and anesthesia.

Summary Recommendations

Preoperative

- Recommend OSA screening for all patients prior to elective outpatient surgery
- Preoperative CPAP use is strongly recommended (NIPPV if CPAP is not tolerated)
- Patients should bring their home CPAP/NIPPV device for perioperative use as needed
- Due to the increased difficulty with airway management, the ASA recommends all patients with known or suspected OSA to be treated as a potential difficult airway

Intraoperative

- OSA patients are exquisitely sensitive to the sedating and respiratory-depressant effects of volatile anesthetics, opioids, benzodiazepines, and sedatives. The anesthetic plan should focus on limiting the use of these medications, multimodal analgesia, and regional anesthesia when applicable.

- Regional or local anesthesia with mild sedation should be strongly considered when applicable, to minimize or eliminate perioperative opioid requirements.
- Regional anesthesia (under MAC) is associated with decreased unplanned admissions after ambulatory surgery
- Consider using CPAP/NIPPV during sedation in patients with known moderate-severe OSA (under MAC).
- Continuous ETCO2 monitoring should be used for all OSA patients undergoing sedation, due to the higher incidence of airway collapse and apnea.
- If general anesthesia is indicated, a secured airway with cuffed ETT should be utilized over nonsecure devices such as LMA's
- Unless contraindicated, sleep apnea patients should be extubated awake, and in semirecumbent position.
- Multimodal analgesics (NSAIDS, acetaminophen, ketamine, IV-magnesium, lidocaine) should be used when applicable to reduce opioid requirements.

Postoperative

- Continuous monitoring of oxygenation/ventilation in PACU due to increased sensitivity of sedating/apneic effects of anesthetic gases, opioids, benzodiazepines, and other sedatives.
- Supplemental oxygen should be given for all OSA patients once in the recovery room, until saturation is able to be maintained on room air while unstimulated.
- Patients who routinely use a CPAP/NIPPV at home should be encouraged to do so in PACU
- OSA patients should not be discharged to an unmonitored location until they are no longer at risk of respiratory depression.

Additional Sources

1. Ambulatory & Non–Operating Room Anesthesia. Morgan & Mikhail's Clinical Anesthesiology, 6e Eds. John F. Butterworth IV, et al. New York, NY: McGraw-Hill. http://accessmedicine.mhmedical.com.proxy.library.vcu.edu/content.aspx?bookid=2444&sectionid=193563339.
2. American Society of Anesthesiologists Task Force on Perioperative Management of Patients with Obstructive Sleep Apnea. Practice guidelines for the perioperative management of patients with obstructive sleep apnea. Anesthesiology. 2014;120:268. [PubMed: 24346178].
3. Chung F, Memtsoudis S, Ramachandran S, et al. Society of Anesthesia and Sleep Medicine guidelines on preoperative screening and assessment of adult patients with obstructive sleep apnea. Anesth Analg. 2016;123:452. [PubMed: 27442772].
4. Joshi G, Ankichetty S, Gan T, Chung F. Society for Ambulatory Anesthesia consensus statement on preoperative selection of adult patients with obstructive sleep apnea scheduled for ambulatory surgery. Anesth Analg. 2012;115:1060.
5. Fouladpour N, Jesudoss R, Bolden N, et al. Perioperative complications in obstructive sleep apnea patients undergoing surgery; a review of the legal literature. Anesth Analg. 2016;122:145. [PubMed: 26111263].
6. White P, Tang J, Wender R, et al. The effects of oral ibuprofen and celecoxib in preventing pain, improving recovery outcomes and patient satisfaction after ambulatory surgery. Anesth Analg. 2011;112:323. [PubMed: 21156974].
7. Chung S, Yuan H. ChungF. A systemic review of obstructive sleep apnea and its implications for anesthesiologists. Anesth Analg. 2008;107:1543. [PubMed: 18931212].
8. Elvir-Lazo O, White P. The role of multimodal analgesia in pain management after ambulatory surgery. Curr Opin Anesthesiol. 2010;23:697.
9. NagappaM, WongDT, CozowiczC, RamachandranSK, MemtsoudisSG, ChungF. Is obstructive sleep apnea associated with difficult airway? Evidence from a systematic review and meta-analysis of prospective and retrospective cohort studies. PLoS One. 2018;13(10):e0204904. Published 2018 Oct 4. https://doi.org/10.1371/journal.pone.0204904.(https://www.ncbi.nlm.nih.gov/pmc/articles/PMC6171874/) "OSA Difficult Airway 2018)"
10. Nagappa M, Subramani Y, Chung F. Best perioperative practice in management of ambulatory patients with obstructive sleep apnea. Curr Opin Anaesthesiol. 2018;31(6):700–6. https://doi.org/10.1097/ACO.0000000000000661.
11. Bonsignore MR, Baiamonte P, Mazzuca E, et al. Obstructive sleep apnea and comorbidities: a dangerous liaison. Multidiscip Respir Med. 2019;14:8. https://doi.org/10.1186/s40248-019-0172-9.
12. Salviz EA, Xu D, Frulla A, Kwofie K, Shastri U, Chen J, Shariat AN, Littwin S, Lin E, Choi J, Hobeika P, Hadzic A. Continuous interscalene block in patients having outpatient rotator cuff repair surgery. Anesth Anal. 2013;117(6):1485–92. https://doi.org/10.1213/01.ane.0000436607.40643.0a.
13. Gorlin AW, Rosenfeld DM, Ramakrishna H. Intravenous sub-anesthetic ketamine for

perioperative analgesia. J Anaesthesiol Clin Pharmacol. 2016;32(2):160–7. https://doi.org/10.4103/0970-9185.182085.
14. Riddell JM, Trummel JM, Onakpoya IJ. Low-dose ketamine in painful orthopaedic surgery: a systematic review and meta-analysis. Br J Anaesth. 2019;123(3):325–34. https://doi.org/10.1016/j.bja.2019.05.043.
15. Preoperative Gabapentinoids Increase Risk of Postoperative Opioid-Related Respiratory Depression in Adult Patients Undergoing Total Hip and Knee Arthroplasties Sean Moore, TetsuOhnuma, KarthikRaghunathan, John Whittle, Raquel R. Bartz, Srinivas Pyati, Alan Ellis, William E. Bryan, Marc Pepin, Vijay Krishnamoorthy (IARS –2019).
16. Kharasch ED, Clark JD, Kheterpal S. Perioperative gabapentinoids: deflating the bubble. Anesthesiology. 2020; No Pagination Specified.; https://doi.org/10.1097/ALN.0000000000003394.
17. Chung F, Liao P, Yegneswaran B, Shapiro CM, Kang W. Postoperative changes in sleep-disordered breathing and seep architecture in patients with obstructive sleep apnea. Anesthesiology. 2014;120(2):287–98. https://doi.org/10.1097/ALN.0000000000000040.

22 Special Considerations: Management of Pediatric Pain in an Ambulatory Setting

Ellise Cappuccio and Veronica P. Carullo

Abstract

Ambulatory surgery centers have quickly become a preferred site for pediatric outpatient elective surgeries for a variety of reasons. There are many benefits to providing surgery and anesthesia that allow a pediatric patient to recover in the comfort of their own home; therefore, provision of optimal pain management to help facilitate recovery at home is a crucial aspect of ambulatory surgical care. Advances in regional anesthesia and multimodal pain management strategies can allow for this to occur with minimal or no exposure to opioid analgesics. Given that we are in the midst of a national opioid crisis, it has become even more important to utilize multimodal strategies including thoughtful utilization of regional anesthesia to optimize management of ambulatory surgical pain in children and adults.

E. Cappuccio
Montefiore Medical Center, Department of Anesthesiology, Bronx, NY, USA

V. P. Carullo (✉)
University of Mississippi Medical Center, Jackson, MS, USA
e-mail: vcarullo@umc.edu

Introduction

Ambulatory surgery centers are the favored site for pediatric outpatient elective surgeries in a select population of pediatric patients. With appropriate utilization of procedure and patient selection criteria, anesthesia and postoperative analgesia for ambulatory surgery can be provided safely, efficiently, and efficaciously to infants and children [1, 2]. Providing surgery and anesthesia that allows a pediatric patient to recover at home can lead to improved outcomes; this includes reduced cost of surgical care, decreased risk of nosocomial infections, decreased disruption to families, and increased patient and parent satisfaction [2].

Pharmacologic Therapy and Multimodal Analgesia

There are several special considerations in the pediatric population that are important to understand. Developmental differences in drug pharmacokinetics, pharmacodynamics, and pharmacogenomics must be taken into consideration for appropriate determination of drug, dosing, and interval [3]. For example, delayed maturation of hepatic enzyme systems and decreased glomerular filtration rate in neonates and infants affect drug conjugation and clearance of most analgesics including nonsteroidal anti-

K. Rajput et al. (eds.), *Pain Control in Ambulatory Surgery Centers*,
https://doi.org/10.1007/978-3-030-55262-6_22

inflammatory drugs (NSAIDs), opioids, and local anesthetics. Furthermore, decreased plasma concentration of alpha-1 acid glycoprotein in neonates and infants can result in higher concentrations of unbound amino-amide local anesthetic (i.e., lidocaine, bupivacaine, ropivacaine) resulting in potential for drug toxicity. Another important consideration is the need to respond to parental, patient, and provider concerns raised by the current opioid crisis, particularly since there seems to be a higher potential for misuse and adverse effects among adolescents [4–6]. While opioids can be safe and effective when prescribed and used appropriately, limiting the number of doses prescribed is one important strategy to mitigate the current opioid crisis. Utilizing nonopioid analgesics, such acetaminophen and NSAIDs, along with regional anesthesia techniques for treatment of pain can significantly reduce or prevent the need for opioid utilization. While studies on the efficacy of regional anesthesia in pediatrics are limited, a large multi-institutional study by the Pediatric Regional Anesthesia Network (PRAN), has established that regional anesthesia is safe in the pediatric population [7].

Table 22.1 summarizes the most commonly utilized intravenous and oral analgesics in the pediatric population. Of note, most analgesics used in the pediatric population are used off-label given the lack of appropriate randomized controlled studies in this population. However, their use is recommended by experts in the field as part of a multimodal approach [8], and they have been used safely and efficaciously for several decades in the pediatric population.

Adenotonsillectomy is one of the most common ambulatory pediatric surgeries, second only to myringotomy and tubes, and presents a variety of pain management challenges [9]. Post-tonsillectomy pain varies with surgical technique and is frequently moderate to severe, yet the use of postoperative opioids has been found to be associated with significantly increased risk of

Table 22.1 Intravenous and Oral Analgesics

Medication	IV	PO
Acetaminophen	Children ≥2–12 yrs and adolescents <50 kg: 15 mg/kg/dose Q 6 hours, or 12.5 mg/kg Q 4 hours to a maximum of 75 mg/kg/day Adolescents >50 kg: 1000 mg every 6 hours or 650 mg every 4 hours to a maximum of 4000 mg per day	<50 kg: 10–15 mg/kg/dose Q 4 hours, not to exceed 75 mg/kg/day (60 mg/kg/day for term neonates and infants). ≥50 kg: 500–650 mg Q 4 hours or 975 mg Q 6 hours, not to exceed 4 grams daily
Ibuprofen	6 mo-12 yrs: 10 mg/kg over 10 minutes to a maximum single dose of 400 mg Q 4–6 hours 12–17 yrs: 400 mg over 10 minutes Q 4–6 hours Maximum daily dose: lesser of 40 mg/kg/day or 2400 mg/day	6 mo-12 yrs: 6–10 mg/kg/dose Q 6–8 hours to a maximum dose of 40 mg/kg/day >12 yrs: 400–600 mg Q 6–8 hours to a maximum of 2400 mg/day
Ketorolac[a]	1–16 yrs and <50 kg: 0.5 mg/kg/dose Q 6 hours to a maximum single dose of 30 mg; >16 yo and >50 kg: 15–30 mg Q 6 hours	For children >50 kg: 10 mg PO Q 4–6 hours
Naproxen	N/A	6–10 mg/kg/dose Q 8–12 hours Maximum single dose: 375 mg/dose
Fentanyl	1–3 mcg/kg/dose Q 1–2 hours as needed to a maximum initial dose of 50 mcg	N/A
Morphine[a]	0.05–0.1 mg/kg Q 3–4 hours as needed to a maximum initial dose of 4 mg	0.15–0.3 mg/kg Q 4–6 hours as needed
Oxycodone[a]	N/A	0.1–0.2 mg/kg/dose Q 4 hours as needed to a maximum initial dose of 5 mg
Hydrocodone[a]	N/A	0.1–0.15 mg/kg/dose Q 4 hours as needed to a maximum initial dose of 7.5 mg
Dexmedetomidine[a]	0.5–1 microgram/kg/dose	N/A

[a]Off-label use in pediatrics

morbidity and mortality due to complications associated with obstructive sleep apnea syndrome and CYP450 2D6 polymorphisms [10]. In 2013, following multiple deaths associated with codeine use post-tonsillectomy, the FDA issued a black box warning cautioning against the use of codeine to relieve pain after tonsillectomy or adenoidectomy in children [11]. However, pharmacogenomic differences do not fully account for opioid risk in this population as postoperative treatment with morphine, which is not metabolized by the 2D6 pathway, was found to be associated with increased frequency of desaturation events when compared with ibuprofen [12]. The updated clinical practice guideline developed by the American Academy of Otolaryngology-Head and Neck Surgery Foundation therefore recommends the routine administration of a single intraoperative dose of intravenous dexamethasone and postoperative administration of oral acetaminophen and ibuprofen, and strongly advises clinicians not to administer or prescribe codeine after tonsillectomy to children under 12 years of age [13]. Intravenous acetaminophen and intravenous ibuprofen are both available in the U.S. and FDA approved in children since 2010 and 2015, respectively. However, higher cost of the intravenous formulations compared with their oral counterparts presents a significant barrier to their routine use in clinical practice. In a 2018 survey of anesthesiologist members of the Society for Pediatric Anesthesia, 85% of respondents reported that they never use IV ibuprofen for pediatric tonsillectomy cases citing the two most common reasons as lack of availability at their institutions and concern for increased bleeding [14], although a recent large, retrospective analysis found that the observed bleeding rate after pediatric tonsillectomy was not statistically different in patients who received intraoperative IV ibuprofen versus those who did not receive this medication [15]. The national opioid crisis has challenged us to reconsider the use of opioids as primary analgesics for perioperative pain management. Through quality improvement methodology, it is possible to develop effective anesthesia and analgesia protocols that minimize opioids and provide effective pain relief without increasing recovery times or reoperation rates [16]. Moreover, a combination of dexmedetomidine, nonsteroidal anti-inflammatory drugs, and regional anesthesia can help minimize perioperative opioids for pediatric ambulatory surgeries without compromising patient outcomes or value [17].

Nonpharmacologic Therapies

It is very important to consider and optimize the use of nonpharmacologic interventions for pain management in an ambulatory surgery setting. For infants, the act of sucking with or without a sucrose-containing liquid and/or breastfeeding can provide soothing relief for procedural pain [18].

Another effective nonpharmacologic treatment for both pain and anxiety is distraction therapy. Newer techniques which require patient participation, including guided imagery and immersive virtual reality (VR) are gaining popularity as they are effective without the potential side effects of pharmacologic therapies. There is a growing body of evidence demonstrating the efficacy of VR for reduction in anxiety and procedural pain in a variety of settings including venipuncture, laceration repair, burn dressing changes, vaccinations, and physical therapy [19, 20].

Other active distraction techniques, such as arts and crafts, digital games, and pretend play, are often used with success to help with perioperative anxiety and pain. In addition to active distraction, passive distraction, such as watching TV and music therapy, can also be a helpful adjunct in the perioperative setting. This can be especially useful for children whose level of distress may be too high to effectively participate in any activity [21].

Other holistic modalities widely used in the treatment of pediatric chronic pain, such as heat and cold therapy, massage therapy, and acupuncture may also have benefits in a perioperative setting. Cold packs are not only used to reduce postoperative swelling, but can also help treat acute pain. Heat and massage therapy can be useful for postoperative muscle spasms associated with various orthopedic procedures.

In addition to acute pain and anxiety, postoperative nausea and vomiting is important to consider and avoid, as patients cannot be discharged home until they are tolerating PO intake. Acupuncture has been widely used for a variety of medical conditions, such as pain, anxiety, and headaches. While more randomized controlled studies are needed in the pediatric population, there is evidence to suggest that acupuncture is an effective treatment for postoperative nausea and vomiting after pediatric tonsillectomy [22].

Peripheral Regional Anesthesia/Analgesia

Moving away from opioid-based techniques to utilizing a multimodal approach that includes the use of peripheral regional anesthetic techniques is fundamental to current pediatric ambulatory practice, and its use will continue to increase as the emphasis on improved patient outcomes and improved patient satisfaction also increases [23, 24]. In particular, patients undergoing orthopedic and urologic ambulatory surgeries are excellent candidates for peripheral regional anesthesia to optimize postoperative pain control and minimize opioid use. Lower extremity peripheral nerve blocks such as femoral nerve, adductor canal, or sciatic nerve blocks can be utilized to help reduce opioid requirements and facilitate discharge home with minimal pain following lower extremity surgeries such as ACL repairs and knee arthroscopy [25]. In addition, ultrasound-guided pudendal nerve blocks are being utilized more frequently for pediatric circumcisions as well as hypospadias repairs as an alternative to caudal analgesia [26–28].

The most commonly utilized peripheral nerve blocks in infants, children, and adolescents with common indications are summarized below [29]. Data from the Pediatric Regional Anesthesia Network not only demonstrated the safety of pediatric regional blockade under general anesthesia or sedation, but also actually reported fewer adverse events in children under anesthesia; therefore, it is has become the standard of care to perform pediatric regional blocks under anesthesia [30].

Upper Extremity Blocks

Supraclavicular Nerve Block

Local anesthetic injected around the trunks and divisions of the brachial plexus.

- Indications: Shoulder, arm, elbow, forearm, and hand surgery
- Ultrasound-guided technique: The patient should be placed supine with the head turned away from the arm being blocked. The probe is placed above the clavicle in a transverse plane. The brachial plexus can be identified as a "cluster of grapes" lateral and sometimes superior to the subclavian artery. After identifying these important landmarks, a needle is inserted in-plane with the ultrasound probe and advanced to the inferior lateral corner of the subclavian artery. With full visualization of the needle and after gentle aspiration, local anesthetic is injected. The brachial plexus should appear to move superiorly and peel away from the subclavian artery. The proximal part of the medial side of the arm, which corresponds to the distribution of the intercostobrachial nerve (T2), is usually spared and can be blocked by injecting local anesthetic subcutaneously distal to the axilla.

Interscalene Nerve Block

Local anesthetic injected around the C5, C6, and C7 nerve roots of the brachial plexus.

- Indications: Shoulder or upper arm surgery
- Ultrasound-guided technique: The patient should be placed supine with the head turned away from the arm being blocked. The probe is placed above the clavicle in a transverse plane to identify the brachial plexus at the supraclavicular level. After identifying the important landmarks, the probe is moved cephalad until the "cluster of grapes" disappears and the nerve roots are visible. Often, a "streetlight" is identified as the C5, C6, and C7 nerve roots. The needle should be inserted in-plane with

the ultrasound probe and advanced until the tip is in between the C5 and C6 nerve roots. With full visualization of the needle and after gentle aspiration, local anesthetic is injected.

Lower Extremity Blocks

Femoral Nerve Block (FNB) Versus Adductor Canal Block (ACB)

- Indications: Knee arthroscopy, ACL repair, foot/ankle surgery (in combination with sciatic nerve block)
- Ultrasound-guided techniques:
- For a femoral nerve block, the probe is placed in a transverse position just below the inguinal ligament. The structures identified from medial to lateral include the femoral vein, femoral artery, and femoral nerve. Utilizing an in-plane technique, local anesthetic is injected adjacent to the femoral nerve, the hyperechoic structure just lateral to the femoral artery.
- For an adductor canal block, the probe is placed at the midthigh, anteromedially, and local anesthetic is injected around the saphenous nerve deep to the sartorius muscle and lateral to the femoral artery.

Quadriceps weakness following FNB has been reported, potentially putting patients at risk for falls, by causing weakness in the pectineus muscle. The ACB is a predominantly sensory nerve block, while it has been shown to also cause some quadriceps weakness; studies have shown that it is to a lesser degree than the FNB which facilitates better ambulation. For this reason, the ACB has gained more popularity, especially in an ambulatory setting [31].

Sciatic Nerve Block

- Indications: Foot and ankle surgery, and as an adjunct to ACB for ACL repair.
- Ultrasound-guided technique: Several different approaches have been described, including popliteal, subgluteal, and anterior. Because the anterior approach can be performed supine, it is used often in patients that cannot tolerate being positioned laterally. For the anterior approach, place the probe on the anterior proximal thigh just below the inguinal crease until the sciatic nerve is identified. Utilizing an out-of-plane technique, inject local anesthetic around the sciatic nerve between the adductor magnus muscle and biceps femoris muscle.

Truncal Nerve Blocks/Other Peripheral Nerve Blocks

Rectus Sheath Block

- Indications: Umbilical hernia repair, other umbilical surgeries
- Ultrasound-guided technique: The probe is placed in a transverse orientation just lateral to the umbilicus and the rectus abdominis muscle is identified, located medial to the aponeurosis of the external and internal oblique and the transversus abdominis muscle. The needle is inserted in-plane in a lateral to medial direction until the tip of the needle is visualized at the posterior aspect of the rectus muscle just between the rectus muscle and its posterior rectus sheath. After negative aspiration, 1–2 mL of saline or local anesthetic is injected ("hydrodissection") to confirm appropriate spread along the posterior aspect of the rectus muscle. Once confirmed, a large volume of dilute local anesthetic is injected slowly and incrementally until spread is visualized along the entire posterior aspect of the rectus muscle.

Transversus Abdominis Plane Block (TAP)

- Indications: Laparoscopic appendectomy or other laparoscopic procedures involving multiple port sites
- Ultrasound-guided technique: The probe is placed in a transverse orientation, lateral to the umbilicus, and moved laterally until

three muscle layers (i.e., external oblique, internal oblique, and transverse abdominus) are visualized. The needle is inserted from either the lateral or medial aspect of the probe using an in-plane technique, and advanced between the internal oblique and transversus abdominis muscles into the TAP. Local anesthetic is injected slowly and incrementally between the fascia with intermittent aspiration separating the internal oblique and transversus abdominis muscle layers.

Quadratus Lumborum Block (QLB)

- Indications: Upper and lower abdominal surgeries

The QLB is a novel abdominal truncal block which is gaining popularity although it is technically more difficult to perform than the TAP block. There are four different approaches described, all with the goal of providing local anesthetic spread to the thoracic paravertebral space. It has been shown to provide longer and more effective postoperative analgesia as compared to the TAP block [32, 33].

Pudendal Nerve Block (PNB)

- Indications: Circumcision, hypospadias repair
- Ultrasound-guided technique: The transperineal approach is easily done with ultrasound guidance [21]. With the patient in frog leg position, the ischium on one side is palpated before the ultrasound probe is placed in a transverse plane. The probe is then moved medially so that the ischial ischium and rectum are both in view (see Fig. 22.1). Visualization of the pudendal artery (neurovascular bundle) is helpful to determine correct needle placement. Using an out-of-plane technique, the needle is inserted into the ischiorectal fossa and local anesthetic injected and visualized surrounding the neurovascular bundle. The same technique is repeated on the contralateral side to block the pudendal nerve bilaterally. The goal is to block the pudendal nerve as it enters the lesser sciatic foramen.

A recent study evaluating the efficacy of PNB versus caudal block for hypospadias repair reported improved pain control and longer duration of analgesia in patients randomized to pudendal nerve blocks [23]. Additionally, PNB avoids the risk of temporary urinary retention and

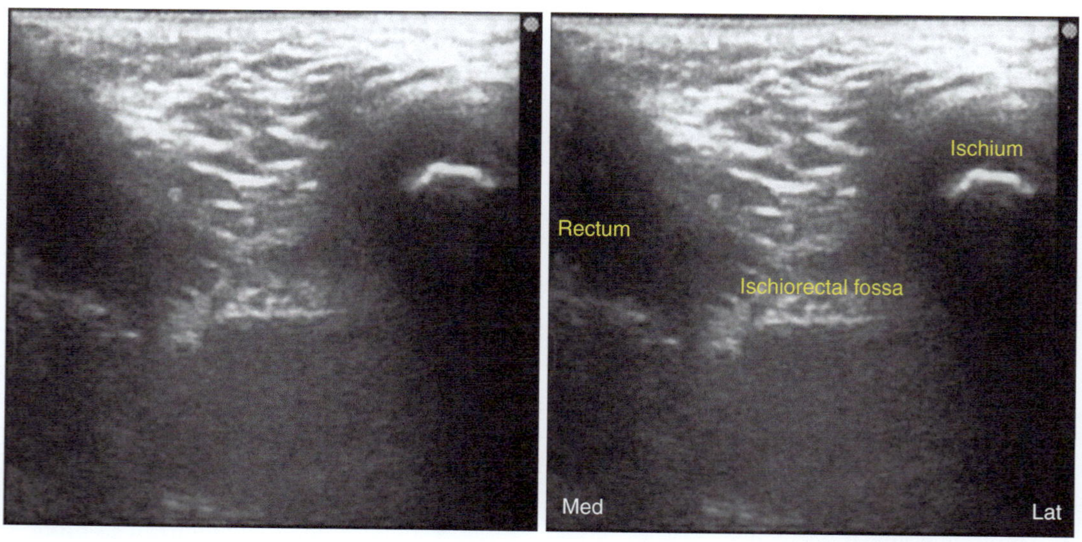

Fig. 22.1 Right-sided ultrasound-guided pudendal nerve block in a child (left – unlabeled, right – with labels)

lower extremity weakness associated with caudal block [34].

Local Anesthetic Dosing and Adjuncts

For peripheral nerve blocks, ropivacaine or bupivacaine are both good choices; however, due to a greater risk for severe cardiotoxicity with bupivacaine in the case of intravascular injection, ropivacaine is more widely utilized. Furthermore, ropivacaine is known to produce less motor blockade when compared with bupivacaine. Table 22.2 summarizes local anesthetic dosing for peripheral blocks in children.

Additionally, adjuncts such as clonidine, dexmedetomidine, and dexamethasone have been used to augment the intensity and prolong the duration of blockade, although studies evaluating these agents in pediatric regional blocks are limited [35, 36]. Due to concerns for neurotoxicity associated with off-label use of perineural injection of dexamethasone, many studies have tried to identify the efficacy of systemic administration of dexamethasone as an adjuvant for prolonging the analgesic effect of a peripheral nerve block. According to a recent meta-analysis, perineural dexamethasone prolongs the duration of the nerve block without an increase in adverse events; however, it is unclear whether this increase in duration is clinically significant to the overall postoperative pain experience and whether it should be used routinely versus intravenous administration [37].

Table 22.2 Local anesthetic dosing for pediatric regional blockade

Location of block	Local anesthetic	Dose
Upper extremity blocks	Ropivacaine 0.2% Bupivacaine 0.25%	0.2–0.4 mL/kg
Lower extremity blocks	Ropivacaine 0.2% Bupivacaine 0.25%	0.2–0.3 mL/kg
Truncal nerve blocks		
Rectus Sheath TAP Quadratus lumborum	Ropivacaine 0.2% Bupivacaine 0.25% vs. 0.125%	0.1–0.2 mL/kg per side 0.2–0.4 mL/kg per side 0.3–0.5 mL/kg
Pudendal nerve block	Ropivacaine 0.2% Bupivacaine 0.25%	0.2 mL/kg per side

Pain Assessment

Depending on the procedure, pain after surgery is an expected occurrence. In an ambulatory surgery center, in particular, a patient's pain must be adequately controlled without the need for treatment with multiple doses of intravenous medications, given the inability to admit a patient for pain control. In order to assess a patient's readiness for discharge, adequate assessment of pain is crucial to avoid undertreatment of pain and subsequent prolonged PACU stays or unplanned inpatient admission. There are many challenges and potential barriers for the proper and accurate assessment of pain in the pediatric population including but not limited to developmental and cognitive delays which are obstacles that health care providers must overcome when assessing a child's pain [38].

In the case of infants and nonverbal children, use of physiological parameters and behavioral observation are used; however, standard physiologic parameters, such as blood pressure, heart rate, and respiratory rate, alone have not been found to be reliable sources. While certain behaviors that are associated with pain and discomfort have been described, this may not be sufficient for accurate assessment. As such, observational scales, such as FLACC (face, legs, activity, cry, consolability) have been created. Observational scales are typically used in infants and children from 2 months to 7 years of age. As development and cognition progress, children as young as 3-years old may be able to successfully use self-report pain assessment tools, such as the Faces Pain Scale, to describe their level of pain. Later, depending on the child's level of language development, they may be able to use words to describe what hurts and the severity of the pain. Older children, typically over the age of 8 years old, who have the cognitive ability to understand the concept of serial numbers and greater or less than, are able to use the visual analog scale (VAS) or numerical rating scale (NRS) to describe the severity of their pain [39].

When assessing pain, it is very important to continuously assess pain, particularly after an intervention to determine the effectiveness of therapy. For each patient, using the same pain assessment tool to trend pain scores is important to ensure reliable and consistent results.

While self-reported pain scores are considered the gold standard for pain assessment in children, regular assessment of pain using a combination of approaches, including self-reported measures, behavioral observation, and assessment of cognitive and emotional factors must be considered to ensure optimal pain management.

Summary

In conclusion, a multimodal analgesic approach with an emphasis on available nonopioid pharmacologic and nonpharmacologic therapies and including thoughtful utilization of ultrasound-guided peripheral regional techniques can optimize management of ambulatory surgical pain in children, reduce costs, facilitate home recovery, and improve outcomes and satisfaction in ambulatory pediatric surgical care.

References

1. Nordin AB, Shah SR, Kenney BD. Ambulatory pediatric surgery. Semin Pediatr Surg. 2018;27(2):75–8. https://doi.org/10.1053/j.sempedsurg.2018.02.003.
2. Deer JD, Sawardekar A, Suresh S. Day surgery regional anesthesia in children: safety and improving outcomes, do they make a difference? Curr Opin Anaesthesiol. 2016;29(6):691–5. https://doi.org/10.1097/ACO.0000000000000403.
3. van den Anker J, Reed MD, Allegaert K, Kearns GL. Developmental changes in pharmacokinetics and pharmacodynamics. J Clin Pharmacol. 2018;58(Suppl 10):S10–25. https://doi.org/10.1002/jcph.1284.
4. Razdan R, Stevens L, Ritchie M, Kennedy T, Carr MM. Parents' attitudes toward post-operative narcotic use in pediatric patients. Int J Pediatr Otorhinolaryngol. 2019;124:173–8. https://doi.org/10.1016/j.ijporl.2019.06.006.
5. McCabe SE, West BT, Veliz P, McCabe VV, Stoddard SA, Boyd CJ. Trends in medical and nonmedical use of prescription opioids among US adolescents: 1976-2015. Pediatrics. 2017;139(4):e20162387. https://doi.org/10.1542/peds.2016-2387.
6. Yaster M, McNaull PP, Davis PJ. The opioid epidemic in pediatrics: a 2020 update. Curr Opin Anaesthesiol. 2020;33(3):327–34. https://doi.org/10.1097/ACO.0000000000000865.
7. Polaner DM, Taenzer AH, Walker BJ, et al. Pediatric Regional Anesthesia Network (PRAN): a multi-institutional study of the use and incidence of complications of pediatric regional anesthesia. Anesth Analg. 2012;115(6):1353–64.
8. Chou R, Gordon DB, de Leon-Casasola OA, et al. Management of postoperative pain: a clinical practice guideline from the American Pain Society, the American Society of Regional Anesthesia and Pain Medicine, and the American Society of Anesthesiologists' Committee on Regional Anesthesia, Executive Committee, and Administrative Council [published correction appears in J Pain. 2016 Apr;17(4):508-10. Dosage error in article text]. J Pain. 2016;17(2):131–57. https://doi.org/10.1016/j.jpain.2015.12.008.
9. Lerman J. Pediatric ambulatory anesthesia: an update. Curr Opin Anaesthesiol. 2019;32(6):708–13. https://doi.org/10.1097/ACO.0000000000000787.
10. Tan GX, Tunkel DE. Control of pain after tonsillectomy in children: a review. JAMA Otolaryngol Head Neck Surg. 2017;143(9):937–42. https://doi.org/10.1001/jamaoto.2017.0845.
11. Kuehn BM. FDA: no codeine after tonsillectomy for children. JAMA. 2013;309(11):1100. https://doi.org/10.1001/jama.2013.2403.
12. Kelly LE, Sommer DD, Ramakrishna J, et al. Morphine or Ibuprofen for post-tonsillectomy analgesia: a randomized trial. Pediatrics. 2015;135(2):307–13. https://doi.org/10.1542/peds.2014-1906.
13. Mitchell RB, Archer SM, Ishman SL, et al. Clinical practice guideline: tonsillectomy in children (update)-executive summary. Otolaryngol Head Neck Surg. 2019;160(2):187–205. https://doi.org/10.1177/0194599818807917.
14. Patel J, Hsieh H, Bottalico D, Cappuccio E, et al. Use of intravenous Ibuprofen in pediatric tonsillectomy cases. In: Society for pediatric anesthesia; March 15–17. Houston; 2019.
15. Patel NK, Shah SJ, Lee NK, Gao Q, Carullo VP, Yang CJ. Intraoperative intravenous ibuprofen use is not associated with increased post-tonsillectomy bleeding. Int J Pediatr Otorhinolaryngol. 2020;133:109965. https://doi.org/10.1016/j.ijporl.2020.109965.
16. Franz AM, Dahl JP, Huang H, et al. The development of an opioid sparing anesthesia protocol for pediatric ambulatory tonsillectomy and adenotonsillectomy surgery-A quality improvement project. Paediatr

Anaesth. 2019;29(7):682–9. https://doi.org/10.1111/pan.13662.

17. Franz AM, Martin LD, Liston DE, Latham GJ, Richards MJ, Low DK. In pursuit of an opioid-free pediatric ambulatory surgery center: aquality improvement initiative [published online ahead of print, 2020 Apr 10]. Anesth Analg. 2020; https://doi.org/10.1213/ANE.0000000000004774.
18. Stevens B, Yamada J, Ohlsson A, Haliburton S, Shorkey A. Sucrose for analgesia in newborn infants undergoing painful procedures. Cochrane Database Syst Rev. 2016;7(7):CD001069. Published 2016 Jul 16. https://doi.org/10.1002/14651858.CD001069.pub5.
19. Arane K, Behboudi A, Goldman RD. Virtual reality for pain and anxiety management in children. Can Fam Physician. 2017;63(12):932–4.
20. Iannicelli AM, Vito D, Dodaro CA, et al. Does virtual reality reduce pain in pediatric patients? A systematic review. Ital J Pediatr. 2019;45:171. https://doi.org/10.1186/s13052-019-0757-0
21. Abdelmoniem SA, Mahmoud SA. Comparative evaluation of passive, active, and passive-active distraction techniques on pain perception during local anesthesia administration in children. J Adv Res. 2016;7(3):551–6. https://doi.org/10.1016/j.jare.2015.10.001.
22. Shin HC, Kim JS, Lee SK, et al. The effect of acupuncture on postoperative nausea and vomiting after pediatric tonsillectomy: a meta-analysis and systematic review. Laryngoscope. 2016;126(8):1761–7. https://doi.org/10.1002/lary.25883.
23. Stein AL, Baumgard D, Del Rio I, Tutiven JL. Updates in pediatric regional anesthesia and its role in the treatment of acute pain in the ambulatory setting. Curr Pain Headache Rep. 2017;21(2):11. https://doi.org/10.1007/s11916-017-0614-z.
24. Kaye AD, Green JB, Davidson KS, et al. Newer nerve blocks in pediatric surgery. Best Pract Res Clin Anaesthesiol. 2019;33(4):447–63. https://doi.org/10.1016/j.bpa.2019.06.006.
25. Schloss B, Bhalla T, Klingele K, Phillips D, Prestwich B, Tobias JD. A retrospective review of femoral nerve block for postoperative analgesia after knee surgery in the pediatric population. J Pediatr Orthop. 2014;34(4):459–61.
26. Gaudet-Ferrand I, De La Arena P, Bringuier S, et al. Ultrasound-guided pudendal nerve block in children: a new technique of ultrasound-guided transperineal approach. Paediatr Anaesth. 2018;28(1):53–8. https://doi.org/10.1111/pan.13286.
27. Tutuncu AC, Kendigelen P, Ashyyeralyeva G, et al. Pudendal nerve block versus penile nerve block in children undergoing circumcision. Urol J. 2018;15(3):109–15. https://doi.org/10.22037/uj.v0i0.4292.
28. Kendigelen P, Tutuncu AC, Emre S, et al. Pudendal versus caudal block in children undergoing hypospadias surgery: *a randomized controlled trial*. Reg Anesth Pain Med. 2016;41:610–5.
29. Suresh S, Sawardekar A, Shah R. Ultrasound for regional anesthesia in children. Anesthesiol Clin. 2014;32(1):263–79. https://doi.org/10.1016/j.anclin.2013.10.008.
30. Taenzer AH, Walker BJ, Bosenberg AT, Martin L, et al. Asleep versus awake: does it matter?: pediatric regional block complications by patient state: a report from the Pediatric Regional Anesthesia Network. Reg Anesth Pain Med. 2014;39:279–83.
31. Jæger P, Nielsen ZJK, Henningsen MH, Hilsted KL, Mathiesen O, Dahl JB. Adductor canal block *versus* femoral nerve block and quadriceps strength: a randomized, double-blind, placebo-controlled, crossover study in healthy volunteers. Anesthesiology. 2013;118(2):409–15. https://doi.org/10.1097/ALN.0b013e318279fa0b.
32. Hussein MM. Ultrasound-guided quadratus lumborum block in pediatrics: trans-muscular versus intramuscular approach. J Anesth. 2018;32(6):850–5. https://doi.org/10.1007/s00540-018-2563-z.
33. Öksüz G, Bilal B, Gürkan Y, et al. Quadratus lumborum block versus transversus abdominis plane block in children undergoing low abdominal surgery: a randomized controlled trial. Reg Anesth Pain Med. 2017;42(5):674–9. https://doi.org/10.1097/AAP.0000000000000645.
34. Hecht S, Piñeda J, Bayne A. Ultrasound-guided pudendal block is a viable alternative to caudal block for hypospadias surgery: a single-surgeon pilot study. Urology. 2018;113:192–6. https://doi.org/10.1016/j.urology.2017.11.006.
35. Lundblad M, Trifa M, Kaabachi O, et al. Alpha-2 adrenoceptor agonists as adjuncts to peripheral nerve blocks in children: a meta-analysis. Paediatr Anaesth. 2016;26(3):232–8. https://doi.org/10.1111/pan.12825.
36. Leurcharusmee P, Aliste J, Van Zundert TC, et al. A multicenter randomized comparison between intravenous and perineural dexamethasone for ultrasound-guided infraclavicular block. Reg Anesth Pain Med. 2016;41:328–33.
37. Chong MA, Berbenetz NM, Lin C, Singh S. Perineural versus intravenous dexamethasone as an adjuvant for peripheral nerve blocks: a systematic review and meta-analysis. Reg Anesth Pain Med. 2017;42(3):319–26. https://doi.org/10.1097/AAP.0000000000000571.
38. Walker SM. Pain in children: recent advances and ongoing challenges. Br J Anaesth. 2008;101(1):101–10. https://doi.org/10.1093/bja/aen097.
39. McGrath PA, Gillespie J. Pain assessment in children and adolescents. In: Turk DC, Melzack R, editors. Handbook of pain assessment. New York: The Guilford Press; 2001. p. 97–118.

23 Pain Management in Former Addicts on Medication-Assisted Treatment (MAT) Program

Kanishka Rajput, Gopal Kodumudi, and Nalini Vadivelu

Abstract

There has been resurgence in heroin abuse in recent times as opioid prescriptions have declined, especially with federal and state efforts to curb the opioid epidemic. Despite widespread efforts, only a fraction of patients in the general population are on Medication-Assisted Treatment for opiate addiction (MAT). Opiate addiction is related to genetic, environmental, and pharmacologic risk factors. Medication-assisted treatment (MAT) has the strongest evidence to maintain patients in remission, with three drugs currently approved by the Food and Drug Administration (FDA) for this purpose - methadone, buprenorphine, naltrexone. This chapter reviews the mechanism of action of the three commonly used drugs and unique perioperative concerns when these patients present for ambulatory surgery. We discuss optimal perioperative pain management strategies and considerations for discharge planning, to ensure adequate pain relief, while minimizing the risk of withdrawal and relapse.

Background

Opioid addiction continues to be a major public health problem in the United States, with an estimated 10.3 million Americans aged 12 and older having misused opioids in 2018, including 9.9 million prescription opioid abusers and 808,000 heroin users [1]. Deaths related to opiate analgesic overdose now exceed those caused by motor vehicle accidents and both heroin and cocaine combined [2]. Opioid use disorder (OUD) is a maladaptive use of opioids, prescribed or illicit, resulting in two or more criteria as defined by the Diagnostic and Statistical Manual of Mental Disorders that reflect impaired health or function over a 12-month period [3]. OUD is scaled according to severity (mild/moderate/severe) and does not require physiological tolerance or dependence in order to be considered a substance use disorder [4] (Table 23.1).

Historically, use of opioids for chronic noncancer pain started to increase sharply in the mid- to late 1990s [5], when pain was referred to as the fifth vital sign. Use of opiates for noncancer pain

K. Rajput (✉)
Department of Anesthesiology and Pain Medicine, Yale University School of Medicine, New Haven, CT, USA
e-mail: kanishka.rajput@yale.edu

G. Kodumudi
Department of Anesthesiology, Louisiana State University Health Shreveport, Shreveport, LA, USA
e-mail: gkodumud@tulane.edu

N. Vadivelu
Department of Anesthesiology, Yale University School of Medicine, New Haven, CT, USA

K. Rajput et al. (eds.), *Pain Control in Ambulatory Surgery Centers*,
https://doi.org/10.1007/978-3-030-55262-6_23

Table 23.1 DSM-5 Criteria for Opioid Use Disorder (OUD)

1. Opioids are often taken in larger amounts or over a longer period than was intended.
2. There is a persistent desire or unsuccessful efforts to cut down or control opioid use.
3. A great deal of time is spent in activities necessary to obtain the opioid, use the opioid, or recover from its effects.
4. Craving, or a strong desire or urge to use opioids.
5. Recurrent opioid use resulting in a failure to fulfill major role obligations at work, school, or home.
6. Continued opioid use despite having persistent or recurrent social or interpersonal problems caused or exacerbated by the effects of opioids.
7. Important social, occupational, or recreational activities are given up or reduced because of opioid use.
8. Recurrent opioid use in situations in which it is physically hazardous.
9. Continued opioid use despite knowledge of having a persistent or recurrent physical or psychological problem that is likely to have been caused or exacerbated by the substance.
10. Exhibits tolerance.
11. Exhibits withdrawal.

Severity scaling is determined by the number of criteria that are met. 2–3 = mild, 4–5 = Moderate, >6 = severe

was not only encouraged but also cited to be safe without significant adverse effects; the problem being compounded by aggressive marketing from pharmaceutical companies [6]. Shortly thereafter, nonmedical opioid use also started to increase significantly, reaching a peak of 2.7 million new users in 2002 [7]. From 1999 to 2011, hydrocodone use increased more than two-fold, oxycodone use more than five-fold [8], and the mortality rate of opioid-related overdose almost four-fold [9]. In more recent years, national initiatives to reduce opioid prescribing have modestly decreased the number of prescription opioids dispensed [10]. However, many people who otherwise would have been using prescription opioids have transitioned to heroin use, with one study reporting that about 80 percent of current heroin users began with prescription opioids [11]. This resulted in a three-fold increase in heroin-involved overdose deaths from 2010 to 2014 [12]. The overall frequency of heroin deaths has further accelerated since 2015 due to heroin supplies being laced with fentanyl. Data from DEA strategic intelligence section note that drug traffickers mix fentanyl into local heroin supplies in order to respond to users' demand for high quality heroin. Instead of supplying a purer product, demand can be satisfied with fewer costs, and charged at a higher price by supplying heroin adulterated with enough fentanyl to provide customers the high they seek, all while maintaining stable heroin purity. This new development however, has put users at greater risk of overdose and death [13].

Who Is at Risk of Developing Opiate Addiction?

Above evidence associating nonmedical use of pain relievers with subsequent heroin use [11] highlights the link between licit and illicit drug use and the importance of addressing both as a continuum of the same epidemic. Little is known about why only certain individuals develop OUD following recurrent opioid exposure, although the risk for developing opiate addiction seems to be a complex interaction between genetics, environmental factors, and the pharmacological effects of opiates [14]. Human family and twin studies have not only identified increased genetic risk for addiction in first degree relatives of addicts but also that the genetic risk specific to opiate addiction is second only to that for alcoholism [15, 16]. Population studies in patients receiving opioid analgesics identify co-occurring substance use and mental illness as risk factors for developing OUD [17]. A recent meta-analysis suggests that the rs1799971 polymorphism of the OPRM1 gene, the gene that codes for the mu-opioid receptor, may confer vulnerability to OUD following exposure to either heroin or prescription opioids [18].

Environmental factors such as availability of opiates, perceived risk of opiate use, psychosocial stressors, and learned coping strategies; all influence the risk of developing opiate addiction. For example, the incidence of opiate addiction has paralleled increased availability of opiates. While 75% of high school seniors perceive using heroin once or twice as dangerous, only 40% perceive similar use of prescription opiates as dangerous [19]. Traumatic lifetime experience may increase the risk for opiate addiction. In rodent models, maternal separation early in life increases vulnerability to opiate addiction for both the pup and the dam and, in humans; weak parental bonds increase the risk for illicit drug use during adulthood [20–22]. In humans, there is an association between post-traumatic stress disorder and opiate addiction with an over-representation in prevalence of this disorder in opiate addicts compared to the general population and to those with other substance use disorders [23].

The euphoria and abuse liability of an opiate similarly may be a risk factor. Opiate receptors are present throughout the brain with highest density in areas that modulate pain and reward (e.g., thalamus, amygdala, anterior cingulate cortex, and striatum). Receptor activation initiates a cascade of effects related to reward. In turn, the risk of repeated opiate use is elevated due to the heightened saliency of drug-related cues and the incubation of drug craving [24, 25]. Human imaging studies have identified ongoing reductions in dopamine D2 receptor-binding potential in opiate addicts and this reduction correlates with the duration of opiate use [26, 27]. Repeat opiate administration induces tolerance and imparts the potential for a withdrawal syndrome upon cessation. The unpleasant physical and psychological symptoms of withdrawal produce negative reinforcement, so the user continues to use opiates at escalating doses to avoid these adverse symptoms [28]. Furthermore, short-acting opiates cause dysregulation of the stress-responsive pathways and promote stress-induced negative reinforcement. This stress dysregulation can continue long after a person has discontinued opiates and, thereby, is a contributing factor to the risk for relapse during stress.

The interaction between genes, environment, and drugs forms the hypothesized foundation for the persistence of addiction vulnerability even in those who have discontinued drug use and is the primary reason for utilization of long-term relapse prevention strategies that include both environmental and pharmacological interventions beyond the immediate period of withdrawal [14].

Medication-Assited Treatment (MAT) and Its Availability

Medication-assisted treatment of opioid use disorder with physiological dependence at least doubles the rates of opioid-abstinence outcomes in randomized controlled trials comparing psychosocial treatment of opioid use disorder with medication versus with placebo or no medication. The Food and Drug Administration (FDA) has approved three medications for stabilization/maintenance treatment of OUD and for preventing opioid relapse: methadone, buprenorphine and naltrexone. The evidence strongly supports the use of agonist therapies to reduce opioid use and to retain patients in treatment, with methadone maintenance being the gold standard of care [29]. Combined buprenorphine/naloxone, however, also demonstrates significant efficacy and favorable safety and tolerability in multiple populations, including youth and prescription opioid-dependent individuals, as buprenorphine monotherapy does in pregnant women. The evidence for antagonist therapies is weak. Oral naltrexone demonstrates poor adherence and increased mortality rates, although the early evidence looks more favorable for extended-release naltrexone, which has the advantages that it is not subject to misuse or diversion and that it does not present a risk of overdose on its own [4].

Of the 10.3 million Americans addicted to opiates, only fractions (1,172,371) are enrolled in medication-assisted treatment programs. The breakdown of numbers from SAMSHA from 2018 is methadone (450,247), buprenorphine (648,864), and naltrexone (73,260) [30]. Although we have a long way to go, these numbers reflect ongoing efforts at national and state levels to increase the number of opioid treatment programs (OTPs) available to dispense these treatments to patients that need it the most. The number of OTPs have increased from approximately 1100 in 2003 to almost 1500 by the end of 2016 from results of a recent survey. The number of clients receiving methadone on this survey increased from 227,000 in 2003 to over 350,000 in 2015. The percentage of OTPs offering buprenorphine similarly increased from 11 percent in 2003 to 58

Table 23.2 FDA-Approved Medications for Treatment of OUD

Medication	Mu-opioid receptor activity	Mechanism of action	Side effects
Methadone	Full Mu agonist + NMDA antagonist	Reduced opioid craving and withdrawal. Reduction of reinforcing effects of other opioids.	Opioid-class effects: dose-dependent sedation, constipation, sweating, neurocognitive impairment, and sexual dysfunction. Early phase treatment euphoria abates with dose stabilization
Buprenorphine	Partial Mu agonist + kappa antagonist	Reduced opioid craving and withdrawal. Competitive blockade/reduction of reinforcing effects of other opioids.	Sedation constipation and diaphoresis. "Ceiling effect" on respiratory depression and euphoria [32]
Naltrexone	Mu Antagonist	Competitive blockade of reinforcing effects of other opioids.	Insomnia, injection site reactions, mild transaminase elevation, hypertension, nasopharyngitis, and influenza [33]

percent in 2015; the percentage of facilities without OTPs offering buprenorphine increased from 5 percent in 2003 to 21 percent in 2015. The percentage of OTPs offering extended-release, injectable naltrexone also increased from 11 percent in 2011 to 23 percent in 2015; the percentage of facilities without OTPs offering extended-release, injectable naltrexone increased from 8 percent in 2011 to 16 percent in 2015 [31].

A significant number of these patients may be expected to present for emergency or elective surgery, although data regarding the incidence of MAT use in perioperative surgical populations are lacking.

These three drugs used in MAT programs are ligands that bind to central mu-opioid receptors as the molecular target for their therapeutic activity; however, they differ significantly in their respective actions at the mu-opioid receptor, their pharmacokinetic and pharmacodynamic properties (with effects on efficacy and toxicity), and the mechanisms by which they confer relapse-prevention protection to treated individuals. Table 23.2 summarizes mechanism of action of these drugs and their relevant side effects.

Unique Preoperative Concerns

Guidelines on the management of perioperative pain recommend that preoperative patient evaluation and preparation include a thorough history of prior chronic pain complaints, opioid use and abuse, other substance use, identifying any medications whose cessation may lead to withdrawal, and assessing for psychiatric and other Substance Abuse Disorder comorbidities, along with a complete physical examination [34, 35]. To further appreciate anesthetic implications, specifically influencing perioperative pain management in the presence of MAT drugs, it is important to review the basic pharmacology of these drugs.

A. *PHARMACOLOGY*

(i) *Methadone:* Methadone is a pure mu-opioid agonist with NMDA receptor antagonism, the latter effect contributing to its effects on neuropathic pain and mitigation of opioid-induced tolerance [36]. The degree of NMDA antagonism produced by methadone is similar to that of ketamine [37]. It also causes some inhibition of reuptake of serotonin and norepinephrine and when combined with other SNRIs could be a risk factor for serotonin syndrome. Methadone has high oral bioavailability of 85%, around three that of morphine with a high volume of distribution in humans (4.2–9.2 L/kg in opioid addicts and 1.7–5.3 L/kg in chronic pain patients). At physiological pH, 86% of methadone is bound to plasma proteins, predominately to α1-acid glycoprotein (AAG). Biotransformation of methadone is via conjugation in the liver by the CYP3A4 and CYP2D6 enzymes. The activities of these cytochrome enzymes, especially

CYP3A4, can be induced or inhibited by other drugs or by the methadone itself, accounting for the large individual variations in methadone pharmacology. At daily doses less than 55 mg, the majority of metabolites, that are inactive, are cleared via the fecal route. Methadone does not accumulate in patients with renal failure and is poorly removed by hemodialysis. Methadone undergoes a biphasic pattern of elimination: slow distribution or α-elimination phase (8–12 hr) and a ß-elimination phase (30–60 hr). The α-elimination correlates with the duration of analgesia that is typically 6–8 hours. The plasma level in the ß-elimination phase is subanalgesic but is sufficient to prevent withdrawal symptoms. Thus, it accounts for the three or four times daily dosing typically needed when prescribed for analgesia compared to the once a day dosing used in MAT.

(ii) *Buprenorphine:* Buprenorphine is a partial agonist at mu receptors and an antagonist at kappa receptors. This combination of partial mu-receptor agonism and kappa-receptor antagonism makes buprenorphine useful as an analgesic while also providing some abuse deterrence. Suboxone®, is a combination of the partial opioid agonist-antagonist buprenorphine and the opioid antagonist naloxone. Naloxone is added to buprenorphine to further enhance abuse deterrence to prevent intravenous or intramuscular injection. Because of buprenorphine's high-lipid solubility, it has exceptional sublingual bioavailability; however, the naloxone component displays no sublingual absorption and very little oral absorption. As a result, the naloxone component only takes affect when a patient attempts to abuse Suboxone® via intravenous or intramuscular injection.

(iii) *Naltrexone*: Naltrexone is a pure opioid antagonist that competes with and displaces opioids at opioid receptor sites with greatest affinity for the μ-opioid receptor. Although useful to reverse the effects of an opioid overdose, naltrexone is also used to prevent relapse of both opioid and alcohol dependence by reducing cravings in patients who have completed detoxification programs [38]. Newer formulations, such as an extended-release, once-monthly injectable form of naltrexone (XR naltrexone), are also available as an alternative to daily oral dosing. Its efficacy is mediated through interactions between dopamine and the endogenous opioid neuropeptide systems, also involved in the expression of reinforcing effects of alcohol. Being a pure antagonist, maintenance on naltrexone makes patients resistant to the effects of opioids. After discontinuation however, patients may be more sensitive to the effects of opiates secondary to opioid receptor upregulation from chronic antagonism [39]. The new once-monthly extended-release formulation of injectable naltrexone prevents the relapse to opioid dependence following detoxification [33]. Although methadone remains the gold standard for MAT, number of patients on naltrexone especially of the once-monthly injection, are increasing.

B. *ANXIETY and Fear of being judged/ hesitation to get exposed to opioids given prior history*

Surgery is a stressful period for any individual, especially for patients with a prior history of OUD who are now stable on MAT. These patients often worry the effect of re-exposure to opioids on their risk of relapse. Individuals with OUD also fear that they will face unfair treatment and adverse judgment by medical providers during their hospital stay. Shame and self-stigma are common among individuals with SUDs and known to confound their help seeking [40]. These patients worry about receiving inadequate pain relief, experiencing opioid withdrawal symptoms, and relapsing. It is imperative to establish a good rapport with these patients, who appreciate honesty and a clear description of expectations both from the surgical service and the nurse as well as a direct line of communication with the Acute Pain Service whom they see as a valued resource. In addition, screening for high-risk comorbid psychiatric conditions can help guide perioperative pain management. Anxiety and catastrophic thinking have been associated with higher risk of opioid misuse in chronic pain patients and those with a history of SUDs [41, 42]. The Pain Catastrophizing Scale is a reliable and valid scale that can help identify those who may experience significant helplessness and catastrophic thinking about their pain and inform decisions related to pain management [43]. Negative affect such as anxiety is known to trigger drug craving [44]. Pain Catastrophizing Scale can be a useful tool to screen patients with OUD for anxious, catastrophizing thinking before a surgical procedure. The Opioid Risk Tool identifies those with chronic pain who may be at high risk if opioid analgesics are prescribed and can help guide postoperative pain management [45]. The anxiety surrounding surgery and postoperative pain are significant stressors and can easily elicit a conditioned response, trigger powerful memories of drug use, and ultimately result in drug cravings [46].

C. *Opioid tolerance/To hold or continue*

The difficulties in controlling pain for this special population have been reported previously. Patients with OUD have been shown to have lowered pain thresholds, increased sensitivity to pain secondary to opioid induce hyperalgesia, and comorbid chronic pain conditions compared to that of opioid-naive control groups [47, 48]. A detailed history regarding dose of MAT, frequency of ingestion, time of last dose, and level of stability (as indicated by take-home dose level), should be obtained. This information helps in the assessment of opioid tolerance. MAT patients may be able to recount successful analgesia regimes from previous admissions for surgery and reviewing old charts may assist in determining how opioid-tolerant these patients have been.

(i) *Methadone:* For patients on stable doses of methadone for OUD, consensus recommendations are to continue the usual dose during the perioperative phase. Patients should be instructed to take their normal dose of methadone on the morning of surgery with a small sip of water. If the patient forgets to or is unable to take their dose orally, they may be administered IV methadone intraoperatively. Traditional oral to IV conversion for methadone is 2:1. Unfortunately, a minority of patients may be diverting some or all of their methadone for sale or trade. In questionable cases, a portion of the MAT dose may be given parenterally with induction of anesthesia after application of full ASA monitors. If IV methadone is not available in the ambulatory setting, equianalgesic dose of morphine may be used. Unfortunately, methadone conversion is often challenging since conversion calculations are not bidirectional (i.e., the morphine-to-methadone conversion ratio may not be the same as the methadone-to morphine ratio). Since methadone is metabolized by CYP450, pharmacokinetic parameters and polymorphism of CYP450 enzymes may result in large interpatient variability in the equianalgesic conversion ratio and half-life variation (up to 150 hours) [49]. Moreover, some drugs such as antidepressants (selective serotonin reuptake inhibitors [SSRIs], amitriptyline), antifungals (fluconazole, ketoconazole), and macrolide antibiotics (erythromycin, clarithromycin) may increase methadone concentrations, by inhibiting CYP3A4 metabolism. Conversely, other drugs such as antiepileptics (carbamazepine, phenobarbital, phenytoin), antipsychotics (risperidone), antiretrovirals (nevirapine, ritonavir), antitubercular (rifampin) may decrease methadone concentrations [50]. When converting from high doses of opiates to methadone, less methadone will be required. Conversely, converting from methadone to other opioids is an area of limited research but of increasing importance. In one study, the estimated dose ratio for IV methadone to oral Morphine Equivalent Dose (MED) has been found to be 13.5 and that for oral methadone to oral MED is 4.7 [51]. When oral methadone is converted to IV methadone, the estimated dose ratio is 2:1. This difference between IV and oral methadone, in terms of MED, is not expected based on methadone's high oral bioavailability, but it appears to be clinically important and likely due to presystemic (first pass) elimination. However, this ratio may vary depending on patient metabolism. Table 23.3 gives a broad guideline from the CDC when converting from methadone to oral morphine equivalents, using extra caution as the conversion factor increases at higher doses. For example, a patient on 30 mg methadone daily would need approximately 240 mg morphine in a 24-hour period, based on the conversion table below. However, it is always recommended to reduce the dose by 25–75% when converting between different opioids to account for incomplete cross tolerance. One would therefore start at a dose of approximately 120 mg of PO morphine equivalents in divided doses over a 24-hour period.

(ii) *Buprenorphine:* While there are several different schools of thought on how best to control acute pain in patients on buprenorphine maintenance therapy, clinical evidence remains limited and experts remain divided on the best approach in the perioperative period. Earlier approaches recommended eliminating the partial blockade of buprenorphine, by discontinuing the medication 72 h prior to surgery and converting to a full agonist preoperatively, especially if surgery was expected to cause severe pain. The patient is then continued on a full mu agonist for pain control upon discharge. Subsequently, induction/reconversion to buprenorphine maintenance therapy will need to be performed after the patient recovers from acute pain related to surgery [53]. However, it is imperative to weigh the risks and benefits of discontinuing buprenorphine/naloxone, since patients view this treatment as a lifesaving therapy. Discontinuing a stabilizing medication, coupled with the preoperative anxiety and anticipation of pain, can be unbearable and lead to stress-triggered relapse [54]. Given the accumulating evidence of tolerability and favorable outcomes of patients receiving buprenorphine/naloxone and adjunct opioid therapy perioperatively, automatically discontinuing buprenorphine/naloxone 2–5 days before surgery does not seem to be supported by high-level evidence and may be unsafe given the increased risk of mortality on treatment cessation [55]. An alternate method therefore is to continue buprenorphine perioperatively, especially for less painful surgeries and supplement it via a multimodal analgesic approach with an emphasis on nonopioids. If necessary, additional buprenorphine can be used as well, since buprenorphine has strong analgesic properties itself. Despite conflicting expert opinions on the best method to manage patients on Suboxone®, there is consensus that a multimodal analgesic regimen be employed along with the use of nonopi-

Table 23.3 Calculating morphine milligram equivalents (MME) [52]

Opioid (dose in mg/day)	Conversion factor
Morphine	1
Methadone	
1–20 mg/day	4
21–40 mg/day	8
41–60 mg/day	10
>= 61–80 mg/day	12

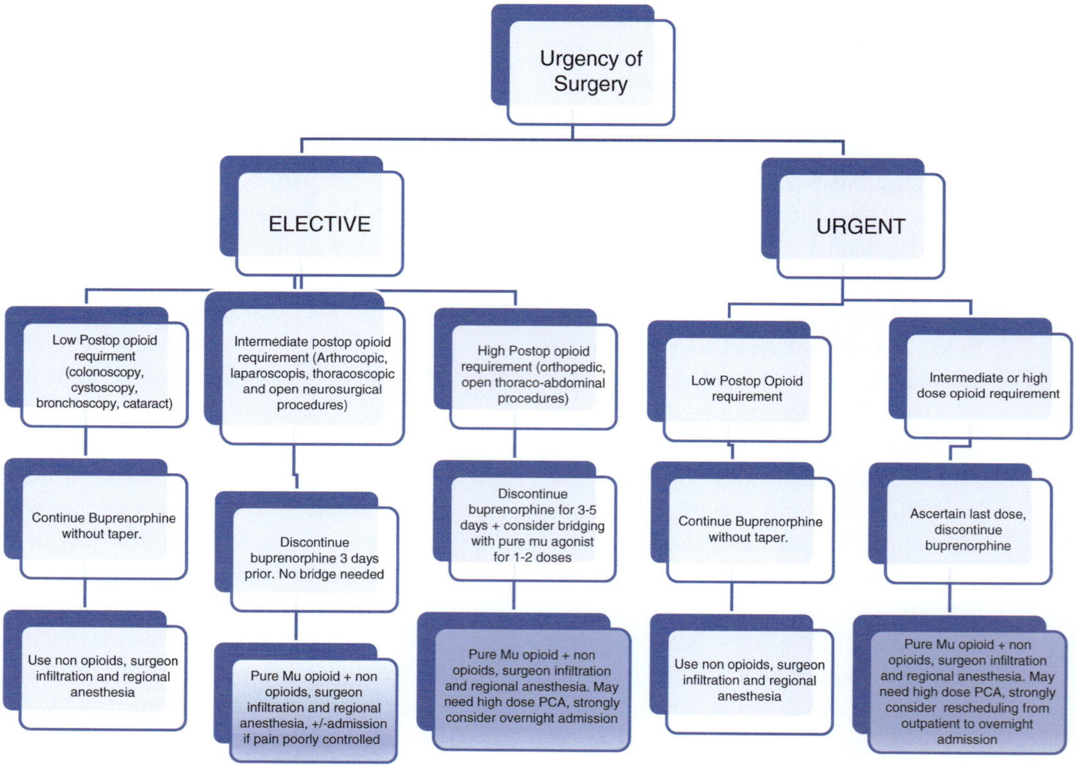

Fig. 23.1 Best practice strategies on perioperative pain management in patients on buprenorphine undergoing ambulatory surgery

oid adjuncts and regional anesthesia if applicable [56]. Figure 23.1 is a simplified version of best practice strategies for perioperative pain management in patients on buprenorphine undergoing ambulatory surgery, based on the expected postoperative opioid requirement [57].

(iii) *Naltrexone:* Few data are available on perioperative management of patients under maintenance naltrexone treatment. These patients represent a challenge for anesthesiologists for perioperative pain control, since naltrexone may cause reduced sensitivity to opioids or precipitate withdrawal symptoms, when redosing naltrexone soon after opioid use [38]. For oral once daily regimen, naltrexone should be discontinued 24–72 hours prior to elective surgery. The once-monthly extended release formulation should be held for 3–4 weeks prior to elective surgery that should be planned during the fourth week [39]. In case of emergency, a risk versus benefit discussion between the surgeon, anesthesiologist, and patient should precede the decision to perform the surgery in an ambulatory setting. This is due to the fact that much higher doses of opioids may be needed perioperatively (identified by titration) and a prolonged period of observation may be required for these patients in the postoperative care unit. There should be a low threshold for overnight admission for patients who have been on maintenance naltrexone due to risk of rebound opioid sensitivity.

D. *UDS - Coexistent smoking/marijuana use/alcohol use*

Many patients use medical marijuana for a wide range of indications including chronic pain. Coexistent smoking, alcohol, and ongoing use of other illicit substances may have anesthetic implications and should be specifically asked about. A urine toxicology screening specifically testing for methadone, buprenorphine, fentanyl in addition to other drugs such as benzodiazepines can be helpful to gather objective information in high-risk cases, who are relatively unstable. A history of recent benzodiazepine use can be helpful to prevent a potentially complicated postoperative sedative withdrawal syndrome from occurring. Online prescription drug monitoring program databases should be reviewed for controlled substance prescriptions.

E. *Prolonged QTc*

Of the three drugs used for MAT, methadone is the only one associated with QTc prolongation. The risk of prolonged QTc with methadone (associated with Torsades de pointes, which has an estimated 10–17% risk of sudden death due to cardiac arrhythmia) is dose-dependent [58]. It has been seen at doses as low as 29 mg/day, but most literatures suggest that this is dose-dependent. It is the levacetylmethadol metabolite that affects cardiac repolarization. Since methadone is a long-acting drug, this metabolite would be present at once daily (e.g., 40 mg daily) or 4 times a day (e.g., 10 mg q 6 hours) regimen. Overall high dose would be a risk for QTC prolongation [59].

Other risk factors for QTc prolongation include parenteral administration of methadone, oral administration of doses greater than 200 mg/day, and medical conditions or medications that predispose patients to QTc interval prolongation. Medications relevant to the perioperative period include ondansetron, chlorpromazine, clarithromycin, disopyramide, erythromycin, haloperidol, amiodarone, and some of the other antiarrhythmic agents that are known to increase QT interval. Although screening baseline QTc intervals have not yet been shown to assist risk management during methadone maintenance, a baseline EKG in the preoperative period is recommended [60]. Neither buprenorphine nor naltrexone is associated with QTc prolongation.

F. *Coexistent HIV, Hep B, Hep C*

Patients with prior history of opiate and substance abuse may have coexistent HIV, Hep B, and Hep C infections, with or without hepatic sequelae. Cumulative, lifetime HCV seroprevalence estimates among injection-drug users is up to 90% with high seroconversion rates attributable to both sharing syringes/needles and sharing drug preparation equipment (e.g., drug cookers and spoons, filtration cottons, vehicle fluids) [61, 62]. Routine labs including LFTs and tests for synthetic function including coagulation studies may be indicated for moderate to high-risk surgery in patients with above history.

G. *Difficult IV access/Airway evaluation/ Poor dentition*

Prior history of opiate abuse in the form of prescription drugs or heroin may be associated with sclerosing of veins, making IV access particularly challenging in some cases. Anesthesiologists should anticipate difficulty and have back up equipment such as infrared vein finders and portable ultrasound available. Only the most-experienced staff should try to obtain IV access, given very limited options. In extreme cases, IV access team may have to be consulted for placing a PICC line. As with any other preoperative evaluation, the importance of airway evaluation cannot be stressed enough. Special note should be made of poor or missing dentition.

Intraoperative Management

A. *Intraoperative Opiates:*

Studies suggest that opioid-tolerant patients may require approximately three to four times as much opioid during the perioperative period compared to their opioid-naïve counterparts [63, 64]. Possible explanations for this include associated tolerance, physical dependence, psychological disorders, such as concomitant anxiety, depression, etc., all of which alone or in combination may diminish opioid-analgesic effectiveness [65]. It is therefore recommended to use a multimodal analgesic approach, including the use of non-opioid adjuncts and regional anesthesia when possible.

(i) *Methadone*: Given opioid tolerance, the usual daily dose of methadone for OUD is insufficient to provide adequate perioperative analgesia [56, 60]. Additional opioids may be titrated intraoperatively based on vital signs. The adequacy of intraoperative opioid dosing may be gauged by allowing spontaneous ventilation towards the end of the case, after reversing neuromuscular blockade. Patients with respiratory rates greater than 20 breaths/min and exhibiting slight to markedly dilated pupils generally require additional opioids. IV boluses of morphine, fentanyl, or hydromorphone may be titrated as needed to maintain a rate of 12–14 breaths/min and a slightly miotic pupil [65]. In addition to continuing the usual methadone dose, nonpharmacological interventions and nonopioid medications depending on the surgery and severity of acute pain are recommended as per the Guidelines on the Management of Postoperative Pain [66]. Commonly used nonopioid adjuncts include acetaminophen, COX2-inhibitors, antidepressants, and anticonvulsants (such as gabapentinoids), all of which are considered a part of multimodal pre-emptive analgesia. Many of these patients have neurological deficits and sedentary lifestyles that are associated with complications of perioperative management and adverse events attributed to side effects, drug interactions, and problems with tolerance, all which needs close monitoring in the perioperative period [67]. Partial opioid agonist such as butorphanol and buprenorphine should be avoided as they may precipitate withdrawal symptoms. For moderate to severe pain, peripheral, regional, and neuraxial analgesia is recommended.

(ii) *Buprenorphine*: If a decision is made to continue buprenorphine for MAT, a different opioid may be used for analgesia, by titrating an oral short-acting (immediate release [IR] morphine or oxycodone) or IV opioid analgesic (morphine or fentanyl) to the desired analgesic effect (continuous infusions are not recommended, knowing that higher doses of opioids could be necessary for competing with buprenorphine). Alternatively, if a patient is taking a low-maintenance dose of buprenorphine (e.g., 2–8 mg per day), it may be used as analgesic itself. The daily dose of the buprenorphine maintenance therapy could be administered at the same or a higher dose, if necessary, given every 6–8 hours to take advantage of its analgesic properties, by increasing its plasma blood level.

Finally, for major surgery, when postoperative pain is expected to be high and to require opioid therapy, consider that buprenorphine could act as an antagonist on MOR, due to its high affinity and its ceiling effect, and prevent the analgesic activity of the full opioid agonist. Moreover, buprenorphine has kappa-opioid receptor antagonist activity that may interfere with the actions of other opioids.

(iii) *Naltrexone*: Opioid antagonists should be discontinued at least 24–72 hours preoperatively. After abrupt discontinuation, a selective up-regulation of mu receptors with enhanced opioid sensitivity may develop. Perioperative opioids must be therefore titrated carefully to avoid excessive sedation or respiratory depression in this setting [65]. Perioperative analgesia should include use nonopioid analgesics, such as NSAIDs and acetaminophen, corticosteroids, ketamine, and regional analgesic techniques, when indicated. Postoperative administration of opioid antagonists should be similarly avoided to prevent precipitating withdrawal symptoms in patients who are dependent on potent opioids.

B. *Regional Anesthesia:*

Expert opinion suggests that opioid-tolerant patients should be offered regional anesthesia whenever possible, especially for orthopedic procedures [53, 68–71]. Advantages of a regional anesthetic/analgesic approach include reduction in parenteral/oral opioid requirements, improvement in distal perfusion from the sympathetic blockade and the ability to be discharged home with indwelling brachial plexus catheters and local anesthetic infusions for up to 48 hours via disposable pumps. Other interventions that are often used include injection of local anesthetics and opioids into the knee and other articular joints and injections of local anesthetics into disc spaces or the iliac crest for spinal surgery. The goal is to minimize pain perception and reduce, although not completely eliminate, the use of oral or parenteral opioids for baseline requirements in opioid-dependent patients. Considerations specific for peripheral nerve blocks and neuraxial anesthesia are covered in a subsequent chapter.

C. *NonOpioid Adjuncts:*

Nonopioid adjuvants such as acetaminophen, NSAIDS, and ketamine may help reduce opioid requirements and provide multimodal analgesia, although relatively few evaluations have been performed in opioid-tolerant patients. Nonopioid analgesics including acetaminophen, nonselective nonsteroidal anti-inflammatory drugs and more specific cyclooxygenase-2 inhibitors have been shown to minimize inflammatory pain [72, 73]. Low-dose ketamine may antagonize NMDA receptor activation and has been studied more so in the chronic pain population.

Ketamine is an NMDA antagonist with intense analgesic efficacy that has received considerable interest particularly, for patients on chronic opioid therapy or chronic illicit drug users, especially in major surgeries. While anesthetic doses of ketamine can cause hallucinations and dissociative side effects similar to PCP, in subanesthetic doses, the drug's NMDA antagonist properties may accentuate perioperative analgesia.

The use of perioperative ketamine has been summarized in a systematic review by Laskowski et al. involving 4701 patients concluded that intravenous ketamine is an effective adjunct for postoperative analgesia in a variety of surgeries, but they concluded that it may not be particularly beneficial for surgeries associated with mild pain (VAS-equivalent <40% of the maximum score on any pain scale). By surgical site, ketamine was not efficacious for tonsillectomy, dental or head, and neck surgery, but it had significant analgesic benefit for those procedures involving the upper abdomen and thorax. Timing of administration (pre or postincision) and size of dose had no influence, and there was no pre-emptive effect identified [74]. For ambulatory surgeries, low-dose ketamine has been studied in outpatient arthroscopic knee and shoulder surgeries with conflicting results. Menigaux et al. in their study on outpatient arthroscopic meniscectomy concluded that adding low-dose ketamine (0.15 mg/kg IV just after the induction of anesthesia) to a multimodal analgesic regimen improved postoperative analgesia and functional outcome, without affecting time to awakening and discharge [75]. Schotola et al., on the other hand studied a single dose of ketamine (albeit a higher dose 1 mg/kg) in outpatient arthroscopic shoulder surgery and concluded that not only did ketamine fail to reduce postoperative pain severity, but it also increased surgical time, time to emergence, postoperative vomiting, and PACU length of stay [76]. The orthopedic studies including mildly painful arthroscopic surgery showed no benefit from ketamine and the authors suggested that more painful surgeries such as total joint replacements should be studied further [74].

There seems to be therefore, a relative dearth of literature on the use of low-dose ketamine in the ambulatory setting, especially in the opiate tolerant population, that includes patients on MAT. Due to the variability of ketamine's effects and side effect profile, monitoring of the patient's vitals, respiratory status, analgesia, sedation, and muscle stiffness is indicated, which may not be necessarily possible in ambulatory surgery centers. However, given its significant opiate-sparing effect especially in the opiate-tolerant population, it certainly could be a consideration for hospital-based outpatient surgeries where patients have the option of being admitted for 23 hours for further monitoring, if needed.

From an administration standpoint, a low-dose ketamine infusion will be more applicable if the period of administration is going to be longer than 2 or 3 h. In short cases for the ambulatory setting, serial bolus administration is a reasonable approach. Gorlin et al. [77] recommend an IV bolus of 0.1–0.3 mg/kg with induction for short cases lasting <60 minutes, with a repeat bolus every 30–60 minutes for cases lasting more than an hour. These authors recommend avoiding a repeat-bolus dose within 30 minutes of emergence to avoid delayed awakening.

For longer cases where ketamine infusions may be more appropriate, recommended doses are commonly in the range of 0.1–0.2 mg/kg/h (2 mcg/kg/min is a common infusion dose as well). Psychosensory effects increase at doses above 0.3 mg/kg, so this can be considered a soft upper limit for bolus doses in awake patients. In obese patients, ideal body weight should be used for dose calculation [77].

Postoperative Management in Recovery Room

In the postanesthesia care unit, recommendations for opioid-tolerant patients on MAT is to initially administer IV boluses of short-acting, potent-opioid analgesics, such as fentanyl or sufentanil, with close monitoring of vital signs. A longer than usual monitoring period may be indicated for patients needing excessively high doses of opioids in the PACU.

Discharge Planning

There are several issues with regards to postoperative pain control that need to be considered prior to discharging patients on MAT. These include effective relief of postoperative pain, prevention of withdrawal, prevention of relapse, and addressing associated social, behavioral, and psychiatric issues with appropriate referrals to ensure long-term care, if needed [78].

Opioid tolerant patients could require greater amounts of postoperative analgesia and for longer periods of time than opioid-naïve patients [64, 79].The pain could also take longer to subside. It is well known that there could be ongoing issues with polydrug or opioid abuse in patients enrolled in substitution programs [80, 81]. Several risk factors for unintended opioid overdose have been identified and remain an important consideration when discharging patients on MAT with additional opioids for postoperative pain [4]. These include misuse of heroin and opioids, misuse of diverted buprenorphine and methadone, having multiple prescribers or pharmacies filling prescriptions, being prescribed doses equivalent to more than 100 mg morphine, opioid ingestion along with alcohol or use of other sedatives/hypnotics (with synergistic effects on respiratory depression), receipt of public subsidy income providing access to drug purchase and binge drug use, suboptimal methadone-induction practices in relation to both pain management and addiction, opioid-analgesic switching, previous overdose history, loss of opioid tolerance among OUD due either to extended abstinence during incarceration or to treatment-related abstinence, and older age, with smoking status and co-occurring medical conditions likely contributing to fatalities [82–86].

The overdose risk is also dose-dependent with a higher opioid dose associated with higher overdose risk [82, 87–91]. In the absence of above risk factors, patients on methadone maintenance may be instructed to continue taking their usual dose after being discharged, with additional opioid analgesics prescribed at the lowest effective dose and for a limited time period preferably less than a week [92]. If severe pain is present for over a week, the frequency of follow-ups should be increased. Patients on methadone sometimes need last methadone dose verification letter (if administered at the hospital) for follow-up with the MAT clinic [54].

Patients on buprenorphine maintenance preoperatively may continue their usual buprenorphine if it was never discontinued. These patients similarly need additional alternative opioid for analgesia in addition to their daily dose of buprenorphine [56]. However, if it was discontinued for 3–5 days prior to more painful surgery and pain control was obtained with pure mu-opioid agonists, bup-nx treatment will need reinduction with the outpatient OAT program. Patients should have a follow-up with their bup-nx provider as soon as possible.

Patients with naltrexone similarly will need to have a follow-up with their outpatient naltrexone prescriber after being weaned off of perioperative opiates for therapy reinduction to prevent relapse.

To avoid relapse, goals of treatment should be established with patients and risk and benefits of opioid prescription for postoperative use should be explained and discussed to prevent potential relapse and overdose [90]. In addition to educating the patient and family, cognitive behavioral approaches may be employed to manage anxiety, craving, and pain. After discharge, facilitating self-help group attendance, involving sponsor and/or a peer support, when applicable, and collaboration with patient's current mental health or SUD clinician are some of the other strategies to increase support and mitigate risk of relapse.

Discharge planning should also include safe medication use and storage and disposal of all unused opioids. A responsible support person should be involved to hold/dispense the opioid-analgesic medications. Due to the loss of tolerance during abstinence, relapse can lead to overdose and death. Overdose prevention education and nasal naloxone prescription (OPENP), the opioid-receptor antagonist to reverse opioid overdose, should be considered. Effective strategies to prevent relapse while providing adequate pain relief requires further research; however, identifying those who are at risk for relapse is crucial [54].

Weaning Plan

An extremely important need in caring for these patients is a plan for weaning off of opioids prescribed for acute pain after ambulatory surgery. This is feasible by means of a mutually agreed upon tapering plan between the patient and the prescribing physician. This is important since there is a greater chance of long-term use of opioids when opioids are prescribed for acute pain [93, 94].

Experts recommend that opioid-tolerant patients, including those on MAT should be offered regional analgesia whenever possible, especially for orthopedic procedures, with the advantage of being discharged with local anesthetic infusion pumps. Baseline requirements for oral opioids after ambulatory surgery usually need supplementation with additional medication (generally 20–50% increases above baseline) as regional analgesia wears off. Oral opioids should then be down-titrated slowly over 3–7 days as the intensity of acute pain diminishes [53]. When opioids can be reduced or discontinued by patient request, tapering should be slow to avoid opioid withdrawal. Tapering can begin with a 10 percent per week decrease in dose of additional opioids being used [92]. These patients therefore may need a 2-week prescription of opioids postoperatively as opposed to only 7–10 days, with clear instructions on weaning down as suggested above. As opioids are tapered, the use of nonpharmacological therapies such as exercise therapy, cognitive behavioral therapy, and multimodal analgesics including the use of nonopioid pain medications such as antidepressants, anticonvulsants, nonsteroidal anti-inflammatory drugs, and acetaminophen should be considered [92, 95, 96]. These patients would need more frequent follow-ups with their surgeon and outpatient OAT program to further assist in the weaning process.

Summary

In summary, safe and effective pain control after ambulatory surgery is possible with a multidisciplinary collaborative approach [78]. The need to address several underlying issues such as psychosocial comorbidities, depression, homelessness, psychiatric disorders, medical comorbidities such as infections, nonopioid substance abuse disorders, cannot be overemphasized. The discharging service should consider early involvement of pain specialist, primary care physician, and patients' MAT program to assist in the perioperative management [4, 97]. It is also important to reinforce safe storage and disposal of unused opioids, in addition to overdose prevention education and nasal naloxone prescription.

References

1. Rachel N.Lipari EP-L. Key substance use and mental health indicators in the United States: results from the 2018 National Survey on Drug Use and Health. Substance abuse and mental health 2018.
2. Mack KA, Jones CM, Paulozzi LJ. Vital signs: overdoses of prescription opioid pain relievers and other drugs among women—United States, 1999–2010. MMWR Morb Mortal Wkly Rep. 2013;62:537.
3. Association AP. Diagnostic and statistical manual of mental disorders (DSM-5®). Arlington: American Psychiatric Pub; 2013.
4. Connery HS. Medication-assisted treatment of opioid use disorder: review of the evidence and future directions. Harv Rev Psychiatry. 2015;23:63–75.
5. VolkowND. America's addiction to opioids: heroin and prescription drug abuse. Senate Caucus on International Narcotics Control 2014;14.
6. Manchikanti L, Helm S 2nd, Fellows B, Janata JW, Pampati V, Grider JS, Boswell MV. Opioid epidemic in the United States. Pain Physician. 2012;15:ES9–ES38.
7. Kolodny A, Courtwright DT, Hwang CS, Kreiner P, Eadie JL, Clark TW, Alexander GC. The prescription opioid and heroin crisis: a public health approach to an epidemic of addiction. Annu Rev Public Health. 2015;36:559–74.
8. Jones C. Trends in the distribution of selected opioids by state, US, 1999–2011 National Meeting Safe States Alliance Baltimore: National Center for Injury Prevention and Control, 2013.
9. Chen LH, Hedegaard H, Warner M. Drug-poisoning deaths involving opioid analgesics: United States. NCHS Data Brief. 1999-2011;2014:1–8.
10. Dart RC, Surratt HL, Cicero TJ, Parrino MW, Severtson SG, Bucher-Bartelson B, Green JL. Trends in opioid-analgesic abuse and mortality in the United States. N Engl J Med. 2015;372:241–8.
11. Muhuri P, Gfroerer J, Davies C. Associations of nonmedical pain reliever use and initiation of heroin use in the United States. CBHSQ data review. Substance Abuse and Mental Health Services Administration https://www.samhsa.gov/data/sites/default/files/DR006/DR006/nonmedical-pain-reliever-use-2013 htm. Published August 2013.
12. Compton WM, Jones CM, Baldwin GT. Relationship between nonmedical prescription-opioid use and heroin use. N Engl J Med. 2016;374:154–63.
13. section Dsi. National Drug Threat Assessment. 2019.
14. Bart G. Maintenance medication for opiate addiction: the foundation of recovery. J Addict Dis. 2012;31:207–25.
15. Merikangas KR, Stolar M, Stevens DE, Goulet J, Preisig MA, Fenton B, Zhang H, O'Malley SS, Rounsaville BJ. Familial transmission of substance use disorders. Arch Gen Psychiatry. 1998;55:973–9.
16. Tsuang MT, Lyons MJ, Meyer JM, Doyle T, Eisen SA, Goldberg J, True W, Lin N, Toomey R, Eaves L. Co-occurrence of abuse of different drugs in men: the role of drug-specific and shared vulnerabilities. Arch Gen Psychiatry. 1998;55:967–72.
17. Sehgal N, Manchikanti L, Smith HS. Prescription opioid abuse in chronic pain: a review of opioid abuse predictors and strategies to curb opioid abuse. Pain Physician. 2012;15:ES67–92.
18. Haerian BS, Haerian MS. OPRM1 rs1799971 polymorphism and opioid dependence: evidence from a meta-analysis. Pharmacogenomics. 2013;14:813–24.
19. Ahmed MB. OPIATE ADDICTION. ثناتبخلا مهئلاء م, زخيو تابو 201441: لإخيو(طلا مهنا).
20. Brook JS, Brook DW, Zhang C, Cohen P. Pathways from adolescent parent-child conflict to substance use disorders in the fourth decade of life. Am J Addict. 2009;18:235–42.
21. Kalinichev M, Easterling KW, Holtzman SG. Long-lasting changes in morphine-induced locomotor sensitization and tolerance in long-Evans mother rats as a result of periodic postpartum separation from the litter: a novel model of increased vulnerability to drug abuse? Neuropsychopharmacology. 2003;28:317–28.
22. Vazquez V, Giros B, Daugé V. Maternal deprivation specifically enhances vulnerability to opiate dependence. Behav Pharmacol. 2006;17:715–24.
23. Mills KL, Teesson M, Ross J, Peters L. Trauma, PTSD, and substance use disorders: findings from the Australian National Survey of Mental Health and Well-Being. Am J Psychiatr. 2006;163:652–8.
24. Pickens CL, Airavaara M, Theberge F, Fanous S, Hope BT, Shaham Y. Neurobiology of the incubation of drug craving. Trends Neurosci. 2011;34:411–20.
25. Volkow ND, Wang G-J, Fowler JS, Tomasi D, Telang F. Addiction: beyond dopamine reward circuitry. Proc Natl Acad Sci. 2011;108:15037–42.
26. Wang G-J, Volkow ND, Fowler JS, Logan J, Abumrad NN, Hitzemann RJ, Pappas NS, Pascani K. Dopamine D2 receptor availability in opiate-dependent subjects before and after naloxone-precipitated withdrawal. Neuropsychopharmacology. 1997;16:174–82.

27. Zijlstra F, Booij J, van den Brink W, Franken IH. Striatal dopamine D2 receptor binding and dopamine release during cue-elicited craving in recently abstinent opiate-dependent males. Eur Neuropsychopharmacol. 2008;18:262–70.
28. Koob GF, Volkow ND. Neurocircuitry of addiction. Neuropsychopharmacology. 2010;35:217–38.
29. Mattick RP, Breen C, Kimber J, Davoli M. Buprenorphine maintenance versus placebo or methadone maintenance for opioid dependence. Cochrane Database Syst Rev. 2014. Issue 2. Art. No.: CD002207.
30. Administration SAaMHS. National Survey on Drug Use and Health (NSDUH). 2018.
31. Alderks CE. Trends in the use of methadone, buprenorphine, and extended-release naltrexone at substance abuse treatment facilities: 2003-2015 (update) The CBHSQ report: Substance Abuse and Mental Health Services Administration (US), 2017.
32. Dahan A. Opioid-induced respiratory effects: new data on buprenorphine. Palliat Med. 2006;20:3–8.
33. Krupitsky E, Nunes EV, Ling W, Gastfriend DR, Memisoglu A, Silverman BL. Injectable extended-release naltrexone (XR-NTX) for opioid dependence: long-term safety and effectiveness. Addiction. 2013;108:1628–37.
34. Apfelbaum J, Connis R, Nickinovich D, Pasternak L, Arens J, Caplan R, Fleisher L, Flowerdew R, Gold B, Mayhew J. Practice advisory for preanesthesia evaluation: an updated report by the American Society of Anesthesiologists Task Force on Preanesthesia Evaluation. Anesthesiology. 2012;116:522–38.
35. Management ASoATFoAP. Practice guidelines for acute pain management in the perioperative setting: an updated report by the American Society of Anesthesiologists Task Force on acute pain management. Anesthesiology. 2012;116:248–73.
36. Inturrisi CE. Clinical pharmacology of opioids for pain. Clin J Pain. 2002;18:S3–S13.
37. Ebert B, Thorkildsen C, Andersen S, Christrup LL, Hjeds H. Opioid analgesics as noncompetitive N-methyl-D-aspartate (NMDA) antagonists. Biochem Pharmacol. 1998;56:553–9.
38. Curatolo C, Trinh M. Challenges in the perioperative management of the patient receiving extended-release naltrexone. AA Pract. 2014;3:142–4.
39. Coluzzi F, Bifulco F, Cuomo A, Dauri M, Leonardi C, Melotti RM, Natoli S, Romualdi P, Savoia G, Corcione A. The challenge of perioperative pain management in opioid-tolerant patients. Ther Clin Risk Manag. 2017;13:1163.
40. Matthews S, Dwyer R, Snoek A. Stigma and self-stigma in addiction. JBioeth Inq. 2017;14:275–86.
41. Martel M, Wasan A, Jamison R, Edwards RR. Catastrophic thinking and increased risk for prescription opioid misuse in patients with chronic pain. Drug Alcohol Depend. 2013;132:335–41.
42. Morasco BJ, Turk DC, Donovan DM, Dobscha SK. Risk for prescription opioid misuse among patients with a history of substance use disorder. Drug Alcohol Depend. 2013;127:193–9.
43. Sullivan MJ, Bishop SR, Pivik J. The pain catastrophizing scale: development and validation. Psychol Assess. 1995;7:524.
44. Koob GF, Volkow ND. Neurobiology of addiction: a neurocircuitry analysis. Lancet Psychiatry. 2016;3:760–73.
45. Webster LR, Webster RM. Predicting aberrant behaviors in opioid-treated patients: preliminary validation of the opioid risk tool. Pain Med. 2005;6:432–42.
46. Volkow ND, Koob GF, McLellan AT. Neurobiologic advances from the brain disease model of addiction. N Engl J Med. 2016;374:363–71.
47. Compton P, Charuvastra V, Ling W. Pain intolerance in opioid-maintained former opiate addicts: effect of long-acting maintenance agent. Drug Alcohol Depend. 2001;63:139–46.
48. Wachholtz A, Gonzalez G. Co-morbid pain and opioid addiction: long-term effect of opioid maintenance on acute pain. Drug Alcohol Depend. 2014;145:143–9.
49. Fonseca F, de la Torre R, Díaz L, Pastor A, Cuyàs E, Pizarro N, Khymenets O, Farré M, Torrens M. Contribution of cytochrome P450 and ABCB1 genetic variability on methadone pharmacokinetics, dose requirements, and response. PLoS One. 2011;6:e19527.
50. McCance-Katz EF, Sullivan LE, Nallani S. Drug interactions of clinical importance among the opioids, methadone and buprenorphine, and other frequently prescribed medications: a review. Am J Addict. 2010;19:4–16.
51. Walker PW, Palla S, Pei B-L, Kaur G, Zhang K, Hanohano J, Munsell M, Bruera E. Switching from methadone to a different opioid: what is the equianalgesic dose ratio? J Palliat Med. 2008;11:1103–8.
52. Services USDoHaH. CDC.
53. Vadivelu N, Mitra S, Kaye AD, Urman RD. Perioperative analgesia and challenges in the drug-addicted and drug-dependent patient. Best Pract Res Clin Anaesthesiol. 2014;28:91–101.
54. Ward EN, Quaye AN-A, Wilens TE. Opioid use disorders: perioperative management of a special population. Anesth Analg. 2018;127:539–47.
55. Sordo L, Barrio G, Bravo MJ, Indave BI, Degenhardt L, Wiessing L, Ferri M, Pastor-Barriuso R. Mortality risk during and after opioid substitution treatment: systematic review and meta-analysis of cohort studies. BMJ. 2017;357:j1550.
56. Alford DP, Compton P, Samet JH. Acute pain management for patients receiving maintenance methadone or buprenorphine therapy. Ann Intern Med. 2006;144:127–34.
57. Jonan AB, Kaye AD, Urman RD. Buprenorphine formulations: clinical best practice strategies recommendations for perioperative management of patients undergoing surgical or interventional pain procedures. Pain Physician. 2018;21:E1–e12.

58. Treece JM, Al Madani M, El Khoury G, Khraisha O, Martin JE, Baumrucker SJ, Neglia CA, Paul TK. Comprehensive review on methadone-induced QT prolongation and torsades. J Pharmacol Pharmacother. 2018;9:66.
59. Krantz MJ, Martin J, Stimmel B, Mehta D, Haigney MC. QTc interval screening in methadone treatment. Ann Intern Med. 2009;150:387–95.
60. Peng PW, Tumber PS, Gourlay D. Perioperative pain management of patients on methadone therapy. Can J Anesth. 2005;52:513–23.
61. Palmateer N, Hutchinson S, McAllister G, Munro A, Cameron S, Goldberg D, Taylor A. Risk of transmission associated with sharing drug injecting paraphernalia: analysis of recent hepatitis C virus (HCV) infection using cross-sectional survey data. J Viral Hepat. 2014;21:25–32.
62. Pouget ER, Hagan H, Des Jarlais DC. Meta-analysis of hepatitis C seroconversion in relation to shared syringes and drug preparation equipment. Addiction. 2012;107:1057–65.
63. Carroll IR, Angst MS, Clark JD. Management of perioperative pain in patients chronically consuming opioids. Reg Anesth Pain Med. 2004;29:576–91.
64. Rapp SE, Ready LB, Nessly ML. Acute pain management in patients with prior opioid consumption: a case-controlled retrospective review. Pain. 1995;61:195–201.
65. Mitra S, Sinatra RS. Perioperative management of acute pain in the opioid-dependent patient. Anesthesiology. 2004;101:212–27.
66. Chou R, Gordon DB, de Leon-Casasola OA, Rosenberg JM, Bickler S, Brennan T, Carter T, Cassidy CL, Chittenden EH, Degenhardt E. Management of Postoperative Pain: a clinical practice guideline from the American pain society, the American Society of Regional Anesthesia and Pain Medicine, and the American Society of Anesthesiologists' committee on regional anesthesia, executive committee, and administrative council. J Pain. 2016;17:131–57.
67. Vadivelu N, Kai AM, Kodumudi V, Berger JM. Challenges of pain control and the role of the ambulatory pain specialist in the outpatient surgery setting. J Pain Res. 2016;9:425–35.
68. Hord A, Sinatra RJApm, Yearbook mSLM. Postoperative analgesia in the opioid-dependent patient. In: Acute pain: mechanisms and management. St. Louis: Mosby Yearbook; 1992. p. 390–8.
69. Jage J, Bey TJAP. Postoperative analgesia in patients with substance use disorders: part I. Acute Pain. 2000;3:29–44.
70. May JA, White HC, Leonard-White A, Warltier DC, Pagel PS. The patient recovering from alcohol or drug addiction: special issues for the anesthesiologist. Anesth Analg. 2001;92:1601–8.
71. Pasero C, Compton PJAJN. Pain management in addicted patients. Am J Nurs. 1997;4:17–9.
72. Katz WA. Cyclooxygenase-2-selective inhibitors in the management of acute and perioperative pain. Cleve Clin J Med. 2002;69(Suppl 1):SI65–75.
73. Reuben SS, Connelly NR. Postoperative analgesic effects of celecoxib or rofecoxib after spinal fusion surgery. Anesth Analg. 2000;91:1221–5.
74. Laskowski K, Stirling A, McKay WP, Lim HJ. A systematic review of intravenous ketamine for postoperative analgesia. Can J Anaesth. 2011;58:911–23.
75. Menigaux C, Guignard B, Fletcher D, Sessler DI, Dupont X, Chauvin M. Intraoperative small-dose ketamine enhances analgesia after outpatient knee arthroscopy. Anesth Analg. 2001;93:606–12.
76. Schotola H, Kirsch KC, Hocker J, Egan M, Buttner B, Wiese C, Mansur A, Hinz JM, Bergmann I. Ketamine in outpatient arthroscopic shoulder surgery: effects on postoperative pain, hemodynamic stability and process times. Open Med (Wars). 2015;10:297–305.
77. Gorlin AW, Rosenfeld DM, Ramakrishna H. Intravenous sub-anesthetic ketamine for perioperative analgesia. J Anaesthesiol Clin Pharmacol. 2016;32:160–7.
78. Huxtable C, Roberts L, Somogyi A, MacIntyre P. Acute pain management in opioid-tolerant patients: a growing challenge. Anaesth Intensive Care. 2011;39:804–23.
79. Chapman CR, Donaldson G, Davis J, Ericson D, Billharz J. Postoperative pain patterns in chronic pain patients: a pilot study. Pain Med. 2009;10:481–7.
80. Boscarino JA, Rukstalis M, Hoffman SN, Han JJ, Erlich PM, Gerhard GS, Stewart WF. Risk factors for drug dependence among out-patients on opioid therapy in a large US health-care system. Addiction. 2010;105:1776–82.
81. Reid MC, Engles-Horton LL, Weber MB, Kerns RD, Rogers EL, O'Connor PG. Use of opioid medications for chronic noncancer pain syndromes in primary care. J Gen Intern Med. 2002;17:173–9.
82. Baumblatt JAG, Wiedeman C, Dunn JR, Schaffner W, Paulozzi LJ, Jones TF. High-risk use by patients prescribed opioids for pain and its role in overdose deaths. JAMA Intern Med. 2014;174:796–801.
83. Chou R, Weimer MB, Dana T. Methadone overdose and cardiac arrhythmia potential: findings from a review of the evidence for an American Pain Society and College on problems of drug dependence clinical practice guideline. J Pain. 2014;15:338–65.
84. Darke S. Opioid overdose and the power of old myths: what we thought we knew, what we do know and why it matters. Drug Alcohol Rev. 2014;33:109–14.
85. Wikner BN, Öhman I, Seldén T, Druid H, Brandt L, Kieler H. Opioid-related mortality and filled prescriptions for buprenorphine and methadone. Drug Alcohol Rev. 2014;33:491–8.
86. Zlotorzynska M, Milloy MJS, Richardson L, Nguyen P, Montaner JS, Wood E, Kerr T. Timing of income assistance payment and overdose patterns at a Canadian supervised injection facility. Int J Drug Policy. 2014;25:736–9.
87. Bohnert AS, Logan JE, Ganoczy D, Dowell D. A detailed exploration into the association of prescribed opioid dosage and overdose deaths among patients with chronic pain. Med Care. 2016;54:435.

88. Bohnert AS, Valenstein M, Bair MJ, Ganoczy D, McCarthy JF, Ilgen MA, Blow FC. Association between opioid-prescribing patterns and opioid overdose-related deaths. JAMA. 2011;305:1315–21.
89. Dunn KM, Saunders KW, Rutter CM, Banta-Green CJ, Merrill JO, Sullivan MD, Weisner CM, Silverberg MJ, Campbell CI, Psaty BM. Opioid prescriptions for chronic pain and overdose: a cohort study. Ann Intern Med. 2010;152:85–92.
90. Gomes T, Mamdani MM, Dhalla IA, Paterson JM, Juurlink DN. Opioid dose and drug-related mortality in patients with nonmalignant pain. Arch Intern Med. 2011;171:686–91.
91. Zedler B, Xie L, Wang L, Joyce A, Vick C, Kariburyo F, Rajan P, Baser O, Murrelle L. Risk factors for serious prescription opioid-related toxicity or overdose among Veterans Health Administration patients. Pain Med. 2014;15:1911–29.
92. Dowell D, Haegerich TM, Chou R. CDC guideline for prescribing opioids for chronic pain—United States, 2016. JAMA. 2016;315:1624–45.
93. Alam A, Gomes T, Zheng H, Mamdani MM, Juurlink DN, Bell CM. Long-term analgesic use after low-risk surgery: a retrospective cohort study. Arch Intern Med. 2012;172:425–30.
94. Webster BS, Verma SK, Gatchel RJ. Relationship between early opioid prescribing for acute occupational low back pain and disability duration, medical costs, subsequent surgery and late opioid use. Spine. 2007;32:2127–32.
95. Kamper SJ, Apeldoorn A, Chiarotto A, Smeets R, Ostelo R, Guzman J, Van Tulder M. Multidisciplinary biopsychosocial rehabilitation for chronic low back pain: Cochrane systematic review and meta-analysis. BMJ. 2015;350:h444.
96. Lee C, Crawford C, Swann S. Multimodal, integrative therapies for the self-management of chronic pain symptoms. Pain Med. 2014;15:S76–85.
97. Donroe JH, Holt SR, Tetrault JM. Caring for patients with opioid use disorder in the hospital. CMAJ. 2016;188:1232.

24 The Impact of Marijuana and Other Drugs of Abuse on Pain Control in Ambulatory Anesthesia

Clifford Gevirtz

Abstract

The large expansion of Marijuana consumption as well as the popularization of other drugs of abuse (Cocaine, methamphetamine) has had a major impact on the conduct of anesthetics. These drugs can affect both the dosing of anesthetic medications, postoperative analgesic choices as well as increase post procedure complications. Vaping is another concern for anesthesiologists where lung injury can complicate otherwise simple anesthetics. Reviewing the pharmacology and pharmacodynamics of these drugs can prevent or better prepare anesthesiologists in managing untoward events. With a rise in proportion of ambulatory surgeries, this knowledge is particularly important for the ambulatory anesthesiologist who may have limited resources in an ASC setting.

Introduction

When taking an initial history from a patient, a question about the use of "drugs of abuse" is the standard of care. However, physicians may have a vastly different perspective on what constitutes a "drug of abuse" than the patient. For example, the daily consumption of edible marijuana, which is legal in many states, may be considered by the patient as nothing special and not worth mentioning. Marijuana and other drugs of abuse as well as their novel route of consumption such as vaping, may have a major impact on the course of an anesthetic and postoperative pain control.

It would be unusual for the anesthesia consultant to order urine or serum toxicology screen preoperatively. If there is a strong concern, then the advice and consent of the surgeon should be obtained. In Table 24.1, drugs of abuse, their detection window, and common medications which can cause False-Positives are reviewed. In patients who have unexplained postoperative complications, the quality assurance function may be better served by obtaining urine toxicology.

Marijuana

The legalization of marijuana has grown throughout the United States and with it a continued expansion in use by the American population. The legalization began with medical marijuana for pain and for diseases which had no effective therapy and has now progressed to legal recreational use. With this expansion, there are an increased number of patients who chronically

C. Gevirtz (✉)
LSU New Orleans, New Orleans, LA, USA

Somnia, Inc, Harrison, NY, USA

K. Rajput et al. (eds.), *Pain Control in Ambulatory Surgery Centers*,
https://doi.org/10.1007/978-3-030-55262-6_24

Table 24.1 Urine Toxicology Detection Windows and Common False-Positive Medications

Drug of Abuse	Detection Window	Common False-Positive Medications
Marijuana	1 day to 30 days (in chronic users)	Sulindac, Dronabinol
Cocaine	12–72 hours	Tonic Water, Quinine, Amoxicillin
Methamphetamine/ Amphetamine	6–48 hours	Ephedrine, Pseudoephedrine, Amantadine, Labetalol
Ecstasy	6–48 hours	Pseudoephedrine
PCP	1–8 days	Ketamine, Tramadol,Dextromethorphan, Venlafaxine, Diphenhydramine
Heroin	1–48 hours	Morphine, Hydromorphone
LSD	***-up to 120 hours by Blood Test only	

enjoy marijuana and CBD products. As of 2020, 11 states and the District of Columbia have legalized the recreational use of marijuana, and 33 states have authorized the use of medical marijuana. The remaining states have yet to legalize either use of the drug. Marijuana can have quite variable effects, both pharmacokinetic and pharmacodynamic and can interact with anesthetic medications which can alter expected outcomes.

Marijuana-Pharmacology

Bridgeman and Abazia [1] reviewed the three most common methods for marijuana administration which include inhalation either by smoking or vaporization, ingestion through edible products, and the use of CBD oils. Each of these methods have widely variable onset, intensity, and duration of effects. Although smoking is the most common form of marijuana use, inhalation by vaporization (vaping) is gaining in popularity and may reduce the exposure of harmful smoking byproducts, carcinogens, and decrease the adverse respiratory effects. CBD [1] can be taken via the oral, rectal, sublingual, or even transdermal routes.

The endocannabinoids are thought to have a homeostatic role and function through the parasympathetic nervous system [1]. Patients with low levels of endocannabinoids have been found to be susceptible to depression, fibromyalgia, irritable bowel syndrome, multiple sclerosis, schizophrenia, and Parkinson's disease. It is for this reason that many patients have sought out medical marijuana prescriptions even though evidence of efficacy is purely anecdotal. However, patients presenting with these diseases should be questioned as to whether they are trialing medical marijuana.

Cannabinoid receptor type 1 (CB_1) is the most abundant endocannabinoid G-protein-coupled receptor. The receptor is found throughout the central nervous system including the substantia nigra, hippocampus, cerebral cortex, cerebellum, and the amygdala. CB_1 is also found diffusely in other areas such as adipocytes, hepatocytes, musculoskeletal tissues, and the gonads. CB_2 is primarily found in immune cells, although it may also be expressed to a lesser degree in the central nervous system.

The most well-known CB ligands are N-arachidonoyl-ethanolamide (anandamide or AEA), also known as the "bliss molecule" and 2-arachidonoyl-glycerol (2-AG). AEA and 2-AG are released from cell membrane phospholipid precursors. This "classic" CB system has expanded with the discovery of secondary receptors, ligands, and ligand metabolic enzymes. For example, AEA, 2-AG, and the smoked cannabinoids Δ^9-THC and CBD may also bind as ligands at GPR55, GPR18, and several other transient receptor potential ion channels (e.g., TRPV1) that have actions similar to capsaicin. This diverse mixture of receptors makes for complicated and somewhat unpredictable pharmacology.

Unlike THC, CBD does not attach to the CB1 and CB2 receptors but is thought to control endocannabinoid levels by decreasing the uptake of the endocannabinoid anandamide, without any direct psychotropic effects [2]. CBD has the potential for use as an antiepileptic, anti-inflammatory, anxiolytic, antipsychotic and may have neuroprotective effects. It is believed that the anti-inflammatory and immunosuppressive effects of CBD are modulated through serotonin and adenosine receptors. Finally, CBD has shown to be a DNA transcriptional repressor and may regulate cell proliferation and differentiation by DNA methylation [2]. Again, many patients are trying CBD as an over the counter solution to their infirmities.

The Role of THC as an Antiemetic

THC has been utilized to prevent postoperative nausea and vomiting (PONV). Kleine-Brueggeney et al. [3] conducted a randomized, double blind placebo-controlled study to evaluate if the utilization of intravenous (IV) THC could prevent PONV. They hypothesized that IV THC would diminish PONV by 25%. Forty patients were included in this study and received either a placebo or 0.125 mg/kg IV THC before emergence from anesthesia. The primary outcome measure was whether or not the patient experienced PONV within the first 24 hours after the administration of anesthesia [3].

They found a 12% reduction in PONV in the group who received IV THC. However, Kleine-Brueggeney et al. [3] concluded that THC was not clinically useful as compared to other conventional PONV rescue treatments. Although the PONV incidence was decreased, there were critical side effects experienced. These side effects include prolonged sedation, increased confusion, mood changes, hallucinations, and increased anxiety postoperatively. They found that patients who had received IV THC took much longer to emerge from anesthesia and had increased sedation scores in the postanesthesia care unit (PACU) as well as statistically longer discharge times. While IV THC may be useful in alternative settings, such as with chemotherapy-induced PONV, Kleine-Brueggeney et al. [3] concluded that IV THC has no place in the perioperative setting at this time.

Advocates for the use of THC in an ambulatory anesthesia setting have cited the Australian Government Department of Health [4] "Guidance for the use of Medicinal Cannabis for the Prevention or Management of Nausea and Vomiting." This guideline discusses the management of nausea and vomiting and how medicinal marijuana can help. But this guidance specifically does not address medicinal marijuana use as related to general anesthesia and notes there is a lack of research. The guideline specifically states medicinal cannabis for nausea and vomiting should only be used after traditional clinical medications have been trialed.

The Adverse Effects of Marijuana Consumption

A case report by Karam et al. [5] asserts that marijuana deleteriously affects the central nervous system, respiratory system, and the cardiovascular system. They found that small doses of marijuana increase sympathetic activity leading to tachycardia, but at the same time, decrease the parasympathetic activity, which depresses cardiac output. With larger doses of marijuana, there is inhibition of the sympathetic nervous system, which can lead to reduced blood pressure and bradycardia. They postulate that THC synergistically affects medications which cause cardiac depression, thus leading to myocardial depression and possible myocardial infarction. They further state that the inhalation of marijuana can cause airway irritation and lead to upper airway edema, laryngospasm, and bronchospasm. Sputum production has been noted to be 144% greater in marijuana smokers, as compared to nonsmokers [5].

Dickerson [6] and Mallat [7] both put forth an untenable suggestion: that all anesthesias should be avoided in a patient who has utilized marijuana within 72 hours before elective surgery. Clearly, this recommendation would lead to wide-spread cancellation of cases and while it may present the absolute safest course, it is just not economically viable in any modern practice. It is important to recognize that patients with chronic marijuana use may have an unpredictable anesthesia course and that abstaining from the use of marijuana before surgery should be recommended. Additional informed consent about the increased risks associated with anesthesia and surgery with chronic marijuana use is appropriate.

Smoking marijuana will mimic the damage to the lungs in a similar manner to tobacco [8]. Adverse effects to be anticipated in a chronic marijuana smoker include increased airway reactivity, bronchial edema, and bronchospasm. Beaulieu [8] has warned that there is an increase in risk for myocardial infarction after the first hour of marijuana use due to the increased myocardial oxygen demand, increased cardiac output, elevated catecholamine levels, as well as an increase in carboxyhemoglobin levels in the blood.

In patients with acute marijuana use before general anesthesia, there is an increase in the anesthetic medication effects and prolonged somnolence [8]. This may interfere with rapid discharge in the ambulatory setting as well as make pain management more challenging. In a chronic marijuana user, increased doses of propofol and opiates may be required for placement of an LMA. Chronic users also have a more unpredictable response to medicines used for induction of anesthesia. Marijuana is metabolized by the cytochrome P450 CYP3A4 and CYP2C9 isozymes. Thus, marijuana may interfere with medications which are also metabolized by CYP2C9, including warfarin, clopidogrel, and nonsteroidal anti-inflammatory drugs (e.g., naproxen, celecoxib). Similarly, medications metabolized by CYP3A4 such as codeine, fentanyl, and oxycodone may also show an increased plasma level with prolonged duration of effect. A higher incidence of respiratory depression should be expected.

CBD is an inhibitor of the enzymes CYP3A4 and CYP2D6. CYP3A4 inhibition by CBD may increase blood concentrations of calcium channel blockers, benzodiazepines, and antihistamines. The enzyme CYP2D6 metabolizes SSRIs, beta blockers, narcotics, and tricyclic antidepressants, and increased plasma levels and prolongation of duration of action of these medications is to be expected. A similar increased risk of respiratory depression exists as above.

Another method of consuming marijuana is to eat it via edibles such as cookies, brownies, lozenges, and beverages. Barrus et al. [9] concluded that edibles are a safer alternative to inhaling marijuana, as it does not cause the harmful effects to the pulmonary system. The most significant difference between inhalational and ingestible marijuana is the delayed onset of effects [9]. Currently, there is extraordinarily little-published research on therapeutic and subjective effects of edibles and the safety of this method of consumption. Edibles are more readily associated with overconsumption than inhalation marijuana due to the delay in onset and impatience of users. Edibles are absorbed from the gastrointestinal tract and the THC is taken up by the portal system and travels to the liver. In the liver, THC goes through the first pass effect through the cytochrome P450 system and is transformed into 11-hydroxytetrahydrocannabinol, a more potent psychotropic form than THC. Because of this metabolism, it is hypothesized that edibles are stronger and longer lasting then inhaled marijuana, which may also explain their increasing popularity.

Cocaine

Carl Koller first utilized cocaine as a local anesthetic in 1884 for eye surgery. It was subsequently used by Matas for spinal anesthesia. While it has been utilized by the Incas as a stimulant to keep slaves productive, its abuse in the United States dates to the early 1900s where it was incorporated into patent medicines and elixirs. Today, its powder and crystalline (crack) forms are still extremely popular.

Cocaine is an ester anesthetic and is metabolized by tissue and plasma esterase [10] into both active (e.g., cococaine, norcocaine) and inactive metabolites that are eventually excreted in the urine. The onset and duration of cocaine's hemodynamic effects depend on its route of use. In general, the intravenous and inhaled (i.e., smoked) routes have a very rapid onset of action (measured in seconds) and short-lived duration (approximately 30 min) compared with the mucosal absorption (e.g., oral, nasal [i.e., snorted], rectal, and vaginal routes).

Cocaine's hemodynamic effect is dose-dependent; the early phase of toxicity results in heart rate and blood pressure (BP) elevation (typically a 10% to 25% increase from the baseline); as toxic levels increase there will be further elevations in heart rate and BP, although BP may drop precipitously in sustained tachyarrhythmias. At very high levels, a significant myocardial depressive effect is evidenced, with profound bradycardia and hypotension. Importantly, because some cocaine metabolites such as norcocaine continue to be active, they can exert cardiovascular effects similar to those of the drug itself long after the cocaine has been completely metabolized.

Evidence for a potential induction of chronic hypertension in cocaine abusers is abundant [11]; cocaine produces endothelial damage and vascular fibrosis. Furthermore, hypertrophic cardiomyopathy and kidney mesangial fibrosis were demonstrated [12] in autopsies of cocaine abusers.

The mechanism behind cocaine-induced myocardial ischemia includes increased myocardial oxygen consumption as a result of increased chronotropy and inotropy, which is inappropriately accompanied by coronary artery vasoconstriction. Cocaine abusers have accelerated coronary atherosclerosis as demonstrated in an autopsy study [13] comparing nonabusers with cocaine abusers who died from an acute coronary artery thrombosis.

The cocaine-induced heightened sympathetic tone increases the risk of cardiac arrhythmias. When combined with the production of myocardial ischemia and prolongation of QT interval, this heightened sympathetic tone can induce ventricular ectopy, torsade de pointes, and ventricular fibrillation. An electrocardiogram should be obtained to look for QTc abnormalities as well as any evidence of ischemia and an echocardiogram can be useful in patients who inhale the drug. There was theoretical concern [14] in using beta blockers alone or labetalol in hypertensive cocaine users because of unopposed alpha adrenergic action, but clinical experience has demonstrated the safety of beta blockade to treat hypertension and tachycardia in these patients.

Hyperthermia as a result of cocaine abuse is another important systemic effect of the drug. In humans, cocaine-induced hyperthermia occurred at "clinically relevant" doses of 2 mg/kg and was worsened with increasing dosage. Active cooling may be required in the perioperative period.

Although authoritative texts [15, 16] suggest waiting for 48 hours after cocaine ingestion to perform elective procedures, the metabolites may be present for up to a week and so the anesthesiologist must be vigilant for tachyarrthymias and myocardial ischemia even if the patient has abstained for 48 hours. Absent acute intoxication, most practitioners will proceed with elective cases.

Methamphetamine

Stimulant abuse, particularly methamphetamine, use has increased dramatically. In addition, many adolescents and adults are prescribed amphetamine derivatives for attention deficit disorder and narcolepsy, which they may abuse or divert. The acute physiologic effects of supratherapeutic dosages are similar to that of cocaine, with sympathetic system activation during periods of acute intoxication and significant risk of psychosis with long-term use. Chronic use is suspected to lead to a depletion of catecholamines and decreased response to vasopressors (e.g., ephedrine). Neuraxial blockade may be complicated by more frequent and more difficult to treat hypotension due to catecholamine depletion in the chronic nonintoxicated abuser.

An electrocardiogram should be obtained to look for QTc abnormalities as well as any evidence of ischemia and an echocardiogram can be useful in patients who inhale the drug. Inhaled methamphetamine may lead to pulmonary toxicity including emphysematous changes and arteriole fibrosis which can lead to pulmonary hypertension.

The oropharynx can be damaged by chronic use of methamphetamine. "Meth mouth" is caused by the combination of poor oral hygiene, xerostomia, and an inadequate diet. This combination can lead to damaged teeth and extensive periodontal disease which makes teeth prone to dislodgement during intubation and extubation. Like cocaine, intranasal use can lead to septal necrosis and extra care should be taken when placing nasogastric tubes. Just as with chronic cocaine usage, the patient may become hypertensive or hypotensive during induction, depending on the levels of circulating catecholamines. The continuation of prescription amphetamines during the perioperative period to prevent further instability has been reviewed by Fisher et al. [17] and they concluded that it is safe to continue these medications. In addition, methamphetamine has been associated with cardiomyopathy, and myocardial ischemia, and the clinician should be aware of marked hemodynamic instability in the patient who has not undergone a thorough preoperative work-up. Methamphetamine withdrawal peaks at 24 hours after last ingestion and is characterized by somnolence, hyperphagia, and depression symptoms, all of which may prolong discharge. There is no consensus on the treatment of methamphetamine withdrawal; although psychosocial support and medical treatments have been suggested. Postoperative analgesia needs to be adjusted depending on the timing of the consumption of the last dose. Patients who are more than 24 hours from last ingestion will most likely need less analgesics because of the somnolence. In contrast, patients who have large amounts still in the system, may require much larger amounts of analgesics.

Ecstasy

MDMA or Ecstasy is a new derivative of an old drug, amphetamine. It was first manufactured in the early 1900s and then was "re-discovered" as a club drug. One of the major problems in dealing with this drug is that it is very difficult to screen for using immunoassays. In acute MDMA toxicity, the patient may be hyperthermic with profuse sweating and hyponatremic from consuming large amounts of water. Patients with severe hyponatremia may require fluid restriction or 3% saline to correct the problem. Hyperthermia should be treated with active cooling. Agitation can be managed with sedation with benzodiazepines. Postoperative analgesia should be slowly titrated as the synergic effect of opiates and benzodiazepines may be more pronounced. Analgesia with nonopiates may be a better choice.

Bath Salts

The abuse of "bath salts" is a fairly new trend among adolescents [18]. These substances, which are sold under various brand names, contain a mixtures of several synthetic cathinones such as 3,4-methylenedioxypyrovalerone (MDPV). These patients may present with delusions, hallucinations, severe psychomotor agitation, and various other physiological effects. It is important to note that routine drug screens will not detect these in the urine and special screens need to be ordered to detect these substances. Management is mostly supportive and has involved the use of benzodiazepines, antipsychotics, and general anesthesia in extreme cases. There is a concern with the use of beta blockers to treat hypertension as dangerous paradoxical increases in blood pressure have occurred. Postoperative pain management may be very difficult due to the drug induced delirium. Abusers of bath salts make poor candidates for ambulatory anesthesia.

Vaping

While nicotine is not considered a drug of abuse, the use of E-cigarettes (EC) has significant anesthetic implications as multiple other drugs aside from nicotine are consumed using this technology. E-cigarettes entered the U.S. marketplace in 2008 and they have become the most commonly used tobacco product among teenagers. In addition to nicotine, the vapor that users inhale and exhale from e-cigarettes can potentially expose both themselves and second hand smokers to multiple other harmful substances, including heavy metals, volatile organic compounds, and small particles that can be inhaled deeply into the lungs.

Vaping using E-cigarettes has led to a new syndrome "E-cigarette vaping associated lung injury" (EVALI) first noted in 2019 [19]. While little long-term health hazard data are available, both the mechanical components of the EC and resultant volatile products of e-cigarettes may harm the respiratory system. Propylene glycol and glycerin are humectants (water-retaining excipients) that when vaporized produce a wide range of pulmonary irritants and carcinogenic carbonyl compounds (e.g., formaldehyde, acetaldehyde, and acrolein). The metals contained in the heating elements and cartridge casings may leach into the vapor produced. These toxic metals include a wide range of aluminum, chromium, iron, lead, nickel, as well as tin compounds. A very wide range of flavoring agents are specifically marketed to appeal to teenagers (e.g., bubblegum). However, while these flavorings are approved by the FDA for oral ingestion there is absolutely no safety data for inhalational exposure. Diacetyl, a common buttery-tasting flavoring agent commonly used on popcorn, was previously known to produce pulmonary toxicity when there is inhalational exposure leading to bronchiolitis obliterans. Clusters of lung injury associated with e-cigarette vaping use were first identified in Wisconsin and Illinois. This syndrome has now been identified in all 50 states and territories.

Based on data obtained in the investigation of EVALI since August 2019, the CDC [20] recommends that all persons to not use THC-containing e-cigarette, or vaping products. Vitamin E acetate has been strongly linked to the EVALI outbreak; it has been detected in product samples tested by FDA and state laboratories and in lung fluid samples from patients tested by CDC from geographically diverse states. In addition, the CDC recommends that substances not intended by the manufacturer should not be added to e-cigarette, or vaping products, including to products purchased through retail establishments. However, the evidence is not sufficient to rule out the contribution of other chemicals of concern, including chemicals in either THC- or non-THC-containing products, as reported in some EVALI cases.

Patients with EVALI should be treated as pulmonary cripples, and analgesics that do not suppress respiratory drive should be used preferentially.

Summary

Marijuana and other drugs of abuse pose a great challenge to providing analgesia to the Anesthesiologist in the postoperative setting. One is often faced with an incomplete or less than truthful history and a patient who may have significant pathology that induction agents will unmask. Postoperative analgesia may, similarly, be very challenging. Slow titration of multimodal analgesia may be the best approach using medications such as NSAIDs and aminoacetophenone. Vigilance before, during, and after the case is often the only remedy.

References

1. Bridgeman MB, Abazia DT. Medicinal Cannabis: history, pharmacology, and implications for the acute care setting. P T. 2017;42(3):180–188. PMID: 28250701; PMCID: PMC5312634.
2. Morales P, Reggio PH. CBD: a new hope? ACS Publications. Washington, DC; 2019. p. 694–5.
3. Kleine-Brueggeney M, Greif R, Brenneisen R, Urwyler N, Stueber F, Theiler LG. Intravenous Delta-9-tetrahydrocannabinol to prevent postoperative nausea and vomiting: a randomized controlled trial. Anesth Analg. 2015;121(5):1157–64. https://doi.org/10.1213/ANE.0000000000000877.
4. Australian Government: Department of Health. Guidance for the use of medicinal cannabis for the prevention or management of nausea and vomiting in Australia. Therapeutic Goods Administration, 2017. Retrieved from https://www.tga.gov.au/sites/default/files/guidance-use-medicinal-cannabis-prevention-or-management-nausea-and-vomiting-australia.pdf.
5. Karam K, Abbasi S, Khan FA. Anaesthetic consideration in a cannabis addict. J Coll Physicians Surg Pak. 2015;25(Suppl 1):S2–3.
6. Dickerson SJ. Cannabis and its effect on anesthesia. AANA J. 1980;48:526–8.

7. Mallat A, Roberson J, Brock-Utne JG. Preoperative marijuana inhalation—an airway concern. Can J Anaesth. 1996;43:691–3.
8. Beaulieu P, Boulanger A, Desroches J, Clark A. (2016). Medical cannabis: considerations for the anesthesiologist and pain physician. Can J Anesth. 2016;63:608–24. https://doi.org/10.1007/s12630-016-0598-x.
9. Barrus D, Capogrossi K, Cates S, Gourdet C, Peiper N, Novak S, Lefever T, Wiley J. Tasty THC: promises and challenges of cannabis edibles. Methods Rep (RTI Press). 2016; https://doi.org/10.3768/rtipress.2016.op.0035.1611.
10. Inaba T, Steward DJ, Kalow. Metabolism of cocaine in man. Clin Pharmacol Ther. 1978;23:547–56.
11. Hoffman RS. Cocaine. In: Goldfrank LR, Flomenbaum NE, Hoffman RS, et al., editors. Goldfrank's toxicological emergencies. 8th ed. New York: McGraw-Hill Medical Publishing; 2006. p. 1133–9.
12. Kim ST, Park T. Acute and chronic effects of cocaine on cardiovascular health. Int J Mol Sci. 2019;20(3):584. Published 2019 Jan 29. https://doi.org/10.3390/ijms20030584.
13. Dressler FA, Malekzadeh S, Roberts WC. Quantitative analysis of amounts of coronary narrowing in cocaine addicts. Am J Cardiol. 1990;65:303–11.
14. Richard JR, Garber D, Laurin EG, et al. Treatment of cocaine cardiovascular toxicity: a systematic review. Clin Toxicol (Phila). 2016;54:345–60. Epub 2016 Feb 26
15. Wijeysundera DN, Finlayson E. Chapter 31 preoperative evaluation in Miller's anesthesia. In: Gropper MA, editor. . 9th ed. Philadelphia: Elsevier; 2020. p. 982–3.
16. Marschall KE, Hines RL. Chapter 29 psychiatric diseases, substance abuse and drug overdose. In: Hines RL, Marschall KE, editors. Stoelting's anesthesia and co-existing disease. 7th ed. Philadelphia: Elsevier; 2019. p. 623–4.
17. Fischer SP, Schmiesing CA, Guta CG, et al. General anesthesia and chronic amphetamine use: should the drug be stopped preoperatively? Anesth Analg. 2006;103(1):203–6.
18. Airuehia E, Young Walker L, Nittler J. A review of "Bath Salts": evolving designer drugs of abuse. J Child Adolesc Subst Abuse. 2015;24(4):186–90. https://doi.org/10.1080/1067828X.2013.803942.
19. Hartnett KP, Kite-Powell A, Patel MT, et al. Syndromic surveillance for e-cigarette, or vaping, product use-associated lung injury. N Engl J Med. 2019; https://www.nejm.org/doi/10.1056/NEJMsr1915313
20. Krishnasamy VP, Hallowell BD, Ko JY, et al. Update: characteristics of a Nationwide outbreak of E-cigarette, or vaping, product use–associated lung injury — United States, August 2019–January 2020. MMWR Morb Mortal Wkly Rep. 2020;69:90–4. https://doi.org/10.15585/mmwr.mm6903e2

25 Special Considerations – Indwelling Spinal Cord Stimulators and Intrathecal Pumps

Colin Beals, Robert Chow, Nalini Vadivelu, and Kanishka Rajput

Abstract

With an increase in the number of ambulatory surgeries, anesthesiologists now encounter an increasing number of chronic pain patients with implanted devices such as spinal cord stimulators (SCS) and intrathecal (IT) pumps. This unique subset of patients may exhibit central sensitization, with or without opioid tolerance. There is a paucity of literature to guide best practice in the perioperative management of patients with implanted SCS and IT pumps. For patients with implanted SCS, guidelines recommend turning the SCS down to minimal settings prior to surgery, avoidance of both electrocautery and neuraxial anesthesia, encouraging regional anesthesia, maximizing multimodal analgesia including acetaminophen and NSAIDs, as well as postoperative interrogation of the SCS before resuming normal function. IT pumps should generally be left infusing during surgery, and long acting or continuous opioid use should be avoided. Damaged IT pumps should be turned off and the patient transitioned to systemic medications. IT clonidine and baclofen pump dysfunction is an emergency as withdrawal can be fatal. Postoperatively, patients with IT pumps and SCS should have an appointment with their pain physician within 2 weeks or as soon as feasible.

C. Beals · R. Chow · N. Vadivelu
Department of Anesthesiology, Yale University School of Medicine, New Haven, CT, USA

K. Rajput (✉)
Department of Anesthesiology and Pain Medicine, Yale University School of Medicine, New Haven, CT, USA
e-mail: kanishka.rajput@yale.edu

Introduction

Spinal Cord Stimulation (SCS) is an increasingly common modality used for treating a variety of chronic pain conditions, most common being Failed Back Surgery Syndrome (FBSS) and Complex Regional Pain Syndrome (CRPS). After initial success, its use has expanded to other indications including neuropathic pain, axial back pain, and refractory angina [1–3].

Spinal cord stimulation involves implanting electrical leads into the epidural space that are then attached to a subcutaneously implanted generator, although some systems offer an external generator that communicates wirelessly with the leads. The SCS works by delivering electrical stimulation to the epidural space overlying the dorsal column of the spinal cord [2]. Electrical impulses preferentially activate large-diameter axons through changes to membrane potentials [4]. This generates orthodromic and antidromic

K. Rajput et al. (eds.), *Pain Control in Ambulatory Surgery Centers*,
https://doi.org/10.1007/978-3-030-55262-6_25

action potentials along the activated pathways. Recruited fibers usually span only a few spinal segments [3]. The mechanisms by which the generated potentials attenuate and alleviate chronic pain are still being investigated. One of the first proposed mechanisms that led to initial use of spinal cord stimulation for chronic pain was the Melzack Gate Control Theory (GCT) [4]. Melzack theorized that non-painful stimuli acting on nerves can "gate" them, shutting off the transmission of painful impulses [5]. However, with advances in SCS technology, there are now modes of stimulation that do not produce results that are concordant with those expected from a pure GCT mechanism of action [2]. More recent investigations into spinal cord stimulation's mechanism of pain relief indicates that wide dynamic range neuron inhibition in the dorsal horn, increased inhibitory neurotransmitter activity, cortical processing changes, and glial modulation have roles in the SCS' impact in modulating the chronic pain experience [2–4, 6–9].

SCS implants for FBSS and CRPS have been found to be more cost-effective than pure medical management in the long term, mainly through decreased healthcare utilization and decreased adverse effects from opiates [9]. With good efficacy and cost-effectiveness, it is not surprising that SCS implantation has doubled from an estimated 27,000 yearly cases in 2007 to 50,000 estimated implantations in 2017 [4, 10]. That number will likely continue to increase, given the large population of patients with chronic pain and the thrust toward reducing chronic opioid use.

Intrathecal (IT) pumps deliver medications directly into the intrathecal space and are also being used more frequently. Guidelines regarding IT therapy are evolving in favor of earlier use and for a broader variety of syndromes [11]. Initially used as salvage therapy for patients with cancer pain on high-dose systemic opiates, IT pumps are now being used for other chronic pain syndromes, spasticity, and as initial therapy for some cancer pain patients [12–15]. Medications commonly delivered intrathecally include opiates, ziconotide, and baclofen [11]. Administering medications intrathecally avoids systemic effects from medications that do not cross the blood–brain barrier while significantly reducing required doses of opiates by a factor of 10-100x, thereby decreasing adverse effects and addiction risk [13]. In 2018 alone, Medicare paid for new implantation of around 2300 IT pumps according to the Medicare Physician/Supplier Procedure database [16]. As the indications and comfort with use increase, the number of patients in the population with these implanted devices is likely to keep increasing as well.

As implanted spinal cord stimulators and intrathecal pumps become increasingly prevalent in the community with more being implanted every year, these patients are likely to present for outpatient procedures at an ambulatory surgical center (ASC). ASCs now provide over 60% of the surgical volume in the USA, with their cost-effectiveness driving an increase in the diversity of operations being performed [17, 18]. Paralleling this increased growth in volume and financial savings is the pressure to treat patients with higher levels of acuity in the ASC. These patients have increased body mass indices, higher ASA categorical scores, and a greater likelihood of baseline chronic pain along with receiving opioid therapy [19]. Not all ASCs are well equipped with specialty services to manage complex patients and there is some evidence pointing to a lack of oversight on quality control for care provided at ASCs [20, 21].

Unfortunately, there is a dearth of literature to guide optimal perioperative management of patients with indwelling SCS or IT pumps in an outpatient setting [22]. The concept of an ambulatory pain physician has been suggested to provide oversight of perioperative pain management for these complex patients, but that role does not exist currently at most ASCs [19]. Caring for these patients may be challenging even in the inpatient hospital setting with access to specialist consultants. In this chapter, we endeavor to provide guidelines for the anesthesiologist/perioperative care specialist and the surgeon to optimally care for patients with an implanted SCS or IT pump in an ambulatory surgical setting.

General Perioperative Concerns

Perioperative management of a patient with an implanted SCS or IT pump needs to take several aspects into consideration, the most important of which are the patient's opioid and pain tolerance, and invasiveness of the planned surgery. Specifically, for patients with indwelling IT pumps, an inquiry into the exact medication regimen infusing through the pump is extremely important to guide perioperative management. Communication with the patient, outpatient pain physician, surgeon, and medical device company representative is essential for both SCS and IT pumps, not only to understand the patient's pain history but also to formulate a plan for optimal periprocedural pain control.

Patients with SCS suffer from chronic pain and may be on a multiple analgesics, including opioids [23]. Outpatient chronic opioid use leads to increased dosing requirements in the perioperative period [19]. The specific management of an opioid-tolerant patient in an ambulatory setting is discussed elsewhere in this book.

Patients suffering from chronic pain may also exhibit a wide variety of central neuroplastic changes, including increased sensitization to noxious stimuli, neuroinflammation, and decreased tolerance to situations where they expect to feel pain, leading to a phenomenon of "pain intolerance" [24]. There is evidence to suggest that although SCS can modulate this neuroplasticity to an extent, the neuromodulation is usually not enough to consider these patients as having a "normal" pain tolerance [25]. Therefore, when managing patients with SCS, it is important to consider both their pain intolerance and their likely opioid tolerance when formulating a perioperative plan. Both phenomena can lead to a need for increased doses of opioids, which in turn increases the risk of medication-related morbidity and adverse events [19]. These phenomena should not be construed as "drug-seeking" behavior. Administering high doses of opioids for intraoperative and postoperative surgical pain has a high rate of adverse drug events for all comers [26]. Patients with SCS and IT pumps should be considered especially at risk, and hence presumed to require a longer period of post-op monitoring in the recovery room. Scheduling these cases earlier during the day helps to avoid after-hours discharge from the ambulatory surgery center. Another factor unique to SCS and IT pumps is the physical location of the components of these systems. If regional techniques such as a subarachnoid or transverse abdominal plane block are used, strong consideration to the use of fluoroscopy is necessary. Some regional techniques may accidentally violate these components, particularly the soft and flexible silastic intrathecal catheter.

In addition to these issues, identification of the drug infusion through the IT pump is imperative. As of the 2017 Polyanalgesic Consensus Conference (PACC) guidelines, there are four categories of medications delivered through IT pumps for pain: opioids, ziconotide, clonidine, and local anesthetics. Baclofen is used for neurogenic spasticity, specifically in patients with Parkinson's [11]. Ziconotide and morphine are first-line agents for IT delivery for cancer-related pain syndromes. Ziconotide, a potent and selective N-type calcium channel blocker, is typically started at 0.5 mcg/day and has a max dose of 19.2 mcg/day. This is almost a 1000-fold reduction compared to dosing for morphine. Dosing for some of the other drugs used as intrathecal therapy is shown in Table 25.1. Other first-line options for cancer-related pain include hydromorphone, and combinations of morphine or hydromorphone with bupivacaine. Second-line regimens include morphine/hydromorphone in addition to clonidine or ziconotide. Third-line

Table 25.1 Commonly used IT pump medications and their recommended starting and maximum doses [11]

Medication	Intrathecal dosing (starting dose – max dose)
Ziconotide	0.5–19.2 mcg/day
Morphine	0.1–15 mg/day
Hydromorphone	0.01–10 mg/day
Bupivacaine	0.01–20 mg/day
Clonidine	20–600 mcg/day
Fentanyl	25–1000 mcg/day
Sufentanil	10–500 mcg/day
Baclofen	50–1000 mcg/day [27]

agents are usually triple therapies of an opioid + bupivacaine + clonidine or ziconotide and combinations of ziconotide + bupivacaine or clonidine. In these infusions, only one drug is a rate-limiting step for the pump rate of delivery. Regimens for non-cancer-related pain, nociceptive, or neuropathic pain differ somewhat. These regimens include fentanyl and sufentanil as first- and third-line agents, respectively [11].

It is important to verify the drug regimen and dosing of medications when providing anesthesia for a patient with an IT pump. While IT pumps should generally be left on and functioning during surgery, it is critically important that IT pumps delivering clonidine (serious withdrawal with abrupt discontinuation) and baclofen (abrupt withdrawal may be fatal) continue to function as normal throughout the case [13].

Management of Patients with Indwelling Spinal Cord Stimulator

Preoperative

Preoperative anesthesia planning should prepare for these patients to be pain intolerant as well as possibly opioid tolerant, and therefore likely to require larger perioperative opioid doses. These patients should therefore be closely monitored for inadequate analgesia throughout the intra and postoperative period [24]. In addition, a preoperative pain consult may help tailor an optimized postoperative pain management plan for discharge, based on the invasiveness of surgery and specific patient characteristics.

In general, an implanted SCS should be programmed at the lowest possible amplitude, placed in a bipolar mode (relevant for old SCS systems), and then switched off prior to surgery [28, 29]. Turning the device off reduces the chance of device reprogramming via interference generated during the case or device interference with ECG monitoring. The additional step of turning the device to the lowest amplitude before turning it off reduces the risk of any stimulation delivered if the device is accidentally turned on during surgery [22]. For device-specific recommendations, the anesthesia team should consult the relevant manufacturer's instructions and call the device help line prior to surgery, if needed [29]. The manufacturer's representative may also be helpful in turning the device down to the lowest setting before turning it off for the patient. The surgery team should be alerted to the presence of an implanted SCS and advised to avoid monopolar electrocautery, if possible during the case [30].

Intraoperative

Electrocautery A discussion about electrocautery use should be held with the surgical team before the case begins. Ideally, no electrocautery should be used for patients with an implanted SCS. However, in cases where electrocautery is necessary, bipolar is preferred over monopolar as the energy transfer is confined to between the tips of the bipolar forceps [30]. Cases where monopolar cautery has to be used and bipolar is not feasible, the monopolar grounding pad should be distal to the SCS leads and placed such that the path between the pad and the surgical site avoids the implanted generator [22]. Generally, the implanted generator is one on side of the body such as the posterior buttock or anterior abdomen.

Opioids Intraoperative opioid dosing should be based on the patient's opioid tolerance. Standard doses of opioids may be sufficient in opioid-naïve patients, while patients on chronic opioids may require up to 3-4x as much to achieve the same level of analgesia [31, 32]. SCS patients in general are expected to have high inter-patient variability regarding opioid needs and require close monitoring for inadequate pain control. Even opioid-naïve patients may require additional opioid for similar pain stimuli due to central sensitization and the relative "pain intolerance" [24]. A conservative initial approach is to administer half of the estimated required dose up front and deliver the other half over the course of the case based on vital signs. Toward the end of the case, spontaneous respiratory rate >20 breaths/minute and dilated pupils are both signs that more opioids are required. Miotic pupils, spontaneous respiratory rates of 12–14 breaths/minute, and heart rate are reasonable targets for titration of additional opioids [33].

Another possible approach, especially for patients with chronic opioid use, is to slowly give a large dose of equianalgesic opioid as soon as full monitoring and supplemental oxygen are in place. Doses can usually be adjusted down when providing parenteral opioids as the first-pass metabolism is bypassed. Although less conservative, the latter approach may be beneficial in patients who have a history of poor analgesia with prior surgeries. The importance of reviewing past anesthesia records and obtaining a thorough pain history including patient recollection of analgesic regimens that have worked historically and expectations with perioperative pain control cannot be overemphasized. Notably, some surgeons ask pain physicians to help wean their elective surgical patients off of opioids ahead of time. If these practices gain traction, the anesthesiologist may have to consider these patients to be opioid naïve. Another regulatory hurdle not yet expected of perioperative specialists, but routine for pain physicians, is cross checking prescription monitoring programs (PMP). Virtually, all states in the USA have these systems in place to reduce "doctor shopping" and drug diversion. In the ASC, checking the PMP will allow the practitioner to fact check the correct dose of chronic opioids that the patient is taking on a regular basis.

Non-opioid analgesia Expert guidelines recommend acetaminophen and NSAIDs as adjunct pain medications that are appropriate for use in most cases. NSAIDs minimize the inflammatory component of pain and both NSAIDs and acetaminophen have been shown to have an opioid-sparing effect [34, 35].

The use of ketamine as an analgesic in outpatient surgery is a more nuanced discussion. Ketamine is an NMDA antagonist, which at higher doses induces dissociation and hallucinations and at subanesthetic doses acts as an analgesic. However, there is a paucity of research regarding use of ketamine as an analgesic in a purely outpatient setting. A review by Lancoste et al. that included 39 clinical trials of ketamine infusions found only 6 trials that limited ketamine use to intraoperative period (most infusions were continued for 48 hrs postoperatively) and of those only 4 showed an opiate-sparing effect [36]. However, in all of these 4 trials, patients were admitted to the hospital postoperatively.

Ketamine has been investigated as an adjunct for pain control in few outpatient orthopedic surgeries, although with mixed results. For example, ketamine improved post-op analgesia in arthroscopic meniscectomy, but not in arthroscopic shoulder surgery. In fact, in the latter study, ketamine use was associated with longer surgical time and increased adverse medication effects [37, 38]. Overall, ketamine may have a role for more painful surgeries such as abdominal and thoracic surgery [39].

Given the lack of strong data regarding ketamine use as an adjunct analgesic in an outpatient setting, and the significant side-effect profile with higher doses; the benefits of ketamine for strictly ambulatory surgery must be weighed against the risk of side effects and potential for a longer recovery room stay. It may therefore be reasonable to limit ketamine infusions for surgeries expected to cause at least moderate to severe pain.

If the decision is made to utilize a ketamine infusion, there is no good data to support specific infusion strategies [40]. However, recommendations by Himmelseher and Durieux as well as Gorlin et al. support IV ketamine bolus dosing of 0.1–0.3 mg/kg ideal body weight (psychosensory effects increase above 0.3 mg/kg) at the beginning of the case, followed by repeat boluses every 30–60 minutes for shorter cases. Infusions at subanesthetic doses of 0.1–0.2 mg/kg IBW/hr may be considered for cases lasting >3 hrs [40, 41]. It is recommended to avoid ketamine administration (bolus or infusion) within 30 minutes of expected emergence to prevent recovery room delays.

Regional and Neuraxial Anesthesia In general, upper or lower extremity regional anesthesia should be considered to augment analgesia for patients with indwelling SCS. However, there is a lack of research regarding safety of lumbar plexus or paravertebral blocks in these patients.

The literature is currently silent regarding neuraxial anesthesia for general OR cases in patients with SCS. Investigations into epidural anesthesia in obstetric patients with implanted SCS suggest that it is feasible to provide neuraxial anesthesia in some cases [42, 43]. However, obstetric anesthesia requires placement of the epidural catheter much lower in the spine than neuraxial anesthesia required for general abdominal surgery, which typically requires T6-T10 dermatomal coverage. This is also the most common level of SCS lead placement for low back and leg pain. Therefore, current recommendations are to avoid neuraxial anesthesia for patients with implanted SCS devices or strongly consider the use of fluoroscopy as stated above [22].

Postoperative

Postoperatively, SCS devices should be interrogated and then restarted [22]. Interrogation does not need to happen immediately post-op but should occur before the device is restarted to ensure that it is functioning as it was, before the case. The device manufacturer's representative again, may be able to assist in interrogating the device before turning it back on. However, since the patient may be under the influence of perioperative sedatives and analgesics and needs to be functionally ambulatory on discharge, restarting the SCS could conceivably wait 24 hours.

Otherwise, patient care should be governed by similar principles as care for the general postoperative patient. As alluded to earlier, SCS patients may require higher or more frequent opioid dosing due to central sensitization and a potentially longer postoperative monitoring period should be expected.

Management of Patients with Indwelling Intrathecal Pumps

Preoperative

Similar to patients with a SCS, patients with IT pumps should be thought to be pain intolerant and those with opioids delivered intrathecally will have some opioid tolerance as well [13]. A preoperative pain consult involving the outpatient pain physician and surgeon may be extremely helpful to tailor the pain plan to unique patient characteristics and invasiveness of the surgery. IT pumps should generally be left on and functioning as usual for surgery. The medication(s) and dose(s) should be verified and taken into account when formulating an anesthetic plan.

Intraoperative

Per ASRA guidelines, providers should utilize caution when administering opioids to patients with IT opioid infusions running [44]. It is safest to use only short-acting opioids in conjunction with acetaminophen and NSAIDs for analgesia in these patients. As discussed in the SCS section, ketamine infusion is reasonable to consider but the adverse effects and risks may outweigh the benefits in a purely ambulatory setting, especially for less painful surgeries.

The use of regional anesthesia should be maximized as another avenue for providing optimal pain control. However, experts generally recommend against neuraxial anesthesia. Per ASRA recommendations, lumbar epidural access should only be attempted with image guidance in patients with IT pumps [44].

Should the IT pump be damaged during surgery, it should be turned off and the patient transitioned to systemic opioids postoperatively until such time as the pump is functioning again. For baclofen and clonidine pumps, acute withdrawal can be fatal, and a damaged pump is an emergency [13, 45]. If a patient's IT baclofen or clonidine pump is damaged, the pump should be shut off and they should be transitioned to oral baclofen or IV clonidine and admitted postoperatively until such time as their pump can be replaced and intrathecal administration restarted [45].

Postoperative

Postoperative pain control for a patient with an IT pump faces the same issues of central sensitization and opioid tolerance as for a patient with SCS. Additionally, administering systemic opioids on top of preexisting intrathecal opioids can induce respiratory depression [46]. Long-acting opioids should be avoided, including continuous infusion through PCAs. Experts recommend continuous pulse oximetry, apnea monitoring, and a plan for a longer than usual postoperative monitoring period. The patient should follow up with their primary pain physician within 2 weeks postoperatively or as soon as feasible, for continued management of their chronic and any new postoperative pain [44].

Discharge Planning

Ideally, the perioperative pain management plan should include a plan for postoperative discharge as well, guided by the invasiveness of surgery, expected pain, and patient's preoperative opioid tolerance. A preoperative pain consult ensures clear understanding of expectations postoperatively and can aid in tailoring a structured pain plan in collaboration with the patient and the surgeon. In general, a short course (not more than 7 day supply) of short-acting opioids may be prescribed at discharge to control acute postoperative pain. Multimodal and regional analgesia should be maximized as much as possible. Opioid-tolerant patients are usually advised to continue their usual home dose of opioid and use the prescribed short-acting opiates for breakthrough pain control. It is extremely important for patients with implanted intrathecal pumps or spinal cord stimulators to schedule a follow-up with their outpatient pain physician as soon as feasible, ideally in the first 2 weeks following discharge.

In addition to a postoperative pain plan, all patients including those with indwelling SCS and IT pumps need to meet standardized discharge criteria. Post anesthesia discharge scoring system (PADS) is a commonly employed scoring system that requires pain and nausea to be adequately controlled, vital signs and activity level to be consistent with preoperative baseline, and surgical bleeding to be minimal before discharge.

Summary

In summary, perioperative management of patients with indwelling SCS and IT pumps in the outpatient surgical setting can be optimized by a well-thought-out perioperative plan. Goals for these patients include adequate perioperative pain management as well as avoidance of complications and unplanned admissions. Planning needs close collaboration with the patient's outpatient pain physician, primary care physician, and surgeon, with an active role played by the patient. Coordination of patient and care teams in the perioperative period reduces the risk of adverse events faced by a patient presenting with an indwelling device, and a postoperative meeting with the outpatient pain physician closes the loop on postoperative pain and device function.

References

1. Rock AK, et al. Spinal cord stimulation. Neurosurg Clin N Am. 2019;30:169.
2. Dones I, Levi V. Spinal cord stimulation for neuropathic pain: current trends and future applications. Brain Sci. 2018;8(8):138.
3. Shah RV, Kaye AD, Urman RD. Emerging concepts in the closed-loop spinal cord stimulation system: preliminary results of the Avalon study. Ann Palliat Med. 2020;9:1272.
4. Sdrulla AD, Guan Y, Raja SN. Spinal cord stimulation: clinical efficacy and potential mechanisms. Pain Pract. 2018;18(8):1048–67.
5. Melzack R, Wall PD. Pain mechanisms: a new theory. Science. 1965;150(3699):971–9.

6. Bentley L, et al. Brain activity modifications following spinal cord stimulation for chronic neuropathic pain: a systematic review. Eur J Pain. 2016;20(4):499–511.
7. Kapural L, et al. Comparison of 10-kHz high-frequency and traditional low-frequency spinal cord stimulation for the treatment of chronic back and leg pain: 24-month results from a multicenter, randomized, controlled pivotal trial. Neurosurgery. 2016;79(5):667–77.
8. Sun FT, Morrell MJ. Closed-loop neurostimulation: the clinical experience. Neurotherapeutics. 2014;11(3):553–63.
9. Oklahoma City O, Grider J. Effectiveness of spinal cord stimulation in chronic spinal pain: a systematic review. Pain Physician. 2016;19:E33–54.
10. Prager J. Estimates of annual spinal cord stimulator implant rises in the United States. Neuromodulation: Technology at the Neural Interface. 2010;13(1):68–9.
11. Deer TR, et al. The Polyanalgesic Consensus Conference (PACC): recommendations on intrathecal drug infusion systems best practices and guidelines. Neuromodulation: Technology at the Neural Interface. 2017;20(2):96–132.
12. Lake W, Shah H. Intrathecal baclofen infusion for the treatment of movement disorders. Neurosurg Clin. 2019;30:203.
13. Bruel BM, Burton AW. Intrathecal therapy for cancer-related pain. Pain Med. 2016;17(12):2404–21.
14. Ver Donck A, et al. Intrathecal drug administration in chronic pain syndromes. Pain Pract. 2014;14(5):461–76.
15. Deer TR, et al. Intrathecal therapy for chronic pain: a review of morphine and ziconotide as firstline options. Pain Med. 2019;20(4):784–98.
16. Physician-Supplier Procedure Summary, C.f.M.M. Services, Editor, 2020.
17. Chung F, Ritchie E, Su J. Postoperative pain in ambulatory surgery. Anesth Analg. 1997;85(4):808–16.
18. Steiner CA. et al. Statistical brief# 223, 2017.
19. Thomas D-A, et al. Concept of the ambulatory pain physician. Curr Pain Headache Rep. 2017;21(1):7.
20. Quality oversight of Ambulatory Surgery Centers: a system in neglect, D.o.H.a.H. Services, Editor. Department of Health and Human Services Report, 2002.
21. Schaefer MK, et al. Infection control assessment of ambulatory surgical centers. JAMA. 2010;303(22):2273–9.
22. Harned ME, et al. Anesthetic considerations and perioperative management of spinal cord stimulators: literature review and initial recommendations. Pain Physician. 2017;20(4):319–29.
23. Pollard EM, et al. The effect of spinal cord stimulation on pain medication reduction in intractable spine and limb pain: a systematic review of randomized controlled trials and meta-analysis. J Pain Res. 2019;12:1311.
24. Ji R-R, et al. Neuroinflammation and central sensitization in chronic and widespread pain. Anesthesiology. 2018;129(2):343.
25. Campbell CM, et al. Dynamic pain phenotypes are associated with spinal cord stimulation-induced reduction in pain: a repeated measures observational pilot study. Pain Med. 2015;16(7):1349–60.
26. Golembiewski J, Dasta J. Evolving role of local anesthetics in managing postsurgical analgesia. Clin Ther. 2015;37(6):1354–71.
27. Medtronic, full prescribing information intrathecal Baclofen therapy with LIORESAL® INTRATHECAL (Baclofen Injection), 2019.
28. Nevro. Physician implant data. [Manual] 2015 May 2020]; Available from: accessdata.fda.gov/cdrh_docs/pdf13/P130022d.pdf.
29. BostonScientific. Precision spectra™ spinal cord stimulator system. 2020 May. 2020]; Available from: https://www.controlyourpain.com/safety-information/precision-spectra/.
30. Walsh KM, Machado AG, Krishnaney AA. Spinal cord stimulation: a review of the safety literature and proposal for perioperative evaluation and management. Spine J. 2015;15(8):1864–9.
31. Rapp SE, Ready LB, Nessly ML. Acute pain management in patients with prior opioid consumption: a case-controlled retrospective review. Pain. 1995;61(2):195–201.
32. Carroll IR, Angst MS, Clark DJ. Management of perioperative pain in patients chronically consuming opioids. Reg Anesth Pain Med. 2004;29(6):576–91.
33. Mitra S, Sinatra RS. Perioperative management of acute pain in the opioid-dependent patient. Anesthesiology-Philadelphia Then Hagerstown. 2004;101:212–27.
34. Katz WA. Cyclooxygenase-2-selective inhibitors in the management of acute and perioperative pain. Cleve Clin J Med. 2002;69(1):65–75.
35. Reuben SS, Connelly NR. Postoperative analgesic effects of celecoxib or rofecoxib after spinal fusion surgery. Anesth Analg. 2000;91(5):1221–5.
36. Jouguelet-Lacoste J, et al. The use of intravenous infusion or single dose of low-dose ketamine for postoperative analgesia: a review of the current literature. Pain Med. 2015;16(2):383–403.
37. Menigaux C, et al. Intraoperative small-dose ketamine enhances analgesia after outpatient knee arthroscopy. Anesth Analg. 2001;93(3):606–12.
38. Schotola H, et al. Ketamine in outpatient arthroscopic shoulder surgery: effects on postoperative pain, hemodynamic stability and process times. Open Med. 2015;10(1):297.
39. Laskowski K, et al. A systematic review of intravenous ketamine for postoperative analgesia. Can J Anesth/Journal canadien d'anesthésie. 2011;58(10):911.
40. Himmelseher S, Durieux ME. Ketamine for perioperative pain management. Anesthesiology J Am Soc Anesthesiol. 2005;102(1):211–20.
41. Gorlin AW, Rosenfeld DM, Ramakrishna H. Intravenous sub-anesthetic ketamine for perioperative analgesia. J Anaesthesiol Clin Pharmacol. 2016;32(2):160.

42. Patel S, Das S, Stedman RB. Urgent cesarean section in a patient with a spinal cord stimulator: implications for surgery and anesthesia. Ochsner J. 2014;14(1):131–4.
43. Bernardini DJ, et al. Spinal cord stimulation and the pregnant patient-specific considerations for management: a case series and review of the literature. Neuromodulation: Technology at the Neural Interface. 2010;13(4):270–4.
44. Grider JS, Brown RE, Colclough GW. Perioperative management of patients with an intrathecal drug delivery system for chronic pain. Anesth Analg. 2008;107(4):1393–6.
45. Lee HMD, Ruggoo V, Graudins A. Intrathecal clonidine pump failure causing acute withdrawal syndrome with 'stress-induced' cardiomyopathy. J Med Toxicol. 2016;12(1):134–8.
46. Nadherny W, Anderson B, Abd-Elsayed A. Perioperative and periprocedural care of patients with intrathecal pump therapy. Neuromodulation: Technology at the Neural Interface. 2019;22(7):775–80.

Part V

Discharge Considerations

26

Discharge from Recovery Room in Ambulatory Surgery Centers

Rajeev Dalal, Sadie Smith, Justin Pachuski, David Fanelli, Patrick McQuillan, Alan David Kaye, and Henry Liu

Abstract

Ambulatory surgery has gained tremendous popularity within the last 2–3 decades. More and more surgeries are performed on outpatient basis at ambulatory surgery centers. The understanding of how the postanesthesia care unit (PACU) functions is important in the appropriate care and discharge of the patients. Multiple phases of recovery exist and patients can be triaged based on their emergence from anesthesia. PACU discharge scoring systems have been implemented to progress a patient through the stages of recovery until discharge. The scoring systems initially developed by Aldrete, later modified by Chung and White, are still being used today. Discharge from ambulatory surgery centers has unique concerns when compared with discharge from PACU to hospital wards. This chapter will discuss the special considerations when discharging patients from PACU in ambulatory surgery centers.

R. Dalal · J. Pachuski · P. McQuillan · A. D. Kaye
Department of Anesthesiology and Perioperative Medicine, Penn State Milton S. Hershey Medical Center, Hershey, PA, USA
e-mail: jpachuski1@pennstatehealth.psu.edu; akaye@lsuhsc.edu

S. Smith · D. Fanelli · H. Liu (✉)
Department of Anesthesiology and Perioperative Medicine, Penn State College of Medicine, Milton S. Hershey Medical Center, Hershey, PA, USA
e-mail: ssmith38@pennstatehealth.psu.edu; dfanelli@pennstatehealth.psu.edu

Introduction

Ambulatory surgery centers (ASCs) are facilities that provide same-day surgical care for diagnostic and therapeutic procedures. They function similar to hospital outpatient departments and must comply with federal rules and regulations. Various types of procedures are typically performed in ASCs by specialties of orthopedics, urology, ophthalmology, gastroenterology, plastic surgery, otolaryngology, dentistry, interventional pain, and more. Established in response to challenges in scheduling, operating room availability, and hospital policies, the first freestanding ASC opened in early 1970. The American Society of Anesthesiologists released its very first guideline for postanesthesia care unit (PACU) discharge in ASCs few years later, and a rapid growth in ASCs ensued nationwide [1]. By the mid-1980s, ambulatory surgery accounted for almost 50% of all surgical volume in the nation [2]. Fast forward to the latest decade, around 48.3 million procedures, both surgical and nonsurgical, were performed

K. Rajput et al. (eds.), *Pain Control in Ambulatory Surgery Centers*,
https://doi.org/10.1007/978-3-030-55262-6_26

with almost half occurring in ASCs in 2010. About 95% of those ambulatory surgery patients in hospitals and ASCs were routinely discharged at the same day, while the other 5% were either admitted to the hospital, placed under observation status, or other options [3]. Despite attempting to optimize patients for discharge at ASCs, some patients will need to be transferred for admission to a nearby hospital for further care. Justifications for doing so include acute coronary syndromes, unstable arrhythmias, need for blood transfusions, and other lifesaving interventions. In concordance with the growth of ambulatory centers, the complexity of surgeries and patient comorbidities have been on the rise as well. The essence of ambulatory anesthesia involves rapid but safe discharge and return to daily function, so the anesthesiologists should be cognizant of the process patients face from arrival to discharge [4].

PACU and PACU Discharge

It is the national standard that patients who undergo general anesthesia, regional anesthesia, or monitored anesthesia care receive postanesthesia management in PACU, with the exception of critically ill patients who may go to the intensive care unit (ICU) directly. Upon arrival to the PACU, vital signs immediately monitored include blood pressure, heart rate, oxygen saturation, respiratory rate, and temperature. These vital signs are measured every 5 minutes for the first 15 minutes, then every 15 minutes. Airway patency, level of consciousness, and pain levels, among others, are also important characteristics that are assessed regularly. During this time of transition from anesthesia provider to PACU nurse, a handoff report must be given. This report includes essential perioperative factors; specifically, the preoperative history, intraoperative process and pertinent issues, assessment and report of current status, and postoperative instructions for the patient. Patients emerging from anesthesia require frequent monitoring as complications may arise and lifesaving measures may be required in a timely fashion [5].

In order for patients to receive individualized care following anesthesia, there must be an appropriate triage. Thus, PACU care is often divided into phases which are commonplace between hospitals and ASCs. Phase I represents the immediate recovery of a patient from anesthesia until hemodynamically stable. Specific criteria based on discharge scoring systems must be met before the patient progresses to Phase II. Phase II focuses on preparing patients for discharge along with postoperative education and instructions. At times, a patient may bypass phase I and head directly from the operating room to Phase II, a process referred to as "fast-tracking" [6]. This process improves efficiency in ASCs and allows for faster discharge. Practice models and logistics vary among institutions; Phase I and Phase II may be in the same location or they may be in separate locations. This is important in terms of staffing. Nurses take care of multiple patients simultaneously, so the RN ratio may alter in distinct phases. As well, if the phases are in separate areas, coordination must exist for the patient to be transported and monitored appropriately to the desired location. This creates additional planning in ensuring a smooth process for patients.

The determination of advancing a patient through the stages of the recovery process was initially time-based; in some countries this is still commonly practiced [7]. However, more recently, criteria-based scoring systems have been developed in guiding PACU personnel whether a patient may be discharged from PACU or progress to the subsequent phase of recovery. The first PACU discharge scoring system was developed in the 1970s by Dr. Antonio Aldrete [8]. His goal was to provide objective information on the condition of patients after anesthesia, analogous to the Apgar scoring system. It was called Postanesthetic recovery score (PARS). The following components were identified: activity, respiration, circulation, consciousness, and color (Fig. 26.1). A score of 0, 1, or 2 was given to each category, with a total maximum score of 10. A score of 7 was indicative for further monitoring and scores of 8–9 were acceptable for discharge; an ideal score was 10.

Systematic reviews were conducted to elucidate the reliability of the criteria used in several

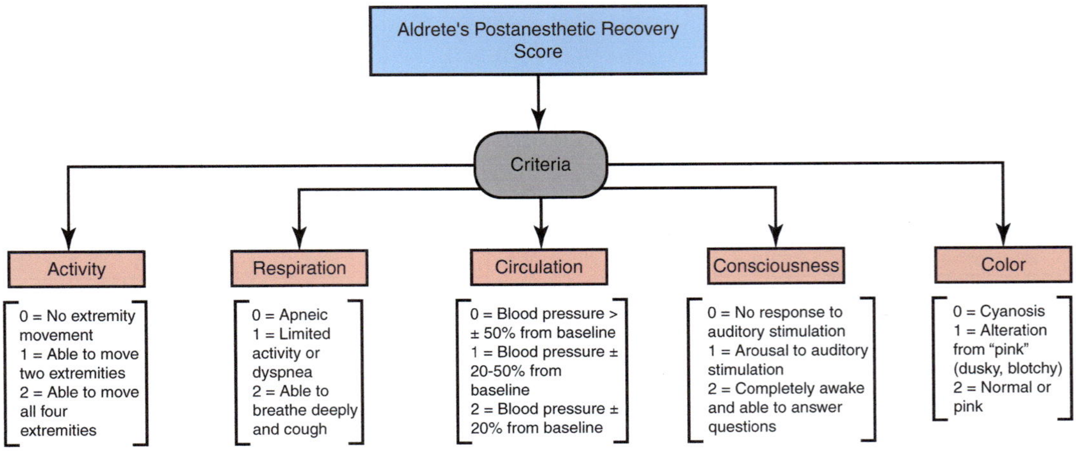

Fig. 26.1 Adapted from Aldrete's Postanesthesia Recovery Score [8]

Table 26.1 ASA Task Force Discharge Protocol

1. Urination before discharge should not be universal and should be evaluated for select patients.
2. Requirement to drink clear fluids should not be universal and should be evaluated for select patients.
3. Every patient should have a responsible individual accompany them home.
4. Observation is needed until patients have no increased risk of cardiorespiratory consequences.
5. A minimum stay is not needed.
6. Discharge criteria should be created in a way to minimize risk of CNS or cardiorespiratory depression following discharge.

ASA American Society of Anesthesiologists, *CNS* Central nervous system

discharge systems. Investigations published in databases in the last 40 years were searched, 8 studies were included. An important recommendation they made was assessing pain, nausea, and vomiting before the patient is discharged. This suggests the original Aldrete scoring system was incomplete as it did not take into account those components. Studies also found that there were limited investigations to validate the criteria used to evaluate PACU discharge readiness [9, 10].

The American Society of Anesthesiologists (ASA) published practice guidelines in 2013 on postanesthetic care. These guidelines addressed the protocol for discharge from the PACU. They were intended to assist the practitioner in making healthcare decisions (Table 26.1).

Difference in Discharge Criteria in ASC

The care of patients at ASCs presents unique challenges throughout the perioperative process. The main goal is to ascertain the patients can be safely discharged to their residence following their scheduled surgical/diagnostic procedure in the ASCs. Since the forthcoming of the original Aldrete's PACU discharge criteria scoring system, there have been various developments and revisions to scoring systems. Dr. Aldrete modified his scoring system in 1995, changing the criteria of color to oxygen saturation. In addition, he also created a PACU discharge score specifically for ambulatory surgery patients due to increased popularity in ambulatory surgery. In this scoring system, specifically designed for PACU in ASCs, five components were added: dressing, pain, ambulation, urine output, and feeding [11]. This system now doubled its criteria, and the recommendation at that time was to discharge patients when their score was 18 or greater.

The Post-Anesthetic Discharge Scoring System (PADSS) is another scoring system developed by Dr. Frances Chung in 1995 [12]. Essential to the creation of this system was the determination of home readiness. The criteria included vital signs, activity, mental status, pain or nausea or vomiting, surgical bleeding, and intake and output. Tolerating

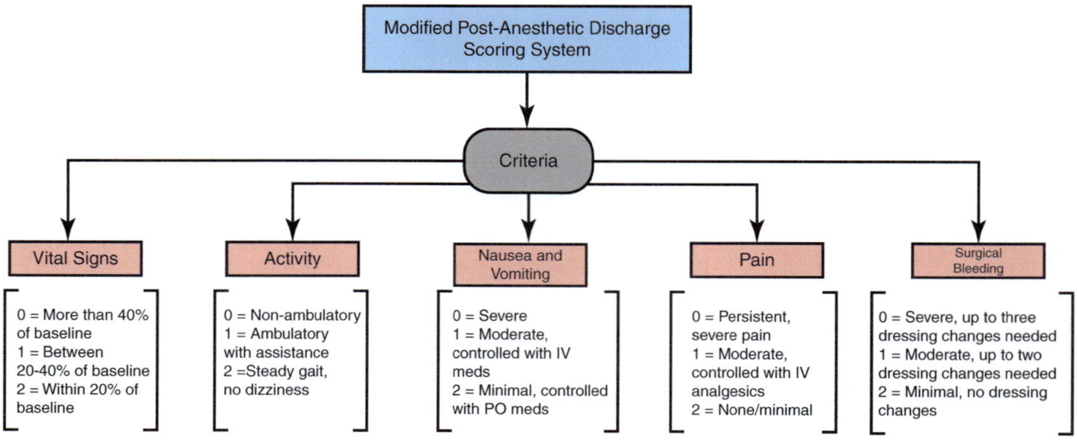

Fig. 26.2 Adapted from Modified Postanesthesia Discharge Scoring System [12]

fluids and ability to void have long been a controversy surrounding discharge, but there is no universal acceptance for these components to be satisfied at the time of discharge. The practice guidelines published by the American Society of Anesthesiologists recommend these criteria should be evaluated on a case-by-case basis. Thus, the PADSS system was later modified (Fig. 26.2). In fact, this scoring system was used to assess home readiness in patients undergoing colonoscopy and concluded that modified PADSS allowed for earlier discharge after the procedure [13].

Understanding modified PADSS can influence how the anesthesiologist devises the perioperative anesthetic plan. Knowledge of the type of surgery and its invasiveness can determine whether certain methods are employed to minimize postoperative pain, such as regional anesthesia. For example, regional anesthesia has been used in the outpatient setting to minimize postoperative pain. Broadly speaking, orthopedic total knee arthroplasties are commonly performed at outpatient centers and peripheral nerve blocks have been shown to reduce postoperative pain [14]. Some factors that come into consideration include using continuously infusing local anesthetic catheters versus single-shot nerve blocks. Single-shot blocks eliminate the requirement of follow-up, but the disadvantage is the relatively short amount of analgesic time. On the other spectrum is nerve catheters that provide analgesia for a few days postoperatively, but the disadvantage is follow-up may be required if complications arise. Neuraxial anesthesia, a form of regional anesthesia, is another option for ambulatory surgeries, but slow recession of the block may preclude strength, mobility, and urination. As with peripheral nerve blocks, some factors that come into consideration include the type of local anesthetic used with or without the addition of opioids. Using opioids improves analgesia with the risk of respiratory depression which can be problematic after discharge. A specific scoring tool called the WAKE score evaluated the needs of regional anesthesia patients and their ability to bypass PACU. It was modeled after the modified Aldrete system and included "zero tolerance criteria," which were pain, PONV, shivering, pruritus, and orthostatic symptoms [15, 16]. This tool may allow fast-tracking of these patients in an outpatient setting. For some patients, even more burdensome than pain is postoperative nausea and vomiting (PONV). Use of the Apfel scoring system has been validated for identifying high-risk patients for PONV [17]. Using alternative methods such as total intravenous anesthesia can be used to minimize risk of prolonged stay from PONV for same-day surgery patients. The last component of modified PADSS is surgical bleeding. Surgical selection is an important factor to consider as intra-abdominal, vascular, and orthopedic surgeries carry higher risk of perioperative bleeding. In certain cases, and in conjunction with the surgeon, the anesthesiologist can give pharmacologic interventions such as tranexamic acid to decrease the risk of bleeding [18]. The caveat is that ASCs might not have the availability to transfuse blood, so appropriate surgical and patient selection must be utilized in outpatient settings. As with managing any patient, risks and benefits must be weighed in the setting of patient comorbidities.

Various other factors can lead to prolonged PACU stay which influences the anesthetic choice, especially in ambulatory surgery patients. A predictive model was utilized to optimize case sequencing and revealed morbid obesity, hypertension, surgical specialty (ENT, gastroenterology), anesthesia type (general), and case duration led to higher odds of prolonged PACU stay [19]. These are not contraindications, but allow for cases involving patients with these risk factors to be performed earlier in the day in anticipation for a prolonged PACU stay. These factors also play a role in the type of anesthetic. For example, for short outpatient procedures in morbid obesity patients, it may be feasible to administer monitored anesthesia care if appropriate to allow for faster discharge home, as opposed to general anesthesia. Overall, physiologic-based scoring systems, anesthetic choice, and unique concerns in the ambulatory surgery patient are all important factors for discharge.

Recent Research

In the current day, discharge criteria for PACUs in the hospital and outpatient ASCs is primarily based on physiological criteria. A recent prospective study compared PACU discharge times based on physiological criteria, using the PARS and PADSS scoring systems by Aldrete and Chung, versus time-based criteria. A statistically significant difference was found to suggest physiological-based criteria enhances the speed of transit of pediatric ambulatory surgery patients through the PACU [20]. Another recent study compared general anesthesia with total intravenous anesthesia with a secondary outcome to compare discharge scoring systems of White's fast-tracking scoring system and the modified Aldrete scoring system. Dr. White created a scoring system in the 1990s in comparison to the modified Aldrete's scoring system with a focus on time to fast-track eligibility. This study revealed the fast track ratio was greater for the patient cohort assigned to the modified Aldrete scoring system [21]. Furthermore, the International Association for Ambulatory Surgery published guidelines quite similar to the modified PADSS. The guidelines stress the importance of vital signs, minimal nausea/vomiting, tolerable pain, micturition especially following neuraxial anesthesia, and more. Recent studies are also being performed about implementing a discharge checklist that informs patients of signs and symptoms post discharge to improve safety [22].

Despite many institutions still utilizing variants of PACU discharge scoring systems, there are select circumstances in which discharge from ASCs may require more than an established protocol. The rise in spine surgery at ASCs has been unprecedented. Given the concern for patient safety, the surgeon, anesthesiologist, and nurses should ultimately dictate the final disposition for these spinal surgery patients, not discharge criteria and safety check points [23].

Lastly, the role of ASCs is quickly evolving. Coronavirus Disease 2019 (COVID-19) has resulted in a global pandemic, affecting many ASCs as elective diagnostic and therapeutic procedures have been delayed. The hospital system nationwide has encountered an unimaginable surge in capacity. ASCs have the potential to assist acute care hospitals in performing urgent and emergent surgeries. Hospital beds for critically ill COVID-19 patients can be conserved if ASCs have the appropriate staffing and resources for performing such procedures. ASCs have adapted to the needs of the current time and now have the potential to serve a greater role [24].

Summary

Since the 1970s, ambulatory anesthesia has become more popular and many surgical and nonsurgical procedures are being performed at ASCs. Many institutions have PACUs with progressive phases of recovery. The first ever PACU discharge scoring system was developed by Dr. Aldrete in order to evaluate patients emerging from anesthesia. Since his creation, modifications and other newly developed discharge scoring systems were studied and implemented. Given the nature of ASCs, discharge criteria had to be streamlined to the needs of patients undergoing same-day surgery. Appropriate hemodynamics and vitals, adequate analgesia, minimal PONV, ambulation, surgical bleeding, and others are some of the factors accounted for in these criteria. Factors that prolong PACU stay such as morbid obesity and type of surgery are also important in the efficiency of discharging patients from ASCs. These discharge criteria systems are still in use today and provide guidelines for anesthesia-trained personnel for safely managing a patient throughout the perioperative process.

References

1. Hedley-Whyte J, Milamed DR. The evolution of sites of surgery. Ulster Med J. 2006;75(1):46–53. PMID 16457404.
2. Pregler JL, Kapur PA. The development of ambulatory anesthesia and future challenges. Anesthesiol Clin North Am. 2003;21(2):207–28. PMID 12812391.
3. Hall MJ, Schwartzman A, Zhang J, Liu X. Ambulatory surgery data from hospitals and ambulatory surgery centers: United States, 2010. Natl Health Stat Report. 2017;(102):1–15. PMID 28256998.
4. Lee JH. Anesthesia for ambulatory surgery. Korean J Anesthesiol. 2017;70(4):398–406. PMID 28794834.
5. Kellner DB, Urman RD, Greenberg P, Brovman EY. Analysis of adverse outcomes in the post-anesthesia care unit based on anesthesia liability data. J Clin Anesth. 2018;50:48–56. PMID 29979999.
6. Duncan PG, Shandro J, Bachand R, Ainsworth L. A pilot study of recovery room bypass ("fast-track protocol") in a community hospital. Can J Anaesth. 2001;48(7):630–6. PMID 11495868.
7. Jain A, Muralidhar V, Aneja S, Sharma AK. A prospective observational study comparing criteria-based discharge method with traditional time-based discharge method for discharging patients from post-anaesthesia care unit undergoing ambulatory or outpatient minor surgeries under general anaesthesia. Indian J Anaesth. 2018;62(1):61–5. PMID 29416152.
8. Aldrete JA, Kroulik D. A postanesthetic recovery score. Anesth Analg. 1970;49(6):924–34. PMID 5534693.
9. Phillips NM, Street M, Kent B, Haesler E, Cadeddu M. Post-anaesthetic discharge scoring criteria: key findings from a systematic review. Int J Evid Based Healthc. 2013;11(4):275–84. PMID 24298921.
10. Hegarty J, Burton A. Post anaesthetic care units in the Republic of Ireland: a survey of discharge criteria. J Perioper Pract. 2007;17(2):58–66. PMID 17319567.
11. Aldrete JA. The post-anesthesia recovery score revisited. J Clin Anesth. 1995;7(1):89–91. PMID 7772368.
12. Chung F, Chan VW, Ong D. A post-anesthetic discharge scoring system for home readiness after ambulatory surgery. J Clin Anesth. 1995;7(6):500–6. PMID 8534468.
13. Trevisani L, Cifalà V, Gilli G, Matarese V, Zelante A, Sartori S. Post-Anaesthetic Discharge Scoring System to assess patient recovery and discharge after colonoscopy. World J Gastrointest Endosc. 2013;5(10):502–7. PMID 24147194.
14. Cullom C, Weed JT. Anesthetic and analgesic management for outpatient knee arthroplasty. Curr Pain Headache Rep. 2017;21(5):23. PMID 28283810.
15. Williams BA. For outpatients, does regional anesthesia truly shorten the hospital stay, and how should we define postanesthesia care unit bypass eligibility? Anesthesiology. 2004;101(1):3–6. PMID 15220763.
16. Williams BA, Kentor ML. The WAKE© score: patient-centered ambulatory anesthesia and fast-tracking outcomes criteria. Int Anesthesiol Clin. 2011;49(3):33–43. PMID 21697668.
17. Weilbach C, Rahe-meyer N, Raymondos K, Weissig A, Scheinichen D, Piepenbrock S. Postoperative nausea and vomiting (PONV) : usefulness of the Apfel-score for identification of high risk patients for PONV. Acta Anaesthesiol Belg. 2006;57(4):361–3. PMID 17236637.
18. Ghadimi K, Levy JH, Welsby IJ. Perioperative management of the bleeding patient. Br J Anaesth. 2016;117(suppl 3):iii18–30. PMID 27940453.
19. Gabriel RA, Waterman RS, Kim J, Ohno-Machado L. A predictive model for extended postanesthesia care unit length of stay in outpatient surgeries. Anesth Analg. 2017;124(5):1529–36. PMID 28079580.
20. Armstrong J, Forrest H, Crawford MW. A prospective observational study comparing a physiological scoring system with time-based discharge criteria in

pediatric ambulatory surgical patients. Can J Anaesth. 2015;62(10):1082–8. PMID 26149598.

21. Çaparlar C, Özhan M, Süzer MA, Yazicioğlu D, Eşkin MB, Şenkal S, et al. Fast-track anesthesia in patients undergoing outpatient laparoscopic cholecystectomy: comparison of sevoflurane with total intravenous anesthesia. J Clin Anesth. 2017;37:25–30. PMID 28235523.
22. Jakobsson JG. Recovery and discharge criteria after ambulatory anesthesia: can we improve them? Curr Opin Anaesthesiol. 2019;32(6):698–702. PMID 34125193.
23. Witiw CD, Wilson JR, Fehlings MG, Traynelis VC. Ambulatory surgical centers: improving quality of operative spine care? Global Spine J. 2020;10(1 Suppl):29S–35S. PMID 31934517.
24. Rajan N, Joshi GP. COVID-19: role of ambulatory surgery facilities in this global pandemic. Anesth Analg. 2020;131(1):31–6. PMID 32243288.

27 Recovery Room Protocols for Nursing in Ambulatory Surgery Centers (ASCs) and Hospital Outpatient Departments (HOPDs)

Jill Zafar, Nalini Vadivelu, Kanishka Rajput, and Paul Fontanez

Abstract

Outpatient surgeries have increased dramatically over the last three decades. Recovery Room protocols for nursing in ambulatory settings can improve quality of care through standardization of practice to follow evidence-based guidelines. Protocols should be developed using a multidisciplinary team. Fast-track protocols, where patients are able to bypass phase I of recovery, can lead to decreased length of stay and are an economically efficient model. Pain assessment scales are important for the development of pain management protocols that should employ a multimodal approach to pain management. Postoperative nausea and vomiting is a common cause of delayed discharge and unplanned admissions. Nursing protocols for postoperative nausea and vomiting that rely on nurse assessments, communication, and protocolized treatments may further improve quality of care. Hypothermia protocols should similarly be developed to correct hypothermia aggressively due to associated risks including impaired wound healing, adverse cardiac events, altered drug metabolism, and coagulopathies.

Introduction

Ambulatory surgery, either in an Ambulatory Surgery Center (ASC) or a Hospital Outpatient Department (HOPDs), has increased dramatically in the last three decades. In 2010, 28.6 million ambulatory surgery visits and 48.3 million ambulatory procedures were performed [1]. As of 2011, outpatient procedures represented over 60% of all surgeries in the United States, up from 19% in 1988 [2]. Changes in insurance reimbursement have disproportionately redirected many outpatient surgeries to ambulatory surgery centers. Ambulatory surgery centers are viewed as less expensive, more efficient, and more convenient for patients [2].

Nursing Recovery Room protocols in Ambulatory Surgery Centers (ASCs) or Hospital Outpatient Departments (HOPDs) help standardize postoperative care of patients with the goal of obtaining the fastest recovery from anesthesia, while providing adequate pain control with mini-

J. Zafar (✉) · N. Vadivelu
Department of Anesthesiology, Yale University School of Medicine, New Haven, CT, USA
e-mail: jill.zafar@yale.edu

K. Rajput
Department of Anesthesiology and Pain Medicine, Yale University School of Medicine, New Haven, CT, USA

P. Fontanez
Yale New Haven Hospital, Perioperative Services, New Haven, CT, USA
e-mail: paul.fontanez@ynhh.org

K. Rajput et al. (eds.), *Pain Control in Ambulatory Surgery Centers*,
https://doi.org/10.1007/978-3-030-55262-6_27

mal side effects of sedation and nausea or vomiting. Protocols need to be developed using a multidisciplinary team consisting of nursing, anesthesia, and surgery. This chapter recommends several areas where protocols can be developed for nursing in the recovery room as well as several example protocols that can be adapted based on institutional needs.

Fast-Track Protocols

Phase 1 level of care is the immediate post-anesthesia period, while phase 2 is usually reserved as a secondary level of care for outpatients prior to discharge. Fast-track protocols establish criteria to allow a patient to go directly from the operating room or procedural area to phase 2 care. Fast-tracking to phase 2 care allows patients to be discharged home earlier without increased risk of complications [3–6]. Phase 2 care can also be staffed with a higher patient-to-nurse ratio, providing a more efficient and economic model.

Protocols for fast tracking patients directly to phase 2 care should be developed using a multidisciplinary team, taking into consideration the procedure, anesthetic technique, and patient's comorbidities. A patient that goes directly to phase 2 from the procedure or operating room should have already met all phase 1 discharge criteria. There are several criteria in use to determine if a patient can safely bypass phase 1 of post-anesthesia care and be directly transferred to phase 2 recovery. The Modified Aldrete Score, combined with pain and nausea and vomiting, assessments is a widely used scoring system that requires patients to achieve a minimum score before being fast tracked to phase 2 recovery (Table 27.1) [7–10].

Table 27.1 Criteria for fast tracking after ambulatory surgery with general anesthesia

I.	Level of consciousness	
	Awake and oriented	2
	Arousable with minimal stimulation	1
	Responsive only to tactile stimulation	0
II.	Physical activity	
	Able to move all extremities on command	2
	Some weakness in movement of extremities	1
	Unable to voluntarily move extremities	0
III.	Hemodynamic stability	
	Blood pressure ± 15% of baseline	2
	Blood pressure ± 30% of baseline	1
	Blood pressure ± 50% of baseline	0
IV.	Respiratory stability	
	Respiratory rate 10–20 breaths/min, able to breathe deeply	2
	Tachypnea with good cough	1
	Dyspneic with weak cough	0
V.	Oxygen saturation status	
	Maintains value >90% while breathing room air	2
	Requires supplemental oxygen to maintain saturation >90%	1
	Saturation <90% with supplemental oxygen	0
VI.	Postoperative pain assessment	
	No or mild discomfort	2
	Moderate-to-severe pain controlled with intravenous analgesics	1
	Persistent moderate-to-severe pain	0
VII.	Postoperative emetic symptoms	
	No or mild nausea with no active vomiting	2
	Transient vomiting or retching controlled with intravenous antiemetics	1
	Persistent moderate-to-severe nausea and vomiting	0
Total score		14

Reprinted with permission from Ref. [9]

Note: A minimum score of 12 (with no score <1 in any individual category) would be required for a patient to be fast-tracked after general anesthesia

Discharge Protocols

Criteria should be established that direct Recovery Room nurses on when it is appropriate to discharge patients from the Post Anesthesia Care Unit (PACU), including transitioning to phase 2, discharge directly to home, or transfer to an inpatient floor. The American Society of Anesthesiologists state that a physician is responsible for the discharge of patients from the PACU and that any discharge criteria that are developed must be approved by the Department of Anesthesiology and medical staff [11]. Discharge criteria should be developed using a multidisciplinary team and should establish specific discharge criteria that patients must meet prior to going home after a procedure. Using a patient assessment scale (example in Table 27.1) can be helpful. Most institutions use a Modified Aldrete Score greater than 9 as the criteria for a patient to be acceptable for discharge from the Post Anesthesia Care Unit (PACU) (Table 27.2) [7].

Table 27.2 Modified Aldrete Score: a score > 9 is acceptable for discharge from PACU

Criteria	Characteristics	Points
Activity	Moves all extremities on command or voluntarily	2
	Moves two extremities on command or voluntarily	1
	Unable to move	0
Respiration	Breathe deeply and cough	2
	Dyspnea, hypoventilation	1
	Apneic	0
Circulation	BP +/− 20% of baseline	2
	BP > or < 20–50% mmHg baseline	1
	BP > or < 50% mmHg baseline	0
Consciousness	Fully awake	2
	Arousable	1
	Unconscious	0
O_2 saturation	O_2 saturation ≥92% on room air	2
	Need oxygen to maintain O_2 saturation ≥90%	1
	O_2 saturation <90% even with oxygen	0

Discharge criteria may vary depending on discharge location and its monitoring and nursing capabilities.

In order for a patient to be discharged home after a procedure, there are additional criteria that have to be met. Patients must have a responsible adult to accompany them home. This is required due to the prolonged effects of anesthetic medications. Patients should be instructed not to drive for at least 24 hours or longer while still requiring opioid pain medication. It is not a requirement that patients need to void prior to discharge but they should be instructed to call their physician if they still have not voided several hours after discharge. Consumption of food is not required prior to discharge although patients should not be actively vomiting. Patients should have minimal nausea, pain that is well controlled, and no more than expected bleeding from the procedure. The Post Anesthesia Discharge Scoring System (PADS) can help assist in determining a patient's readiness for discharge (Table 27.3) [12].

Discharge after regional anesthesia requires special considerations. Regional anesthesia and peripheral nerve blocks can be beneficial in providing effective pain relief while reducing opioid use, and promoting a quicker discharge. The area

Table 27.3 Post anesthesia discharge scoring system (PADS): a score of 10 is suitable for discharge home after a procedure

Activity	Criteria	Points
Vital signs: stable and consistent with age and preoperative baseline	BP and pulse within 20% of baseline	2
	BP and pulse 20–40% of baseline	1
	BP and pulse >40% of baseline	0
Activity level: able to ambulate at preoperative level	Steady gait, no dizziness, or meets preoperative level	2
	Requires assistance	1
	Unable to ambulate	0
Nausea and vomiting: minimal prior to discharge	Minimal: successfully treated with PO medications	2
	Moderate: successfully treated with IM/IV medications	1
	Severe: continues despite repeated treatment	0
Pain: minimal prior to discharge; acceptable level of pain to the patient; controlled with PO medications; location, type, and intensity consistent with anticipated postoperative discomfort	Yes – acceptable	2
	No	1
Surgical bleeding: consistent with expected blood loss for the procedure	Minimal: does not require dressing change	2
	Moderate: up to 2 dressing changes	1
	Severe: ≥3 dressing changes	0

PO oral

of caution for these patients is that some of these blocks may cause the limb to become immobile with loss of sensation. This must be taken into consideration when using the patient assessment scales and is addressed later on in this chapter in the section on Regional Anesthesia Nursing Protocols. For spinal anesthesia, it is important to ensure that motor, sensory, and sympathetic blocks have resolved. Some criteria to judge when this has occurred include normal perianal (S4–5) sensation, plantar flexion of the foot, and proprioception in the big toe [12]. Specific discharge nursing protocols should be developed that take these considerations into account.

Pain Assessment

Moderate to severe pain occurs in about 30–40% of patients after outpatient surgery, especially in the first 24–48 hours after surgery [13]. Adequate pain control is one of the key requirements to assess readiness for discharge after ambulatory surgery. Patients often have misconceptions about pain and its treatment, such as fears about addiction and potential adverse effects. These misconceptions can lead to under reporting, underdosing, and poor compliance, all of which can result in significant post discharge pain and the potential for development of chronic pain [14].

The groundwork for assessment and management of postoperative pain should ideally be laid in the preoperative period. The preoperative period allows obtaining a thorough pain history and evaluates patients' prior experiences with pain, their attitudes, beliefs, levels of knowledge, and unrealistic expectations, if any. A preoperative strategy geared toward patient education has been shown to reduce anxiety and postoperative pain with a major impact on patient satisfaction [14]. The pain history also provides insight into the coping strategies previously used by the patient and their effectiveness [15].

Patients should be educated preoperatively and provided with both verbal and written information on how their pain will be assessed and managed during the immediate postoperative period. This can be particularly helpful for the pediatric population where preoperative education might help allay parents' anxiety, address parental barriers to appropriate management of postoperative pediatric pain, such as uncertainty regarding how to evaluate pain and reluctance to use pain medication because of fears of addiction [16]. The preadmission period is also the ideal time to discuss the relationship between comfort and functional goals, such as deep breathing and ambulation.

The American Pain Society, the American Society of Regional Anesthesia and Pain Medicine, and the American Society of Anesthesiologists recommend the use of a validated pain assessment tool to track responses to postoperative pain treatments and adjust treatment plans accordingly [16]. A number of pain assessment tools have been validated for detecting the presence of and quantifying the severity of pain. These scales have been tested for intra-patient and inter-rater reliability. The tools use different methods to measure pain, including visual analog scales, numeric or verbal rating scales, symbols, and others [16]. There is insufficient evidence to recommend one type of pain scale over another. The use of one particular pain assessment tool is therefore a matter of clinical or clinician/institutional preference. Optimal results require consistent use of one particular pain assessment tool in a clinical setting; however, it is less important which particular tool is used than that one tool be selected and used consistently [17]. The Joint Commission also requires that hospitals select and use the same pain assessment tools across all departments. This standard suggests providing options among scales such as the Numerical Rating Scale (NRS), the Wong-Baker FACES scale, and a verbal descriptor scale. [15].

An introduction of commonly used pain scales during the preoperative visit ensures that the patient would be familiar with the scale. Once the patient is in the recovery room, pain assessment should be brief and simple to complete.

Pain scales can be divided into three broad categories. (1) Numerical rating scales use a

Table 27.4 Validated pain intensity scales [16]

Name of scale	Rating system
Numeric rating scale (NRS)	Six-point NRS (NRS 0–5) Eleven-point NRS (NRS 0–10) Twenty-one-point NRS (NRS 0–20)
Verbal rating scale (VRS)	Four-point VRS Seven-point graphic rating scale Six-point present pain inventory (PPI)
Visual analog scales	Commonly rated 0–10 cm or 0–100 mm
Pain thermometer	Combines a visual thermometer with verbal descriptions of pain
Faces rating scales	Faces pain scale-revised Wong-Baker FACES pain rating scale Oucher scale

number system to rate a patient's pain. (2) Visual analog scales ask the patient to look at a scale and mark their pain level. (3) Categorical scales use words or pictures often also combined with numbers, colors, or localization. The selection of a particular pain assessment tool is based on factors such as developmental status, cognitive status, level of consciousness, educational level, and cultural and language differences. Examples of validated scoring systems are listed in Table 27.4. As the scale increases in complexity, it gives a more accurate description of the patient's pain but at the cost of additional time required to complete. With a patient recovering from anesthesia in the recovery room, it may be difficult to have the patient participate in a comprehensive pain assessment.

The NRS and VAS scales are most often used in cognitively intact adults. In children, the Pediatric Initiative on Methods, Measurement, and Pain Assessment in Clinical Trials group suggests the use of the Face, Legs, Arms, Cry, Consolability (FLACC) and Parents Post-operative Pain Measure for assessing acute pain in preverbal and nonverbal children on the basis of the reliability, validity, and ease of use [16, 18]. Elderly patients with advanced dementia similarly require behavioral observation to determine the presence of pain; tools such as the PAIN-AD are available for this patient population [19]. Figure 27.1 depicts the FACES, Oucher, and Wong-Baker FACES pain rating scales.

In addition to a pain score, location and quality of pain are important elements to help determine etiology and more effectively manage pain. Patients may experience pain in areas other than the surgical site, the pain experienced may be chronic (e.g., headache, low-back pain) or it may be related to the positioning and padding used during the procedure. The quality of pain can be assessed using instruments such as the McGill Pain Questionnaire [20] that contains a variety of verbal descriptors that help distinguish between musculoskeletal and nerve-related pain. Typically, patients describe deep tissue pain as dull, aching, and cramping, while nerve-related pain tends to be more sporadic, shooting, or burning [21].

Since pain is inherently subjective, patient self-report is the primary basis of all pain assessments. For patients who cannot adequately report their pain because of cognitive deficits, sedation, developmental stage, or other factors, clinicians might need to use behavioral assessment tools as described above and solicit input from caregivers to assess pain [22]. In all cases, clinicians should not rely solely on "objective" measures such as pain-related behaviors or vital signs in lieu of patient self-report to determine the presence of or intensity of pain because such measures are neither valid nor reliable. At similar levels of pain, pain behaviors may vary markedly between individuals. Therefore, although assessments of pain behaviors might supplement information from self-reported pain, it is important to interpret behavioral observations cautiously. Nevertheless, behavioral cues indicating pain include splinting, grimacing, moaning or grunting, distorted posture, and reluctance to move. Physiological responses of sympathetic activation such as tachycardia, increased respiratory rate, and hypertension may also indicate that pain is present. However, a lack of physiological responses or an absence of behaviors indicating pain may not mean the patient is not experiencing pain and hence should not be solely relied upon.

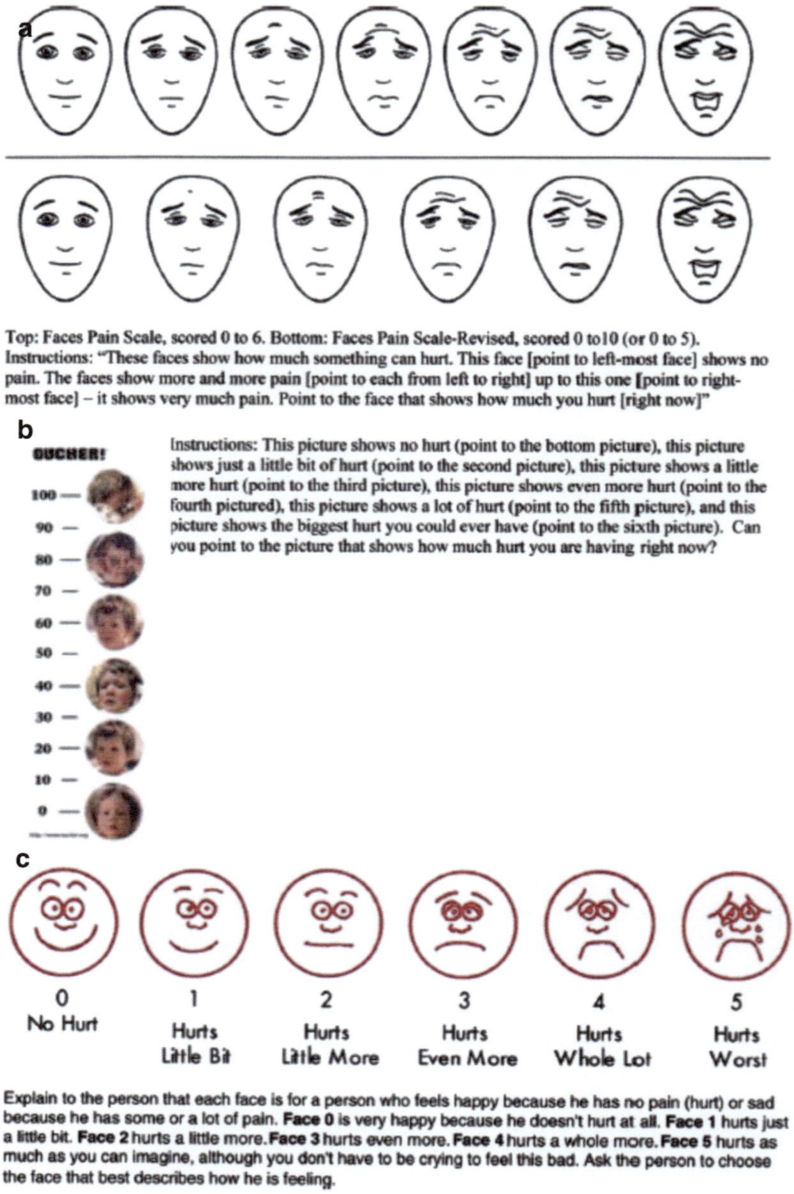

Fig. 27.1 Examples of FACES rating pain assessment scales. (**a**) Wong-Baker FACES pain scales; (**b**) Oucher scale; (**c**) Wong-Baker FACES pain rating scale. (Reprinted with permission from Ref. [18])

Pain Management Protocols

Pain management regimens are complex and based on patient's comorbidities as well as the surgical procedure, making standardized nursing protocols challenging to create. Nursing should be involved in the development of patient care pathways and should raise their concerns when physician decisions vary from standardized care. Nursing should also be educated on multimodal pain management including regional anesthesia, the various classes of medications used to control pain in the immediate postoperative period, as well as their side effects and synergistic affects [23].

An important concept to understand is the difference between time of onset and time of peak effect. When repeat doses of medications are administered over a short time period, there is potential to create additive effects if enough time has not elapsed between repeat doses. This is particularly concerning with respect to side effects of respiratory depression and hypotension, especially in the elderly and opioid naïve population.

Table 27.5 provides route of administration, onset time, time to peak effect, and duration of commonly used opioid pain medications in the recovery room [24, 25].

Non-opioid pain medications used as part of a multimodal analgesic regimen can have several advantages. Their opioid-sparing effects result in less respiratory depression and nausea which is particularly desirable in an ambulatory setting to promote a faster discharge. Typical postoperative non-opioid pain medications include acetaminophen, nonsteroidal anti-inflammatory drugs (NSAIDs), and gabapentinoids.

Acetaminophen is available in intravenous, oral, or rectal formulations and can provide effective pain relief alone for mild to moderate pain, as well as synergistic pain relief for severe pain. Acetaminophen should be used with caution in patients with liver disease. NSAIDs are available in intravenous and oral formulations and can provide similar and synergistic pain relief with acetaminophen. NSAIDs affect the clotting pathway and can theoretically increase postoperative bleeding, although this has not been proven to be significant [26]. NSAIDs should be used with caution in patients with renal dysfunction.

Gabapentinoids, including gabapentin and pregabalin, are similarly effective in reducing overall opioid requirement in the perioperative period and are often used as part of a "pre-emptive analgesic regimen." However, caution needs to be exercised especially when large doses are used, given their synergistic effect of respiratory depression when combined with opioids [27]. If patients are planned to be discharged home on a short course of gabapentinoids, nursing staff should educate the patients on the importance of tapering these medications over a period of several days.

Figure 27.2 is an example of a recovery room pain pathway for nursing using a multimodal approach.

Table 27.5 Opioid pain medication pharmacokinetics for adult opioid-naive patients

Opioid	Route	Dose	Time of onset (min)	Peak	Duration of action	Recommended recovery room dosing intervals
Fentanyl	IV	25–100 μg	1–2	3–5 min	30–60 min	Q5 min
Morphine	IV	2–5 mg	5–10	30–60 min	3–4 h	Q10 min
Hydromorphone	IV	0.25–1 mg	5–10	10–20 min	2–3 h	Q10 min
Oxycodone	PO	5–10 mg	10–20	0.5–1 h	3–6 h	Q4–6 h
Codeine	PO	30–60 mg	30–60	1–1.5 h	4–8 h	Q4–6 h
Tramadol	PO	25–50 mg	30–60	1.5 h	3–7 h	Q6 h
Hydrocodone	PO	5–10 mg	10–20	1–3 h	4–8 h	Q4–6 h

h hours, *Q* every, *IV* intravenous, *PO* oral, *min* minutes

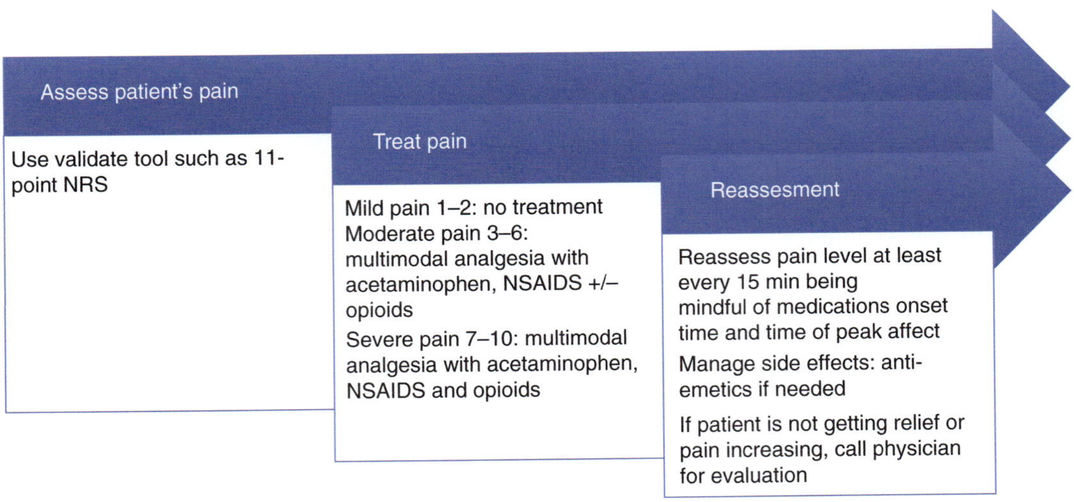

Fig. 27.2 Example of nursing pain management recovery room pathway

Postoperative Nausea and Vomiting Protocols

Despite advances in anesthetic drugs and pharmacology, postoperative nausea and vomiting (PONV) remains extremely common, with approximately 30% of surgical patients experiencing postoperative vomiting and 50% of patients experiencing postoperative nausea [28–30]. PONV can be extremely uncomfortable for patients and many patients fear PONV more than postoperative pain. PONV increases PACU length of stay and increases the cost of care. PONV can also lead to unplanned hospital admissions, which can be challenging for an Ambulatory Surgery Center [29].

In phase 1 of post-anesthesia care, a patient should be assessed for nausea and/or vomiting at least every 15 minutes along with other nursing assessments. Specific nursing protocols for nausea and vomiting are difficult to create as one must consider multiple factors in prescribing anti-emetic medications including the patient's history, home medications, and comorbidities, as well as concurrently given medications. Although it is out of the nursing scope of practice to prescribe anti-emetic medications, the nurse can have a tremendous impact on patient's postoperative nausea and vomiting. The nurse should focus on informing the perioperative team of the patient's nausea and vomiting risk preoperatively, as well as focus on multimodal pain control options that limit opioids [29].

This assessment begins in the preoperative period for recognizing patients who may have a high risk for PONV. A history of PONV, female gender, nonsmoking status, postoperative opioids, and emetogenic surgery are all well-known risk factors for PONV (Fig. 27.3). Timely communication with the perioperative team can potentially lead to different anesthetic techniques to be used intraoperatively to reduce PONV, as well as prophylaxis treatment with anti-emetic medications preoperatively and intraoperatively. Figure 27.3 provides an example of an algorithm to prevent and treat PONV.

Nurses should be knowledgeable of the different classes of anti-emetic medications and their risks and benefits. This will allow them to help the perioperative team choose the best pharmacologic treatments for the patient. Typically, repeated doses or multiple medications from the same drug class are not recommended. If rescue PONV medications are necessary, consideration should be given to other classes of medications or other treatment modalities as described in Fig. 27.3 [29, 31].

Hypothermia Nursing Protocols

Perioperative hypothermia, defined as a temperature less than 36 °C, is associated with impaired wound healing, adverse cardiac events, altered drug metabolism, and coagulopathies [32–34]. In cardiac patients undergoing noncardiac surgery, hypothermia is associated with increased cardiac morbidity [35]. Hypothermia has also been linked to impaired wound healing and increased postoperative surgical site infections [36, 37]. Furthermore, hypothermia is associated with impaired platelet function and reduces clotting factor enzyme function [38]. Preventing perioperative hypothermia has also been shown to reduce blood loss and transfusion requirement [39, 40]. Maintaining normothermia is now part of many Enhanced Recovery After Surgery (ERAS) protocols that take a multimodal approach to maintain preoperative organ function and reduce the profound stress response following surgery [41–44]. Hypothermia in the postoperative period is also associated with increased recovery room length of stay which has operational and economic implications [45, 46].

The American Society of Peri Anesthesia Nurses (ASPAN) developed an Evidence-Based Clinical Practice Guideline for the Promotion of Perioperative Normothermia [47]. These guidelines acknowledge that obtaining core body temperature (e.g., pulmonary artery, distal esophagus, nasopharynx, tympanic membrane [via thermistor]) is not always feasible in the postoperative period and that the oral temperature may best approximate the core temperature. This guideline also states that temporal artery measurements can also be used. The guidelines do

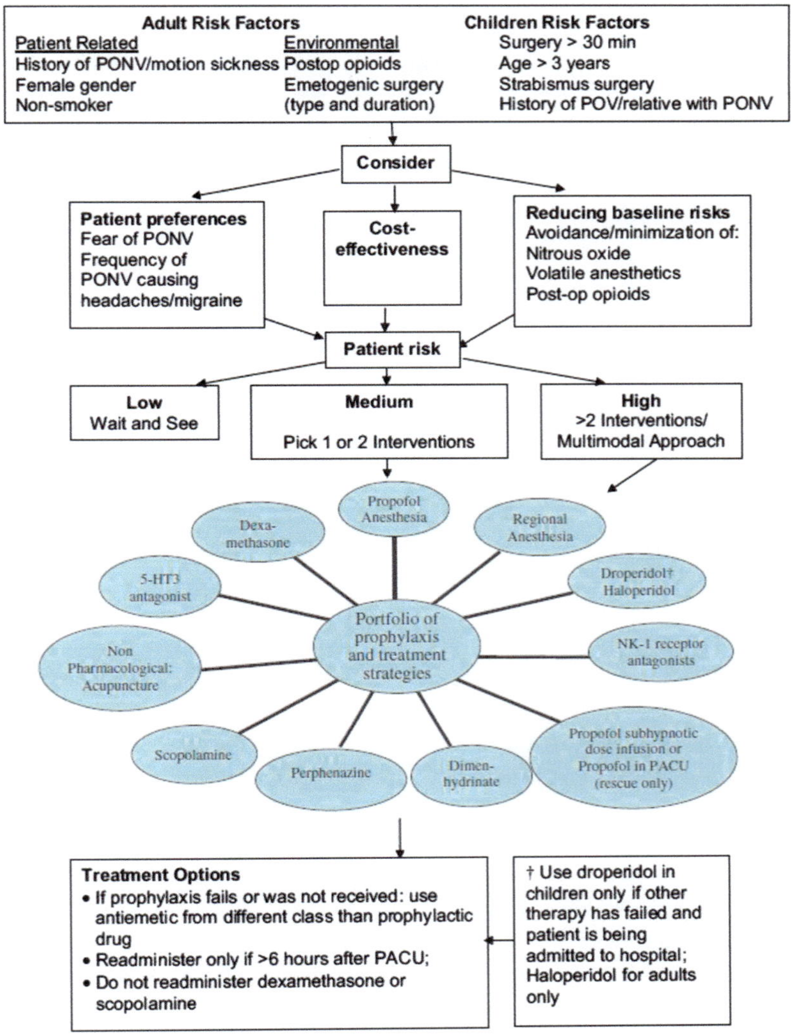

Fig. 27.3 Algorithm for prevention and treatment of postoperative nausea and vomiting. (Reprinted with permission from Ref. [29])

not recommend using Infrared tympanic thermometry as providing accurate temperature measurements in the perioperative period. Nursing assessments should include temperature monitoring as well as identifying signs and symptoms of hypothermia, including shivering, determining the patient's risk for hypothermia (Table 27.6), determining patient's thermal comfort level, and communicating assessment to the perioperative team.

If a patient's body temperature is less than 36 °C, passive and active warming measures should be initiated. Passive warming measures include blankets, head coverings, and increasing the ambient room temperature. Active warming measures include the application of a forced air convection warming system, as well as circulating-water mattresses, resistive heating blankets, radiant warmers, negative-pressure

Table 27.6 Patient risk factors for postoperative hypothermia

Extremes of age
Systolic blood pressure less than 140 mmHg
Female gender
High level of spinal block
BMI below normal
Body surface/wound area uncovered
Longer anesthesia/procedural duration
History of diabetes with autonomic dysfunction

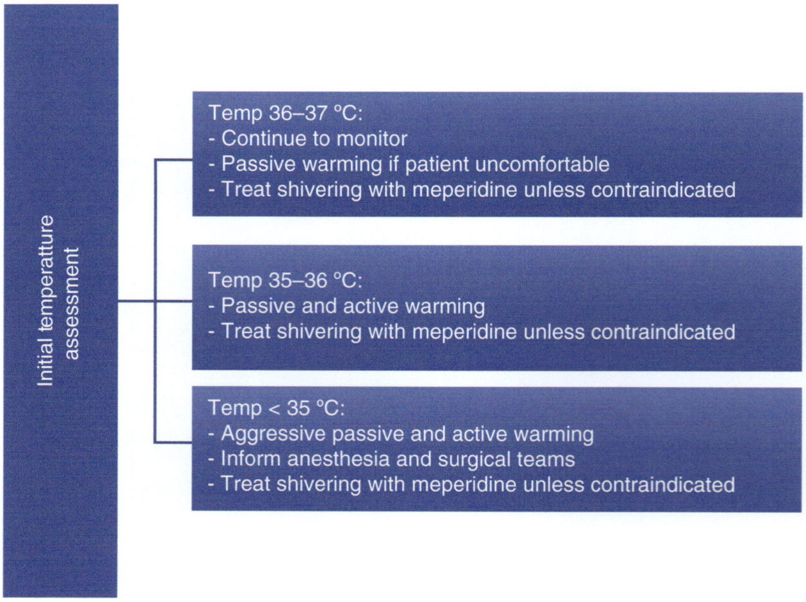

Fig. 27.4 Hypothermia recovery room nursing protocol

warming systems, and warmed humidified inspired oxygen. Temperature assessments should be done at least every 15 minutes during phase 1 of recovery and should be assessed prior to discharge. Figure 27.4 is an example of a recovery room nursing protocol for management of hypothermia.

Shivering can be a sign of hypothermia although it may also occur as a sign of emergence from anesthesia. Shivering increases oxygen consumption by up to 500% and should be treated aggressively, especially in patients with cardiovascular comorbidities [48]. Active warming if the patient is hypothermic is appropriate. Oxygen should be considered, particularly for comorbid patients. Pharmacologic treatment can be considered with physician consultation, including meperidine, clonidine, and doxapram [48], although some of these agents have fallen out of disrepute due to significant side effects.

Regional Anesthesia Nursing Protocols

Recent advances in regional anesthesia with the use of ultrasound guidance have increased the use of regional anesthesia in outpatient surgery. Several advantages of regional anesthesia have been described in the literature. These include faster Phase 1 post anesthesia care unit (PACU) discharge and cost savings [49, 50]. Regional anesthesia has been associated with a decrease in complications while improving analgesia. Patients who have undergone neuraxial or regional anesthesia such as lower extremity or upper extremity nerve block such as femoral, popliteal, interscalene block, etc., might not be able to achieve the >9 score on the Modified Aldrete Score for PACU bypass [51–54]. A useful bypass/discharge scoring system for patients undergoing regional anesthesia in outpatient surgery is the WAKE© score. The WAKE© score is modeled after the Modified Aldrete Score with additional "Zero Tolerance Criteria" [50, 55]. The "Zero Tolerance Criteria" include patients not requiring any intravenous interventions for the treatment of pain, nausea, vomiting, pruritus, shivering, or hypotension/orthostasis/lightheadedness. Pain should be well controlled and less than 3–4 out of 10. Patients who score 8 or above and meet these additional criteria are acceptable for phase I discharge or bypass.

It is well known that regional anesthesia can lead to decreased use of short-term opioids and avoidance of volatile anesthetics in outpatient surgery. Regional anesthesia along with the use of suitable recovery criteria, multimodal analgesia, multimodal postoperative nausea and vomiting prophylaxis, and multimodal sedation-hypnosis makes bypass of phase 1 post anesthesia care unit care possible and allows expedited discharge from same-day surgery [56]. In spite of the advantages, widespread use of regional anesthesia is not prevalent. The utilization of regional anesthesia in outpatient surgery has a surprisingly low frequency of only about 3%. Further studies to understand its limited use are needed.

Summary

Nursing Recovery Room protocols in ASCs and HOPDs can improve the quality of care for patients undergoing outpatient procedures. Protocols should be developed using a multidisciplinary team, including surgeons, nurses, and anesthesiologists. This chapter includes several areas where nursing protocols can be developed, including fast tracking, discharge, pain management, postoperative nausea and vomiting, and hypothermia. Nursing Recovery Room protocols can be developed in other areas by using a similar multidisciplinary approach.

References

1. Hall MJ, Schwartzman A, Zhang J, Liu X. Ambulatory surgery data from hospitals and ambulatory surgery centers: United States, 2010. Natl Health Stat Rep. 2017;(102):1–15.
2. American Hospital Association. Trends in hospital financing. Table 4.4: Aggregate hospital payment-to-cost ratios for private payers, medicare and medicaid, 1989–2009. In: TrendWatch chartbook: trends affecting hospitals and health systems. Washington, DC: American Hospital Association; 2011. p. 37–44.
3. Williams BA, Kentor ML, Williams JP, Vogt MT, DaPos SV, Harner CD, et al. PACU bypass after outpatient knee surgery is associated with fewer unplanned hospital admissions but more phase II nursing interventions. Anesthesiology. 2002;97(4):981–8.
4. White PF, Song D. New criteria for fast-tracking after outpatient anesthesia: a comparison with the modified Aldrete's scoring system. Anesth Analg. 1999;88(5):1069–72.
5. Lubarsky DA. Fast track in the post-anesthesia care unit: unlimited possibilities? J Clin Anesth. 1996;8(3):S70–S2.
6. Duncan PG, Shandro J, Pharma RB, Ainsworth L. A pilot study of recovery room bypass ("fast-track protocol") in a community hospital. Can J Anesth. 2001;48(7):630.
7. Aldrete J. The post-operative recovery score revisited. J Clin Anesth. 1995;7(1):89–91.
8. Aldrete JA, Kroulik D. A postanesthetic recovery score. Anesth Analg. 1970;49(6):924–34.
9. Watkins AC, White PF. Fast-tracking after ambulatory surgery. J Perianesth Nurs. 2001;16(6):379–87.
10. White P. Criteria for fast-tracking outpatients after ambulatory surgery. J Clin Anesth. 1999;11(1):78.
11. American Society of Anesthesiologists Standards for Postanesthesia Care. American Society of Anesthesiologists Annual Meeting, 23 Oct 2019.
12. Marshall SI, Chung F. Discharge criteria and complications after ambulatory surgery. Anesth Analg. 1999;88(3):508–17.
13. Beauregard L, Pomp A, Choiniere M. Severity and impact of pain after day-surgery. Can J Anaesth. 1998;45(4):304–11.
14. Kamming D, Chung F, Williams D, McGrath BM, Curti B. Pain management in ambulatory surgery. J Perianesth Nurs. 2004;19(3):174–82.
15. Wells N, Pasero C, McCaffery M. Improving the quality of care through pain assessment and management. In: Patient safety and quality: an evidence-based handbook for nurses. Rockville: Agency for Healthcare Research and Quality (US); 2008.
16. Chou R, Gordon DB, de Leon-Casasola OA, Rosenberg JM, Bickler S, Brennan T, et al. Management of postoperative pain: a clinical practice guideline from the American Pain Society, the American Society of Regional Anesthesia and Pain Medicine, and the American Society of Anesthesiologists' committee on regional anesthesia, executive committee, and administrative council. J Pain. 2016;17(2):131–57.
17. Kuusniemi K, Pöyhiä R. Present-day challenges and future solutions in postoperative pain management: results from PainForum 2014. J Pain Res. 2016;9:25–36.
18. Young KD. Assessment of acute pain in children. Clin Pediatr Emerg Med. 2017;18(4):235–41.
19. Warden V, Hurley AC, Volicer L. Development and psychometric evaluation of the Pain Assessment in Advanced Dementia (PAINAD) scale. J Am Med Dir Assoc. 2003;4(1):9–15.
20. Melzack R. The short-form McGill pain questionnaire. Pain. 1987;30(2):191–7.
21. Bouhassira D, Attal N, Alchaar H, Boureau F, Brochet B, Bruxelle J, et al. Comparison of pain syndromes associated with nervous or somatic lesions and development of a new neuropathic pain diagnostic questionnaire (DN4). Pain. 2005;114(1–2):29–36.
22. Herr K, Coyne PJ, McCaffery M, Manworren R, Merkel S. Pain assessment in the patient unable to self-report: position statement with clini-

cal practice recommendations. Pain Manag Nurs. 2011;12(4):230–50.
23. Apfelbaum J, Ashburn M, Connis R, American Society of Anesthesiologists Task Force on Acute Pain Management. Practice guidelines for acute pain management in the perioperative setting: an updated report by the American Society of Anesthesiologists Task Force on Acute Pain Management. Anesthesiology. 2012;116:248–73.
24. Lee JS, Solt K. Intravenous and inhalation anesthetics. In: Pino RM, editor. Clinical anesthesia procedures of the Masschusetts General Hospital. 9th ed. Philadelphia: Lippincott Williams & Wilkins; 2016. p. 162–76.
25. Fukuda K. Opioids. In: Gropper MA, editor. Miller's anesthesia, vol. 1. 9th ed. Philadelphia: Elsevier; 2020. p. 680–741.
26. Warltier DC, Marret E, Flahault A, Samama C-M, Bonnet F. Effects of postoperative, nonsteroidal, antiinflammatory drugs on bleeding risk after tonsillectomy meta-analysis of randomized, controlled trials. Anesthesiology. 2003;98(6):1497–502.
27. Cavalcante AN, Sprung J, Schroeder DR, Weingarten TN. Multimodal analgesic therapy with gabapentin and its association with postoperative respiratory depression. Anesth Analg. 2017;125(1):141–6.
28. Odom-Forren J, Hooper V, Moser DK, Hall LA, Lennie TA, Holtman J, et al. Postdischarge nausea and vomiting: management strategies and outcomes over 7 days. J Perianesth Nurs. 2014;29(4):275–84.
29. Hooper VD. SAMBA consensus guidelines for the management of postoperative nausea and vomiting: an executive summary for perianesthesia nurses. J Perianesth Nurs. 2015;30(5):377–82.
30. Odom-Forren J, Jalota L, Moser DK, Lennie TA, Hall LA, Holtman J, et al. Incidence and predictors of postdischarge nausea and vomiting in a 7-day population. J Clin Anesth. 2013;25(7):551–9.
31. Gan TJ, Diemunsch P, Habib AS, Kovac A, Kranke P, Meyer TA, et al. Consensus guidelines for the management of postoperative nausea and vomiting. Anesth Analg. 2014;118(1):85–113.
32. Early A. Clinical guideline for the prevention of unplanned perioperative hypothermia. J Perianesth Nurs. 2001;16(5):305–14.
33. Brown C. Maintaining intraoperative normothermia: a meta-analysis of outcomes with costs. AANA J. 1999;67(2):155.
34. Sessler DI. Complications and treatment of mild hypothermia. Anesthesiology. 2001;95(2):531–43.
35. Frank SM, Fleisher LA, Breslow MJ, Higgins MS, Olson KF, Kelly S, et al. Perioperative maintenance of normothermia reduces the incidence of morbid cardiac events: a randomized clinical trial. JAMA. 1997;277(14):1127–34.
36. Beilin B, Shavit Y, Razumovsky J, Wolloch Y, Zeidel A, Bessler H. Effects of mild perioperative hypothermia on cellular immune responses. Anesthesiology. 1998;89(5):1133–40.
37. Flores-Maldonado A, Medina-Escobedo CE, Ríos-Rodríguez HM, Fernández-Domínguez R. Mild perioperative hypothermia and the risk of wound infection. Arch Med Res. 2001;32(3):227–31.
38. Rohrer MJ, Natale AM. Effect of hypothermia on the coagulation cascade. Crit Care Med. 1992;20(10):1402–5.
39. Schmied H, Reiter A, Kurz A, Sessler D, Kozek S. Mild hypothermia increases blood loss and transfusion requirements during total hip arthroplasty. Lancet. 1996;347(8997):289–92.
40. Rajagopalan S, Mascha E, Na J, Sessler DI. The effects of mild perioperative hypothermia on blood loss and transfusion requirement. Anesthesiology. 2008;108(1):71–7.
41. Gustafsson U, Scott M, Schwenk W, Demartines N, Roulin D, Francis N, et al. Guidelines for perioperative care in elective colonic surgery: Enhanced Recovery After Surgery (ERAS®) Society recommendations. World J Surg. 2013;37(2):259–84.
42. Cerantola Y, Valerio M, Persson B, Jichlinski P, Ljungqvist O, Hubner M, et al. Guidelines for perioperative care after radical cystectomy for bladder cancer: Enhanced Recovery After Surgery (ERAS®) society recommendations. Clin Nutr. 2013;32(6):879–87.
43. Morgan KA, Lancaster WP, Walters ML, Owczarski SM, Clark CA, McSwain JR, et al. Enhanced recovery after surgery protocols are valuable in pancreas surgery patients. J Am Coll Surg. 2016;222(4):658–64.
44. Soffin E, YaDeau J. Enhanced recovery after surgery for primary hip and knee arthroplasty: a review of the evidence. Br J Anaesth. 2016;117(suppl_3):iii62–72.
45. Bissonnette B, Sessler DI. Mild hypothermia does not impair postanesthetic recovery in infants and children. Anesth Analg. 1993;76(1):168–72.
46. Lenhardt R, Marker E, Goll V, Tschernich H, Kurz A, Sessler DI, et al. Mild intraoperative hypothermia prolongs postanesthetic recovery. Anesthesiology. 1997;87(6):1318–23.
47. Hooper VD, Chard R, Clifford T, Fetzer S, Fossum S, Godden B, et al. ASPAN's evidence-based clinical practice guideline for the promotion of perioperative normothermia. J Perianesth Nurs. 2010;25(6):346–65.
48. Kranke P, Eberhart LH, Roewer N, Tramèr MR. Pharmacological treatment of postoperative shivering: a quantitative systematic review of randomized controlled trials. Anesth Analg. 2002;94(2):453–60.
49. Williams BA, Kentor ML, Vogt MT, Vogt WB, Coley KC, Williams JP, et al. Economics of nerve block pain management after anterior cruciate ligament reconstruction: potential hospital cost savings via associated postanesthesia care unit bypass and same-day discharge. Anesthesiology. 2004;100(3):697–706.
50. Williams BA, Kentor ML. The WAKE© score: patient-centered ambulatory anesthesia and fast-tracking outcomes criteria. Int Anesthesiol Clin. 2011;49(3):33–43.

51. Gabriel RA, Ilfeld BM. Use of regional anesthesia for outpatient surgery within the United States: a prevalence study using a nationwide database. Anesth Analg. 2018;126(6):2078–84.
52. Ilfeld BM. Continuous peripheral nerve blocks: an update of the published evidence and comparison with novel, alternative analgesic modalities. Anesth Analg. 2017;124(1):308–35.
53. Hadzic A, Arliss J, Kerimoglu B, Karaca PE, Yufa M, Claudio RE, et al. A comparison of infraclavicular nerve block versus general anesthesia for hand and wrist day-case surgeries. Anesthesiology. 2004;101(1):127–32.
54. Hadzic A, Karaca PE, Hobeika P, Unis G, Dermksian J, Yufa M, et al. Peripheral nerve blocks result in superior recovery profile compared with general anesthesia in outpatient knee arthroscopy. Anesth Analg. 2005;100(4):976–81.
55. Williams BA. For outpatients, does regional anesthesia truly shorten the hospital stay, and how should we define postanesthesia care unit bypass eligibility? Anesthesiology. 2004;101(1):3–6.
56. Moore JG, Ross SM, Williams BA. Regional anesthesia and ambulatory surgery. Curr Opin Anesthesiol. 2013;26(6):652–60.

28 Weaning Protocols After Ambulatory Surgery

Nitish Aggarwal, Jill Zafar, Gopal Kodumudi, Nalini Vadivelu, Maxwell Laurans, and Kanishka Rajput

Abstract

Nearly 60% of all surgeries are performed in an outpatient setting with 24 hours or less of hospital care (Latifi, The modern hospital: patients centered, disease based, research oriented, technology driven. Springer, Cham, 2019; Russo et al., Hospital-based ambulatory surgery. HCUP statistical brief #86, February 2010). These surgeries are performed in both hospital-based outpatient departments (HOPDs) and ambulatory surgery centers (ASCs). There has been a marked increase in the number of surgeries being performed in ASCs in recent years, with cost and convenience being cited as contributing factors (Goldfarb et al., J Am Acad Orthop Surg 25:12–22, 2017). The report by US Government Accountability Office demonstrated that it costs 84% less to perform surgeries in ASCs than in HOPDs (United States Government Accountability Office. Medicare: payment for ambulatory surgical centers should be based on the hospital outpatient payment system, 2006). However, there are some long-term costs that are not necessarily quantifiable. More than 80% of patients undergoing surgery complain of postoperative pain, with pain, intractable nausea, and vomiting cited as major causes of unplanned admissions (Gan, Curr Med Res Opin 30:149–160, 2014). The rate of unplanned admissions after ambulatory procedures is 2.2% in orthopedic procedures and 1.42% in all surgeries (Fortier et al., Can J Anaesth 45:612–619, 1998). Optimum control of postoperative pain can lead to a decrease in unanticipated admissions. A majority of these patients are discharged with an opioid prescription, and nearly half of them are at an increased risk of becoming long-term opioid users (Alam et al., Arch Intern Med 172:425–430, 2012). The primary reason for this inadvertent adverse effect is due to not only lack of immediate postoperative follow-up for patients but also lack of effective guidelines to wean off pain medications postoperatively. In this chap-

N. Aggarwal · J. Zafar · N. Vadivelu (✉)
Department of Anesthesiology, Yale University School of Medicine, New Haven, CT, USA
e-mail: Nitish.aggarwal@yale.edu; Jill.Zafar@yale.edu; nalini.vadivelu@yale.edu

G. Kodumudi
Department of Anesthesiology, Louisiana State University Health Shreveport, Shreveport, LA, USA
e-mail: gkodumud@tulane.edu

M. Laurans
Department of Neurosurgery, Yale University School of Medicine, New Haven, CT, USA
e-mail: maxwell.laurans@yale.edu

K. Rajput
Department of Anesthesiology and Pain Medicine, Yale University School of Medicine, New Haven, CT, USA
e-mail: kanishka.rajput@yale.edu

K. Rajput et al. (eds.), *Pain Control in Ambulatory Surgery Centers*,
https://doi.org/10.1007/978-3-030-55262-6_28

ter, we touch upon optimizing perioperative analgesia and discuss protocols for weaning off opioids after ambulatory surgery. Use of multimodal analgesia is covered in-depth elsewhere in this book.

Introduction

Postoperative pain can be classified into acute and chronic pain. Acute pain refers to pain experienced for up to 7 days after surgery, while chronic pain refers to pain lasting for more than 3 months after surgery [8]. In terms of acute pain, most of the severe pain encountered in postoperative period is in the first 24 hours [9]. A third of the patients discharged from ambulatory surgery centers encounters moderate to severe pain in the first 48 hours [10]. The most commonly prescribed analgesics in the postoperative period are opioids (oxycodone, hydrocodone, and hydromorphone) and Nonsteroidal anti-inflammatory drugs (NSAIDs) such as ibuprofen, acetaminophen, and gabapentinoids. Hydrocodone, in combination with NSAIDs or acetaminophen, may not be prescribed as much due to possible concerns of toxicity; furthermore, patients may not disclose taking NSAIDs or acetaminophen concomitantly as well [11]. Furthermore, both oxycodone and hydrocodone in combination with acetaminophen or ibuprofen are equally efficacious and equally abusable [12]. The abuse potential can be extrapolated to ambulatory surgeries where more than 1.5 million patients are at risk of becoming opioid users yearly after surgery and where around 150,000 patients may develop opioid use disorder [13]. In light of the opioid epidemic, it is imperative to decrease opioid use after surgery as much as possible, given an increased risk of chronic use in postsurgical patients [14].

It is of grave importance to prevent such drug misuse and addiction by instituting appropriate weaning protocols and follow-up. In order to minimize the risk of chronic opioid use after surgery and provide optimal pain relief, opioid sparing interventions such as nerve blocks should be used. Furthermore, by employing a multimodal analgesic approach, teams such as Perioperative Surgical Home or Transitional Pain Service may be able to assist in weaning off of opioids and other pain medications in ambulatory setting [15].

Postoperative Pain Prescriptions as a First Exposure

The United States has seen an unprecedented increase in drug-related and opioid overdose deaths in recent times, with most deaths attributable to two commonly prescribed opioids: hydrocodone and oxycodone [16]. The economic costs of prescription opioid-related abuse, dependence, and overdose are staggering, exceeding $78.5 billion annually [17]. Moderate to severe pain occurs in about 30–40% of patients after outpatient surgery in the first 24–48 hours [18]. Postoperative pain after ambulatory surgery is most commonly treated with opioids or nonopioids such as nonsteroidal anti-inflammatory drugs and paracetamol [19]. Opioids continue to be routinely administered in the perioperative period, even with a history of prior opioid-related adverse events. Eighty percent of patients receive prescription opioids after low-risk surgery, and 80% of these opioids are hydrocodone and oxycodone [20]. Postoperative opioid prescriptions are not always necessary and pose the risk of opioid diversion due to overprescribing [21]. In a study on consumption of prescribed opioids after urological surgery, about two thirds of patients had surplus medication from the initial prescription with no instructions for disposal of surplus narcotics. Surplus prescribing of opioids in the perioperative period creates the potential for diversion to unintended users for nonmedical abuse, and nearly 75% of recent heroin users report being introduced to opioids through prescription medications [22]. The risks of misuse, addiction, persistent or chronic opioid use, and overdose with opioids exist in *both opioid-naïve and opioid-tolerant patients* [14, 23].

There is a paucity of literature on outpatient weaning from prescribed opioids after surgery. Hence, appropriate preoperative patient selection and surgeon competency, followed by immediate and adequate perioperative pain control, are the critical steps toward minimizing postoperative reliance on opiates. The routine use of multimodal analgesics and regional/neuraxial anesthesia is recommended, whenever possible. In addition, the widespread practices of opioid overprescribing and resultant leftover pills have led to the adoption of several mitigation strategies. These have been proposed by not only medical but also regulatory bodies to govern the total amount of opioids prescribed on discharge.

Multimodal Analgesics

The concept of multimodal analgesia to provide opioid sparing has been emphasized in an ambulatory setting [24]. The use of several classes of nonopioid medications and regional anesthetic techniques can be employed to provide opioid sparing analgesia. These include nonsteroidal anti-inflammatory drugs (NSAIDs), gabapentinoids, acetaminophen, ketamine, and glucocorticoids. Regional anesthetic techniques for outpatient surgery include peripheral nerve blocks such as sciatic and femoral nerve blocks, transversus abdominal plane [TAP] blocks, paravertebral blocks, and brachial plexus blocks and neuraxial techniques such as spinal and epidural anesthesia. Advances and increased adoption of ultrasound have led to a revolution in new nerve block techniques that have the potential to further enhance multimodal pain control.

In the ambulatory setting, round the clock, NSAIDs and acetaminophen in conjunction with opioids may be shifted to these nonopioid analgesics within a short time frame. Since NSAIDs and acetaminophen have a different mechanism of action from opioids, the total amount of opioids needed for pain control can be decreased due to synergistic analgesia. A systematic review demonstrated the benefit of adding oral NSAIDS, acetaminophen, or COX-2 inhibitors to morphine intravenous patient-controlled analgesia (PCA) in patients recovering from major surgery. These patients receiving the former medications significantly reduced their postoperative 24 hour morphine consumption [25]. There was no clear benefit of COX-2inhibitors, NSAIDS, and acetaminophen, over one another. A meta-analysis on 52 randomized placebo controlled trials covering nearly 5000 adults similarly confirmed a decrease in 24 hour morphine consumption postsurgery after supplementation with multimodal therapy [26].

COX-2 inhibitors, such as Celecoxib, in combination with opioids may similarly help reduce opioid requirements. Celecoxib, being a selective COX 2 inhibitor, has a decreased risk of gastrointestinal bleeding when compared to NSAIDs. Freedman and colleagues investigated the use of celecoxib with hydrocodone versus hydrocodone alone in the management of postoperative pain following augmentation mammoplasty [27]. The combination administration resulted in a statistically significant decrease in pain scores and postoperative opioid use. Overall, NSAIDs, acetaminophen, and celecoxib can be added to postoperative ambulatory surgery pain management in order to reduce the opioid requirement and therefore ease the opioid weaning process. Given the controversy around NSAIDs with respect to bone and wound healing, a discussion with the surgeon may be warranted.

Gabapentinoids have been recommended by several expert groups as part of multimodal analgesic regimens due to their opioid sparing effect. However, the associated respiratory depression especially with high doses may preclude their use in ambulatory surgeries. This issue was highlighted by a 16-year population-based nested case–control study performed on the safety of taking gabapentin in conjunction with opioids [28]. A coprescription of opioids and gabapentin (900 mg or higher daily dose) was associated with increased odds of opioid-related death. Furthermore, in 2019, FDA updated gabapentinoids' drug label to include respiratory depression effects. By itself or in combination with opioids, it is associated with respiratory depression and opioid overdose death [29]. In addition, drug manufacturers were required to conduct clinical trials on the abuse potential of gabapentinoids when used in combination with opioids. If a patient is discharged with a gabapentinoid prescription, then guidance on weaning will be necessary.

The Issue of Leftover Pills

"One size fits all" or a standard prescription analgesic regimen for discharge, often seen after surgery, although convenient to the surgeon, is one of the many factors responsible for overprescribing. *Postoperative pain management needs to be tailored individually, based on the expected severity of pain after surgery and patient characteristics.* In this capacity, anesthesiologists and pain specialists play critical roles. A surgeon may be busy and opt to have their mid-level or nurse write the prescription. In this situation, the anesthesiologist can provide valuable, yet patient-sensitive input. Several studies have highlighted the issue of leftover pills following surgery. One study found that patients who underwent outpatient minimally invasive abdominal surgeries were prescribed a median of 20 oxycodone 5 mg pills, while the reported use was only 4 pills by the first postoperative visit [30]. Another retrospective study showed the median number of prescribed pills postoperatively were 30 tablets, while the median consumption was only 9 tablets [31]. In another study on patients undergoing upper extremity surgery, nearly 75% of patients took less than 15 tablets, while 45% took less than 5 tablets. Ultimately, the higher the total opioid dose and the longer the opioid prescription duration, the greater the risk of misuse and overdose [32, 33]. Furthermore, each prescription refill is associated with nearly 40% increased risk of misuse and 20% risk with each additional week of opioid use. Recently, with the rise in automated solicitation of refills by pharmacies, patients are at risk for receiving more pills [34]. This underscores the importance of the perioperative/anesthesiology consultant in modulating consumption or access to opioids in the postoperative period.

Discharge planning therefore requires careful consideration of risk factors for extreme postoperative pain, type of surgery being performed, prior analgesic use, and risk factors for drug abuse, in addition to comorbidities including age, hepatic or renal impairment, and cardiorespiratory status.

Planning for Discharge

Since pain is a subjective experience, in order to reduce the likelihood of opioid overuse and addiction, it is imperative that patients are taught how to correctly perform self-assessments with a pain scale [35]. It is important to obtain a baseline pain rating and understand what an individual pain rating means to each patient as far as severity is concerned, since one patient's definition of a certain pain rating is likely different from that of another. Furthermore, predicting pain based on the type of procedure can help standardize the amount of pain medication prescribed and, as such, lead to an easier weaning process. For example, McGrath and colleagues conducted a survey on pain severity, 24 hours after ambulatory surgery on 5703 patients. Their study found that the most painful ambulatory procedures, based on the pain scores were: (1) lumbar microdiscectomy, (2) laparoscopic cholecystectomy, (3) shoulder surgery, (4) elbow and hand surgery, (5) knee, (6) ankle surgery, and (7) inguinal hernia surgery [9]. The quantity of opioid analgesics prescribed can be based on type of ambulatory surgical procedure, preexisting comorbidities, and prior history of opioid use/misuse. This strategy may be helpful to guide physicians and prevent overprescribing, possibly resulting in a shorter weaning period with a lower chance of misuse. Most of the moderate to severe pain lasts 48–72 hours after surgery with the worst pain within the first 24 hours. Theoretically, opioids should be employed to mitigate pain from moderate/severe level to mild level, which, in opioid-naïve patients, tends to occur by postoperative day 3 [36]. One strategy may be to aggressively treat pain with opioids in the first 24 hours and then to space out the opioids for the next 24–48 hours. From this point on (72 hours postsurgery), opioids should be discontinued.

Short-Acting Opioids

To address the severe pain in the first 24 hours, short-acting opioids can be prescribed every 4–6 hours, but not less than every 4 hours [13]. Among the short-acting opioids, oxycodone, hydromorphone, or hydrocodone, are preferred. Vicodin™, Vicoprofen™, and similar opioid/ibuprofen or opioid/acetaminophen combinations are prescribed less frequently due to potential toxicity with concomitant ibuprofen or acetaminophen use. Tramadol is another short-acting opioid but has fallen out of favor due to association with higher risk of prolonged opioid use according to an insurance database study [37]. In the United States, tramadol is classified as a controlled substance. Similarly, codeine, a prodrug that converts to morphine, is not prescribed often, due to significant interindividual variability in its pharmacokinetics. In fact, due to this variability and risk of opioid overdose, *codeine has a black box warning in pediatric population from the Food and Drug Administration.*

Based on the severity of pain expected after common outpatient procedures, weaning protocols can be suggested for less painful versus more painful surgeries. The following section gives broad examples of two such protocols. These protocols are based on expert recommendations and should only be used as a starting guide. Treatment may need to be individualized on a case by case basis guided by underlying comorbidities and extent of preoperative opiate tolerance.

Example of low opioid requirement based on surgery:

- *Weaning Protocol#1*
  - Postoperative Day 1: Oxycodone 5 mg q4–6 hours PRN, Ibuprofen 600 mg q6 hours scheduled, AND Acetaminophen 1000 mg q8 hours scheduled.
  - Day 2–3: Oxycodone 5 mg q8 hours PRN, Ibuprofen 600 mg q6 hours scheduled, AND Acetaminophen 1000 mg q8 hours scheduled.
  - Day 4–7: Ibuprofen 600 mg q6 hours PRN AND Acetaminophen 1000 mg q8 hours PRN.
  - Day 8–14: Ibuprofen 200 mg q6–8 hours PRN AND Acetaminophen 500 mg q8 hours PRN.
  - Continue tapering and eventually discontinue all medications.

Example of high opioid requirement based on surgery, with or without opioid tolerance: Patients with preexisting opioid tolerance present a unique challenge, especially following surgeries expected to cause moderate to severe postoperative pain. These patients often require two to three times their home dose of opioid to treat acute pain and may need a longer weaning period than their opioid-naïve counterparts. One caveat about opioid tolerant patients is that they may have an opioid agreement with their outpatient prescribing doctor or pain specialist. In this scenario, the perioperative team should communicate their recommended weaning protocols to the pain physician and to the pharmacist. The perioperative team may have to indicate acute pain/breakthrough pain on the prescription. Given the regulatory surveillance from state governments with monitoring databases and pharmacy benefit managers, the patient's weaning opioid prescription may be denied. A dedicated staff member at the surgicenter and hospital may have to obtain prior authorization for this weaning protocol.

The patient's existing daily opioid consumption should be converted into morphine equivalents. Then, one can multiply this number by two- to threefold to calculate the starting opioid dose postoperatively. Another simpler approach is to simply take the existing chronic pain opioid and use this for postoperative care, as described in the following example. For instance, here is the weaning protocol for a patient who takes moderate doses of opioids at home, e.g., 5 mg oxycodone Q4–6 hours, and undergoes a high-opioid requiring surgery.

- *Weaning Protocol#2*
  - Postoperative Day 1: Oxycodone 10–15 mg q4–6 hours PRN, Ibuprofen 600 mg q6 hours scheduled, and Acetaminophen 1000 mg q8 hours scheduled.
  - Day 2–4: Oxycodone 10 mg q4–6 hours PRN, Ibuprofen 600 mg q6 hours sched-

uled, and Acetaminophen 1000 mg q8 hours scheduled.

- Day 5–7: Oxycodone 7.5 mg q4–6 hours PRN, Ibuprofen 600 mg q6 hours scheduled, and Acetaminophen 1000 mg q8 hours scheduled.
- Continue gradual tapering to home dose opioid, while ensuring an early follow-up with the outpatient pain provider.

Once the period for acute surgical pain has subsided, the goal in a chronic opioid user should be to taper the opioids back to baseline opioid dose within 1–2 weeks. There is paucity of literature regarding acute opioid weaning regimens in postsurgical patients. In nonsurgical chronic pain patients being weaned down on opiates, literature varies and recommends dose reduction of 10–50% every week to every month, as tolerated [38]. In one study, the mean maximum dose reduction in daily opioid dose was 27% per month with a standard deviation of 17% [39]. CDC guidelines advise 10% per week reduction in dose as a reasonable starting point [40]. Overall, according to Dowell et al., "monthly dose reductions of 10% to 40% may be clinically reasonable" [41]. Regarding tapering in a patient who has been on long-term (more than 6 months) opioids, one has a choice between slow and fast tapering. Physicians only recommend fast tapering (25–50% dose reduction every few days) if there is availability of supervised center and closer monitoring for severe withdrawal symptoms [42]. For tapering in patients taking short-term opioids (Between 2 weeks and 6 months), it is imperative to maintain the same interval between the doses and instead decreasing the quantity by 10–20% every 3–4 days [42]. This is because a more significant drop in serum medication level would occur if patient is switched from high-frequency dosing (q4–6h) to low-frequency dosing (TID or BID). As mentioned earlier, chronic opioid users are prone to withdrawal symptoms if weaned off too rapidly. There are several medications used to mitigate withdrawal symptoms such as ondansetron for nausea, loperamide for diarrhea, and an alpha-2 agonist, such as dexmedetomidine or clonidine for autonomic hyperactivity [43].

Extrapolating some of the above recommendations to postsurgical population, patients who have been taking opioids for less than 2 weeks may be able to stop opioids without the effects of withdrawal [42]. For opioid-tolerant patients, assuming the surgery addressed the reason for opioids, one can start tapering the opioids to the patient's presurgery opioid requirements after 24–72 hours with the goal to be back to baseline by 5–10 days postoperatively. Again, to prevent troughs in serum drug levels, which would make weaning harder, dosing should be maintained at the same frequency while decreasing the actual amount. Even other opioids such as fentanyl patches (duration of 72 hours) can be tapered rapidly by either 50% every 6 days or more slowly by 25% every 15 days [44]. However, fentanyl patches are contraindicated in the United States for use in acute or postoperative pain. If further opioid weaning is warranted from baseline, an emphatic discussion should be initiated with the patient stressing that this implies patient is not a suitable candidate to continue opioids, not that pain care would be abandoned [45]. It is imperative that these discussions, if held in a perioperative realm be documented in the patient's chart, effectively communicated with the outpatient team and patient encouraged to schedule a follow-up as soon as feasible after surgery to continue the weaning process.

A graphical representation of an opioid weaning protocol with the use of supplemental analgesics is depicted below.

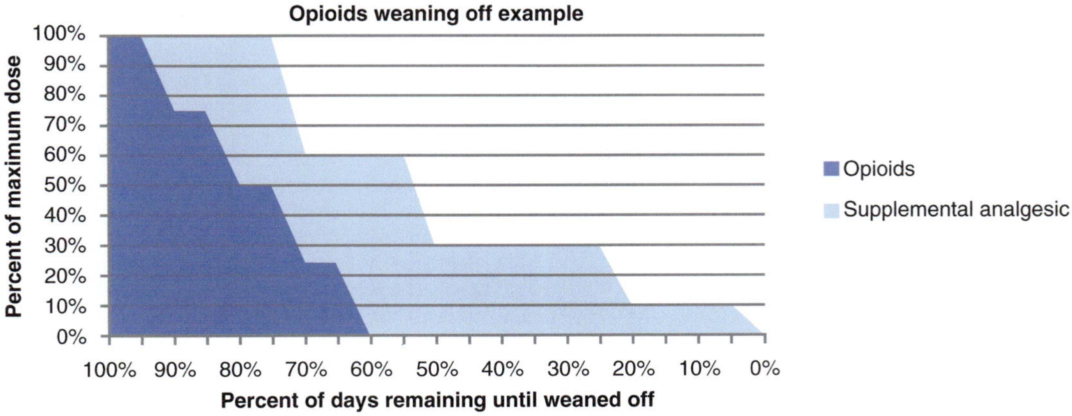

Postoperative Pain Management Service

In the current system, there is no consistent provider managing pain postoperatively. After the first few weeks, pain management falls into the hands of the primary care physician or surgeon, neither of whom is adept at managing postoperative pain. A couple of solutions to this dilemma include establishment of perioperative surgical home (PSH), transitional pain service or telehealth service. Literature suggests improved satisfaction scores and improved clinical outcomes with a PSH [46]. An anesthesiologist managing the PSH can aggressively manage severe acute pain with opioids with full oversight, thereby improving patient outcomes and reducing the risk of opioid misuse. Furthermore, they would be able to educate and empower patients about effective nonopiate analgesia, at the same time avoiding the development of chronic pain. This service is likely better suited for chronic opioid users undergoing ambulatory surgery with the aim of tapering opioids even lower from baseline. The PSH model also allows for faster tapering due to close monitoring by physicians and healthcare providers. A similar but more dedicated service, called the Transitional Pain Service, was started at Toronto General Hospital and has been found to alter patients' pain trajectories by "preventing the transition from acute to chronic pain and reducing suffering, disability, and healthcare costs" [15]. In the latter system, high-risk patients are identified before the procedure and are provided with comprehensive care for up to 6 months after surgery. This type of service would be perfect for opioid de-escalation in an acute postsurgical environment as it satisfies the three fundamental aspects of balancing adequate pain control with patient satisfaction: expectation management, clear algorithm of care, and early involvement of expert resources [47]. A lower-cost alternative to these could be telehealth services. It has been safely used as a substitute for postoperative clinic visits with great patient satisfaction [48]. A seamless coordination between the surgeon and anesthesiologist for such postoperative telehealth visit can be resource-conserving, yet satisfactory with great results, as this circumvents the issue of a lack of immediate postoperative follow-up. This in turn may lead to decreased long-term opioid use. A blueprint for this can be found in the Veterans Health Administration (VA hospitals) where a telemonitoring program successfully conducted multidisciplinary pain consultations [49]. Telehealth also allows an opportunity for education and support by multidisciplinary healthcare providers to reduce dependence on opioids [50]. All of these, if viable to the hospital, require extensive resources, but are a great asset for pain control in postsurgical patients and the community. There are caveats, however, which need to be addressed. In the postoperative setting, the surgeon may be the best judge to determine if the postoperative pain is normal or abnormal. Hence, an anesthesiologist in the postoperative setting, with limited contact with the patient prior to surgery, is posed with legal ramifications. A chain of custody, wherein the surgeon is the first point of contact, may be necessary to ensure that the postoperative pain is not indicative of a surgical complication. Furthermore, payment models in this postsurgical home model must be aligned with the high regulatory and malpractice risk faced by an anesthesiologist or pain specialist [51].

Summary

Despite the fact that over 60% of surgeries are currently performed in an ambulatory setting, there is a dearth of literature to guide optimal postoperative pain management at discharge. Overprescribing of opiates, even after low-risk surgeries, continues to contribute to the issue of leftover pills, which in turn is related to risks of long-term use and abuse. A significant proportion of surgeries performed in an outpatient setting needs intense opioid analgesia only for the first 24–72 hours, after which period most pain can be managed with nonopioid analgesics. Weaning protocols help primary teams prescribe the right amount of opioids, in order to reduce the number of unused pills, while adequately managing acute pain. Alternatively, a perioperative surgical home or transitional pain service may be an asset to provide close follow-up for weaning patients off of opiates, especially those who are opiate tolerant and need assistance to wean down to their baseline dose. However, as alluded to earlier, there are caveats to this approach given malpractice and regulatory risks faced by the prescribing or opioid managing physician in the postoperative period.

References

1. Latifi R. The modern hospital: patients centered, disease based, research oriented, technology driven. Cham: Springer; 2019.
2. Russo CA, Elixhauser A, Steiner C, Wier L. Hospital-based ambulatory surgery. HCUP statistical brief #86. February 2010. Available from: http://www.hcupus.ahrq.gov/reports/statbriefs/sb86.pdf.
3. Goldfarb CA, Bansal A, Brophy RH. Ambulatory surgical centers: a review of complications and adverse events. J Am Acad Orthop Surg. 2017;25(1):12–22.
4. United States Government Accountability Office. Medicare: payment for ambulatory surgical centers should be based on the hospital outpatient payment system. Report No.: GAO-07-86. 2006. Available from: http://www.gao.gov/products/GAO-07-86.
5. Gan TJ, et al. Incidence, patient satisfaction, and perceptions of post-surgical pain: results from a US national survey. Curr Med Res Opin. 2014;30(1):149–60.
6. Fortier J, Chung F, Su J. Unanticipated admission after ambulatory surgery – a prospective study. Can J Anaesth. 1998;45(7):612–9.
7. Alam A, et al. Long-term analgesic use after low-risk surgery: a retrospective cohort study. Arch Intern Med. 2012;172(5):425–30.
8. Gupta A, et al. Clinical aspects of acute post-operative pain management & its assessment. J Adv Pharm Technol Res. 2010;1(2):97–108.
9. McGrath B, et al. Thirty percent of patients have moderate to severe pain 24 hr after ambulatory surgery: a survey of 5,703 patients. Can J Anaesth. 2004;51(9):886–91.
10. Jafra A, Mitra S. Pain relief after ambulatory surgery: progress over the last decade. Saudi J Anaesth. 2018;12(4):618–25.
11. Kenan K, Mack K, Paulozzi L. Trends in prescriptions for oxycodone and other commonly used opioids in the United States, 2000-2010. Open Med. 2012;6(2):e41–7.
12. Marco CA, et al. Comparison of oxycodone and hydrocodone for the treatment of acute pain associated with fractures: a double-blind, randomized, controlled trial. Acad Emerg Med. 2005;12(4):282–8.
13. Pino CA, Covington M, Wakeman SE. Prescription of opioids for acute pain in opioid naïve patients. UpToDate Online. 2020.
14. Hah JM, et al. Chronic opioid use after surgery: implications for perioperative management in the face of the opioid epidemic. Anesth Analg. 2017;125(5):1733–40.
15. Katz J, et al. The Toronto General Hospital Transitional Pain Service: development and implementation of a multidisciplinary program to prevent chronic postsurgical pain. J Pain Res. 2015;8:695–702.

16. Rudd RA, et al. Increases in drug and opioid overdose deaths – United States, 2000-2014. MMWR Morb Mortal Wkly Rep. 2016;64(50–51):1378–82.
17. Florence CS, et al. The economic burden of prescription opioid overdose, abuse, and dependence in the United States, 2013. Med Care. 2016;54(10):901–6.
18. Beauregard L, Pomp A, Choiniere M. Severity and impact of pain after day-surgery. Can J Anaesth. 1998;45(4):304–11.
19. Rawal N. Postoperative pain treatment for ambulatory surgery. Best Pract Res Clin Anaesthesiol. 2007;21(1):129–48.
20. Wunsch H, et al. Opioids prescribed after low-risk surgical procedures in the United States, 2004-2012. JAMA. 2016;315(15):1654–7.
21. Bates C, et al. Overprescription of postoperative narcotics: a look at postoperative pain medication delivery, consumption and disposal in urological practice. J Urol. 2011;185(2):551–5.
22. Compton WM, Jones CM, Baldwin GT. Relationship between nonmedical prescription-opioid use and heroin use. N Engl J Med. 2016;374(2):154–63.
23. Rodgers J, et al. Opioid consumption following outpatient upper extremity surgery. J Hand Surg Am. 2012;37(4):645–50.
24. Kaye AD, et al. Multimodal analgesia as an essential part of enhanced recovery protocols in the ambulatory settings. J Anaesthesiol Clin Pharmacol. 2019;35(Suppl 1):S40–5.
25. Maund E, et al. Paracetamol and selective and non-selective non-steroidal anti-inflammatory drugs for the reduction in morphine-related side-effects after major surgery: a systematic review. Br J Anaesth. 2011;106(3):292–7.
26. Elia N, Lysakowski C, Tramer MR. Does multimodal analgesia with acetaminophen, nonsteroidal antiinflammatory drugs, or selective cyclooxygenase-2 inhibitors and patient-controlled analgesia morphine offer advantages over morphine alone? Meta-analyses of randomized trials. Anesthesiology. 2005;103(6):1296–304.
27. Freedman BM, Balakrishnan TP, O'Hara EL. Celecoxib reduces narcotic use and pain following augmentation mammaplasty. Aesthet Surg J. 2006;26(1):24–8.
28. Gomes T, et al. Gabapentin, opioids, and the risk of opioid-related death: a population-based nested case-control study. PLoS Med. 2017;14(10):e1002396.
29. FDA. 2019. Available from: https://www.fda.gov/news-events/fda-brief/fda-brief-fda-requires-new-warnings-gabapentinoids-about-risk-respiratory-depression.
30. Tan WH, et al. Opioid medication use in the surgical patient: an assessment of prescribing patterns and use. J Am Coll Surg. 2018;227(2):203–11.
31. Howard R, et al. Association of opioid prescribing with opioid consumption after surgery in Michigan. JAMA Surg. 2019;154(1):e184234.
32. Brat GA, et al. Postsurgical prescriptions for opioid naive patients and association with overdose and misuse: retrospective cohort study. BMJ. 2018;360:j5790.
33. Shah A, Hayes CJ, Martin BC. Factors influencing long-term opioid use among opioid naive patients: an examination of initial prescription characteristics and pain etiologies. J Pain. 2017;18(11):1374–83.
34. CMS. Control practices to improve medicaid program integrity and quality patient care—Booklet 4: Billing practices. 2015.
35. Kamming D, et al. Pain management in ambulatory surgery. J Perianesth Nurs. 2004;19(3):174–82.
36. Ruan X, Chiravuri S. Time to onset of sustained post-operative pain relief (SuPPR): evaluation of a new systems-level metric for acute pain management. Clin J Pain. 2016;32(7):643.
37. Thiels CA, et al. Chronic use of tramadol after acute pain episode: cohort study. BMJ. 2019;365:l1849.
38. U.S. Department of Veterans Affairs. Tapering and discontinuing opioids. 2013. Available from: http://www.healthquality.va.gov/guidelines/Pain/cot/OpioidTaperingFactSheet23May2013v1.pdf.
39. Fenton JJ, et al. Trends and rapidity of dose tapering among patients prescribed long-term opioid therapy, 2008-2017. JAMA Netw Open. 2019;2(11):e1916271.
40. Centers for Disease Control and Prevention. Pocket guide: tapering opioids for chronic pain. 2016. Available from: https://www.cdc.gov/drugoverdose/pdf/clinical_pocket_guide_tapering-a.pdf.
41. Dowell D, Haegerich TM, Chou R. CDC guideline for prescribing opioids for chronic pain – United States, 2016. JAMA. 2016;315(15):1624–45.
42. Dave VH. A patient's guide to opioid tapering. 2018. Available from: https://www.hss.edu/conditions_patient-guide-opioid-tapering.asp.
43. Mackey S, Lahidji S, Schonwald G, Newmark J. Safe opioid prescribing and risk evaluation and mitigation strategies. 2015. Available from: http://online.stanford.edu/course/opioid-prescribing-cme-sp2014.
44. Kral LA, Jackson K, Uritsky TJ. A practical guide to tapering opioids. Ment Health Clin. 2015;5(3):102–8. https://doi.org/10.9740/mhc.2015.05.102.
45. Newmark JL. Chapter 6: Tapering opioids. 2019. Available from: https://www.practicalpainmanagement.com/resource-centers/opioid-prescribing-monitoring/when-how-wean-patients-opioids.
46. Kwon MA. Perioperative surgical home: a new scope for future anesthesiology. Korean J Anesthesiol. 2018;71(3):175–81.
47. Souzdalnitski D, et al. Patient satisfaction. In: Chronic pain management for the hospitalized patient. New York: Oxford University Press; 2016.
48. Hwa K, Wren SM. Telehealth follow-up in lieu of post-operative clinic visit for ambulatory surgery: results of a pilot program. JAMA Surg. 2013;148(9):823–7.
49. Frank JW, et al. Evaluation of a telementoring intervention for pain management in the Veterans Health Administration. Pain Med. 2015;16(6):1090–100.
50. Vaughn IA, et al. Multispecialty opioid risk reduction program targeting chronic pain and addiction management in veterans. Fed Pract. 2019;36(9):406–11.
51. Warner R, Deer TR. Malpractice and the practice of pain medicine: an Attorney's perspective. Pain Med. 2008;9(suppl_1):S137–41.

Role of a Focused Ambulatory Pain Physician

29

Anand M. Prem and Suwarna Anand

Abstract

As surgeries in Ambulatory Surgery Centers continue to rise, increasingly complex procedures are performed, requiring greater expertise among anesthesiologists practicing at these centers. With uncontrolled pain and nausea being the two most important factors accounting for delayed discharge from the PostAnesthesia Care Unit, it is incumbent upon these centers to address these issues to remain viable as cost-effective providers of quality care. Untreated postoperative pain has been shown to adversely affect morbidity and mortality, delay early mobilization, and lead to chronic pain states requiring long-term opioid therapy with its attendant risks of dependence, addiction, and even death from opioid use disorder. There is ample evidence that multimodal pain treatment strategies can effectively treat pain reducing the dependence on opioids and improve patient satisfaction and outcomes while keeping cost down. An Ambulatory Pain Physician well-versed in these techniques can coordinate care throughout the perioperative phase optimizing patient care.

A. M. Prem (✉) · S. Anand
Department of Anesthesiology, University of Mississippi Medical Center, Jackson, MS, USA
e-mail: aprem@umc.edu; sanand2@umc.edu

Introduction

The vast majority of patients who have surgery report acute postoperative pain, of which 75% report moderate to severe pain [1, 2]. Studies suggest that of these patients, only half report adequate pain relief with traditional pain management strategies. While good pain relief is often the most important factor determining patient satisfaction, inadequately treated pain adversely impacts early mobilization and recovery of function, length of hospital stay, risk of postsurgical complications, prolonged postsurgical pain leading to chronic pain states, and overall quality of life [2, 6, 10].

With recognition that the treatment of acute postoperative pain is vital to the physical and emotional well-being of the patient, multiple preoperative, intraoperative, and postoperative strategies are now available to manage pain in the perioperative period. In 2016, the American Pain Society (APS) with input from the American Society of Anesthesiologists (ASA) released clinical guidelines for the Management of Postoperative Pain based on the recommendations of an interdisciplinary expert panel, taking into account available evidence and best clinical practices in the absence of such evidence [2]. These guidelines support the need for safe and effective pain management that begins in the preoperative period by assessment of individual needs based on prior pain experience and planned

K. Rajput et al. (eds.), *Pain Control in Ambulatory Surgery Centers*,
https://doi.org/10.1007/978-3-030-55262-6_29

surgery, continues with the use of multimodal analgesic regimens and techniques in all phases of the perioperative period, and concludes with a patient-centered postoperative plan to ensure optimal recovery. The role of formulating and coordinating all these strategies to optimize patient throughput in an Ambulatory Surgery Center could easily be assumed by an Anesthesiologist with additional expertise in Pain Management. This leads to the evolving concept of an Ambulatory Pain Physician, elevating the traditional role of the Anesthesiologist to that of a Perioperative physician with the ability to impact patient outcome well beyond the immediate postoperative period.

Rise of the ASCs

When the first Ambulatory Surgery Center was established in 1970, few could have predicted the significant impact they would have on the Healthcare landscape in the United States. Over the past five decades, there has been an exponential increase in the number of Ambulatory Surgical Centers (ASCs) throughout the country, both freestanding and those that are part of a larger hospital system but geared toward outpatient surgery [3–5]. These centers are typically able to offer the same surgical procedure at 35–50% savings compared to hospital systems. A lower co-pay and the convenience of easy access in a patient-friendly environment make them preferable for patients as well. As healthcare costs continue to rise, there is significant pressure on the industry to move toward more outpatient care, saving an estimated 40 billion a year [3]. In 2018, 5700 ASCs were operational in the United States accounting for 23 million procedures and 35 billion in revenue. This accounted for 50% of all outpatient surgeries in 2017, up from only 32% in 2005. Research by Bain and Company predicts a continued growth of 6–7% annually over the next 2 years.

When ASCs were initially conceptualized, the typical patient catered to was an American Society of Anesthesiologists (ASA) Class 1 or 2 patient undergoing a relatively minor surgical procedure. Over the past few decades, as anesthesia has become safer with improved monitoring capabilities, the advent of newer and better anesthetic drugs, less invasive surgical techniques, and the emphasis on cost containment, ASA Class 3 and 4 patients with multiple comorbidities are having their surgeries performed in outpatient surgical centers. As the number of surgeries in ASCs increases, the pressure to optimize the "patient experience" in the perioperative period has become paramount. As reimbursement is increasingly being linked to quality and cost of care, "patient experience" is a valued and frequently reported index in hospital surveys. A key determinant of this patient satisfaction in the perioperative period is effective pain management. With 50–70% patients reporting moderate to severe pain following surgery, ASCs must devote adequate resources and personnel to combating postoperative pain to remain competitive and viable [7].

Management of Acute Postoperative Pain

Untreated pain has been shown to adversely affect patient morbidity and mortality after surgery through cardiac and respiratory complications (Table 29.1). Ineffective pain control and nausea/vomiting related to commonly used analgesics are the commonest reasons for patient dissatisfaction after surgery [8, 9, 12].

The primary objective of perioperative pain management is to minimize patient suffering, allay anxiety, facilitate early postoperative mobilization, reduce hospital length of stay, optimize patient satisfaction, and prevent the transition of acute postoperative pain to a chronic pain state [6, 10]. While medical care is increasingly moving toward the establishment of "standardized protocols" to deal with disease states, nowhere is the need to individualize care more apparent than in Pain Management. Every pain management strategy to be effective has to take into account patients' prior experience with pain, current comorbidities, psychological condition, level of anxiety, nature of surgical procedure, severity of

Table 29.1 Consequence of ineffective management of acute postoperative pain in the ambulatory setting

1. Increased postoperative morbidity and mortality from pulmonary and cardiovascular complications: hypoventilation, atelectasis, pneumonia, and myocardial infarction.
2. Increased opioid use in PACU leading to undesirable side effects of nausea, vomiting, respiratory depression, itching, urinary retention, constipation, delirium, and sedation, all of which can negatively impact patient experience [2, 27].
3. Poor patient satisfaction.
4. Delayed mobilization and inability to participate in rehabilitation.
5. Delayed discharge from PACU and unplanned hospital admission.
6. Increase in Emergency Room visits and calls to surgeon for pain control issues.
7. Increased opioid prescriptions in the postoperative period increasing community supply, chronic opioid use, and potential for diversion [13].
8. Transition from acute to chronic pain states, especially after thoracotomy, mastectomy, and inguinal herniorrhaphy.
9. Increased healthcare costs from all the reasons listed above.

postoperative pain anticipated, and response to treatment modalities in addition to patient preference [2].

While traditionally postoperative pain management was primarily opioid dependent, the past decade has seen a significant shift toward a "multimodal strategy" incorporating nonnarcotic analgesics, local anesthetic infiltration, regional anesthetic techniques, and even complementary modalities such as TENS and acupuncture to reduce the dependence on opioids [6, 7]. The recognition that the United States is in the midst of an "opioid crisis" has accelerated the adoption of these alternative modalities and development of multiple Enhanced Recovery After Anesthesia (ERAS) protocols. As the Opioid crisis unfolded, mass media attention over the past 4 years has often highlighted the plight of hundreds of patients who succumbed to opioid abuse after their initial exposure to opioids followed an otherwise routine surgery [6].

While there are several stakeholders who can impact the patient's course during the crucial perioperative period such as primary care physicians, anesthesiologists, surgeons, perioperative nurses, and pain physicians, there has to be a "captain" to harness all these resources and deliver the most effective care. The best person to take on this challenge in an ASC would be an "Ambulatory Pain Physician" who is an anesthesiologist who besides taking care of the patient in the intraoperative phase is able to assess the pain control needs of the patient preoperatively and devise an efficient, coordinated plan to manage pain in the postoperative period as well [8, 9].

Against this background, this chapter will highlight the need for a focused Ambulatory Pain Specialist who can take charge and execute an aggressive pain management strategy throughout the perioperative period to optimize patient outcome, utilizing a multimodal approach.

Challenges of Managing Pain in the Ambulatory Setting

Multiple factors are responsible for increasingly complex surgeries moving out of the Inpatient surgical centers to ASCs.

1. Traditionally, ASCs have been able to reduce cost of surgical care by being lean, well-managed facilities that are able to offer patients the same surgery at 35% cost savings compared to hospital systems, saving the US healthcare system about 40 billion dollars annually [3].
2. Insurance companies and payors have increased reimbursement to ASCs and decreased patient co-pays further encouraging the shift of highly profitable surgical procedures to lower cost healthcare settings. This has prompted many Hospital systems to acquire ASCs to recapture lost business [3, 5].
3. ASC-based physicians and administrators are more price conscious than their hospital-based peers.
4. Patients find these smaller centers to be more accessible and user friendly with often decreased co-pay costs compared to traditional hospitals.

5. As anesthetic care has become increasingly safer with newer drugs and advanced monitoring capabilities and surgical techniques have become less invasive, the emphasis has shifted away from prolonged postoperative stays to returning the patient home as early as possible, significantly impacting cost of care [7, 22].
6. Surgeons prefer ASCs due to the potential to own equity, have control of their own schedules, and having to deal with significantly lesser bureaucracy than in traditional hospitals [3].

Caring for sicker patients undergoing more complex surgeries in ASCs has placed the onus on these centers to offer more specialized care than in the past. With effective perioperative pain management being a key driver of patient satisfaction, more emphasis is being placed on offering the most advanced pain treatment strategies in the outpatient setting as well.

The Ambulatory Surgery Center setting presents several unique challenges to the management of pain in the perioperative period [8–10].

1. As the emphasis is to move patients quickly through the postoperative recovery phase, anesthesiologists have a limited amount of time to optimize pain management for patients.
2. Early mobilization and rehabilitation requirements render traditional neuraxial techniques of pain management such as Epidural and intrathecal anesthesia impractical, as return of motor function and bladder control are key factors determining patient discharge from the hospital.
3. As more complex surgeries are being performed, the likelihood of more severe postoperative pain increases as well, requiring more advanced pain treatment modalities and greater physician expertise.
4. Patients with significant comorbidities may not be good candidates for both opioid and nonopioid analgesics as well as some regional techniques, all of which are effective pain control modalities in healthier patients. For example, Opioids may need to be used more sparingly in patients with Obstructive sleep apnea and Chronic Obstructive Pulmonary Disease (COPD), while Renal disease and gastrointestinal and bleeding issues may obviate the use of Nonsteroidal anti-inflammatory drugs (NSAIDS). Interscalene blocks for postoperative analgesia are not a good option in patients with compromised preoperative respiratory function due to the potential for temporary hemidiaphragmatic paresis leading to further loss of pulmonary reserve.
5. Patients with preexisting chronic pain on long-term opioid therapy, Opioid Use Disorder (OUD), and medication-assisted treatment (MAT) for substance abuse may also present to ASCs [8, 9, 14, 17–19]. These patients typically have higher levels of pain in the postoperative period, making it more difficult to control and greater level of dissatisfaction with their care. This requires physicians to have more expertise in the field of Pain management to device an effective and comprehensive treatment plan.

While the onus for a smooth perioperative course largely depends on the Anesthesiology care team, the move away from a primarily opioid-dependent strategy toward a more multimodal one requires greater knowledge of Regional anesthesia, pain pharmacology, and acute and chronic pain concepts than in the past. This clearly emphasizes the need for an Ambulatory Pain Physician to be involved in the care of surgical patients in an ASC, now more than ever [8, 9].

Role of the Ambulatory Pain Specialist

Beyond the traditional role of providing anesthesia for the scheduled surgery, the Ambulatory Pain specialist by virtue of their training and expertise can impact every aspect of the treatment of perioperative pain by their critical role in each of the different phases of the anesthetic management of the patient.

Preoperative Phase

1. Preoperative assessment of patients to determine patient's prior pain experience, exposure to opioids, allergies, and contraindications to regional techniques.
2. Allay patient anxiety/fear through education regarding anticipated pain level based on surgical procedure and available pain treatment strategies with the use of patient education materials, videos [2].
3. Set appropriate patient expectations regarding postoperative pain, outlining the potential complications of overzealous treatment of pain.
4. Device a cost-effective multimodal strategy for perioperative pain management – set up clearly defined protocols with leeway to individualize therapy based on specific patient needs.
5. Train nursing staff and other physicians on appropriate pain assessment, protocol adherence, potential benefits, and pitfalls and periodically update them on changes
6. Oversee administration of appropriate preoperative medications at the right time in the Preoperative holding area to ensure optimum analgesia.
7. Consult with patient's Chronic Pain Physicians on the perioperative management of patients with Spinal cord stimulators or Intrathecal pumps.

Intraoperative Phase

8. Implement intraoperative elements of planned multimodal strategy: intraoperative regional blocks, planned local anesthetic infiltration by surgeons, and Lidocaine and Ketamine infusions.
9. Judicious use of opioid and nonopioid analgesics.
10. Appropriate antiemetic prophylaxis.

Postoperative Phase

11. Rescue strategies if initial analgesic plan fails – supplement failed regional blocks with "rescue blocks", alternative medications, and complementary pain treatment modalities.
12. Rescue antiemetic use in patients with PONV.
13. Advise surgeon on discharge medications for pain: choice of appropriate medication at the lowest effective dose and an appropriate number of pills for the expected duration of pain. Overprescription of narcotics following surgery beyond what is required is often cited as a reason for the higher opioid supply in the community, leading to diversion, experimental use in children, dependence, and addiction.
14. Discharge teaching should include plans for safe use and discontinuation of narcotics as pain and function improve, as long-term opioid use often begins with opioids initiated for treating acute pain.
15. Advise patient on safe disposal of residual narcotics.
16. Follow up call to evaluate effectiveness of pain control regimen, provide oversight to assess and address complications, and gauge overall patient satisfaction.
17. Serve as an effective liaison for patients who fail the pain treatment plan and may require admission to the inpatient service for more involved pain therapy, consult with the acute pain service, or initiate follow-up with a chronic pain physician.
18. Develop Quality improvement initiatives and quality-of-care indicators to track unplanned admissions, optimum operating room (OR) utilization, adequacy of staffing, quality of care, and assessment outcomes [8, 28].
19. Revise protocols periodically based on analysis of these outcome measures.

A thorough preoperative consultation with the patient can go a long way in ensuring optimum pain control and patient satisfaction by setting expectations for the likely intensity and duration of pain and educating the patient about pain treatment goals, benefits of multimodal analgesia, and specific modalities available to the patient for their type of surgical procedure [2, 6]. Patient education can occur through one-on-one interaction in the Preoperative clinic or by providing them printed materials, videos, or Web-based content depending on the patient's level of education and other social factors. Patients can also be advised on general principles of optimizing postoperative recovery such as early ambulation, deep breathing and coughing, incentive spirometry, and participation in rehabilitation protocols.

An Ambulatory Pain specialist may be especially invaluable in certain special Situations:

1. Patients with history of prior severe allergic reactions to commonly used analgesics.
2. History of poor pain control after previous surgery.
3. Patients scheduled for more complicated surgical procedures with potential for severe pain. Certain surgeries such as thoracotomy, mastectomy, amputation, urological procedures, and inguinal herniorrhaphy are particularly prone to transitioning into chronic pain syndromes [6, 24, 25].
4. Patients on chronic opioid therapy for pain prior to current surgery.
5. Patients on Medication Assisted Treatment (MAT) for Opioid use disorder – on Methadone or Buprenorphine.

In these situations, the Ambulatory Pain Physician recognizes the need for a more individualized regimen to optimize care. If specific medications are to be avoided, Regional anesthesia and complementary modalities may assume a more important role.

While the concept of preemptive analgesia has been validated in animal studies, it has not been replicated consistently in humans. However, the concept of "Preventive Analgesia" is gaining ground [6]. Administering appropriate analgesics in the preoperative period, prior to surgical incision, has been shown to decrease postoperative opioid requirements. Oral or intravenous Acetaminophen, anticonvulsants such as Gabapentin and Pregabalin, Cox 2 inhibitors such as Celecoxib and intravenous Decadron are all components of an effective premedication regimen geared toward reducing need for opioids in the intraoperative and postoperative periods [6–11, 14]. The Ambulatory Pain Physician can determine the appropriate doses for each patient and decide when and who administers it. Educating the nurses in the preoperative holding area about the benefits of each of these medications and their adverse effects can help prepare them to be more effective caregivers.

Expertise in Regional anesthetic techniques is a cornerstone of Multimodal analgesia regimens and ERAS protocols. The field is ever expanding with newer ultrasound guided techniques evolving at a rapid pace, and the onus is on the Pain physician to keep abreast with these developments to provide the patient with the best care available. Facilities should have clearly defined policies in place for monitoring and competency-based training of other personnel involved in the care of the patient as well. Proctoring other anesthesia providers during acquisition of these newer skills is another critical role. The timing of preoperative Regional blocks is another key component of ensuring smooth throughput of the patient, on-time surgical starts, and preventing surgical delays further encouraging "buy in" from the surgeons as well.

A well-conceived preoperative plan will fail without proper execution by all members of the anesthesia and surgical teams. By establishing protocols for each phase of care, the Ambulatory Pain Physician can clearly communicate his/her expectations to every stakeholder involved in the care of the patient, without being individually responsible for its execution at every level. IV Lidocaine and Ketamine infusions are common components of multimodal intraoperative regimens with favorable evidence for decreased postoperative opioid requirements and improved analgesia [6, 14]. Judicious use of opioids intraoperatively, considering all other adjunctive pain treatment modalities in play further improves chances for successful pain control. The surgeon often depends on the expertise of the Pain physician to determine doses of local anesthetics for surgical wound infiltration, and this may be especially important in patients who have had preoperative regional anesthetic blocks.

In the Postoperative phase, the responsibility of prompt recognition of a failure of the established preoperative plan also falls on the Ambulatory Pain Physician. A thorough knowledge of regional anesthesia often comes in handy in these situations. The use of "rescue blocks" in addition to alternative opioid and nonopioid medications and complementary modalities has to be initiated early to optimize pain control and prevent having to play "catch up," which often requires higher doses of analgesics and consequently more adverse reactions. Postoperative nausea and vomiting may further limit opioid use. Surgeon preference may preclude the use of NSAIDs in some orthopedic procedures and in situations where postsurgical bleeding is a concern. Anxiolytics in conjunction with analgesics may work synergistically to control pain, especially in patients with preoperative chronic pain or psychological comorbidities. Education of PACU nurses by the pain physician is vital to correct longstanding misconceptions regarding pain and analgesics [2]. Some of these include the belief that pain is to be expected after surgery and treatment is warranted only after extreme expressions of pain by the patient, that opioids are always indicated to manage pain, and that use of opioids will inevitably cause addiction especially in patients with prior history of substance abuse. Frequent reassessment of pain is an essential component of optimizing pain management, particularly in the "difficult" patient. Often, the presence of a physician who shows concern and is ready to intervene has a positive impact on the patient, improving satisfaction scores.

Another essential role of the Ambulatory Pain Physician is in formulating an effective discharge strategy for the patient. Consultation with the surgeon may help determine the appropriate analgesic prescription at the lowest effective dose for the expected duration of pain based on the surgery [2]. In the past, it has been common practice among surgeons to prescribe narcotics, well in excess of required amounts for the average patient, and this has led to long-term opioid use, dependence, and addiction besides the potential for diversion. Data suggests 1 in 30 patients continue to use opioids 90 days after surgery and 1 in 15 opioid-naïve patients becomes addicted to prescription opioids. With the national opioid crisis front and center, it is especially vital to limit overprescription of narcotics to limit the community supply of opioids.

There are no consensus guidelines on opioid tapering after surgery, though the need is well recognized. This is due to significant interindividual variability in the pain experience (old vs young and +/− comorbidities), differences in surgical techniques (invasive vs noninvasive), and anticipated recovery times as well as differences in metabolism based on prior opioid exposure (opioid naive vs tolerant). As a result, there is wide variability in opioid prescribing practices among surgeons, even for the same surgery. One study showed 83% of patients discharged home after mastectomy and thoracotomy consumed less than half their prescribed opioids [26]. Unused opioids are often not discarded appropriately and could end up in the hands of family members and even children, significantly increasing the risk of opioid overdose and death. There is a dearth of good research available to guide us on the best methods and outcomes of discharge planning. Appropriate patient education at discharge and coordination of transition to outpatient care can lead to better patient outcomes. Such discharge planning often involves an interdisciplinary approach involving nurses, physicians, physical therapists, and pharmacists. Instructions to the patient should be clear regarding follow-up and as to who will address specific questions the patient may have, until they are ready to transition back to their primary care provider.

Multimodal Analgesia

Historically, opioids have been the mainstay of treatment in postoperative pain in both the inpatient and outpatient setting. It is common knowledge that opioids cause nausea, vomiting, dysphoria, itching, constipation, sedation, and respiratory depression, all of which are undesirable side effects in the postoperative patient but could also potentially lead to serious morbidity and mortality in the unmonitored setting [6, 24]. Many opioid-naïve patients have their first exposure to narcotics in the immediate postoperative period, which, according to recent literature, can lead to long-term opioid use, opioid use disorder, and even death [6, 13].

As the variety and complexity of surgical procedures performed in ASCs increase, the need for an individualized approach to postoperative pain care is paramount to ensure optimal patient outcome. "Balanced" or "Multimodal" analgesia is the practice of using two or more pharmacological agents or modalities acting at two or more different sites/receptors or through different mechanisms to provide analgesia, with the intent of maximizing the benefits of each agent while minimizing their adverse effects [7, 15, 16, 19, 21]. By preventing and treating pain with regimens that incorporate Regional anesthetic techniques in combination with opioid and nonopioid analgesics, each acting at different centers in the Central and Peripheral nervous system, one can improve analgesia by their synergistic actions while decreasing the use of any one agent and minimizing the associated side effects, particularly opioids. This has been proven to result in improved postoperative analgesia, decreased opioid requirements and related side effects, earlier mobilization, and higher patient satisfaction [15, 23].

As Enhanced Recovery After Anesthesia (ERAS) protocols in the Ambulatory setting continues to evolve, opioids are increasingly being used more as "rescue analgesics" rather than the first choice in the management of pain [24]. As per the ASA taskforce guidelines on acute postoperative pain management, Regional anesthetic techniques, Acetaminophen, NSAIDS, Gabapentinoids, Ketamine, Lidocaine, Local anesthetic surgical wound infiltration, and Alpha-2 agonists are rapidly being adopted as part of a Multimodal analgesic regimen well supported by emerging evidence. Nonpharmacological approaches such as Acupuncture, Mindfulness, Guided Meditation, Biofeedback, Behavioral Pain Management, and Transcutaneous Electrical Stimulation (TENS) are more often being considered as complementary modalities particularly in the more complex "difficult to treat" patients undergoing ambulatory surgery [24].

For a long time, research has focused on the addition of a single modality or drug to an existing analgesic regimen and evaluating its potential therapeutic benefits [11]. However, over the past decade this has changed with a surge in research evaluating multimodal regimens showing improved postoperative outcomes and patient satisfaction, accounting for their increased acceptance worldwide.

Multimodal Analgesia is rapidly becoming the "standard of care" in Ambulatory centers worldwide to deal with acute postoperative pain.

Managing the Chronic Pain Patient with Acute Postoperative Pain

A focused Ambulatory Pain Physician can especially be useful when dealing with a patient who is on chronic opioid therapy coming in for surgery. These opioid tolerant patients may have a history of particularly rocky postoperative courses if their higher pain medication requirements are not adequately addressed [20]. These patients often have greater fear and anxiety related to the anticipated pain following surgery. While there is widespread societal acceptance of chronic opioid use in Cancer pain, patients who are on chronic opioid therapy for noncancer pain often feel misunderstood and stigmatized when they encounter newer healthcare providers. During preoperative evaluations, they may downplay their opioid use to avoid being labeled a "difficult" patient. It is common for PACU nurses to be less empathetic to these patients. Often an Anesthesiologist familiar with chronic pain patients may be able to gain their confidence and reassure them that their pain will be managed effectively.

Managing the Patient with Opioid Use Disorder and Substance Abuse

Methadone and Buprenorphine are effective opioid agonists routinely used in the medication assisted treatment (MAT) of Opioid use disorder (OUD). Postoperative pain is particularly challenging in these patients because of high cross-tolerance to other opioids, heightened pain sensitivity due to opioid-induced hyperalgesia (OIH), illicit drug use, and societal misconceptions regarding pain treatment in the patient with history of substance abuse [6, 14, 17]. Very few studies address the concern that opioid use in the perioperative period in these patients may lead to relapse to drug use. A small retrospective study on patients on chronic methadone MAT did not show greater risk of relapse after exposure to postoperative opioids compared to matched controls who did not undergo surgery or receive additional opioids. Patients on buprenorphine present an even greater challenge as it has greater affinity for the mu opioid receptor and dissociates from it slower making them more resistance to standard opioids used in postoperative pain. At present, there is no consensus or good evidence of optimal strategy for continuing buprenorphine use and acute pain management in these patients [8, 14, 17]. While some protocols suggest continuation of buprenorphine, the University of Michigan protocol suggests discontinuation for at least 5 days prior to elective surgery and substituting it with short course of opioids. However, there is consensus among physicians in the need for increased use of multimodal pain treatment strategies including regional anesthesia, local anesthetic infiltration, membrane stabilizers, NSAIDs, and acetaminophen, with the recognition that should opioids be indicated, requirements may be higher. Recent evidence points to more favorable outcomes and better patient tolerance with the use of adjunct opioid therapy while continuing buprenorphine in the perioperative period. Hence, routine discontinuation prior to surgery is not supported by high level of evidence and in fact may even be unsafe based on the increased risk of mortality with treatment cessation [14, 17, 18].

The Ambulatory Pain Physician plays a crucial role in the treatment of patients with a history of substance abuse. Adequate treatment of pain should not be withheld from patients with history of substance abuse due to the fear that it can worsen addiction or precipitate a relapse. Besides violating ethical standards, inadequately treated pain can often trigger a relapse [18]. Instead, preoperative planning and an effective perioperative regimen with generous use of Multimodal analgesia with regional techniques, NSAIDs, and nonopioid analgesics like ketamine and lidocaine can limit the need for opioids in the postoperative period. When opioids are used, preoperative education of the patient and family and use of cognitive and behavioral approaches to manage anxiety, craving, and pain can be very useful in preventing relapse. Preemptive prescription of nasal naloxone to combat potential overdose and engaging the patient's family to monitor the patient are an additional safety net, until opioids are weaned according to an individualized, clearly documented tapering strategy [18]. Consultation with Psychiatry and patients' Addiction Specialist to deal with chemical dependency issues and its underlying causes can help achieve a successful postoperative outcome [14, 18].

Considerations for the Future

As ERAS protocols evolve and newer ultrasound-guided regional anesthesia techniques are defined and refined, the options for perioperative pain management are ever expanding. Just as intravenous Acetaminophen has been widely accepted in the preoperative period as an effective analgesic, injectable NSAIDs are being developed. Pharmacotherapeutic advances such as liposomal local anesthetic preparations will likely be expanded to even more regional techniques, affording patients extended duration of pain relief without the need for continuous catheter-based techniques. Transdermal drug delivery systems without painful injections are closer to reality than ever before, potentially allowing the option for patient-controlled analgesia (PCA) at home, without infusion pumps or even parenteral access. Transitional pain clinics will likely expand from the few tertiary centers they are currently in, as their value is recognized in decreasing the conversion of acute poorly treated pain to more chronic pain conditions, saving the healthcare system significant resources. As newer drugs and techniques suitable for ambulatory anesthesia are developed, due consideration must be paid to the cost-effectiveness of such treatment in addition to improving the patient experience in the perioperative period [28]. Future studies must reconcile the increase in cost of these advances with the potential financial savings from reduced length of PACU stay, earlier discharge from the hospital, reduced hospital admissions and emergency room visits, and earlier return to work [10, 11].

Summary

Untreated or poorly treated pain is a key factor delaying discharge from the PACU, adversely affecting the patient's ability to ambulate early and participate in rehabilitation activities, which in turn negatively impacts healthcare costs as well as surgical outcomes and patient satisfaction. Preventive strategies to treat pain are more effective than reactive treatment strategies, and early initiation of pain treatment preoperatively with effective intraoperative and postoperative follow-up is key to achieving adequate pain control.

In the era of Evidence-Based Medicine, Multimodal analgesia is here to stay, gaining global acceptance on the basis of emerging scientific evidence showing clear benefits of using both nonopioid and opioid analgesics in combination with Regional Anesthesia and complementary modalities to treat acute perioperative pain. The reduction of opioid use and its adverse effects without compromising analgesia, shortening hospital length of stay, and improving postoperative outcomes and patient satisfaction is an obvious step in the right direction to curb the opioid epidemic.

Surgeons are increasingly "buying in" to the concept of Anesthesia-led Multimodal pain protocols to optimize patient care in the perioperative period. The onus is clearly on Anesthesiology as a specialty to rise to the occasion to facilitate the best possible postoperative care in a cost-effective and time sensitive manner, contributing to improved patient outcomes as well as satisfaction.

The Ambulatory Pain Specialist can effectively lead this charge, consistently implementing multimodal strategies individualized to specific patient needs and providing an added dimension to value-based quality care of the patient throughout the perioperative period in Ambulatory Care Centers worldwide.

References

1. Apfelbaum JL, et al. Postoperative pain experience: results from a national survey suggest postoperative pain continues to be undermanaged. Anesth Analg. 2003;97(2):534–40. Table of contents.
2. Chou R, Gordon DB, de Leon-Casasola OA, et al. Management of postoperative pain: a clinical practice guideline from the American Pain Society, the American Society of Regional Anesthesia and Pain Medicine, and the American Society of Anesthesiologists' Committee on Regional Anesthesia, Executive Committee, and Administrative Council [published correction appears in J Pain. 2016 Apr;17(4):508–10. Dosage error in article text]. J Pain. 2016;17(2):131–57. https://doi.org/10.1016/j.jpain.2015.12.008.
3. van Biesen T, Johnson T. Ambulatory surgery center growth accelerates: is MedTech ready? 2019.
4. Cullen KA, Hall MJ, Golosinskiy A. Ambulatory surgery in the United States, 2006. Natl Health Stat Report. 2009;11:1–25.
5. Manchikanti L, Parr AT, Singh V, Fellows B. Ambulatory surgery centers and interventional techniques: a look at long-term survival. Pain Physician. 2011;14(2):E177–215.
6. Mariano ER, Fishman S, Crowley M. Management of acute perioperative pain. In: UpToDate, Post TW(Ed), Waltham, MA, UpToDate Inc. 2021.
7. Crews J. Multimodal pain management strategies for office based and ambulatory procedures. Clinician's corner. JAMA. 2002;288(5):629–32.
8. Vadivelu N, Kai AM, Kodumudi V, Berger JM. Challenges of pain control and the role of the ambulatory pain specialist in the outpatient surgery setting. J Pain Res. 2016;9:425–35. Published 2016 Jun 17. https://doi.org/10.2147/JPR.S86579.
9. Thomas DA, Chang D, Zhu R, Rayaz H, Vadivelu N. Concept of the ambulatory pain physician. Curr Pain Headache Rep. 2017;21(1):7. https://doi.org/10.1007/s11916-017-0611-2.
10. Jafra A, Mitra S. Pain relief after ambulatory surgery: progress over the last decade. Saudi J Anaesth. 2018;12(4):618–25. https://doi.org/10.4103/sja.SJA_232_18.
11. White PF. Multimodal analgesia: its role in preventing postoperative pain. Curr Opin Investig Drugs. 2008;9(1):76–82.

12. Pavlin DJ, et al. A survey of pain and other symptoms that affect the recovery process after discharge from an ambulatory surgery unit. J Clin Anesth. 2004;16(3):200–6.
13. Calcaterra SL, et al. Opioid prescribing at hospital discharge contributes to chronic opioid use. J Gen Intern Med. 2016;31(5):478–85.
14. Vadivelu N, Kai AM, Kodumudi V, Zhu R, Hines R. Pain management of patients with substance abuse in the ambulatory setting. Curr Pain Headache Rep. 2017;21(2):9. https://doi.org/10.1007/s11916-017-0610-3.
15. Schug SA, Chong C. Pain management after ambulatory surgery. Curr Opin Anaesthesiol. 2009;22(6):738–43. https://doi.org/10.1097/ACO.0b013e32833020f4.
16. Elvir-Lazo OL, White PF. The role of multimodal analgesia in pain management after ambulatory surgery. Curr Opin Anaesthesiol. 2010;23(6):697–703. https://doi.org/10.1097/ACO.0b013e32833fad0a.
17. Ward EN, Quaye AN, Wilens TE. Opioid use disorders: perioperative management of a special population. Anesth Analg. 2018;127(2):539–47. https://doi.org/10.1213/ANE.0000000000003477. PMID: 29847389; PMCID: PMC6523021.
18. Sordo L, Barrio G, Bravo MJ, et al. Mortality risk during and after opioid substitution treatment: systematic review and meta-analysis of cohort studies. BMJ. 2017;357:j1550. Published 2017 Apr 26. https://doi.org/10.1136/bmj.j1550.
19. Dickerson DM. Acute pain management. Anesthesiol Clin. 2014;32(2):495–504. https://doi.org/10.1016/j.anclin.2014.02.010.
20. Rapp SE, Ready LB, Nessly ML. Acute pain management in patients with prior opioid consumption: a case-controlled retrospective review. Pain. 1995;61(2):195–201.
21. Chauvin M. State of the art of pain treatment following ambulatory surgery. Eur J Anaesthesiol Suppl. 2003;28:3–6.
22. Fosnot CD, Fleisher LA, Keogh J. Providing value in ambulatory anesthesia. Curr Opin Anaesthesiol. 2015;28(6):617–22. https://doi.org/10.1097/ACO.0000000000000255.
23. Moore JG, Ross SM, Williams BA. Regional anesthesia and ambulatory surgery. Curr Opin Anaesthesiol. 2013;26(6):652–60. https://doi.org/10.1097/ACO.0000000000000011.
24. Tan M, Law LS, Gan TJ. Optimizing pain management to facilitate Enhanced Recovery After Surgery pathways. Can J Anaesth. 2015;62(2):203–18. https://doi.org/10.1007/s12630-014-0275-x.
25. Perkins FM, Kehlet H. Chronic pain as an outcome of surgery. A review of predictive factors. Anesthesiology. 2000;93:1123–5.
26. Bartels K, et al. Opioid use and storage patterns by patients after hospital discharge following surgery. PLoS One. 2016;11(1):e0147972.
27. Oderda GM, Evans RS, Lloyd J, Lipman A, Chen C, Ashburn M. Cost of opioid related adverse drug events in surgical patients. J Pain Symptom Manag. 2003;25:276–83.
28. Frezza EE, Girnys RP, Silich RJ, Coppa GF. Commentary: quality of care and cost containment are the hospital-based ambulatory surgery challenges for the future. Am J Med Qual. 2000;15(3):114–8. https://doi.org/10.1177/106286060001500305.

30 Inclusion of Pain Management Services in Ambulatory Surgical Centers

Aimee Pak

Abstract

The inclusion of pain management services would be an organic expansion of perioperative care at ambulatory surgery centers. Clinical evidence and research have promoted the need for acute perioperative pain control. The current trajectory within the United States healthcare system also increasingly supports the addition of perioperative pain services through regulatory agencies and economic factors. If well designed and implemented, pain management services may provide multifaceted benefits to all stakeholders – patients, local community, physicians, clinical providers, administrators, owners, and investors.

Introduction

A growing body of research is providing evidence against poorly controlled acute, postoperative pain. We will discuss the clinical aspects of acute postoperative pain, pain management, and associated financial considerations within the economic and regulatory framework of the United States healthcare system.

Pain After Surgery

Since the 1980s, the numbers of ambulatory surgeries and procedures have increased [1]. An estimated 48.3 million surgical and nonsurgical outpatient procedures were performed in 2010, of which 22.5 million occurred at ambulatory surgery centers based on National Hospital Ambulatory Medical Care Survey data [2]. A focus on cost-containment, improvements in anesthetic techniques, and development of minimally invasive procedures continues to push the growth of outpatient surgery [2, 3]. This expansion is troubling when contextualized with another statistics: 30–40% of patients suffer from moderate to severe pain in the first 48 hours after ambulatory surgery [4, 5]. The latter information is based on survey data from the 1990s but can be extrapolated to current times even with heightened attention to postoperative pain [6, 7]. A 2014 survey by Gan et al. found that 80% of patients reported pain in the immediate postoperative period in the outpatient setting and, of that, nearly 60% reported moderate, severe, or extreme pain [7]. Given the potential magnitude, poorly controlled postoperative pain will be harder to ignore in the era of accountable care.

A. Pak (✉)
Department of Anesthesiology, The University of Oklahoma Health Sciences Center, Oklahoma City, OK, USA
e-mail: aimee-pak@ouhsc.edu

K. Rajput et al. (eds.), *Pain Control in Ambulatory Surgery Centers*,
https://doi.org/10.1007/978-3-030-55262-6_30

The Problem with Acute Pain

Acute pain is directly and indirectly responsible for numerous healthcare problems. Poorly controlled postoperative pain adversely affects patients, healthcare systems, and society and has serious economic ramifications. The financial effect of acute postoperative pain, on hospitals and ambulatory surgery centers, will be discussed separately in this chapter.

Patient Morbidity

Acute postoperative pain contributes to both short-term and long-term patient morbidity. Physiological sequelae of uncontrolled postoperative pain span multiple systems: (1) a sustained sympathetic response may cause coronary ischemia and myocardial infarction (cardiovascular); (2) respiratory splinting leading to atelectasis and pneumonia (pulmonary); (3) hypomotility may lead to nausea, vomiting, and ileus (gastrointestinal); (4) urinary retention and oliguria (renal); and (5) a reduced immune response (immune) [8]. Side effects from escalating opioid doses to treat acute pain may compound this clinical scenario. These include an altered mental status, hyperalgesia, respiratory depression, nausea, vomiting, constipation, and pruritis. Furthermore, overall well-being and quality of life are worsened when acute postoperative pain is not controlled adequately [8]. Psychological distress leading to anxiety and depression may be caused or exacerbated in the postoperative period [7, 9]. Sleep, mood, and physical function are negatively affected with severe postoperative pain [10, 11].

Opioid use that continues beyond 90 days after surgery, particularly in young, opioid-naïve patients, is a known postsurgical risk. The incidence is approximately 6% for both major and minor surgeries [12, 13]. A related concern includes the development of chronic postsurgical pain. Chronic postsurgical pain is estimated to have an incidence of 10–50% depending on type of procedure, including commonly performed outpatient surgery, of which 2–10% have severe debilitating pain [14]. A study published by Sun et al. found an increased risk for chronic opioid use after common surgeries compared to nonsurgical patients: open or laparoscopic cholecystectomy, open appendectomy, simple mastectomy, cesarean delivery, total knee arthroplasty, and total hip arthroplasty; the odds ratios range from 1.28 to 5.10 [15]. Both scenarios may have long-term individual and societal ramifications.

Societal Ramifications

Opioid dependence and abuse have been labeled a public health crisis. Overdose deaths in the United States have risen steadily since 2000; in 2017, prescription opioids caused over 17,000 fatalities [16]. The societal cost of opioid fatal and nonfatal abuse was estimated at over $78.5 billion US dollars in 2013 for health care, substance abuse treatment, lost productivity, and criminal justice expenses [17]. The bulk of this financial burden fell on the American public, through spending via government agencies and lost tax revenue [17].

Meanwhile, chronic pain has been estimated at $560–635 billion USD in 2010, including healthcare cost and lost productivity [18]. The widespread impact of opioid dependence and abuse on society is detrimental, costly, and ongoing.

The significant and widespread ramifications of pain and opioid dependence have been well-documented in literature. The contribution toward these problems specifically by acute postoperative pain is concerning and certainly needs greater mitigation efforts. Furthermore, acute postoperative pain in the broader context of the evolving U.S. healthcare system warrants further discussion in the next section.

Section Key Points: Broader Concerns Regarding Postoperative Pain

- A large percentage of postsurgical patients experience moderate to severe postoperative pain.
- Significant short-term and long-term patient morbidities have been well-described with poorly controlled acute pain.

- Persistent opioid dependence and abuse have created a larger societal and economic crisis.
- Better postoperative pain management is a focus within the changing U.S. healthcare system.

Ambulatory Surgery

The problems arising from acute pain management must be considered in the larger context of the state of American health care. Health care in the United States has been the source of long-standing national debate and criticism. From the 1950s to present, bloating costs, poor quality of care, and inadequate coverage plagues the healthcare system. The following section will explore pertinent issues and changes in recent healthcare history that has led to the outward migration toward ambulatory surgery.

U.S. Health Care and the Legislation Driving Change

National health expenditure has increased 4.6% to $3.6 trillion USD in 2018 and accounts for 17.7% of the Gross Domestic Product (GDP) [19]. It was $2.4 trillion in 2008 and 16.3% of the GDP a decade earlier [19, 20]. In 2014, The Commonwealth Fund placed the U.S. health system the lowest in efficiency, equity, outcomes, and overall ranking, but highest in national spending on health care compared to 11 other industrialized nations [20]. Its 2017 update reiterated the bottom placement in access, equity, outcomes, and overall ranking for the U.S. and second to last placement for administrative efficiency [21]. In his 2016 publication in *JAMA*, then-President Barack Obama cited that 1 in 7 Americans were uninsured, which was 49 million in 2010 [22]. On these criticisms, the highly controversial Patient Protection and Affordable Care Act (ACA, also referred to as Obamacare) was passed in 2010 with the arching goals of expanding coverage, controlling cost, and improving quality.

Expanding Coverage

With the enactment of the ACA, the number of uninsured Americans declined from 49 million in 2010 to 29 million in 2015 [22]. Insurers must offer coverage with guaranteed renewal to all applicants and prohibition on medical underwriting and exclusion based on preexisting conditions [20]. The ACA also mandated nonexempt individuals to obtain minimum essential coverage or pay a tax penalty and limits on open enrollment to defray costs from high-utilizing consumers with healthy, low-risk individuals [23]. With this rapid addition of 20 million (primarily Medicaid) insured patients as of 2016 [22] with access to surgical and medical procedures, including preventative measures (i.e. screening colonoscopies), the patient volume demands on all healthcare providers, including anesthetic providers, have increased.

Controlling Cost

The national health expenditure is projected to be nearly $6 trillion dollars, 19.4% of the GDP, or $16,907 per capita by 2027 [19]. Prior to the ACA, a "fee-for-service" (FFS) payment model was used, which rewarded quantity rather than quality of care delivered. The ACA made several changes to the healthcare payment system to slow the ballooning rate including:

1. Changes in rates paid by Medicare, which also influences the private insurance sector,
2. Detecting and penalizing fraud,
3. Implementing value-based payments for Medicare FFS,
4. Price transparency, and
5. Implementing alternative payment models (APM) based on outcomes such as bundled payment models and accountable care organizations [20, 22].

The result of these payment structures drives certain clinical care decision and practice as will be discussed further. The rate of Medicare spending is seemingly reduced at approximately −1% mean annual growth in per enrollee spending between 2010 and 2014 from a mean annual growth in per enrollee spending of 4.7% between

2000 and 2005, with private insurers mirroring this trend [22]. Whether this is directly due to the ACA legislation or other causes (i.e., recession economy, increased consumer cost sharing, avoidance, inability for consumers to engage with medical care, etc.) is still hotly contested and outside the scope of this chapter.

Improving Quality
The high price of American health care has not necessarily translated into better patient outcomes. It has been characterized by fragmentation and disorganization, with hospital-acquired morbidity and mortality adding to the poor care and costs [22]. The ACA sought to tie compensation with value to incentivize quality. However, the resultant expansion of regulations and overseeing agencies, promotion of mandatory electronic health record systems, and increased volume of nonclinical administrative tasks seem to offset productivity and gains in quality, which has drawn heavy criticism [20].

The Push Out of Hospitals and Into Ambulatory Surgery Centers

Outpatient procedures, which do not need overnight hospitalization (also referred to as ambulatory surgery or the same day surgery), may be performed in ambulatory surgery centers (ASC), hospital outpatient departments (HOPD), and, in certain cases, physician offices. This chapter will focus on ASC. ASCs are separate entities that may be independently owned ("freestanding") or hospital owned. Recently, the growth and demand for ASCs have increased: ASC growth over 1 year in 2016–2017 was 2.4% from 1.0% during the prior 4 years in 2012–2016 for Medicaid beneficiaries [3].

There are many contributing reasons for ASC growth, primarily

1. Cost containment,
2. Advancements in surgical and anesthetic techniques, and
3. Demand.

Data from 2007 published by the Healthcare Cost and Utilization Project reported a lower average charge for ambulatory surgery at $6100 compared to inpatient surgery at $39,000 [24]. Healthcare payment structures (i.e., Medicare Outpatient Prospective Payment System) have encouraged outpatient surgeries over the more expensive inpatient setting [24]. Between the two outpatient options, costs were lower and surgery visits were shorter in ASCs compared to HOPDs: cataract surgery with intraocular lens insertion was $977 in ASCs versus $1917 in HOPDs in 2019 [2, 3]. Overall, the paradigm shift in health care toward value-based and cost reduction has increased interest in ASCs by hospital systems, insurers, and private equity firms [3].

Improvements in operative techniques and technology as well as in anesthesia and analgesia have contributed to the expansion of available surgeries in ambulatory settings. There has been increasing proficiency and availability of minimally invasive (i.e., laser surgery, laparoscopy, and endoscopy) surgery, reducing blood loss, and risk for infection with smaller incision [2, 3, 25]. Newer anesthetic agents allowing for more rapid wake up, widespread adoption of ultrasound-guided regional anesthesia, and emphasis on multimodal analgesia and postoperative nausea and vomiting (PONV) prophylactic measures have improved recovery and discharge [25, 26].

There is an indisputable increase in new ASCs and increased volume of ASC surgical services, which begs the question: where is this growth from? Notably, there is evidence that physician-owned ASCs have increased procedural volume, which may create a financial rather than medical drive for utilization and potentially lead to inappropriate patient selection [3, 27]. Analysis by Hollenbeck et al. suggests that ASCs offload surgical volume from the more-expensive hospital settings due to a lower cost per care episode and that ASCs likely generate overall surgical volume in the local health market from existing unmet need [3, 27, 28]. While the concerns of induced demand are possible (most ASCs have some degree of physician ownership) [3] and warrants oversight, the extent of this influence may not be as dramatic as anticipated and without negatively affecting mortality or admission rates [27, 28]. Additionally, the Medicare Payment Advisory Commission attributes ASC growth to several other factors including easier scheduling and lower coinsurance for beneficiaries and autonomy and efficiency for physician proceduralists [3]. Overall, further utilization of ASCs may offer a safe, cost-efficient means to satisfy increasing demand.

Most ambulatory invasive surgeries were performed on the eye, ear, nose, mouth, and pharynx, followed by muscle, tendon, and soft tissue surgery (e.g., rotator cuff and trigger finger release) [24]. Lens and cataract surgeries have consistently been the top surgery performed in ASCs [3, 24]. Nonsurgical procedures most frequently involved endoscopy, colonoscopy, and spinal pain procedures [3]. Other common procedures are performed on the neurological, cardiovascular, musculoskeletal, abdominal, integumentary, urogenital, and gynecological systems [24].

However, there is a continued economic push to move higher-risk, traditionally inpatient procedures (e.g., spine surgery, total joint arthroplasty, and craniotomy) toward the outpatient setting via fast-track or enhanced recovery models and minimally invasive techniques [26, 29–33]. Increasingly patients with medical comorbidities are being selected for outpatient surgery, which makes the practice of ambulatory anesthesia more challenging [25]. To further complicate matter, patients with opioid-tolerant histories are becoming more frequent in the ambulatory setting and this poses difficulties with pain management [34]. The current and future healthcare environment is moving toward performing more complex surgeries on increasingly challenging patients with payment delivery based on value and cost efficiency.

Aligning Provider Payment with Value-Based Health Care

Fee-for-service (FFS) payment structures dominate anesthesia economics. From 1992 to 2016, anesthesia charge was simply calculated by the base unit plus time unit plus any modifiers all multiplied by the conversion factor rate [35]. The base unit was the value for a specific procedure, captured by a Current Procedural Terminology (CPT) code, which would account for the intensity and complexity of care in the perioperative period including resuscitation and noninvasive monitor interpretation [35]. The time unit starts when anesthetic care begins in the operating room or equivalent location and ends in the post-anesthetic care unit (PACU) or recovery area, often in 15-minute increments [35]. Modifiers may include physical status, extremes of age, and emergency nature of surgery [35]. The conversion factor rate was determined by the Centers for Medicare and Medicaid Services (CMS) [35]. Additional billing would apply for invasive monitors and postoperative pain procedures [35]. Voluntary reporting of quality measures began in 2007 through the Physician Voluntary Reporting Program and later incentivized to encourage reporting, with subsequent addition of a financial penalty to discourage not reporting [35]. This became the Physician Quality Reporting System (PQRS) [35].

In 2015, the Medicare Access and CHIP Reauthorization Act (MACRA) legislation consolidated many of the existing quality programs, including PQRS, under the Quality Payment Program (QPP), which (1) produced the Merit-based Incentive Payment System (MIPS) and (2) provided bonus payment for participation in eligible alternative payment models (APM) [36].

CMS Value-Based Payment Model: MIPS

If a clinician is eligible for MIPS, Medicare payment is made based on four metrics weighted annually by CMS for a total of 100% or 100 points. As of 2020, the weighted categories were:

1. Quality (45%),

   For the *Quality* category, at least six quality measures in certain percentages of patients must be reported [36, 37]. However, the specific quality measures reported depend on which of the six available collection types is utilized: (1) Qualified Clinical Data Registry by the National Anesthesia Clinical Outcomes Registry (NACOR) supported by the Anesthesia Quality Institute (AQI) of the American Society of Anesthesiologists, (2) Electronic Clinical Quality Measures (eCQM), (3) MIPS Clinical Quality Measures (CQM) via a Qualified Registry, (4) Medicare Part B Claims measures, (5) CMS Web Interface measures, or (6) the Consumer Assessment of Healthcare Providers and Systems (CAHPS) for MIPS survey [36, 37]. The explicit queries related to perioperative pain management and patient experience [36] are areas directly addressed by pain management services.

2. Promoting Interoperability (25%),

   Anesthesia providers in hospital and ambulatory settings are usually exempt from the *Promoting Interoperability* category, and so the weighting is added to the Quality category for a total of 70% [37].

3. Improvement Activities (15%)

   For full credit in the *Improvement Activities*, 40 total points must be achieved by performing 10-point medium weighted or 20-point high-weighted activities, which would improve care coordination, Medicare beneficiary engagements, and patient safety. The Perioperative Surgical Home and Enhanced Recovery After Surgery protocols would be medium weighted [36].

4. Cost (15%)

   For *Cost*, the clinician or group's performance is compared with an established benchmark, usually the Medicare Spending Per Beneficiary measure, a population-based cost measure [37].

It is a budget neutral process, and so payments may be adjusted from −9% to +27% with 45 of 100 points as the benchmark [36]. Though convoluted, MIPS has opportunity for positive payment adjustments through attention to its weighted metrics. Pain management services may provide additional benefit by addressing components of MIPS, most directly through the Quality metric, which will be discussed in the next section.

CMS Value-Based Payment Model: APM

APMs reward eligible clinicians or practices for assuming more than nominal financial risk related to patients' outcomes, either by specific clinical condition, for the duration of a care episode, or by a patient population [38]. There are three APM pathways at the time of this publication:

1. Advanced APMs (AAPM),

   Though potentially risky, AAPMs would be excluded from certain MIPS reporting and its potential negative adjustments and can receive an attractive payout though a lump sum bonus and a higher annual fee schedule [36, 38, 39]. Pain management services may be beneficial to certain AAPMs, such as Comprehensive Care for Joint Replacement payment model.

2. All-Payer Combination Advanced APMs

   As of 2019, the All-Payer Combination AAPM would be available to eligible providers or groups who qualify as an AAPM participant and meet AAPM criteria from other payers after review by CMS [38, 39]. As with AAPMs, participants will receive an APM incentive payment and would not need to fulfill MIPS reporting requirements or undergo its adjustments [38, 39].

3. MIPS APMs

   Finally, MIPS APMs are an option for MIPS-eligible providers who participate in an APM that does not qualify as an AAPM. Like MIPS, there are categories for Quality, Improvement Activities, Promoting Interoperability, and Cost, but the weighting and reporting requirements differ from MIPS (50%, 20%, 30%, and 0%, respectively, as of 2019 and 2020) [38, 39]. MIPS APMs will not receive the APM bonus but will not be required to have full participation in the MIPS program [38]. Like MIPS, pain management services can influence the Quality component.

Shift Toward Value-Based Health Care in ASCs

Even though ASCs receive payment through a separate program, the physicians and advanced practice providers (e.g., certified registered nurse anesthetist, CRNA, or anesthesia assistants, AA), working in ASCs, are subject to MACRA for professional payments like their hospital-based counterparts [36].

For the MIPS Quality component, there are several measures applicable for the ASC setting as of Performance Year 2020. It is important to note the continuous presence of pain management and patient experience reporting in the heavily weighted Quality measures: Multimodal Pain Management (MIPS #477), Patient-Reported Experience with Anesthesia (AQI 48), which includes a question on postoperative pain management, Use of Neuraxial Techniques and/or Peripheral Nerve Blocks for Total Knee Arthroplasty (AQI 56), and Obstructive Sleep Apnea: Mitigation Strategies (AQI 68), which may be satisfied with documented use of neuraxial anesthesia or peripheral nerve block and multimodal analgesia [36, 40]. Patient experience also appears in the MIPS *Improvement Activities* through participation in Consumer Assessment of Healthcare Providers and Systems (CAHPS) surveys [37]. Pain management and patient satisfaction are recurring components linked to professional compensation.

One APM garnering much interest is bundled payment (also referred to as the episodic payment model, EPM). In this model, predetermined target price covers all costs incurred during an episode of care, such as diagnostics and testing, all provider and facility fees, postacute care, ancillary services, and physical therapy, usually within a specified time frame (generally 60–90 days) [35, 41, 42]. Participating providers assume some financial risk if total expenditures are above the target price due to redundancies or complications [41]. However, provider coordination, care efficiency, and efforts to avoid complications may prove lucrative if costs are minimized [41]. Bundles can be adjusted to account for additional risks based on beneficiary age, behavioral factors, and comorbidities [41]. The bundled payment scheme is designed to incentivize high-quality care at reduced costs.

Given its higher efficiency, lower cost, and increasing demand, the bundled payment model may present a unique financial opportunity for ASCs that is advantageous to all stakeholders [31, 42, 43]. This is predicated on appropriate patient selection and preoperative risk stratification [43], and reduction of any postoperative complications that would erode into narrow profit margins.

Avoiding Costly Complications of Ambulatory Surgery

Avoidance of prolonged PACU recovery, Emergency Department (ED) visits, and hospital admission after discharge from ambulatory surgery have been the subject of much interest and published studies. However, in the era of value-based care, inadequate analgesia, uncontrolled nausea or vomiting, and patient dissatisfaction after discharge are costly complications that should be minimized in an ASC setting.

Pain

Pain is a frequent reason for additional acute care after discharge from surgery. Curtin et al. reported a 9% readmission rate within 30 days postprocedure in over 18,000 patients undergoing open or closed reduction or external fixation of a primary distal radius fracture, of which 69% of the open reduction (68% of cohort) readmission involved pain control [44]. Liu et al. looked at over 100,000 outpatient arthroscopic shoulder surgery and found 1.8% required acute care within 7 days postprocedure most commonly (23.78%) for musculoskeletal pain and most frequently (43.49%) by the first postoperative day [45]. In a separate study, Liu et al. identified 3.90% rate of acute care after outpatient anterior cruciate ligament repair surgery, of which the most common reason (28.9%) was pain followed by infection (10.1%) usually within the first postoperative day [46]. Average ED visit charges have been reported at $1951 (±$2578) [46]. Literature consistently supports the use of multimodal analgesia [26, 47] and regional technique to improve postoperative pain control [26, 47–49]. Poorly controlled pain also correlates strongly with patient dissatisfaction [10, 48].

PONV

PONV is the most common complaint after receiving general anesthesia. The incidence may be as high as 80% in high -risk populations with a history of PONV or motion sickness [25]. PONV is also associated with postoperative pain, female sex, and general anesthesia [48]. The incidence of PONV is markedly reduced when regional anesthesia is used over general anesthesia [49, 50]. Other techniques to reduce PONV include avoidance of nitrous oxide, total intravenous anesthesia multimodal analgesia with emphasis on nonopioid options in addition to regional anesthesia, and multiple antiemetic therapies [48]. Like uncontrolled pain, poorly controlled nausea correlates strongly with patient dissatisfaction [10, 48].

Dissatisfaction

Patient satisfaction is complex and multifactorial. Satisfaction is subjective, prone to biases, and difficult to measure; yet, it is still a driving force in hospital and ambulatory surgery practices that is linked to financial compensation. The relationship between satisfaction and pain control is intertwined, which creates yet another potential benefit for good pain management, which will be explored in section "Advantages of Pain Management Services".

Arising from the lack of information regarding consumers' experiences with health care, CMS and AHRQ developed the Consumer Assessment of Health Providers and Systems (CAHPS) surveys as a tool to collect and compare data on healthcare experience and quality [51, 52]. Various types of CAHPS surveys are available through certified vendors depending on patient population, such HOPDs or ASCs (CAHPS Outpatient and Ambulatory Surgery Survey, OAS CAHPS). CAHPS survey results are available free of charge to the public to help improve healthcare quality, provide comparable data across facilities, and support informed decision-making in consumers' selection of health care institution [52]. Notable organizations, including the National Committee for Quality Assurance, Veterans Health Administration, and Department of Defense, utilize CAHPS results to determine payment incentives and accreditation [52]. As mentioned earlier, the HCAHPS survey is one of the *Quality* component measures for MIPS reimbursement [36, 37].

Developed initially in 2012, the OAS CAHPS (see Fig. 30.1) has initiated voluntary reporting in January 2016 and reported its first dataset in 2018 [53, 54]. Notably, there are questions specifically pertaining to postoperative pain and pain management (Question 15–16), PONV (Questions 17–18), and overall satisfaction (Questions 23–24). At the time of this publication, the OAS CAHPS survey is not mandatory for Medicare-certified HOPDs and ASCs but may conceivably become a requirement in the future.

With quality targets and economic stakes invested in patient satisfaction, there is much interest in identifying the factors that influence patient satisfaction or dissatisfaction. Dissatisfaction comes from irreconcilable differences between experience and expectation [51].

Trinh et al. categorized nonmodifiable and modifiable factors affecting patient experience. Nonmodifiable factors were usually patient factors, such as demographics, health status, and educational level; while modifiable factors included providers' communication skills, information provision to patients, patient engagement with care, patient reported symptoms and perceived attention to symptoms, physician skills and behaviors, operational function of the perioperative environment, and interdisciplinary care [51]. Delving further into some of these factors may provide insight and opportunity for high-yield improvements.

Not surprisingly, better satisfaction occurred with less postoperative complications: infection, inflammation, nausea and vomiting, anxiety, and pain [7, 10, 48, 49, 51]. Pain is a common patient reported symptoms, which is affected by physician skill and perceived provider care. Patient satisfaction appears to be higher with physicians

a

SURVEY INSTRUCTIONS

Answer all the questions by checking the box to the left of your answer.

You are sometimes told to skip over some questions in this survey. When this happens you will see an arrow with a note that tells you what question to answer next, like this:

☐ Yes
☑ No → **If No, go to #1**

This survey asks about your experience at the facility named in the cover letter. For this survey, we use the term "procedure" for diagnostic, surgical or other procedures. We refer to "facility" as the place where you had your procedure.

Please answer these questions only for the procedure(s) you had on the date included in the cover letter. Do not include any other procedures in your answers.

I. BEFORE YOUR PROCEDURE

The first few questions are about getting ready for your procedure. **Include any information you received before and on the day of your procedure.**

1. Before your procedure, did your doctor or anyone from the facility give you all the information you needed about your procedure?
   1 ☐ Yes, definitely
   2 ☐ Yes, somewhat
   3 ☐ No

2. Before your procedure, did your doctor or anyone from the facility give you easy to understand instructions about getting ready for your procedure?
   1 ☐ Yes, definitely
   2 ☐ Yes, somewhat
   3 ☐ No

II. ABOUT THE FACILITY AND STAFF

The next questions ask about the day of your procedure.

3. Did the check-in process run smoothly?
   1 ☐ Yes, definitely
   2 ☐ Yes, somewhat
   3 ☐ No

4. Was the facility clean?
   1 ☐ Yes, definitely
   2 ☐ Yes, somewhat
   3 ☐ No

5. Were the clerks and receptionists at the facility as helpful as you thought they should be?
   1 ☐ Yes, definitely
   2 ☐ Yes, somewhat
   3 ☐ No

6. Did the clerks and receptionists at the facility treat you with courtesy and respect?
   1 ☐ Yes, definitely
   2 ☐ Yes, somewhat
   3 ☐ No

Fig. 30.1 OAS CAHPS Survey. This survey measures patient experiences at HOPDs and ASCs based on communication and care provided by health care providers and office staff, preparation for the surgery or procedure, and preparation for discharge and recover: (**a**) Page 1, (**b**) Page 2, (**c**) Page 3, (**d**) Page 4, and (**e**) Page 5. Note added modification of colored box to highlight specific text: Questions 15–16 (postoperative pain; pink), Questions 17–18 (PONV; green), and Questions 23–24 (patient satisfaction; blue). The survey is available in public domain at https://oascahps.org/

b

7. Did the doctors and nurses treat you with courtesy and respect?

   [1] ☐ Yes, definitely
   [2] ☐ Yes, somewhat
   [3] ☐ No

8. Did the doctors and nurses make sure you were as comfortable as possible?

   [1] ☐ Yes, definitely
   [2] ☐ Yes, somewhat
   [3] ☐ No

III. Communications About your Procedure

As a reminder, please include any information you received before and on the day of the procedure.

9. Did the doctors and nurses explain your procedure in a way that was easy to understand?

   [1] ☐ Yes, definitely
   [2] ☐ Yes, somewhat
   [3] ☐ No

10. Anesthesia is something that would make you feel sleepy or go to sleep during your procedure. Were you given anesthesia?

   [1] ☐ Yes
   [2] ☐ No → **If No, go to #13**

11. Did your doctor or anyone from the facility explain the process of giving anesthesia in a way that was easy to understand?

   [1] ☐ Yes, definitely
   [2] ☐ Yes, somewhat
   [3] ☐ No

12. Did your doctor or anyone from the facility explain the possible side effects of the anesthesia in a way that was easy to understand?

   [1] ☐ Yes, definitely
   [2] ☐ Yes, somewhat
   [3] ☐ No

13. Discharge instructions include things like symptoms you should watch for after your procedure, instructions about medicines, and home care. Before you left the facility, did you get written discharge instructions?

   [1] ☐ Yes
   [2] ☐ No

IV. Your Recovery

14. Did your doctor or anyone from the facility prepare you for what to expect during your recovery?

   [1] ☐ Yes, definitely
   [2] ☐ Yes, somewhat
   [3] ☐ No

Fig. 30.1 (continued)

c

15. Some ways to control pain include prescription medicine, over-the-counter pain relievers or ice packs. Did your doctor or anyone from the facility give you information about what to do if you had pain as a result of your procedure?

   1 ☐ Yes, definitely
   2 ☐ Yes, somewhat
   3 ☐ No

16. At any time after leaving the facility, did you have pain as a result of your procedure?

   1 ☐ Yes
   2 ☐ No

17. Before you left the facility, did your doctor or anyone from the facility give you information about what to do if you had nausea or vomiting?

   1 ☐ Yes, definitely
   2 ☐ Yes, somewhat
   3 ☐ No

18. At any time after leaving the facility, did you have nausea or vomiting as a result of either your procedure or the anesthesia?

   1 ☐ Yes
   2 ☐ No

19. Before you left the facility, did your doctor or anyone from the facility give you information about what to do if you had bleeding as a result of your procedure?

   1 ☐ Yes, definitely
   2 ☐ Yes, somewhat
   3 ☐ No

20. At any time after leaving the facility, did you have bleeding as a result of your procedure?

   1 ☐ Yes
   2 ☐ No

21. Possible signs of infection include fever, swelling, heat, drainage or redness. Before you left the facility, did your doctor or anyone from the facility give you information about what to do if you had possible signs of infection?

   1 ☐ Yes, definitely
   2 ☐ Yes, somewhat
   3 ☐ No

22. At any time after leaving the facility, did you have any signs of infection?

   1 ☐ Yes
   2 ☐ No

Fig. 30.1 (continued)

d

V. Your Overall Experience

23. Using any number from 0 to 10, where 0 is the worst facility possible and 10 is the best facility possible, what number would you use to rate this facility?

☐ 0 Worst facility possible
☐ 1
☐ 2
☐ 3
☐ 4
☐ 5
☐ 6
☐ 7
☐ 8
☐ 9
☐ 10 Best facility possible

24. Would you recommend this facility to your friends and family?

1 ☐ Definitely no
2 ☐ Probably no
3 ☐ Probably yes
4 ☐ Definitely yes

VI. About You

25. In general, how would you rate your overall health?

1 ☐ Excellent
2 ☐ Very good
3 ☐ Good
4 ☐ Fair
5 ☐ Poor

26. In general, how would you rate your overall mental or emotional health?

1 ☐ Excellent
2 ☐ Very good
3 ☐ Good
4 ☐ Fair
5 ☐ Poor

27. What is your age?

1 ☐ 18 to 24
2 ☐ 25 to 34
3 ☐ 35 to 44
4 ☐ 45 to 54
5 ☐ 55 to 64
6 ☐ 65 to 74
7 ☐ 75 to 79
8 ☐ 80 to 84
9 ☐ 85 or older

28. Are you male or female?

1 ☐ Male
2 ☐ Female

29. What is the highest grade or level of school that you have completed?

1 ☐ 8th grade or less
2 ☐ Some high school, but did not graduate
3 ☐ High school graduate or GED
4 ☐ Some college or 2-year degree
5 ☐ 4-year college graduate
6 ☐ More than 4-year college degree

Fig. 30.1 (continued)

e

30. Are you of Hispanic, Latino, or Spanish origin?
   - 1 ☐ Yes, Hispanic, Latino, or Spanish
   - 2 ☐ No, not Hispanic, Latino, or Spanish → **If No, go to #32**

31. Which group best describes you?
   - 1 ☐ Mexican, Mexican American, Chicano
   - 2 ☐ Puerto Rican
   - 3 ☐ Cuban
   - 4 ☐ Another Hispanic, Latino, or Spanish origin

32. What is your race? You may select one or more categories.
   - 1 ☐ White
   - 2 ☐ Black or African American
   - 3 ☐ American Indian or Alaska Native
   - 4 ☐ Asian Indian
   - 5 ☐ Chinese
   - 6 ☐ Filipino
   - 7 ☐ Japanese
   - 8 ☐ Korean
   - 9 ☐ Vietnamese
   - 10 ☐ Other Asian
   - 11 ☐ Native Hawaiian
   - 12 ☐ Guamanian or Chamorro
   - 13 ☐ Samoan
   - 14 ☐ Other Pacific Islander

33. How well do you speak English?
   - 1 ☐ Very well
   - 2 ☐ Well
   - 3 ☐ Not well
   - 4 ☐ Not at all

34. Do you speak a language <u>other than English</u> at home?
   - 1 ☐ Yes
   - 2 ☐ No → **If No, go to #36**

35. What is that language?
   - 1 ☐ Spanish
   - 2 ☐ Other Language (PLEASE SPECIFY):

     ____
     (Please print.)

36. Did someone help you complete this survey?
   - 1 ☐ Yes
   - 2 ☐ No → **If No, go to END.**

37. How did that person help you? Check all that apply.
   - 1 ☐ Read the questions to me
   - 2 ☐ Wrote down the answers I gave
   - 3 ☐ Answered the questions for me
   - 4 ☐ Translated the questions into my language
   - 5 ☐ Helped in some other way: (EXPLAIN):

     ____
     (Please print.)
   - 6 ☐ No one helped me complete this survey

END

Fig. 30.1 (continued)

who are knowledgeable about pain management and skilled in postoperative pain control [51]. Interestingly, the inverse relationship between pain and patient satisfaction appears to reverse if physicians and nurses pay attention to pain and discuss pain treatment, which is evident with survey results showing high satisfaction despite high pain scores [49]. Therefore, patient satisfaction may better correlate with the overall experience of postoperative pain management, rather than the presence or severity of pain itself, which would be a potential area for targeted improvement.

Health care delivery has changed dramatically at the start of the twenty-first century through legislative imperative and economic drivers. The result is the shift from hospital-based surgery to ambulatory practice. The increasingly strong emphasis on providing high quality rather than high volume of care in an increasingly complex patient population further demands improvements in anesthetic and surgical technique. As modern health care evolves, the movement toward interdisciplinary cooperation and patient-focused care pathways will continue. Pain management services in ambulatory centers will be explored in the next section as an organic extension of this ongoing health care trend.

Section Key Points: How Health Care Has Influenced the Development of ASCs

- Health care legislation and initiatives have changed the medical care paradigm toward high-quality, cost-efficient health care through quality programs.
- There are many types of payment pathways available to financially incentivize care alignment with this new paradigm.
- Patients are overall receiving more procedural services requiring anesthesia, which is contributing to higher patient volume.
- There is additional economic pressure toward expanding more procedures and complex surgeries to ASCs.
- Quality improvement and financial opportunities may exist by reducing postoperative complications and improving patient satisfaction, which may both be addressed with pain management services.

The Evolution of Pain Management Services

Pain has been a common experience throughout human history. While its ascribed etiology has evolved with time and cultural context, the search for effective pain management is still ongoing. The utilization of opium, the natural precursor of morphine, for acute pain had been documented in early Sumerian culture and throughout Asia and Asia Minor during antiquity [55]. Likewise, evidence of medical topicalization using coca leaves, which derives the ester local anesthetic cocaine, has been found in ancient Peruvian graves [55]. Many modern analgesics and techniques may have surprisingly ancient origins.

By 1805, the first opioid, morphine, was isolated from opium and the early 1900s saw the creation of synthetic and semisynthetic opioids still used today and its widespread analgesic use and routes of administration [55]. Concurrently, there was the discovery of regional anesthesia techniques and development of local anesthetics [55].

History and Evolution of Acute Pain Services

Pain management did not begin to specifically formalize until the 1950s with the establishment of the Bellevue Hospital pain clinic by anesthesiologist Dr. Emery Rovenstine. In 1988, Dr. L. Brian Ready suggested an anesthesiology-based postoperative pain management – an acute pain service (APS) – and subsequently the practice of acute pain medicine developed. Interest further grew with the combined influence of legislative, financial, political, and clinical factors [56]. The adoption and microevolution of these organized anesthesiology-based acute pain services within a hospital system has been generalized in literature.

Many nascent hospital APSs originate from a user-dependent, pseudorandom utilization of regional anesthesia (RA or nerve blocks) as part of the intraoperative anesthetic plan from enthusiastic stakeholders or out of necessity (i.e., higher risk for morbidity or mortality with general anesthesia) [56]. Multimodal analgesic regimens may be incorporated with RA. Eventually, RA becomes the de facto plan and would next lead to formal, protocol-driven RA programs with ability to follow up ("rounding on") patients with the potential assistance of trained nurses [56]. Once this ability and capacity is reached, continuous management of acute pain beyond the operative setting (i.e., using continuous nerve block catheters) can occur [56].

This organized perioperative pain management service has important benefits to the hospital system regarding providing education and policies, lowering cost, improving patient perioperative throughput, and practicing variance reduction [56–58]. The introduction and implementation of enhanced recovery after surgery (ERAS) and other fast-track protocols has additionally cemented the utility of a hospital APS at this stage of its capability and potential direction for a transitional pain service model to manage pain through hospital discharge [57, 58]. An APS may further mature within a hospital system by providing comprehensive acute pain management consultation outside of the perioperative setting and direct pain therapy in cooperation with other specialized disciplines such as addiction medicine, psychiatry and psychology, palliative care, chronic pain, case managers, physical therapy, and rehabilitation [56, 58].

Ambulatory Pain Management

While APSs have been commonly discussed in the context of larger hospital systems or academic medical centers, private practices and ambulatory surgery centers also benefit from adopting pain management services. An ambulatory pain service is an organic extension of the APS concept into the ASC setting with much potential value. This will be explored in more detail in the next section.

Section Key Points: The Evolution of Acute Pain Services

- Acute Pain Services (APS) frequently have a common evolution within a health system.
- When a formalized, protocol-driven APS can sustain system-level efforts, such as Enhanced Recovery After Surgery, significant benefits may be achieved by the hospital and health system.
- A developed and sophisticated APS can drive coordinated, multidisciplinary care in pain management through the hospitalization process and potentially after discharge.
- Acute pain management services may be developed and specialized for ASC settings.

Pain Management Services at ASCs

With the outward migration of procedures to ambulatory sites due to a burgeoning demand and financial influences in health care, good pain control can potentially be a highly valuable provision at ASCs. The benefits gained from mandatory pain management services warrant serious consideration into such an investment.

Advantages of Pain Management Services

The advantages of acute pain management have been described primarily in hospital settings but seem to translate to ASCs as well. The exact model for delivering pain management services, whether utilizing an ambulatory pain specialist or a selected team of anesthesiologists heading the pain efforts, is dependent on several factors specific to the ASC including patient mix, culture, and infrastructure.

Clinical

The clinical advantages of a pain management service in the ASC setting are to address known complex patients, enhanced recovery pathways for routine cases, and patients with unexpected refractory postoperative pain. Furthermore, best practices of multimodal analgesia and regional techniques may be standardized and consistently implemented. Also, centralized pain management care may allow for systematic and appropriate escalations in care.

An increasing body of evidence supports routine use of multimodal analgesic regimens and incorporation of regional anesthesia techniques to produce faster recovery from anesthesia while also decreasing risk of anesthetic adverse effects, which would slow discharge and reducing overall opioid utilization – namely, ERAS programs. A designated ambulatory pain physician or service team would help with consistent implementation of the opioid-sparing mission in ERAS [26, 34].

Besides directing enhanced recovery protocols, the most obvious role of the ambulatory pain physician or team is in managing acute uncontrolled pain, a distressing and problematic postprocedural complication. This goal may be increasingly challenging in today's ambulatory patient population. Identification of patients who are at high risk for uncontrolled pain may be difficult, given the many factors contributing to pain. Additional efforts may be necessary to tailor, coordinate, and execute an effective pain management plan [34]. Further complicating this matter is the increasing prevalence of patients with preexisting chronic pain states, substance abuse, or (not infrequently) a concurrence of these two issues [59].

Chronic pain patients may be managed by multiple other physicians whose inputs may need to be reconciled with the perioperative environment [34]. They may have implanted pain devices or indwelling pain medication infusion that may affect the postoperative pain management plan [59]. Pain patients may also require significantly higher opioid doses compared to opioid-naïve patients, which often causes over-administration or under-administration of opioid medication, and may need evaluation for potential escalation of care (i.e., hospital admission) [59].

Ambulatory patients with a history of active substance abuse or participating in an opioid-deterrence program also require specialized evaluation and planning in their perioperative pain management. Ongoing abuse and illicit behavior would ideally be identified preoperatively. The patient should be encouraged to undergo substance abuse treatment program with drug testing and addiction counseling prior to surgery. Acute intoxication or chronic use can cause various cardiovascular, sympathetic, electrolyte, neurologic or psychological effects, depending on the specific substance abused, which can be worsened with anesthetics administration [60]. Conversely, substance abuse patients who are not optimized may risk withdrawal within the perioperative period [59].

Drug deterrence therapy with methadone or buprenorphine may create issues with pain control and drug interactions. The long and highly variable half-life of methadone may increase risk for respiratory depression [60], particularly with concurrent opioid administration as in the postoperative period. The partial opioid agonism of buprenorphine requires careful titration while bridging with perioperative opioids due to the risk for acute opioid withdrawal [59]. As with opioid-tolerant chronic pain patients, hyperalgesia and increased pain sensitivity make postoperative pain management difficult [59]. In addition, substance abuse frequently coexists with psychiatric and psychologic disorders, which further complicates pain control [59]. Unfortunately, there is also a high concurrence of opioid abuse and chronic pain therapy at 24% [60].

The dual benefit of specialized pain management services would be to provide centralized direction for enhanced recovery protocols as well as management of particularly challenging patient populations. Ambulatory providers are facing increasing number of these complex pain management patients [59].

Financial

There is a financial incentive for improving pain control and patient satisfaction and financial disincentive for costly expenditures or unnecessary additional care. Refer to the previous sections "Aligning provider payment with value-based health care", "Shift towards value-based health care in ASCs", and "Avoiding costly complications of ambulatory surgery" for specific details.

Pain management services in ASCs would be beneficial on multiple levels. Rapid patient throughput with ERAS or fast-track pathways improves efficiency, turnover, and patient volume. Also, reduction of costly expenditures, such as delay in discharge due to uncontrolled pain or postoperative nausea and vomiting from increasing doses of opioids, contributes by maximizing reimbursement payout. An ambulatory pain specialist may also evaluate high-risk patients for preoperative pain optimization or referral for inpatient admission, as well as assess refractory patients for appropriate interventions or to avoid any inappropriate escalations that come at a financial consequence to profit margins [34, 59].

Since reimbursement is tied to patient satisfaction (i.e., CAPHS survey), the financial gains from improved satisfaction and avoidance of dissatisfaction make pain management an important ambulatory service to have. Studies have shown positive effects on patient satisfaction with effective regional anesthesia usage and good pain control [48]. Patient satisfaction is associated with less acute care utilization [51]. Also, patients who had positive experiences with pain management and satisfaction are more likely to refer other potential patients, which creates new sources of revenue [51, 56]. With the current value-based trend in health care, having a robust pain management service incorporated into an ASC workflow would be a sound financial investment.

Educational and Administrative

The educational and administrative role filled by a pain management physician or team is also highly beneficial for ASCs. Patient education improves patient engagement and provides realistic expectations, which helps overall patient satisfaction and adherence to the care plan [51]. In addition, the pain physician or team helps to develop and implement standards of care, provide education to nurses and surgeons, and initiate quality improvement [56, 58, 59].

For complex patients with preexisting pain, opioid tolerance, or dependency issues, the pain management physician can facilitate care with multiple specialists as described above. Moreover, pain management services may also include consultation for assistance with the postoperative opioid weaning process, which can be difficult to navigate and without much established guidelines [61].

Societal

With the ongoing opioid crisis and concern for new opioid dependency, efforts to curb opioid reliance and mitigate conversion of acute to chronic postsurgical pain would be highly beneficial to society. The ASC pain physician can help by implementing opioid-sparing techniques, such as multimodal analgesia and regional options, reduce intraoperative opioid exposure with balanced anesthetic administration, and assist with postoperative opioid weaning.

Improving acute postoperative pain control and identifying patients at risk for prolonged postsurgical pain can further help to stymie the conversion to chronic pain, a significant morbidity and postoperative complication [56, 58, 61].

Although these mitigation efforts arguably have significant value to society and economic relief to health care, direct financial compensation has not been assigned to these endeavors at the current time. Nevertheless, there are still many direct advantages, as detailed above, for incorporation of mandatory pain management services at ASCs.

Considerations when Developing Pain Management Services

Important considerations while establishing pain management services include direct monetary expenses for specialized personnel and materials, indirect costs from time delays, and effort needed for operation restructuring. For patients, there may be additional personal costs and procedural risk.

Expected Direct Expenses

Expected costs for specialized human resources are necessary for pain management services and materials needed for the performance of regional anesthesia (RA). Ideally, an anesthesiologist with specific training in Regional Anesthesia and Acute Pain Management (RA/APM), advanced practice providers with pain management backgrounds, and nurses with block experience would be recruited.

Performance of nerve blocks requires one or several ultrasound machines, depending on RA volume, as well as block needle and kits, perineural catheters and their associated infusion device (if a catheter program is employed), and local anesthetics injected [56, 58]. Additional allocation of standard safety equipment for RA procedural areas may include monitors and resuscitation equipment. Ready availability of lipid emulsion (e.g. Intralipid™) would also be needed specifically for RA area.

Reducing Indirect Costs

Along with the direct expenses for acquiring trained personnel and purchasing equipment, is the need to select a staffing model and space to optimize cost-effectiveness. This depends on the expected RA volume and technical skill set available at the ASC, which requires detailed knowledge of assets and coordinated planning.

One option is for the OR anesthesiologist to perform the nerve blocks, and nerve catheter if applicable, in the operating room. No additional staff or specialist would be needed since the regional anesthesia and operative anesthesia are handled by the same anesthesia team. Unfortunately, surgical delays and schedule inefficiency may occur with this model since the surgery cannot start until the RA is completed and enough onset time is given [62]. In addition to the performing anesthesiologist's procedural skill and comfort level, the implicit and explicit time pressure contributes to failed blocks, which worsens surgeon and OR staff satisfaction with RA [58, 62].

Another staffing model that is popular particularly with high RA volumes is a dedicated RA procedural space ("block room") for RA to be performed in parallel with OR activities by an anesthesiologist trained or well-experienced in regional anesthesia [62]. This can relieve the time pressure and improve block success [56], but costs include allocating space and specialized team of regional anesthesiologist and trained nurses [62]. If well designed and properly resourced, the block room should not be a source of delay and can provide high-quality RA [62].

Having an anesthesiologist dedicated to perioperative RA/APM without billing for operative anesthesia services may be financially impractical in some cases such as smaller physician-only practices [58]; however, an anesthesia care-team approach may allow for more flexibility. Conversely, for high volume centers, a single dedicated RA/APM anesthesiologist may be insufficient, and so assistance from OR anesthesiologists may be needed [59]. The staffing model employed to facilitate RA performance requires understanding of available skills, ability to cross-train personnel, ASC total caseload, and RA volume.

For some ASCs, a nonOR procedural area might be preferred to perform RA (and potentially generate facility fees [62]) but having allocated block room may not be feasible. An alternative option might include a mobile "block cart" stocked with all requisite RA supplies, resuscitation equipment and monitors, and wheelable ultrasound machine [56]. Cross-utilization of space, such as utilizing the postanesthetic care unit (PACU) or preoperative holding area as the "block room" [58] is performed. Outfitting a specialized monitored area for RA and to administer higher doses of opioid or ketamine for complex or refractory pain management patients may be a consideration as well [58], depending on the typical patients served at the ASC (i.e., high frequency of patients with chronic pain, history of substance abuse, opioid deterrence therapy, or otherwise difficult to control pain).

Cost to Patients

Another concern is unexpected medical charges or "surprise" billing, which may place significant financial strain on the patient. Surprise billing may occur from several different scenarios: (1) a patient is taken to an out-of-network emergency room outside of his or her knowledge or control or receives emergency services without ability to confirm insurance coverage ahead of time, (2) a patient with a high deductible or high co-payment plan undergoes in-network services without realizing the high personal cost toward the deductible, and (3) a patient utilizes an in-network surgeon or proceduralist at an in-network facility but is surprised by bills from out-of-network providers associated with the procedure or subsequent complications [63]. The third scenario has garnered increasing media and bipartisan attention in the past decade.

The practice of "balanced billing" occurs when out-of-network clinicians bill the patient directly for the balance remaining for their charge minus the insurance payment [64]. Often these out-of-network providers are not selected by the patient or their involvement may not even be known to the patient prior to the procedure [64]. Approximately 1 in 5 cases receives surprise bills for elective surgeries performed by in-network surgeons and in-network facilities [64, 65]. Anesthesiologists were associated with the most frequent out-of-network claims at 37–39% of episodes [64, 65] along with surgical assistants (i.e., physician assistants, registered nurses, certified surgical assistants, and other surgeons) at 37% of episodes [64]. Surgical assistants had a higher mean potential balance bill than anesthesiologists at $1219 and $3633, respectively [64]. Nonphysician surgical assistants generate the largest potential surprise bill amount [64, 65]. Other sources for surprise charges may come from consultant physicians such as radiologists, pathologists, neurologists, or nonphysician providers such as durable medical equipment providers, physical therapists, and neuromonitoring providers [64, 65]. Surgical complications were associated with a higher risk of balanced billing [64]. The potential for surprise billing has been reported in 8% of episodes at in-network ASCs at an average of $1483 in 2017 [66]. Some health plans, particularly employer self-funded plans, seem to protect their enrolled patients from surprise bills at the collective expense of all enrollees [66].

As anesthesia services tend to be a common cause for out-of-network charges, patients may be at risk for inadvertent exposure to higher surprise charges – both from the operative anesthesia service and pain management services and consultation. Patient dissatisfaction may likely occur over the unexpected charges and subsequent billing reconciliation process. In addition, there is increasing demand for federal regulation of surprise billing, which may bring this practice under control through financial penalty and threat of regulatory auditing [67]. Therefore, efforts should be made to bring all physician and nonphysician practitioners within the ASC in-network to improve overall patient experience and mitigate liability risk to the ASC, especially if definitive legislative measures are passed.

Procedural Risks

There is the expected procedural risk to performing RA. The more serious adverse effects include local anesthetic systemic toxicity, accidental vascular puncture, pneumothorax, respiratory failure, and neurologic injury.

1. Local anesthetic systemic toxicity (LAST)

   LAST is a toxidrome caused by local anesthesia, usually from cumulative overadministration or direct vascular injection. It is characterized classically as a progression of excitatory and then inhibitory symptoms within the cardiovascular and neurologic systems, which may potentially culminate in refractory cardiac arrest and coma at its end stage. Fortunately, the occurrence of LAST is very low at 0.08–0.87 per 1000 based on large, multicentered studies [68, 69]. Ultrasound guidance appears to reduce the risk of LAST [69].

2. Unintended vascular puncture

   This complication may lead to hematoma formation or LAST if enough local anesthetic administration occurs prior to recognition. With ultrasound utilization, the incidence of venous and arterial trauma has been reported at 0.6 and 1.2 per 1000 blocks, respectively [68].

3. Pneumothorax

   Pneumothorax may be a complication of certain approaches to the brachial plexus nerve block or conceivably with any thoracic intervention (i.e., chest wall blocks, paravertebral or paraspinal blocks, or thoracic epidural placement). The incidence is also low at 6.6 per 10,000 peripheral nerve blocks if only considering those blocks with potential to cause pneumothorax [70].

4. Respiratory failure

   Respiratory failure may be a concern usually with central blockade or deep paraspinal blocks. One prospective survey found the incidence of acute respiratory failure at 0.6 per 10,000 nonobstetric spinal anesthetics and 5 per 1000 nonobstetric posterior lumbar plexus block likely from neuraxial spread [71]. Subjective dyspnea may occur with interscalene brachial plexus approaches in some patients [72].

5. Neurological injury

   Neurological injury after peripheral nerve block is another serious concern, which may lead to long-term morbidity. A prospective, multicentered clinical registry reported 0.9 per 1000 for postoperative neurological symptoms lasting beyond 6 months with ultrasound-guided regional anesthesia [68]. Similarly, data from the International Registry of Regional Anesthesia (IRORA) reported all-cause 60-day neurological injury at 8.3 per 10,000 [70].

While the performance of RA may potentially cause serious complication, those risks are fortunately uncommon. Widespread utility of ultrasound guidance in the hands of experienced individuals seems to minimize such risks.

The addition of RA/APM services to an ASC practice involves significant investment of time, money, and effort. It requires specialized personnel, resources, planning, and cooperation. Surgical delay may impede successful delivery of pain management services. However, if properly supported and well-designed, RA/APM services can be very cost-effective and highly beneficial to patients, ASC, and society.

Section Key Points: Pain Management Services in ASCs

- Robust ambulatory pain management services can create much clinical, financial, education, administrative, and societal benefits.
- A dedicated ambulatory pain physician (ideally with RA/APM training) can centralize protocolized care and appropriate necessary clinical interventions or escalations and provide expert management and guidance for complicated cases.
- There is time cost associated with pain management services, but a well-run pain setup should not create significant delay.
- Several factors specific to the ASC needs to be taken into consideration when selecting the staffing model and resource utilization to deliver efficient pain management services.
- Aligning all physician and nonphysician providers within the ASC and the facility itself under the same insurance networks will avoid potential problems arising from surprise medical charges.

Summary

In this chapter, we reviewed the effect of acute pain clinically, economically, and societally. When viewed through the context of U.S. health care, the significant impact of acute postoperative pain cannot be ignored. The continuous rise in patient demand for operative and procedural anesthesia services and emphasis on value-based care will further push increasingly complicated cases into the ambulatory setting. Development and implementation of an efficient pain management service within the ASC provides significant clinical and societal benefits, align with the expected trajectory of American health care, and can offer a great return on investment to all stakeholders.

Acknowledgements The author would like to thank Drs. Eldhose Abrahams, M.D. and Sarah Cartwright, D.N.P, MSN-PH for their assistance in the preparation of this chapter.

References

1. Cullen KA, Hall MJ, Golosinskiy A. Ambulatory surgery in the United States, 2006 [Internet]. Natl Health Stat Rep. 2009;(11):1–25. Hyattsville: National Center for Health Statistics. Available from https://www.cdc.gov/nchs/data/nhsr/nhsr011.pdf.
2. Hall MJ, Schwartzman A, Zhang J, Liu X. Ambulatory surgery data from hospitals and ambulatory surgery centers: United States, 2010 [Internet]. Natl Health Stat Rep. 2017;(102):1–15. Hyattsville: National Center for Health Statistics. Available from https://www.cdc.gov/nchs/data/nhsr/nhsr102.pdf.
3. MedPAC. Chapter 5: Ambulatory surgical center services [Internet]. In: Report to the congress: medicare payment policy. Washington, DC: MedPAC; 2019. Available at http://www.medpac.gov/docs/default-source/reports/mar19_medpac_ch5_sec.pdf?sfvrsn=0.
4. Rawal N, Hylander J, Nydahl PA, Olofsson I, Gupta A. Survey of postoperative analgesia following ambulatory surgery. Acta Anaesthesiol Scand. 1997;41(8):1017–22. https://doi.org/10.1111/j.1399-6576.1997.tb04829.x.
5. Beauregard L, Pomp A, Choinière M. Severity and impact of pain after day-surgery. Can J Anaesth. 1998;45(4):304–11. https://doi.org/10.1007/BF03012019.
6. McGrath B, Elgendy H, Chung F, Kamming D, Curti B, King S. Thirty percent of patients have moderate to severe pain 24 hr after ambulatory surgery: a survey of 5,703 patients. Can J Anaesth. 2004;51(9):886–91. https://doi.org/10.1007/BF03018885.
7. Gan TJ, Habib AS, Miller TE, White W, Apfelbaum JL. Incidence, patient satisfaction, and perceptions of post-surgical pain: results from a US national survey. Curr Med Res Opin. 2014;30(1):149–60. https://doi.org/10.1185/03007995.2013.860019.
8. Gan TJ. Poorly controlled postoperative pain: prevalence, consequences, and prevention. J Pain Res. 2017;10:2287–98. https://doi.org/10.2147/JPR.S144066.
9. Ghoneim MM, O'Hara MW. Depression and postoperative complications: an overview. BMC Surg. 2016;16:5. https://doi.org/10.1186/s12893-016-0120-y.
10. Pavlin DJ, Chen C, Penaloza DA, Buckley FP. A survey of pain and other symptoms that affect the recovery process after discharge from an ambulatory surgery unit. J Clin Anesth. 2004;16(3):200–6. https://doi.org/10.1016/j.jclinane.2003.08.004.
11. Dihle A, Helseth S, Paul SM, Miaskowski C. The exploration of the establishment of cutpoints to categorize the severity of acute postoperative pain. Clin J Pain. 2006;22(7):617–24. https://doi.org/10.1097/01.ajp.0000210905.57546.c1.
12. Brummett CM, Waljee JF, Goesling J, et al. New persistent opioid use after minor and major surgical procedures in US adults. JAMA Surg. 2017;152(6):e170504. https://doi.org/10.1001/jamasurg.2017.0504.
13. Zaveri S, Nobel TB, Khetan P, Divino CM. Risk of chronic opioid use in opioid-naïve and non-naïve patients after ambulatory surgery. J Gastrointest Surg. 2020;24(3):688–94. https://doi.org/10.1007/s11605-019-04265-2.
14. Kehlet H, Jensen TS, Woolf CJ. Persistent postsurgical pain: risk factors and prevention. Lancet. 2006;367(9522):1618–25. https://doi.org/10.1016/S0140-6736(06)68700-X.
15. Sun EC, Darnall BD, Baker LC, Mackey S. Incidence of and risk factors for chronic opioid use among opioid-naive patients in the postoperative period. JAMA Intern Med. 2016;176(9):1286–93. https://doi.org/10.1001/jamainternmed.2016.3298.
16. Centers for Disease Control and Prevention (CDC). Annual surveillance report of drug-related risks and outcomes: United States, 2019 [Internet]. Atlanta: National Center for Injury Prevention and Control, Center for Disease Control and Prevention; 2019. Available from https://www.cdc.gov/drugoverdose/pdf/pubs/2019-cdc-drug-surveillance-report.pdf
17. Florence CS, Zhou C, Luo F, Xu L. The economic burden of prescription opioid overdose, abuse, and dependence in the United States, 2013. Med Care. 2016;54(10):901–6. https://doi.org/10.1097/MLR.0000000000000625.
18. Gaskin DJ, Richard P. The economic costs of pain in the United States. J Pain. 2012;13(8):715–24. https://doi.org/10.1016/j.jpain.2012.03.009.
19. Centers for Medicare & Medicaid Services (CMS). NHE fact sheet. 2020. https://www.cms.gov/Research-Statistics-Data-and-Systems/Statistics-Trends-and-Reports/NationalHealthExpendData/NHE-Fact-Sheet. Accessed 20 Mar 2020.

20. Manchikanti L, Helm Ii S, Benyamin RM, Hirsch JA. A critical analysis of Obamacare: affordable care or insurance for many and coverage for few? Pain Physician. 2017;20(3):111–38.
21. Schneider EC, Sarnak DO, Squires D, Shah A, Doty MM. Mirror, Mirror 2017: international comparison reflects flaws and opportunities for better U.S. Health Care [Internet]. New York: The Commonwealth Fund; 2017. Available from https://interactives.commonwealthfund.org/2017/july/mirror-mirror/assets/Schneider_mirror_mirror_2017.pdf
22. Obama B. United States health care reform: progress to date and next steps. JAMA. 2016;316(5):525–32. https://doi.org/10.1001/jama.2016.9797.
23. Cox C, Semanskee A, Claxton G, Levitt L. Explaining health care reform: risk adjustment, reinsurance, and risk corridors. 2016. https://www.kff.org/health-reform/issue-brief/explaining-health-care-reform-risk-adjustment-reinsurance-and-risk-corridors/. Accessed 20 Mar 2020.
24. Russo A, Elixhauser A, Steiner C, Wier L. Hospital-based ambulatory surgery, 2007 [Internet], Healthcare cost and utilization project. Statistical brief #86. Rockville: Agency for Healthcare Research and Quality (AHRQ); 2010. Available from https://www.hcup-us.ahrq.gov/reports/statbriefs/sb86.pdf
25. Fosnot CD, Fleisher LA, Keogh J. Providing value in ambulatory anesthesia in 2015. Anesthesiol Clin. 2015;33(4):731–8. https://doi.org/10.1016/j.anclin.2015.07.011.
26. Afonso AM, Tokita HK, McCormick PJ, Twersky RS. Enhanced recovery programs in outpatient surgery. Anesthesiol Clin. 2019;37(2):225–38. https://doi.org/10.1016/j.anclin.2019.01.007.
27. Hollenbeck BK, Dunn RL, Suskind AM, Zhang Y, Hollingsworth JM, Birkmeyer JD. Ambulatory surgery centers and outpatient procedure use among Medicare beneficiaries. Med Care. 2014;52(10):926–31. https://doi.org/10.1097/MLR.0000000000000213.
28. Hollenbeck BK, Dunn RL, Suskind AM, Strope SA, Zhang Y, Hollingsworth JM. Ambulatory surgery centers and their intended effects on outpatient surgery. Health Serv Res. 2015;50(5):1491–507. https://doi.org/10.1111/1475-6773.12278.
29. Vaishnav AS, McAnany SJ. Future endeavors in ambulatory spine surgery. J Spine Surg. 2019;5(Suppl 2):S139–46. https://doi.org/10.21037/jss.2019.09.20.
30. Gologorsky Y. Outpatient spine surgery: transition to the ambulatory surgery center. World Neurosurg. 2018;114:369–70. https://doi.org/10.1016/j.wneu.2018.04.119.
31. Cancienne JM, Brockmeier SF, Gulotta LV, Dines DM, Werner BC. Ambulatory total shoulder arthroplasty: a comprehensive analysis of current trends, complications, readmissions, and costs. J Bone Joint Surg Am. 2017;99(8):629–37. https://doi.org/10.2106/JBJS.16.00287.
32. Banerjee S, Hamilton WG, Khanuja HS, Roberts JT. Outpatient lower extremity total joint arthroplasty: where are we heading? Orthopedics. 2017;40(2):72–5. https://doi.org/10.3928/01477447-20170302-02.
33. Nassiri F, Li L, Badhiwala JH, et al. Hospital costs associated with inpatient versus outpatient awake craniotomy for resection of brain tumors. J Clin Neurosci. 2019;59:162–6. https://doi.org/10.1016/j.jocn.2018.10.110.
34. Thomas DA, Chang D, Zhu R, Rayaz H, Vadivelu N. Concept of the ambulatory pain physician. Curr Pain Headache Rep. 2017;21(1):7. https://doi.org/10.1007/s11916-017-0611-2.
35. Stead SW, Merrick SK. Bundled payments and hidden costs. Anesthesiol Clin. 2018;36(2):241–58. https://doi.org/10.1016/j.anclin.2018.01.005.
36. Merrill DG. Value-based payment in ambulatory anesthesia: MACRA, MIPS, and more. Anesthesiol Clin. 2019;37(2):373–88. https://doi.org/10.1016/j.anclin.2019.01.011.
37. American Society of Anesthesiologists (ASA). The Merit-based Incentive Payment System (MIPS). 2020. https://www.asahq.org/macra/qualitypayment-program/mips/. Accessed 20 Mar 2020.
38. American Society of Anesthesiologists (ASA). Alternative payment model (APM). 2020. https://www.asahq.org/macra/qualitypaymentprogram/apms. Accessed 20 Mar 2020.
39. Quality Payment Program (QPP). APMs overview. 2019. https://qpp.cms.gov/apms/overview. Accessed 20 Mar 2020.
40. Anesthesia Quality Institute (AQI). 2020 QCDR measure specifications [Internet], National Anesthesia Clinical Outcomes Registry; Version 1.01. Illinois: American Quality Institute, American Society of Anesthesiologists; 2020. Available from https://www.aqihq.org/files/MIPS/2020/2020%20QCDR%20Measure%20Book.pdf.
41. NEJM Catalyst. What are bundled payments? 2018. https://catalyst.nejm.org/doi/full/10.1056/CAT.18.0247. Accessed 20 Mar 2020.
42. Wilson T, Gollogly S. Bundled payments for ambulatory surgery have the potential to Foster increased transparency, improved outcomes, lower costs, and increased capacity for health care systems. Health Econ Outcome Res. 2017;3:S1–105. https://doi.org/10.4172/2471-268X.1000.S1-105.
43. Makanji HS, Bilolikar VK, Goyal DKC, Kurd MF. Ambulatory surgery center payment models: current trends and future directions. J Spine Surg. 2019;5(Suppl 2):S191–4. https://doi.org/10.21037/jss.2019.08.07.
44. Curtin CM, Hernandez-Boussard T. Readmissions after treatment of distal radius fractures. J Hand Surg Am. 2014;39(10):1926–32. https://doi.org/10.1016/j.jhsa.2014.07.041.

45. Liu J, Flynn DN, Liu WM, Fleisher LA, Elkassabany NM. Hospital-based acute care within 7 days of discharge after outpatient arthroscopic shoulder surgery. Anesth Analg. 2018;126(2):600–5. https://doi.org/10.1213/ANE.0000000000002188.
46. Liu J, Kim DH, Maalouf DB, Beathe JC, Allen AA, Memtsoudis SG. Thirty-day acute health care resource utilization following outpatient anterior cruciate ligament surgery. Reg Anesth Pain Med. 2018;43(8):849–53. https://doi.org/10.1097/AAP.0000000000000839.
47. Elkassabany NM, Wang A, Ochroch J, Mattera M, Liu J, Kuntz A. Improved quality of recovery from ambulatory shoulder surgery after implementation of a multimodal perioperative pain management protocol. Pain Med. 2019;20(5):1012–9. https://doi.org/10.1093/pm/pny152.
48. Malchow RJ, Gupta RK, Shi Y, Shotwell MS, Jaeger LM, Bowens C. Comprehensive analysis of 13,897 consecutive regional anesthetics at an ambulatory surgery center. Pain Med. 2018;19(2):368–84. https://doi.org/10.1093/pm/pnx045.
49. Teunkens A, Vanhaecht K, Vermeulen K, et al. Measuring satisfaction and anesthesia related outcomes in a surgical day care centre: a three-year single-centre observational study. J Clin Anesth. 2017;43:15–23. https://doi.org/10.1016/j.jclinane.2017.09.007.
50. Lin CJ, Williams BA. Postoperative nausea and vomiting in ambulatory regional anesthesia. Int Anesthesiol Clin. 2011;49(4):134–43. https://doi.org/10.1097/AIA.0b013e318216bf9c.
51. Trinh LN, Fortier MA, Kain ZN. Primer on adult patient satisfaction in perioperative settings. Perioper Med (Lond). 2019;8:11. Published 2019 Sep 19. https://doi.org/10.1186/s13741-019-0122-2.
52. Agency for Healthcare Research and Quality (AHRQ). CAHPS: assessing healthcare quality from the patient's perspective [Internet], Agency for Healthcare Research and Quality; Pub. No. 19(20)-M028. Rockville: Agency for Healthcare Research and Quality; 2020. Available from https://www.ahrq.gov/sites/default/files/wysiwyg/cahps/about-cahps/cahps-program-brief.pdf
53. Centers for Medicare & Medicaid Services (CMS). Outpatient and Ambulatory Surgery CAHPS (OAS CAHPS). 2020. https://www.cms.gov/Research-Statistics-Data-and-Systems/Research/CAHPS/OAS-CAHPS. Accessed 20 Mar 2020.
54. Outpatient and Ambulatory Surgery CAHPS Survey. 2020. https://oascahps.org/. Accessed 20 Mar 2020.
55. Sabatowski R, Schäfer D, Kasper SM, Brunsch H, Radbruch L. Pain treatment: a historical overview. Curr Pharm Des. 2004;10(7):701–16. https://doi.org/10.2174/1381612043452974.
56. Upp J, Kent M, Tighe PJ. The evolution and practice of acute pain medicine. Pain Med. 2013;14(1):124–44. https://doi.org/10.1111/pme.12015.
57. Stamer UM, Liguori GA, Rawal N. Thirty-five years of acute pain services: where do we go from here? Anesth Analg. 2020;131(2):650–6. https://doi.org/10.1213/ANE.0000000000004655.
58. Webb CAJ, Kim TE. Establishing an acute pain service in private practice and updates on regional anesthesia billing. Anesthesiol Clin. 2018;36(3):333–44. https://doi.org/10.1016/j.anclin.2018.04.005.
59. Vadivelu N, Kai AM, Kodumudi V, Berger JM. Challenges of pain control and the role of the ambulatory pain specialist in the outpatient surgery setting. J Pain Res. 2016;9:425–35. Published 2016 Jun 17. https://doi.org/10.2147/JPR.S86579.
60. Vadivelu N, Kai AM, Kodumudi V, Zhu R, Hines R. Pain management of patients with substance abuse in the ambulatory setting. Curr Pain Headache Rep. 2017;21(2):9. https://doi.org/10.1007/s11916-017-0610-3.
61. Roth B, Boateng A, Berken A, Carlyle D, Vadivelu N. Post-operative weaning of opioids after ambulatory surgery: the importance of physician stewardship. Curr Pain Headache Rep. 2018;22(6):40. Published 2018 May 3. https://doi.org/10.1007/s11916-018-0694-4.
62. Gray CF, Smith C, Zasimovich Y, Tighe PJ. Economic considerations of acute pain medicine programs. Tech Orthop. 2017;32(4):217–25. https://doi.org/10.1097/BTO.0000000000000241.
63. Sutton JH. Health care networks: surprise billings for surgical patients. Bull Am Coll Surg. 2016;101(7):19–23.
64. Chhabra KR, Sheetz KH, Nuliyalu U, Dekhne MS, Ryan AM, Dimick JB. Out-of-network bills for privately insured patients undergoing elective surgery with in-network primary surgeons and facilities. JAMA. 2020;323(6):538–47. https://doi.org/10.1001/jama.2019.21463.
65. Dekhne MS, Nuliyalu U, Schoenfeld AJ, Dimick JB, Chhabra KR. "Surprise" out-of-network billing in orthopedic surgery: charges from surprising sources. Ann Surg. 2020;271(5):e116–8. https://doi.org/10.1097/SLA.0000000000003825.
66. Duffy EL, Adler L, Ginsburg PB, Trish E. Prevalence and characteristics of surprise out-of-network bills from professionals in ambulatory surgery centers. Health Aff. 2020;39(5):783–90. https://doi.org/10.1377/hlthaff.2019.01138.
67. Relias Media. Legislation aimed at surprise billing could bring liabilities. 2019. https://www.reliasmedia.com/articles/144970-legislation-aimed-at-surprise-billing-could-bring-liabilities. Accessed 25 May 2020.
68. Sites BD, Taenzer AH, Herrick MD, et al. Incidence of local anesthetic systemic toxicity and postoperative neurologic symptoms associated with 12,668 ultrasound-guided nerve blocks: an analysis from a prospective clinical registry. Reg Anesth Pain

Med. 2012;37(5):478–82. https://doi.org/10.1097/AAP.0b013e31825cb3d6.

69. Barrington MJ, Kluger R. Ultrasound guidance reduces the risk of local anesthetic systemic toxicity following peripheral nerve blockade. Reg Anesth Pain Med. 2013;38(4):289–99. https://doi.org/10.1097/AAP.0b013e318292669b.

70. Sites BD, Barrington MJ, Davis M. Using an international clinical registry of regional anesthesia to identify targets for quality improvement. Reg Anesth Pain Med. 2014;39(6):487–95. https://doi.org/10.1097/AAP.0000000000000162.

71. Auroy Y, Benhamou D, Bargues L, et al. Major complications of regional anesthesia in France: the SOS Regional Anesthesia Hotline Service. Anesthesiology. 2002;97(5):1274–80. https://doi.org/10.1097/00000542-200211000-00034.

72. Marhofer P, Anderl W, Heuberer P, et al. A retrospective analysis of 509 consecutive interscalene catheter insertions for ambulatory surgery. Anaesthesia. 2015;70(1):41–6. https://doi.org/10.1111/anae.12840.

31 New Vistas in Ambulatory Postoperative Pain Management

Kunal R. Sinha, Melissa E. Phuphanich, Nirmal Gosalia, Anh L. Ngo, Mitchell C. Fuller, and Alan David Kaye

Abstract

Postoperative analgesia care is a rapidly expanding field of medicine that includes traditional pharmacotherapy as well as many nonpharmacologic approaches. The nonpharmacologic field is an exciting frontier for anesthesiologists to utilize in an attempt to optimize pain control, decrease healthcare costs, and improve patient satisfaction in the new age of patient-centered care. This chapter discusses new and upcoming vistas in this direction.

K. R. Sinha · M. E. Phuphanich
Department of Physical Medicine and Rehabilitation, UCLA/Greater Los Angeles VA Health Care System, Los Angeles, CA, USA

David Geffen School of Medicine at UCLA, University of California, Los Angeles, CA, USA

N. Gosalia
Department of Internal Medicine, AMITA Health Saint Francis Hospital, Evanston, IL, USA

A. L. Ngo
Pain Specialty Group, Newington, NH, USA

M. C. Fuller (✉)
Medical College of Wisconsin, Wauwatosa, WI, USA
e-mail: mfuller@mcw.edu

A. D. Kaye
Departments of Anesthesiology and Pharmacology, Toxicology, and Neurosciences, Louisiana State University Health Shreveport, Shreveport, LA, USA

Postoperative Pain Management

Postoperative pain management is one of the most important and challenging aspects of perioperative care, particularly in ambulatory surgical centers. Up to 80% of patients experience moderate to severe postsurgical pain [1], which is often poorly controlled [2]. This deficit is highly concerning because inadequate postoperative pain control is associated with delayed postoperative discharge [3, 4], increased morbidity, and increased risk of chronic opioid use following surgery [5].

Multimodal Approach to Pain Control

The goals of postoperative pain management are: (1) to achieve adequate pain control and (2) to minimize the adverse side effects of analgesic modalities, such as postoperative nausea and vomiting (PONV) and urinary retention. Postoperative pain has been traditionally managed with opioids using a unimodal approach until a recent confluence of factors led to a paradigm shift. Factors including the current opioid crisis, the multitude of adverse effects associated with opioid use, and the implementation of Enhanced Recovery After Surgery (ERAS) protocols have advanced postoperative pain control to a multimodal approach that minimizes opioid use. Multimodal analgesia is a personalized

K. Rajput et al. (eds.), *Pain Control in Ambulatory Surgery Centers*,
https://doi.org/10.1007/978-3-030-55262-6_31

approach to pain management that combines opioid and nonopioid medications, topical anesthetics, interventional procedures, and nonpharmacologic treatments. The multimodal approach begins well before the surgery and continues into the postoperative recovery phase. Combining various techniques with distinct mechanisms of action not only has a synergistic analgesic effect but also minimizes reliance on any one specific agent, thereby reducing the potential for adverse reactions to that agent [6].

Optimizing Postoperative Analgesia with Liposomal Bupivacaine

Effective postoperative pain management begins prior to surgery with patient education [7, 8] and premedication, as described in detail in previous sections [8]. Liposomal bupivacaine is FDA approved for preoperative interscalene brachial plexus nerve blocks, an efficacious strategy to reduce postoperative pain after shoulder surgery. Liposomal bupivacaine is also used intraoperatively for infiltration of the surgical wound with local anesthetic. In this regard, this long-acting local anesthetic is utilized off label in a variety of settings to extend analgesia postoperatively. These cost-effective techniques have been widely used by surgeons and anesthesiologists to control pain while minimizing the need for systemic anesthesia [9]. There is strong evidence that these nonopiate treatments are as safe and effective as other conventional analgesic modalities [10], though further studies are required to demonstrate superiority [11].

Nonopioid Pain Medications

A variety of nonopioid analgesic medications from different classes are commonly used in the postoperative period. The American Pain Society strongly recommends acetaminophen, nonsteroidal anti-inflammatory drugs (NSAIDs), and gabapentinoids to improve postoperative pain and decrease opioid consumption [8]. Acetaminophen and NSAIDs are more effective when used in conjunction than when used individually [12]. NSAIDs are conveniently available in oral, intramuscular, and (less commonly) intravenous formulations. Intramuscular administration of NSAIDs is discouraged when oral administration is possible [8]. COX-2 selective NSAIDs are more expensive but have a lower risk of gastrointestinal complications [13]. All NSAIDs, including both COX-2 selective and nonselective COX inhibitors, are associated with an increased dose-dependent risk of myocardial infarction [14]. Moreover, the increased risk of bleeding and impaired bone healing [15] with NSAIDs may preclude the use of these agents in selected patients. Of note, gabapentin carries an FDA warning for respiratory depression in the elderly, in patients with chronic pulmonary conditions, and in patients concurrently using other respiratory depressants such as opioids or benzodiazepines [16].

Appropriate Use of Opioids

Despite the shift toward opioid-sparing therapies, opioids remain an important component of postoperative pain management in many cases. Literature shows that in the inpatient setting, if parenteral opioid administration is required, patient-controlled analgesia (PCA) is preferred [8, 17]. A Cochrane review published in 2015 found that patients treated with PCA versus non-PCA opioid analgesia postoperatively demonstrated lower pain scores, higher patient satisfaction scores, and similar rates of serious adverse effects despite higher total opioid consumption [17]. Limited literature exists to review the efficacy of PCA in the ambulatory setting, although moderate to severe postoperative pain could potentially be controlled using a PCA approach in the postsurgical home model with standardized questionnaires (e.g, connect, introduce, communicate, ask, respond, and exit CICARE) [18, 19]. The main concern for transitioning into routine use of PCA opioids in the outpatient setting is the significant risk for respiratory depression, PONV, urinary retention, delayed discharge, and rarely death. Thus, in addition to standardized questionnaires, patients prescribed opioid-based therapies should be thoroughly educated on these risks, be monitored for adverse effects, and be discharged with a clear tapering schedule and follow-up plan [8]. Ultimately, there will always be an appropriate role for judicious opioid administration in the ambulatory surgery center, and repurposing of the PCA entity may cultivate a new future for postoperative home opioids.

Ambulatory Pain Specialists

The aforementioned importance and challenges of effective postoperative pain management, coupled with the increasing number and complexity of ambulatory surgeries performed in the United States, have led to a growing interest in including ambulatory pain specialists in ASCs [20]. Such ambulatory pain physicians coordinate care that is traditionally divided among general anesthetists, regional anesthetists, acute pain specialists, and chronic pain specialists. The responsibilities of these providers include: identifying patients at high risk for increased postsurgical pain and/or opioid dependence, using multimodal analgesia perioperatively, treating postoperative complications of anesthesia, and crucially, implementing a postdischarge follow-up plan that minimizes the risk of opioid dependence [21].

Nonpharmacologic Pain Management and New Vistas

In addition to opioid and nonopioid analgesic medications, nonpharmacologic modalities may be incorporated into a multimodal strategy to control postoperative pain [8, 22]. These interventions are appealing because they are generally considered to be safe, and some have been shown to be useful for treating chronic pain [23]. However, evidence of their effectiveness for treating postoperative pain is mixed [8]. One of the most promising new therapies for postoperative pain involves peripheral nerve stimulation. This builds on the relatively new techniques that have rapidly become common place utilizing ultrasound-guided nerve blocks and described in previous chapters. Peripheral nerve stimulation has been demonstrated in relatively small studies to be highly effective and significantly reduces opioid consumption postoperatively. Several studies at present involving multiple companies that are developing slightly different technologies for peripheral nerve stimulation are ongoing and will dramatically change the way postoperative pain is managed, if proven effective.

Other technologies have been studied and have mixed results in the setting of acute pain management in the postoperative period. The American Pain Society offers a weak recommendation for the use of transcutaneous electrical stimulation (TENS) and cognitive-behavioral therapies; it neither recommends nor discourages acupuncture, massage, or cold therapy [8].

TENS

Transcutaneous electrical nerve stimulation (TENS) delivers small electrical pulses to peripheral nerves via electrodes placed on the skin [24]. These electrical impulses flood the various targets in the central and peripheral nervous systems including mu-opioid receptors and reduce their ability to transmit nociceptive signals to the spinal cord and brain [25]. Research studies show mixed results, but generally support the use of TENS for postoperative pain control [26–28]. TENS is contraindicated in patients with pacemakers or other electrical cardiac devices, and TENS leads should only be placed on intact skin without lymphedema [8].

Cognitive Behavioral Therapies

Cognitive behavioral modalities including guided relaxation, hypnosis, and music therapy are used to reduce pain and anxiety in the perioperative setting. These modalities are generally effective, but there is insufficient evidence to conclude superiority of one specific cognitive behavioral intervention over the others. The safety of these interventions has also not been tested in children [8].

Acupuncture

Acupuncture originates in ancient Chinese medicine and has evolved as a modern alternative medicine used to treat millions of Americans. Needles are inserted at strategic sites of the body, with or without electrical stimulation, to activate nerves. It is thought that the needles act on neurohormonal pathways and lead to the release of various neurotransmitters including beta-endorphins, which increase the pain threshold [29].

Acupuncture is a safe and efficacious treatment for chronic pain in the outpatient setting [23], but evidence for its role in postoperative pain management is less clear. Some studies demonstrate promising results. For example, a recent meta-analysis of 13 randomized controlled trials (RCTs) suggests that various types of acupuncture may reduce acute pain and opiate use in the first postoperative day [30]. However, other RCTs, particularly studies on auricular acupuncture, a form of acupuncture targeting sites only in the ear, were unable to demonstrate this association [31, 32]. Local pain and nausea are among the most common associated adverse effects. Serious complications such as pneumothorax and severe infection are rare [33] and may be prevented with cautious needle placement in the thorax and avoidance of acupuncture in those with active infection, particularly at potential needle insertion sites.

Music Therapy

The theory of complex pain pathways posits that there are both psychologic and physiologic components. While most of the attention is given to physiologic modulation with multimodal analgesia, a new age of interest is being generated around the psychological phenomena. The safety and efficacy of music therapy use as an adjuvant in the postoperative period have been controversially debated in literature review. In a study of 12 subjects, nearly two thirds of the group said they felt music decreased their pain and 11 of the 12 subjects said they would recommend music as adjuvant therapy [34]. Another study investigated 50 subjects undergoing outpatient orthopedic surgery, half acting as a control group without music therapy and half serving as an experimental group exposed to music therapy. This study by Chiodo et al. found no statistically significant difference ($p = 0.94$ for hospital quality scale and $p = 0.88$ for visual analogue scale) between the control and experimental groups [35]. Further research has suggested a modest efficacy and extraordinarily safe profile for adjunctive music therapy, claiming a positive effect on pain relief, anxiety, and depression in both the acute and chronic complex pain settings [36, 37]. The feasibility of including personalized music therapy into the perioperative course remains a limitation, although with a growing evidence, basis future clinical guidelines may incorporate music as a routine adjuvant option.

Other Nonpharmacologic Treatments

A range of additional nonpharmacologic modalities including heat therapy, cryotherapy, bracing, acupressure, meditation, and massage have been investigated, but there is a lack of quality evidence to make formal recommendations [8, 22].

Postsurgical Home Model

Perhaps most critically, it is more imperative than ever for researchers and pain clinicians to incorporate novel SMS texting platforms in order to track and regulate patient satisfaction [38, 39]. A postsurgical home model following rapid patient stabilization and discharge will combat a paradigm of fragmented patient care with the classic "lost to follow-up" by increasing percent response rates, thereby increasing anesthesia accountability for pain control after PACU care. The postsurgical home model will also advance the patient-centered care model by improving patient satisfaction, optimizing patient cost, and maximizing the value of care.

Summary

Postoperative pain control in the ambulatory surgery center setting remains a challenge in the United States. A transformation to opioid sparing multimodal analgesia is well underway; moreover, when opioids are administered, they should be done so under well-controlled guidelines, as with the patient-controlled pump. Additional evidence continues to build in favor of adjuvant nonpharmacologic methods such as TENS, CBT, acupuncture, and music therapy among a myriad of others. There is not yet convincing evidence in favor of nonpharmacologic therapies as a unimodal approach, but there is evidence suggesting their utility as supplemental antinociceptives, anxiolytics, and antidepressants, as well as tremendous tools for limiting chronic complex pain pathways.

References

1. Meissner W, Zaslansky R. A survey of postoperative pain treatments and unmet needs. Best Pract Res Clin Anaesthesiol. 2019;33(3):269–86. https://doi.org/10.1016/j.bpa.2019.10.003.
2. Gan TJ, Habib AS, Miller TE, White W, Apfelbaum JL. Incidence, patient satisfaction, and perceptions of post-surgical pain: results from a US national survey. Curr Med Res Opin. 2014;30(1):149–60. https://doi.org/10.1185/03007995.2013.860019.
3. Pavlin DJ, Chen C, Penaloza DA, Polissar NL, Buckley FP. Pain as a factor complicating recovery and discharge after ambulatory surgery. Anesth Analg. 2002;95(3):627–34. https://doi.org/10.1097/00000539-200209000-00025.
4. Rae A. Reasons for delayed patient discharge following day surgery: a literature review. Nurs Stand. 2016;31(11):42–51. https://doi.org/10.7748/ns.2016.e10292.
5. Gan TJ. Poorly controlled postoperative pain: prevalence, consequences, and prevention. J Pain Res. 2017;10:2287–98. https://doi.org/10.2147/JPR.S144066.
6. Prabhakar A, Cefalu JN, Rowe JS, Kaye AD, Urman RD. Techniques to optimize multimodal analgesia in ambulatory surgery. Curr Pain Headache Rep. 2017;21(5):1–6. https://doi.org/10.1007/s11916-017-0622-z.
7. O'Donnell KF. Preoperative pain management education: a quality improvement project. J Perianesth Nurs. 2015;30(3):221–7. https://doi.org/10.1016/j.jopan.2015.01.013.
8. Chou R, Gordon DB, De Leon-Casasola OA, et al. Management of postoperative pain: a clinical practice guideline from the American pain society, the American society of regional anesthesia and pain medicine, and the American society of anesthesiologists' committee on regional anesthesia, executive commi. J Pain. 2016;17(2):131–57. https://doi.org/10.1016/j.jpain.2015.12.008.
9. Lanitis S, Karkoulias K, Sgourakis G, Brotzakis P, Armoutides V, Karaliotas C. The late effect of intraoperative wound infiltration with local anaesthetic in surgical patients; is there any? A randomized control trial. Int J Surg. 2015;20:35–40. https://doi.org/10.1016/j.ijsu.2015.05.053.
10. Dasta J, Ramamoorthy S, Patou G, Sinatra R. Bupivacaine liposome injectable suspension compared with bupivacaine HCl for the reduction of opioid burden in the postsurgical setting. Curr Med Res Opin. 2012;28(10):1609–15. https://doi.org/10.1185/03007995.2012.721760.
11. Hamilton TW, Athanassoglou V, Mellon S, et al. Liposomal bupivacaine infiltration at the surgical site for the management of postoperative pain. Cochrane Database Syst Rev. 2017;2017(2):CD011419. https://doi.org/10.1002/14651858.CD011419.pub2.
12. Derry CJ, Derry S, Moore RA. Single dose oral ibuprofen plus paracetamol (acetaminophen) for acute postoperative pain. Cochrane Database Syst Rev. 2013;2017(10):CD010210. https://doi.org/10.1002/14651858.CD010210.pub2.
13. Faich G, Goldstein JL, Simon LS, et al. Gastrointestinal toxicity witeh celecoxib vs nonsteroidal anti-inflammatory drugs for osteoarthritis and rheumatoid arthritis. JAMA. 2000;284(10):1247–55.
14. Bally M, Dendukuri N, Rich B, et al. Risk of acute myocardial infarction with NSAIDs in real world use: Bayesian meta-analysis of individual patient data. BMJ. 2017;357:j1909. https://doi.org/10.1136/bmj.j1909.
15. Wheatley BM, Nappo KE, Christensen DL, Holman AM, Brooks DI, Potter BK. Effect of NSAIDs on bone healing rates: a meta-analysis. J Am Acad Orthop Surg. 2019;27(7):e330–6. https://doi.org/10.5435/JAAOS-D-17-00727.
16. FDA warns about serious breathing problems with seizure and nerve pain medicines gabapentin (Neurontin, Gralise, Horizant) and pregabalin (Lyrica, Lyrica CR)|FDA.
17. Mcnicol ED, Ferguson MC, Hudcova J. Patient controlled opioid analgesia versus non-patient controlled opioid analgesia for postoperative pain. Cochrane Database Syst Rev. 2015;2015(6):CD003348. https://doi.org/10.1002/14651858.CD003348.pub3.
18. Chuang CC, Lee CC, Wang LK, et al. An innovative nonpharmacological intervention combined with intravenous patient-controlled analgesia increased patient global improvement in pain and satisfaction after major surgery. Neuropsychiatr Dis Treat. 2017;13:1033–42. https://doi.org/10.2147/NDT.S131517.

19. Assouline B, Tramèr MR, Kreienbühl L, Elia N. Benefit and harm of adding ketamine to an opioid in a patient-controlled analgesia device for the control of postoperative pain. Pain. 2016;157(12):2854–64. https://doi.org/10.1097/j.pain.0000000000000705.
20. Thomas DA, Chang D, Zhu R, Rayaz H, Vadivelu N. Concept of the ambulatory pain physician. Curr Pain Headache Rep. 2017;21(1):7. https://doi.org/10.1007/s11916-017-0611-2.
21. Vadivelu N, Kai AM, Kodumudi V, Berger JM. Challenges of pain control and the role of the ambulatory pain specialist in the outpatient surgery setting. J Pain Res. 2016;9:425–35. https://doi.org/10.2147/JPR.S86579.
22. American Society of Anesthesiologists. Practice guidelines for acute pain management in the perioperative setting: an updated report by the american society of anesthesiologists task force on acute pain management. Anesthesiology. 2012;116(2):248–73. https://doi.org/10.1097/ALN.0b013e31823c1030.
23. Vickers AJ, Cronin AM, Maschino AC, et al. Acupuncture for chronic pain: individual patient data meta-analysis. Arch Intern Med. 2012;172(19):1444–53. https://doi.org/10.1001/archinternmed.2012.3654.
24. Zhu Y, Feng Y, Peng L. Effect of transcutaneous electrical nerve stimulation for pain control after total knee arthroplasty: a systematic review and meta-analysis. J Rehabil Med. 2017;49(9):700–4. https://doi.org/10.2340/16501977-2273.
25. DeSantana JM, Walsh DM, Vance C, Rakel BA, Sluka KA. Effectiveness of transcutaneous electrical nerve stimulation for treatment of hyperalgesia and pain. Curr Rheumatol Rep. 2008;10(6):492–9. https://doi.org/10.1007/s11926-008-0080-z.
26. Elboim-Gabyzon M, Najjar SA, Shtarker H. Effects of transcutaneous electrical nerve stimulation (TENS) on acute postoperative pain intensity and mobility after hip fracture: a double blinded, randomized trial. Clin Interv Aging. 2019;14:1841–50. https://doi.org/10.2147/CIA.S203658.
27. Husch HH, Watte G, Zanon M, et al. Effects of transcutaneous electrical nerve stimulation on pain, pulmonary function, and respiratory muscle strength after posterolateral thoracotomy: a randomized controlled trial. Lung. 2020;198(2):345–53. https://doi.org/10.1007/s00408-020-00335-4.
28. Johnson MI. Transcutaneous electrical nerve stimulation (TENS) as an adjunct for pain management in perioperative settings: a critical review. Expert Rev Neurother. 2017;17(10):1013–27. https://doi.org/10.1080/14737175.2017.1364158.
29. Cabýoglu MT, Ergene N, Tan U. The mechanism of acupuncture and clinical applications. Int J Neurosci. 2006;116(2):115–25. https://doi.org/10.1080/00207450500341472.
30. Wu MS, Chen KH, Chen IF, et al. The efficacy of acupuncture in post-operative pain management: a systematic review and meta-analysis. PLoS One. 2016;11(3):e0150367. https://doi.org/10.1371/journal.pone.0150367.
31. Plunkett A, McCoart A, Howard RS, Dennison E, Bartoszek M. A randomized, single-blind, prospective trial of auricular "battlefield" acupuncture for the reduction of postoperative tonsillectomy pain in adults. Pain Manag. 2018;8(4):287–95. https://doi.org/10.2217/pmt-2018-0007.
32. Deng G, Rusch V, Vickers A, et al. Randomized controlled trial of a special acupuncture technique for pain after thoracotomy. J Thorac Cardiovasc Surg. 2008;136(6):1464–9. https://doi.org/10.1016/j.jtcvs.2008.07.053.
33. Kelly RB, Willis J. Acupuncture for pain. Am Fam Physician. 2019;100(2):89–96.
34. Radcliffe J, Porterfield S. Music therapy and post-operative pain. Florida State University Archives. https://diginole.lib.fsu.edu/islandora/object/fsu%3A550173/. Accessed 4 June 2020.
35. Chiodo CP, Keyser C, Palms D, Malone C, Bluman EM, Smith JT. The impact of music therapy in the postoperative setting on overall patient satisfaction using validated outcome scores. J Perianesthesia Nurs. 2019;34(2):354–8. https://doi.org/10.1016/j.jopan.2018.04.006.
36. Al Wattar BH, Keay SD. Music therapy to optimise postoperative pain management: how much more evidence is needed? BJOG. 2020;127(6):746. https://doi.org/10.1111/1471-0528.16166.
37. Ilan S, Christensen E. Perspectives on Music Imagery and complex chronic pain. Approaches. Music Therapy and Special Education. https://www.forskningsdatabasen.dk/en/catalog/2468230666. Published 2017. Accessed 4 June 2020.
38. Premkumar A, Lovecchio FC, Stepan JG, et al. A novel mobile phone text messaging platform improves collection of patient-reported post-operative pain and opioid use following orthopedic surgery. HSS J. 2019;15(1):37–41. https://doi.org/10.1007/s11420-018-9635-3.
39. Zaccagnino MP, Bader AM, Sang CN, Correll DJ. The perioperative surgical home: a new role for the acute pain service. Anesth Analg. 2017;125(4):1394–402. https://doi.org/10.1213/ANE.0000000000002165.

Index

K. Rajput et al. (eds.), *Pain Control in Ambulatory Surgery Centers*,
https://doi.org/10.1007/978-3-030-55262-6

T

U

V

W

MIX
Papier aus verantwortungsvollen Quellen
Paper from responsible sources
FSC® C105338

If you have any concerns about our products,
you can contact us on
ProductSafety@springernature.com

In case Publisher is established outside the EU,
the EU authorized representative is:
Springer Nature Customer Service Center GmbH
Europaplatz 3, 69115 Heidelberg, Germany

Printed by Libri Plureos GmbH
in Hamburg, Germany